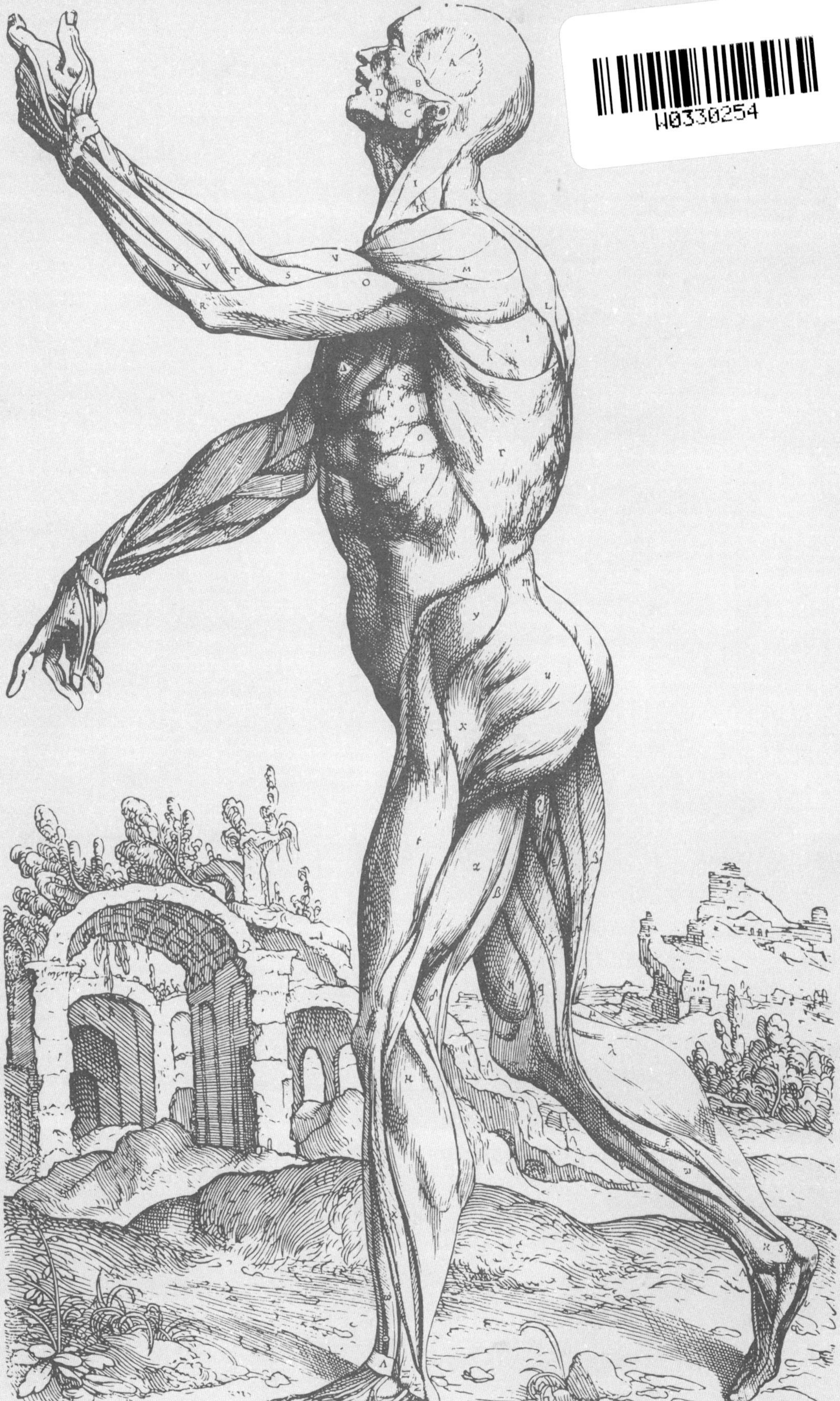

W0330254

Sobotta / Becher · Atlas of Human Anatomy
Vol. 1

Sobotta/Becher

Atlas of Human Anatomy

Original Author Dr. med. J. Sobotta †, Professor of Anatomy and Director of the Anatomical Institute, University of Bonn, Germany

Continued by Prof. Dr. med. and phil. H. Becher, former Director of the Anatomical Institute, University of Münster, Germany

Edited by

Prof. Dr. med. H. Ferner, Director of the Anatomical Institute, University of Vienna, Austria
Prof. Dr. med. J. Staubesand, Director of the Anatomical Institute, University of Freiburg, Germany

Nomenclature in Latin

Vol. 1: Regions, Skeleton, Ligaments, Joints and Muscles

Vol. 2: Visceral Anatomy

Vol. 3: Central and Autonomic Nervous Systems, Peripheral Nerve Pathways, Sense Organs and Skin

Urban & Schwarzenberg · München-Berlin-Wien

Sobotta/Becher

Atlas of Human Anatomy

Edited by
Prof. Dr. med. H. Ferner, Director of the Anatomical Institute, University of Vienna, Austria
Prof. Dr. med. J. Staubesand, Director of the Anatomical Institute, University of Freiburg, Germany

Vol. 1

Regions, Skeleton, Ligaments, Joints and Muscles

365 Illustrations, mostly in colour, Nomenclature in Latin

9th English Edition, based upon the 17th German Edition

Urban & Schwarzenberg · München-Berlin-Wien 1975

The Original Author, Prof. Dr. med. Johannes Sobotta, was born 31. 1. 1869 in Berlin and died 20th of April 1945 in Bonn.

Adresses of the German Editors:

Professor Dr. med. H. Ferner, Vorstand der I. Anatomischen Lehrkanzel der Universität, A-1090 Wien, Währingerstraße 13
Professor Dr. med. J. Staubesand, Director des Anatomischen Instituts der Universität, D-7800 Freiburg, Albertstraße 17

The pictures on the end leaves of the present volume show reproductions of the work of "Andreas Vesalii de corporis humani fabrica libri septem", witch appeared in Basel in 1542. Andreas Vesalius (* Brussels 1514, † 1564) urged and practiced the dissection of human bodies and may be considered to be the founder of Modern Anatomy.

German editions:

1. edition: J. F. Lehmanns Verlag, München 1904
2.–11. edition: J. F. Lehmanns Verlag, München 1913–1944
since 12. edition: Urban & Schwarzenberg, 1948
13. edition: 1953
14. edition: 1956
15. edition: 1957
16. edition: 1967 (ISBN 3-541-02816-5)
17. edition: 1972 (ISBN 3-541-02817-3)

Foreign editions:

Arab. Version
Al Ahram, Cairo/Egypt 1978/1979

English Version (with nomenclature in English)
SOBOTTA/FIGGE, Atlas of Human Anatomy
Urban & Schwarzenberg, München–Berlin–Wien, 9. edition 1974. (ISBN 3-541-06869-8)
1. reprint: Baltimore–Munich 1977

English Version (with nomenclature in Latin–PNA)
SOBOTTA/BECHER, Atlas of Human Anatomy
Urban & Schwarzenberg, München–Berlin–Wien, 9. edition 1975

French Version
Atlas d'Anatomie Humaine
Urban & Schwarzenberg, München–Wien–Baltimore 1977

Greek Version
Gregory Parisianos, Athen 1977

Italian Version
Atlante di anatomia
USES, Firenze 1974

Japanese Version
Igaku-Shoin Ltd., Tokyo 1974

Portuguese Version
Atlas de Anatomia Humana
Editora Guanabara Koogan, Rio de Janeiro 1976

Spanish Version
Atlas de Anatomia
Ediciones Toray, Barcelona 1974

Turkish Version
Insan Anatomisi Atlasi
Urban & Schwarzenberg, München–Wien–Baltimore 1977

© Urban & Schwarzenberg 1975

Publisher: Urban & Schwarzenberg, 8000 München 15, Pettenkoferstraße 18, Germany

No part of this book may be reproduced, in any manner, without written permission from the publisher. 061280

Printed in Germany by Kastner & Callwey, Buch- und Offsetdruckerei, München.

ISBN 3-541-06849-3

Publisher's Preface to the 9th Edition

This atlas of human anatomy with its clear and exact figures has already given untold numbers of medical students the illustrative material needed to supplement a text book and has served physicians as a lasting reference work.

The trend now in many countries to minimize the practical instruction in anatomy makes good illustrative material in this subject more important than ever. For this reason the illustrative part of the atlas has been revised, enlarged and placed in the foreground, whereas the text part has been limited to summaries in table form and to short notes.

The Latin nomenclature (N.A.P.) has been brought up to date and linguistic explanations in the form of a glossary have been placed before the anatomical names. This has been done especially in view of the rising number of students not having an adequate background in the classical languages. The appendix contains an Latin/English and a English/Latin section.

In accordance with the varying requirements in different countries this English edition with Latin nomenclature offers an alternative to the English edition with English nomenclature translated from the German by Frank H. J. Figge and W. Hild.

Preface to the First German Edition

This anatomical Atlas is intended for the medical student and as a reference Atlas for physicians; it is not necessarily for the professional anatomist. For this reason, I have restricted myself to the essentials which I consider necessary to obtain a general knowledge of the anatomy of the human body. The present volume, which is the first of a series, is organized for use during dissection. The method of presentation adheres closely to accepted dissection procedures. Illustrations of dissections, showing the parts of the body in unusual positions, were avoided because this would make orientation more difficult for the beginner.

Brief descriptions on the figures are placed on the text pages opposite the plates. It is thus possible for the student to use the book during the dissection, after reading the text. The myology text is in the form of tables that give the origin, insertion, nerve supply, and function of muscles.

In order to enable the reader to quickly differentiate between the different parts, colors were used in the illustrations: the yellowish tone was used for bones of the joints; red for muscles; various colors for the isolated skull bones and for the articulated skull to show the topographical relationships of parts of the skull. The Basle Nomenclature was used. The publisher has done everything possible to make the volume superior to most of the existing works as to quality of reproduction and number of illustrations.

Würzburg, October 1903 J. Sobotta

Preface to the 17th German Edition

Sobotta's concept of the Atlas has remained the guiding principle for the new editors. In order to emphasize the Atlas character of the work, they have eliminated all text passages. Only the valuable tables on muscles, their origins, insertions, innervation and functions have been retained and – wherever possible – have been coordinated with the corresponding figures.

The planning of a large portion of the new illustrations has still been done by Professor Dr. H. Becher. The accurate execution of the illustrations has been accomplished by the scientific artist, Professor E. Lepier of Vienna.

The repeated request by many students to coordinate figures and captions could be honored in the interest of improved usability by the accommodating attitude of the publishers. To this end, also, the index has been simplified. The nomenclature has been consequently based upon the Nomina Anatomica (Paris 1955) with reference to the latest additional recommendations (New York 1960 and Wiesbaden 1965); (compare: Nomina Anatomica, 3rd Ed. Excerpta Medica Foundation, Amsterdam–New York London Paris–Milan–Tokyo–Buenos Aires 1968).

Medical students Miss G. Adelmann has given valuable help with proofreading. The editors express their appreciation to Mrs. M. Engler for the arrangement of the index.

Special appreciation is due to the publishing house of Urban and Schwarzenberg and their coworkers – especially Dr. R. Degkwitz and Mr. K. Gullath – for the thoughful consideration of the wishes of the editors.

Heidelberg and Freiburg i. Br. H. Ferner
February 1972 J. Staubesand

Table of Contents

Preface . . . . V–VI

The Human Body VIII

General Terms of Direction and Position IX

Abbreviations X

Etymology Meaning and Accentuation of Anatomical Termes . . . . XI–XVI

I. Introduction XI

II. Special Part . . . . XII–XVI

Regions of the Human Body 1– 5

Skeleton—*The Bones of the Human Body*

General Characteristics and Classifications of Bones 7– 11

The Trunk 13– 27

The Skull 29– 63

The Shoulder Girdle and Upper Limb 65– 79

The Pelvic Girdle and Lower Limb 77– 92

The Ligaments Joints and

The Vertebral Column, Thorax, Skull 93–105

The Shoulder Girdle and Upper Limb 107–115

The Pelvic Girdle and Lower Limb 117–137

The Muscles

The Neck, Trunk, and Pelvis 139–166

The Head and Neck 167–188

The Upper Limb 189–224

The Lower Limb 225–259

Index

I. Latin/English 261–276

II. English/Latin 276–293

The Human Body, Corpus humanum

The parts of the human body, *corpus humanum,* which appear externally as the main parts of the entire body, are designated *partes corporis humani;* two unpaired and two pairs of paired components can be distinguished. The unpaired parts are the head, *caput,* and the trunk, *truncus.* The paired parts are the extremities, the upper extremities, *membra superiora,* and the lower extremities, *membra inferiora.* These principal parts of the body are divided in their turn into several named subdivisions. The ventral part of the head is the face, *facies;* the cranial, tapering part of the trunk, which carries the head, is called neck, *collum* (also called *cervix*, especially when used as an adjective). The entire length of the hinder or dorsal surface of the trunk is called the back, *dorsum* (only its most cranial part bordering on the head is designated nape, *nucha*). On the frontal or ventral surface of the trunk two parts are distinguished, the upper part which lies next to the neck, is called breast, *pectus,* while the lower, caudal part is called belly, *abdomen* (or *venter*). The small region between the anus and the genital opening belongs neither to the belly nor to the back and has received the name of *regio perinealis* (see below).

The extremities are subdivided into two principal divisions, the *pars fixa,* which is so intimately incorporated into the trunk that it cannot be seen on inspection from outside, and the *pars libera* which is the free portion of the extremity. Both in the upper and in the lower extremity the pars libera is again divided into three segments; these are in the direction from the trunk to the free end of the membrum superius the upper arm, *brachium,* the arm, *antebrachium,* and the hand, *manus,* and of the membrum inferius the thigh, *femur,* the leg, *crus,* and the foot, *pes.*

The entire outer surface of the human body is covered by the external skin, *integumentum commune;* however, in several places, around the external "true" openings of the body, this general integument suffers an interruption. The true openings of the body are the following: the mouth, *os (rima oris;)* the two nostrils, *nares,* the anal opening, *anus,* the opening of the vagina in the female, *ostium vaginae,* the orifice of the female urethra, *ostium urethrae externum.* While in the female six true ostia are present, in the male body there are only five, since in the male the ostium urethrae externum serves as the outlet of the urins as well as of the sex products. In addition to the true ostia there are two false body openings around which only an invagination but no interruption of the common integument takes place; these are the openings between the eyelids, *rimae palpebrarum,* and the openings of the external duct of the ear, *pori acustici externi.*

The extremities consist only of skeletal parts (bones) with their corresponding joints and ligaments and of muscles (to which are added blood vessels and nerves), while inside the head and trunk the body cavities are present, walled in by bones and (usually) muscles as well, these cavities housing frequently inner organs, *viscera.* These viscera are mainly the organs of digestion respiration and urinary and reproductive function, and furthermore the heart (center of the vascular system) and the central organs of the nervous system, brain and spinal cord.[1]

In each of the parts of the body, described above, there are distinguished again smaller areas, *regiones corporis humani.* Regions which have triangular borders, are called *trigonum;* in cases of distinctly depressed areas the term regio is replaced by the term *fossa.* Some regions are denoted by special terms: palm of the hand, *palma manus,* back of the hand, *dorsum manus,* sole of the foot, *planta pedis,* upper surface of the foot, *dorsum pedis.* Concerning location, boundaries and names of individual regions see Figs. 1 to 5.

[1] The term viscera the etymologic derivation of which is not clear, denoted in the past only the organs of digestion, respiration and urinary and reproductive function, but neither the heart nor the brain. In its form as an adjective, visceralis, it means facing the "viscera" as in the cases of visceral surface of the liver or spleen, visceral leaf of the peritoneum, etc., as contrasted to the term parietalis which means facing the wall (of the abdomen, chest, etc.).

General Terms of Direction and Position

Since the human body is tridimensional in shape, it can be described by three planes (if the body is in erect position, that is, standing erect upon the feet) or more correctly by innummerable planes of three different types; accordingly it has two vertical planes which intersect each other at an angle of 90°, and a third, horizontal plane which intersects both vertical planes at an angle of 90°. Planes of the latter kind are called, also with relation to the human body, horizontal or transverse planes and structures located in such planes are called transversal, *transversus,* or directed transversally, *transversalis.* Of the two kinds of vertical planes those which can be carried through the body from in front backwards (from ventral to dorsal) and which are parallel to the sagittal suture between the two parietal bones of the roof of the cranium, are called sagittal planes (with the adjective *sagittalis*). The second kind of vertical planes, as they intersect the sagittal planes at an angle of 90°, are parallel to the forehead (frontal bone). From this relationship the name frontal planes is derived; and *frontalis* are structures located in that kind of a plane. Among the many possible sagittal planes there is one, the middle one which divides the body into two halves of which the one is the mirror image of the other (embryologically exactly so, later only approximately); this is the median or midsagittal plane. The ventral boundary line of this plane is the *linea mediana anterior,* the dorsal boundary line is the *linea mediana posterior.* Several surface lines parallel to these two lines receive special names, they are: *linea mamillaris,* drawn through the nipple; the *linea parasternalis,* drawn midway between sternal and mamillary lines; *linea axillaris,* dropped from the deepest point of the axilla; and the *linea scapularis,* parallel to the linea mediana posterior, passes through the margo medialis scapulae.

Structures which are closer towards the head are *superior* or *cranialis,* those closer toward the tail end of the body are *inferior* or *caudalis.* A structure which lies closer to the front (when the body is in erect position) is called *anterior* as compared to structures which lie closer to the back and are designated as *posterior.* In the upper extremity of the arm and forearm the surfaces which correspond to the palma manus are termed *anterior* or *palmaris,* those corresponding to the dorsum manus are *posterior* or *dorsalis.* For the foot the terms *anterior* and *posterior* (regions of the foot) together with *plantaris* and *dorsalis* (see above) are in use. For some parts of the head, especially for the brain, the term *rostralis* (from rostrum, the beak) is used in place of cranialis.

Any structure situated in the midsagittal plane is *medianus;* if it is closer to the median plane than to the side it is *medialis;* closer to the side is *lateralis,* between two structures is *medius.* For the purpose of description of the body walls, such as the roof of the cranium or the wall of chest and abdomen, the terms *internus* and *externus* are employed. In other cases again in which there is no layering of a wall to be described, a structure closer to the surface is termed *superficialis* as contrasted to deeper structures which are named *profundus.* In the free extremities a structure closer to the root is termed *proximalis,* while closer to the free end is *distalis.*

Systemata corporis humani

Descriptive anatomy the subject of which it is to describe the "form" of the human body as far as it can be recognized by dissection (= anatomy), is also called systematic anatomy, since it concerns itself with the following systems of the body: 1. *Osteologia,* the bones; 2. *Syndesmologia,* the ligaments and joints *(juncturae ossium);* 3. *Myologia,* the muscles (and bursae); 4. *Angiologia,* the vascular system; 5. *Splanchnologia,* the viscera; 6. *Systema nervosum centrale,* central nervous system (brain and spinal cord); 7. *Systema nervosum periphericum,* the nerves; 8. *Organa sensuum* et *integumentum commune,* sense organs and skin.

Abbreviations

ant.	=	anterior or anterius
a.	=	arteria, aa. = arteriae
art. or artic.	=	articulatio
caud.	=	caudalis, -le
cran.	=	cranialis, -le
dist.	=	distalis, -le
dors.	=	dorsalis, -le
ext.	=	externus, -a, -um
fac.	=	facies
inc.	=	incisura
inf.	=	inferior or inferius
int.	=	internus, -a, -um
lat.	=	lateralis, -le
lig.	=	ligamentum, ligg. = ligamenta
m.	=	musculus, mm. = musculi
med. or medial.	=	medialis, -le
median.	=	medianus, -a, -um
n.	=	nervus, nn. = nervi
obl. or obliq.	=	obliquus, -a, -um
oss.	=	ossis or ossa, ossium
post. or poster.	=	posterior or posterius
proc.	=	processus
prof.	=	profundus
prot.	=	protuberantia
prox.	=	proximalis, -le
r.	=	ramus, rr. = rami
spin.	=	spina, spinae
sup. or super.	=	superior or superius
superfic.	=	superficialis, -le
sut.	=	sutura
transv.	=	transversus, -a, -um
tuberc.	=	tuberculum
tuberos.	=	tuberositas
v.	=	vena, vv. = venae
ventr.	=	ventralis, -le

Etymology, Meaning and Accentuation of Anatomical Termes

I. Introduction

Like any other science anatomy has its own language, a technical nomenclature or terminology; in the case of anatomy it consists of around 5000 terms by which the individual structures of the human body are named. Up to 1935 the anatomical nomenclature internationally in use was the so-called B. N. A. (Basel nomina anatomica) adopted in 1895 at a meeting of the German Anatomical Society in Basel, Switzerland. In order to climinate certain inadequacies of the B. N. A. the German anatomists undertook a revision, known as J. N. A. (Jena nomina anatomica) which was adopted by the German Anatomical Society in 1935 at a meeting in Jena, Germany. This nomenclature was used in the previous English edition of Sobotta. In the new edition the nomenclature is used which was adopted at the International Anatomical Congress held in Paris 1955 and termed the N. A. P. (see also: Preface to the 17th German Edition).

Nearly all the anatomical names date back to the days of antiquity; relatively few were added in more recent times. Most of the anatomical terms are derived from the Latin language; those which are taken from the Greek language were more or less Latinized by the anatomists of the Roman empire. Only very few are derived from oriental (Arabic, Aramaean) languages, but are so completely Latinized that their origin can be barely recognized.

Since now-a-days many medical students are not familiar with Latin and still fewer with Greek, and since a good many Latin terms do not date back to classical Latin but are of late Latin origin, and since finally many Latin words used in anatomy are not a part of the Latin curriculum of high schools and colleges, the following introductory notes, it is hoped, will be a welcome aid in learning and remembering the anatomical terms. Many Greek names which have been a part of the anatomical armamentarium for considerably more than a thousand years, were left unchanged; as they have been, in many instances, Latinized only few of us realize that they were originally Greek words.

Spelling and Accentuation of Names of Greek Origin

Since the Greek alphabet differs in some respects from the Latin alphabet, words of the Greek language will be written with Latin letters in the same way as the old Romans used to write them. The articles, one for each of the three genders, used in the Greek exactly as in the German language (ho, he and to), are omitted in the Latinized words. The Greek kappa (k) is replaced by c; ch stands for chi (ch), ph for phi (ph), ps for psi (ps), x for ksi (x), the for theta (th), h for the spiritus asper; gamma (g) before gamma, kappa, chi and ksi is pronounced like n (for instance, aggeion – angeion, agkos – ankos). Since Greek words beginning with rho (–r) have the spiritus asper over the rho, they must be spelled in Latin with rh, as for instance, rhomboideus, etc. Among the Greek vowels and diphthongs omega (long o) and omikron (short o) are both spelled o, likewise the short epsilon and the long eta are both spelled e; ypsilon, alpha, iota the same as in Greek. The Greek diphthong epsilon-iota is pronounced in the Latinized (as in the modern Greek) word as i, for instance Aristeides (Gr.) in Latin Aristides, or in some instances like e as in tracheia (Greek), trachea (L.). The diphthong omikron-iota is written and pronounced like oe (in English usually like e) as in oikos Gr. = oecus Lat., for instance oeconomy (economy in English); alpha-iota is changed to ae, alpha-ypsilon to au, omikron-ypsilon to u, epsilon-ypsilon to eu. The endings of nouns and adjectives are Latinized (for instance to sternon = sternum, ho isthmos = isthmus; the adjective thorakikos, from thorax, is changed to thoracicus); in most cases the Greek declension is replaced by the Latin, (rarely) the Greek declension is retained; for instance hypophysis, gen. hypophyseos). Frequently, as already customary in Roman times, adjectives are formed from Greek nouns by means of Latin endings (for instance centralis from the Latinized centrum, Gr. to kentron).[1]

Brief Explanation of Anatomical Names

In the pronunciation and accentuation of Greek Latinized names the rules of the Latin language should be applied; for instance Aristides from Aristeides, but Alcibiades from Alkibiádes; Uránia from Gr. Oyranie, but Thalia from Gr. Thaleia. The Greek word for nipple is ho mastos; resembling a nipple is mastoeides, Latinized mastoideus. Mastoideus should have the accent on the second before the last syllable, since the e is short; in this case the old rule "vocalis ante vocalem brevis est" applies, while a vowel taking the place of a Greek diphthong, is long.

1 The Greek adjective from kentron is kentrikos, in Latin centricus (as in eccentric) and is grammatically more correct. Yet central isaccepted by usage.

II. Special Part — Explanation of Individual Names

L = from Latin; G = from Greek

abductor	muscles which pull the bone away from the axis of body or limb
accessorius	adj. to be additional to something (from L. accedere = to be added)
acetábulum	the socket for the head of the femur, likened to a cup-shaped dish for vinegar (L. acetum = vinegar, and the ending bulum which indicates an instrument or utensil)
acromion	highest point of scapula (Gr. akron = summit); adj. acromialis
adductor	muscle which approaches the bone to the axis of body or limb
ala	L. = wing; adj. alaris = wing-like
alvéolus	L. = small cavity, socket for the root of a tooth (also the small vesicles of the lung); adj. alveolaris
amphiarthrosis	union of bones, in which the bones are only slightly movable against each other (Gr. amphi = on both sides, and arthron = joint)
anconaeus	belonging to the elbow (Gr. ankon = elbow)
antebrachium	L. the forearm (incorrectly constructed, should be praebrachium)
anulus	L. a small ring
anus	L. anus = ring; metaphorically for opening of lower bowel; adj. analis
apertura	opening, a late L. word much used in anatomy (from aperire = to uncover, to open)
arcuatus	arched (from L. arcus = arch)
articulatio	L. joint; adj. articularis
atlas	first cervical vertebra (taken from. Gr. mythology: the giant who bears up the heavenly sphere)
auricula	the external ear (from L. auricula = the ear lap); adj. auricularis = belonging to the ear or ear-shaped
basilaris	adj. means at the base (Latinized from Gr. He basis)
biceps	two-headed (L. bis = twice, and caput = head)
brachium	L. arm
brevis	L. short
buccinator	L. the trompeter (with musculus = muscle of the cheek)
bulla	L. capsule, bubble
calcáneus	heel bone (L. calx = heel); adj. calcanearis
calvaria	roof of cranium (from L. calva = scalp)
caninus	adj. as in dens caninus = canine tooth (from L. canis = dog)
capitatum	with a head (L. caput = head)
carotis	with artery = carotid artery (from Gr. He karotis, derivation disputable; perhaps from kar, gen. kratos = head); adj. caroticus
carpus	from Gr. karpos = root of the hand, wrist; adj. carpeus, as f. i. in facies articularis carpęa = joint surface on distal end of radius for articulation with the carpus
cartilago	L. gristle, cartilage
cerebellum	the small brain (diminutive of L. cerebrum) adj. cerebellaris
cerebrum	L. brain; in anatomy it designates the telencephalon (cerebral hemispheres and interbrain); adj. cerebralis
cervix	L. neck or nape; adj. cervicalis
chorda tympani	the tympanic chord, a nerve crossing the tympanic membrane, the only nerve which is not named "nervus" (from Gr. chorde = gutstring)
cingulum	L. girdle
clavicula	clavicle, collarbone (diminutive from L. clavis = key)
clivus	L. a lean-to roof
coccyx	os coccygis, last part of spinal column (from Gr. ho kokkyx = the cuckoo, in allusion to the bill of this bird) adj. coccygeus
collum	L. neck
concha	Gr. konche = (shell of) a mussel
condylus	a bony tubercle bearing a joint-surface (from Gr. kondylos-knuckle); adj. condylaris
conoideus	wedge-shaped (from Gr. konos = wedge)
coracoideus	resembling a raven's beak (Gr. korakoeides, from corax = raven, and eidos – resemblance)
cornu	L. horn; plur. cornua
corona	L. wreath, circle, crown; adj. coronalis and coronarius = circleshaped, encircling as in sutura coronalis = crown suture
coronoideus	shaped like the beak of a crow (Gr. korone = crow and eidos = resembling)
corrugare	L. to wrinkle
costa	L. rib; adj. costalis or costarius
costae spurae	ribs which are joined to the sternum only by intermediation of the cartilage of the seventh rib, or have no connection at all with the sternum (11th and 12th ribs); spurius: L. illegitimate
costae sternales	ribs (first seven) which are joined to the sternum directly by their own cartilages
costae verae	(L. verus: true). same as costae sternales
cranium	Gr. kranion = head
cremaster	with musculus = elevator of the testicle (Gr. suspensor)
cribrosa	adj. as in lamina cribrosa (from L. cribrum = sieve; formed like a sieve)

crista .... L. crest, ridge
crista galli .... L. cock's comb (gallus = cock)
cruciatus .... L. cross-shaped
crus .... L. leg (plural crura; adj. cruralis)
cubitus .... L. elbow
cuneiformis .... wedge-shaped (from L. cuneus = wedge)

decussatus .... crossed or crossing each other (L. of the shape of a X)
deltoideopectoralis . composite adj. from deltoid (Gr.) muscle and L. pectus = breast (adj. pectoralis)
deltoideus .... with muscle = deltoid muscle (from Gr. delta = Greek letter Δ, and eidos = resembling); adj. deltoideus
diaphragma .... sheet-like partition (between thoracic and abdominal cavities); from Gr. dia = across and phragma = wall
diaphysis .... shaft of the long bones between its two ends (from Gr. dia = between, and phyein = to grow)
diarthrosis .... union of bones by freely movable joints (Gr. dia = through and arthron = joint)
digitus .... L. finger (in anatomy digitus manus is the finger, digitus pedis is the toe)
diploe .... ancient name denoting the spongiosa of the bones of the calvaria (Gr. = double) adj. diplóicus
discus .... a disk (Gr. diskos) as the flat discs between individual vertebrae
dorsus .... L. the back

endósteum .... membrane lining inner surface of medullary cavity of bone (from Gr. endon = within and osteon = bone)
epicóndylus .... a projection above a condyle (Gr. epi = above, upon)
epicranius .... resting upon the cranium (Gr. epi = upon, and kranion = head)
epíphysis .... the ends of the long bones (from Gr. epi = upon, on top, and phyein = to grow; physis = growth; i. e. what grows upon the ends of the shaft)
epistrópheus .... second cervical vertebra (from Gr. ho epistropheys = the turner, pivot); N. A. = axis
ethmoideus .... adj. from Gr. ethmoeides = resembling a sieve; as in os ethmoideum = ethmoid bone; adj. ethmoideus = pertaining to the ethmoid bone

facies .... L. a surface; with articularis = a cartilage-covered joint surface
fascia .... denotes the membranous envelops of muscles (L. fascia = band, girth); adj. fascialis
fasciculus .... a small bundle (L. diminutive from fascis)
fascis .... L. bundle
femur .... L. = the thigh (gen. femoris, adj. femoralis) denotes in anatomy the thigh bone (abbreviation for "os femoris")
fibula .... lateral bone of the leg (L. clasp, brooch); adj. fibularis, The fibula was formerly called Gr. he perone; adj. peronaios (peronaeus)
fonticulus .... L. a little spring (denoting the defects or fontanels in the bony cranium of the newborne)
foramen .... L. a hole
fossa .... L. a pit or ditch; in anatomy a deep depression
fovea .... L. a pit, in anatomy a shallow depression
frontalis .... adj. from L. frons = forehead
fundus .... L. = bottom (lowest or deepest part of a sac, depression or recess)

gastrocnemius ..... a muscle belly resting upon the shinbone (Gr. gaster = belly and kneme = shinbone)
gemellus .... paired (L. geminus or gemellus = double, twins)
geniculum .... a little knee (L. dimiuutive from genu = knee)
genioglossus .... with musculus = a muscle of the tongue arising from the chin (Gr. geneion = chin, and glossa = tongue)
genu .... L. knee (genitive = genus)
glabella .... prominent area on the frontal bone above the root of the nose (from L. glaber = beardless, smooth)
gluteus .... from Gr. gloytos = buttock
gracilis .... L. slender
gyrus .... convolution of the cerebral hemisphere (Gr. gyros = circle)

hallux .... L. great toe (gen. hallucis)
hamatus .... with a hook (L. hamus = hook)
hamulus .... a small hook (L. diminutive of hamus = hook)
hiatus .... a gaping opening (from L. hiare = to gape)
humerus .... L. = shoulder, denotes the upper arm bone in anatomy
hyoideus .... with os = hyoid bone (Gr. = resembling a U); adj. hyoídeus
hypochondricus .... with regio, means region caudal to the cartilages of the ribs (Gr. hypo = below; chondros = cartilage)
hypogastricus ..... with regio, means lower abdominal region (Gr. hypo = below; gaster = stomach, belly)
hypoglossus .... together with nervus means the hypoglossal nerve or twelfth cranial N. (from Gr. hypo = below, and glossa = tongue; it is constructed incorrectly, as it should be hypoglossicus
hypophysis .... pituitary gland grown to the under surface of the brain (Gr. hypo = below and physis = growth); Gr. gen. = hypophyseos

ilia .... L. pluraliatantum = the flank; gen. ilium as in os ilium; adj. iliacus
impressio .... L. impression (as in impressio trigemini = impression made by the nervus trigeminus)
incisivus .... L. adj. capble of cutting (from L. incidere = to cut into); with dens = incisor tooth

index .... L. informer, pointer, forefinger (index-finger)
infundibulum ...... L. funnel
inguinalis .... adj. from L. inguen = groin
intertransversarius .. between the transverse processes of the vertebrae
ischium .... from Gr. ischion = buttocks; adj. ischiadicus

jugulum .... the depression between the two clavicles (L. diminutive of jugum = yoke); adj. jugularis
junctura .... L. connection, joint

labium .... L. lip
labyrinthus .... the labyrinth of the inner ear (from Gr. labyrinthos; originally perhaps Egyptian); adj. labyrinthicus
lacer (neuter lacerum) = L. jagged
lambdoideus .... adj. = shaped like the Gr. letter lambda (Λ)
larynx .... Gr. = voice box; adj. laryngeus
latus .... L. broad, wide; superl. latissimus
levator........... elevator, lifter (from L. levere = to raise)
lumbalis .... adj. from L. lumbus = loin
lumbricales .... L. earth worm-shaped
lunatus .... shaped like a half moon (L. luna = moon)

malaris .... adj. from L. mala = cheek
malleolus .... L. a small hammer; denotes the bony projections, one on each side, above the ankle joint; adj. malleolaris
mamma .... L. female breast, also mammary gland (milk-secreting gland; adj. mammarius)
mam(m)illa .... L. nipple (from mamma) a small breast; adj. mamillaris = nipples-haped
mandibula .... lower jaw (from L. mandere = to chew); adj. mandibularis
manubrium .... L. handle of a sword (with sterni = most cranial piece of sternum)
manus .... L. hand
masseter .... masseter muscle (from Gr. = the chewer); adj. massetericus
mastoideus .... adj. with processus = mastoid process of the temporal bone (from Gr. mastos = nipple and eidos = resembling)
maxilla .... upper jaw (L. = jaw)
meatus .... L. passage, opening (from meare = to go)
meniscus .... crescent shaped cartilage between two bones of a joint (Gr. meniskos = a crescent, from mene = moon)
mentum .... L. chin; adj. mentalis
mesogastricus ..... adj., with regio = middle abdominal region (Gr. mesos = middle; gaster = stomach, belly)
metacarpus .... part of the hand, that follows (Gr. meta = after) the carpus
metatarsus .... bones of the foot which follow (Gr. meta = after) the tarsus
multangulum ...... multicornered (L. multus = many, and angulus = corner)
multifidus .... L. cleft into many bundles
musculus .... muscle (L. diminutive of mus = mouse; in old German texts actually called "Mäuslein")
mylohyoideus ...... with musculus = connecting mandible with hyoid bone (mylos = grind stone, grinding tooth; pars pro toto)
myocardium .... the heart muscle (Gr. mys = muscle and kardia = heart)
myologia .... the study of the muscles (Gr. mys = mouse or muscle, and logos = word or study)

navicularis .... L. resembling a boat
nucha .... Latinized from the Arabic, means nape, dorsal region of the neck

obturatus .... stopped up (from L. obturare = to stop up)
occiput .... posterior part of the head (L. from ob = against, and caput = head); adj. occipitalis
olécranon .... from Gr. = elbow, upper end of ulna
omoclavicularis .... pertaining to the shoulder (Gr. omos = shoulder) and to the clavicle (L. clavicula = collar bone)
opticus .... pertaining to vision (Gr. optikos)
orbicularis .... circular (from L. orbis = circle)
orbita .... L. wheel-rut, but used since ancient times for the eye socket
os................ L. bone (gen. ossis, plur. ossa, ossium)
osteologia .... branch of anatomy treating of the bones, from Gr. osteon = bone and logos = word or study

palatum .... L. the palate; adj. palatinus
palma .... L. palm tree; figuratively the palm of the hand; adj. palmaris
parasternalis....... next to the sternum (Gr. para = by the side)
parietalis.......... adj. from L. paries = wall (as in os parietale = parietal bone)
parotideomassetericus. pertaining to parotid gland and masseter muscle
parótis............ with glandula = parotid gland (Gr. next to the ear)
patella .... L. knee cap (an ancien word); adj. patellaris
pecten .... L. = comb, adj. pectíneus
pectus .... L. chest, breast; adj. pectoralis
pelvis .... (from L. pelvis = basin). In osteology the pelvis denotes the girdle of the lower extremity, i. e. both ossa coxae, the sacrum and coccyx
pericranium .... periost of cranium (Gr. peri = around and kranion = head)
perinéum .... Gr. denotes the dam. i. e. region between anus and external genitalia
perióst eum .... membrane investing outer surfaces of bone (Gr. peri = around and osteon = bone)
peronaeus .... related to fibulula (Gr. adj. peronaios; the fibula was formerly called perone)
pes .... L. foot, (Gen. pedis)
petromastoideus .... composite adj. from Gr. petra = a stone (as in petrous portion of

temporal bone) and Gr. mastoeides = nipple shapped (as in mastoid process of temporal bone)

petrosus .... adj. as hard as a rock (from Gr. petra = rock); its use in nervus petrosus is incorrect, but very ancient and means related to the petrous bone

phalanx .... pl. phalanges; because of their arrangement in rows the bones of the fingers are compared with the Greek battle-order

pharyngotympanicus adj. connecting the middle ear with the pharynx (hybr. from pharynx and tympanum)

pharynx .... part of the digestive tube between mouth and esophagus (from Gr. pharynx = throad; gen. pharyngis, adj. pharyngeus)

piriformis .... L. pear-shaped

pisiformis .... pea-shaped (L. pisum = pea)

planta .... sole of the foot

platysma .... cutaneous muscle of neck and pectoral region (Gr. platys = broad)

pneumaticus .... with os = air-containing bone (Gr. pneuma = air)

pollex .... L. thumb (gen. pollicis)

popliteus .... adj. from L. poples = hollow of the knee

porus .... from Gr. poros = passage, path, opening (about the same as the L. meatus)

profundus .... L. deep

promontorium ..... L. promontory (from prominere = to project, not from mons = mountain)

pronate .... L. pronare = to bend forward (to rotate inward)

psoas .... Gr. psoa = loin

pterygoideus .... adj. with processus = pterygoid process of sphenoid bone; (from Gr. pteryx = wing, and eidos = resemblance)

pterygopalatinus ... adj. pertaining to pterygoid process and palate

pubes .... L. = the genitals (gen. pubis)

pulpa .... L. a soft mass inside an organ (f. i. the pulp of a tooth); adj. pulposus

pyramis .... pyramid (from Gr. he pyramis, but originally Egyptian)

quadriceps .... four-headed (from L. quattuor = four, and caput = head)

radius .... lateral bone of forearm (L. spoke of a wheel)

regio .... region; for purposes of ready orientation the entire body is divided into regions named after their chief structures

retinaculum .... a retaining band (from L. retinere = to hold back, to restrain)

rostrum .... L. beak

sacrum .... with os, neuter from L. sacer = sacred. A very ancient anatomical term. but it is unknown why this bone is called sacred (cross-bone in German); adj. sacralis

sagitta .... L. arrow; adj. sagittalis = arrow-shaped, as straight as an arrow

sartorius .... adj. from L. sartor = tailor (musculus sartorius so called because tailors used this muscle when they sat on the table with crossed legs)

scalenus .... uneven, triangular with uneven sides (Gr. skalenos)

scaphoideus .... adj. shaped like a boat (from Gr. skaphe = boat, and eidos = resemblance)

scapula .... L. shoulder blade; adj. scapularis

serratus .... serrated (L. serra = saw)

sesamoideus .... Gr. resembling a sesame seed (with ossa sesamoidea)

sigmoìdeus .... resembling the letter sigma (from Gr. sigmoeides)

sinus .... L. a bay, depression or recess

soleus .... shaped like a sole-fish (L. solea = sole-fish)

sphenoideus .... with os = the sphenoid bone (from Gr. sphen = wedge and eidos = resembling); adj. sphenoideus

sphenomaxillaris ... adj. hybrid from Gr. sphenoides and L. maxilla

spinalis .... adj. from L. spina = thorn, spine; pertaining to the spine (processus spinalis) of a vertebra, but also used, pars pro toto, as pertaining to the whole "spinal" column; as f. i. medulla spinalis = spinal cord; spinal nerve = nerve arising from spinal cord

splenius .... of the shape of a band (from Gr. splenion = plaster, but of recent use)

sqama .... L. = a fish scale; denotes flat scale-shaped bones; adj. squamosus = scaly

sternocleidomastoideus. with musculus = a muscle having attachments to sternum, clavicle and mastoid process (instead of the L. clavis the Gr. kleis = key is used here)

sternum .... breast bone (from Gr. sternon = chest); adj. sternalis

styloideus .... adj. as in processus styloideus (from Gr. stylos = style, and eidos = resembling)

stylomastoideus .... adj. pertaining to styloid and mastoid processes; as in foramen stylomastoideum = an opening located between styloid and mastoid processes

subclavius .... under the clavicula (L. clavis = key, is used instead of clavicula)

sulcus .... L. groove

supercilium .... L. eyebrow; adj. superciliaris

supinate .... to rotate outward (L. supinare = to bend backward)

sura .... L. calf of the leg

sustentáculum ...... L. = support

sutura .... L. a suture (from suere = to sew), denotes a form of union between the skull bones

symphysis .... union of bones by fibrocartilage (Gr. syn = with together, and physis = growth, from phyein = to grow)

synarthrosis .... joining of bones by way of tissues which hold them immovably fixed

	against each other Gr. syn = together and arthron = joint)
synchondrosis	union of two bones by cartilage (Gr. syn = with, together, and chondros = cartilage)
syndesmosis	union of bones by ligaments (Gr. desmos = band and syn = with, together)
synóvia	an artifically constructed word means a joint lubricant
talus	first ankle-bone (L. ankle, heel)
tarsus	the ankle (Gr. tarsos = a wickerwork frame) adj. tarseus
tegmen (synonym of tegmentum).	L. = roof; adj. tegmentalis
temporalis	adj. pertaining to the region of the temples, as os temporale = temporal bone (from L. tempora = temples of the head)
tendo	tendon (medieval L.); adj. = tendíneus
teres	L. elongate round
terminus	L. boundary, end; adj. terminalis
thorax	chest (from Gr. thorax = breast plate, cuirass); gen. thoracis, adj. thoracicus
thyreotdeus	belonging to thyreoid gland (glandula thyreoidea = from Gr. thyreos = shield)
tibia	L. flute, shin-bone (an ancient word)
transversocostalis ...	connecting transverse processes of the vertebrae with the ribs (L. costa = rib)
triceps	threeheaded (L. tres = three, and caput = head)
trigonum	a triangular region of the body
triquetrus	L. triangular
trochanter	each of two prominent bony knobs at the cranial end of the shaft of the femur (Gr. trochanter + a roller, from trochos = wheel)
tróchlea	L. = pulley (originally perhaps Gr.); adj. trochlearis
tuba	a tube-shaped duct (from L. = trompet); adj. tubalis
tuber	L. a bony prominence
tuberculum	a small prominence; L. diminutive from tuber
tuberositas	L. roughness
turcicus	Turkish (late L.)
tympanum	tympanic cavity, cavity of the middle ear (from Gr. tympanon = drum); adj. tympanicus
ulna	medial bone of forearm (L. elbow, ell)
uncinatus	hook-shaped (from L. uncus = hook)
unguis	L. = the nail (adj. = unguicularis)
vagina	L. scabbard or sheath; adj. vaginalis
vastus	L. vast, huge
vertebra	one of the segments of the "vertebral" column; a very ancient name (from L. vertere = to turn); in the English of the 16th century (Thomas Vycarie) whorle-bone designates the vertebral column
vestibulum	L. = antechamber
vomer	L. = plowshare
xiphoid process	caudal tip of sternum (G. xiphos = sword; eidos = resembling); adj. xiphoideus
zygomaticum	adj. with os = zygomatic bone, cheek bone (from Gr. zygon = yoke)

Rules employed in Naming the Joints and Ligaments

Most of the synarthrodial as well as diarthrodial joints are described by composite adjectives which consists of the names of the articulating bones as f. i. *articulatio sacroiliaca,* joint between sacrum and ilium. Similarly, ligaments receive adjectives which are composed of the names of the structures which they connect with each other. Only some of the larger joints have special names as f. i. *articulatio cubiti,* elbow joint; *articulatio coxae,* hip joint; likewise some ligaments have received special names as f. i. *lig. cruciforme atlantis, lig. cruciata* of the knee joint.

Rules employed in Naming the Muscles

All muscles have the generic name *musculus,* only two muscles are excepted from this rule, *platysma* and *diaphragma.* In the selection of adjectives denoting the species of the muscle the following peculiarities are used.

1) **Shape** of the muscle as f. i. *in m. pyramidalis.* If there are several muscles of the same shape, further attributes are used to distinguish them; f. i. *m. rectus abdominis* and *m. rectus capitis.* Since, however, there are several straight muscles of the head, a differentiating adjective is added: *m. rectus capitis posterior* and *m. rectus capitis anterior;* again, there are two dorsal straight muscles of the head; these are distinguished from each other by a fourth attribute, *m. rectus posterior major* and *m. rectus capitis posterior minor.*

2) **Location** of the muscle as f. i. in *m. pectoralis;* again if there are several muscles of the same location, they are distinguished by addition of other adjectives as f. i. *m. pectoralis major* and *m. pectoralis minor.*

3) **Function** of the muscle, together with other criteria if there are several muscles of the same function: *m. abductor pollicis brevis* and *m. abductor pollicis longus; m. adductor brevis, m. adductor longus, m. adductor hallucis* and *m. adductor pollicis.*

4) **Attachments** (origin and insertion): f. i. *m. sternohyoideus, m. sternocleidomastoideus.*

Regions of the Human Body

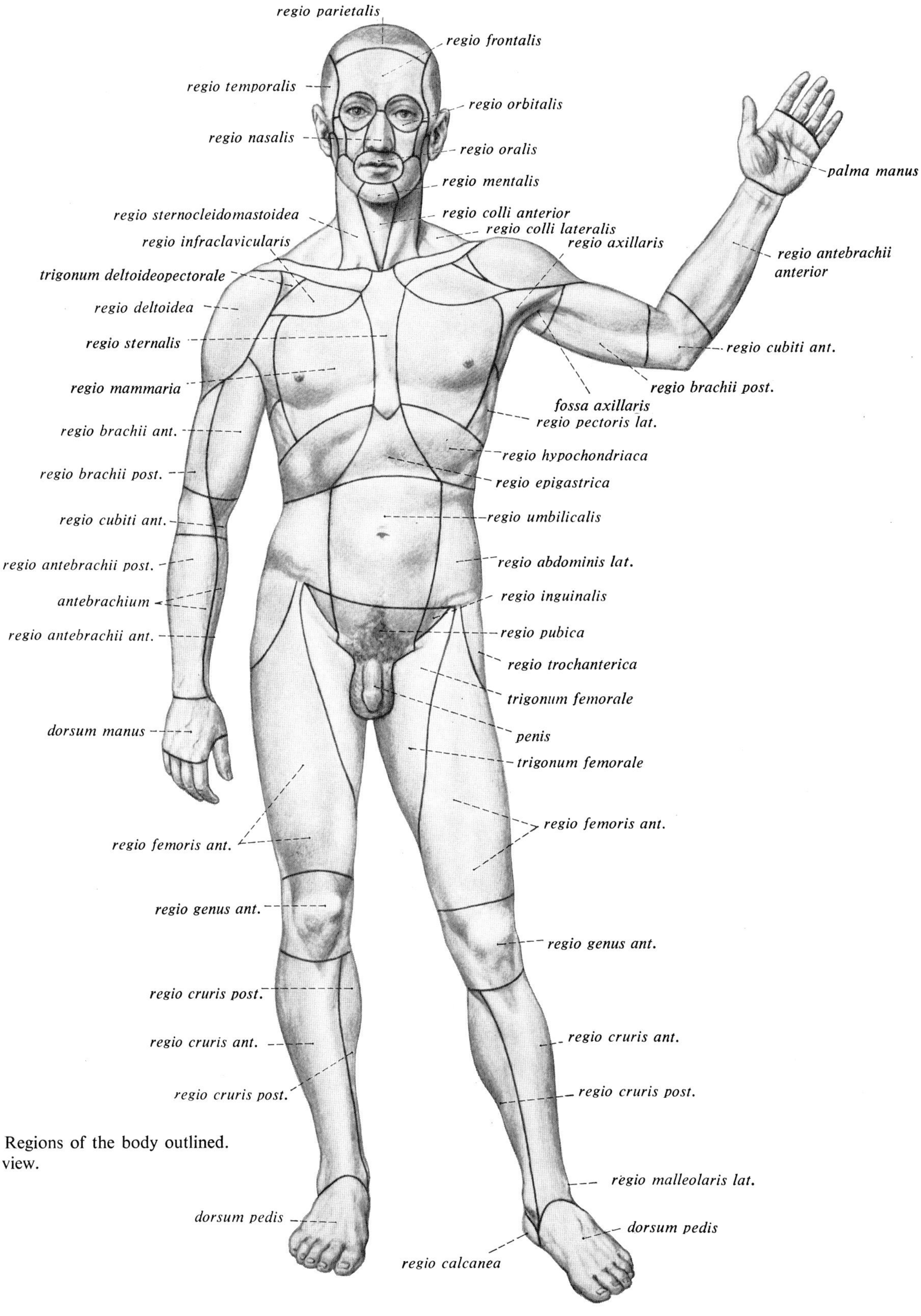
regio parietalis
regio frontalis
regio temporalis
regio orbitalis
regio nasalis
regio oralis
palma manus
regio mentalis
regio sternocleidomastoidea
regio colli anterior
regio colli lateralis
regio infraclavicularis
regio axillaris
regio antebrachii anterior
trigonum deltoideopectorale
regio deltoidea
regio sternalis
regio cubiti ant.
regio mammaria
regio brachii post.
fossa axillaris
regio pectoris lat.
regio brachii ant.
regio hypochondriaca
regio brachii post.
regio epigastrica
regio cubiti ant.
regio umbilicalis
regio antebrachii post.
regio abdominis lat.
antebrachium
regio inguinalis
regio antebrachii ant.
regio pubica
regio trochanterica
trigonum femorale
dorsum manus
penis
trigonum femorale
regio femoris ant.
regio femoris ant.
regio genus ant.
regio genus ant.
regio cruris post.
regio cruris ant.
regio cruris ant.
regio cruris post.
regio cruris post.
regio malleolaris lat.
dorsum pedis
dorsum pedis
regio calcanea

Fig. 1. Regions of the body outlined. Ventral view.

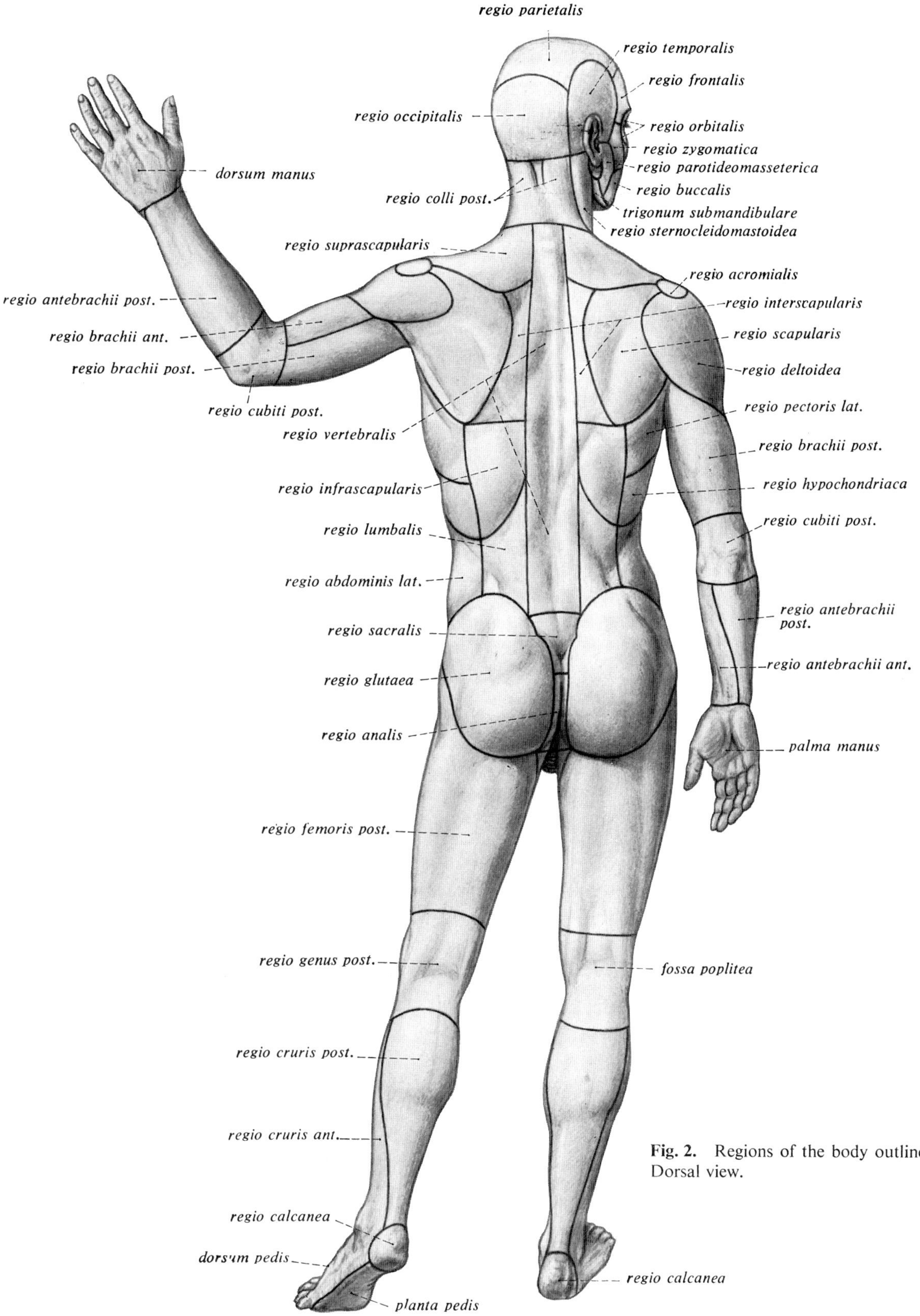
regio parietalis
regio temporalis
regio frontalis
regio occipitalis
regio orbitalis
regio zygomatica
regio parotideomasseterica
dorsum manus
regio buccalis
regio colli post.
trigonum submandibulare
regio sternocleidomastoidea
regio suprascapularis
regio acromialis
regio antebrachii post.
regio interscapularis
regio brachii ant.
regio scapularis
regio brachii post.
regio deltoidea
regio cubiti post.
regio pectoris lat.
regio vertebralis
regio brachii post.
regio infrascapularis
regio hypochondriaca
regio cubiti post.
regio lumbalis
regio abdominis lat.
regio antebrachii post.
regio sacralis
regio antebrachii ant.
regio glutaea
regio analis
palma manus
regio femoris post.
regio genus post.
fossa poplitea
regio cruris post.
regio cruris ant.
regio calcanea
dorsum pedis
regio calcanea
planta pedis

Fig. 2. Regions of the body outlined. Dorsal view.

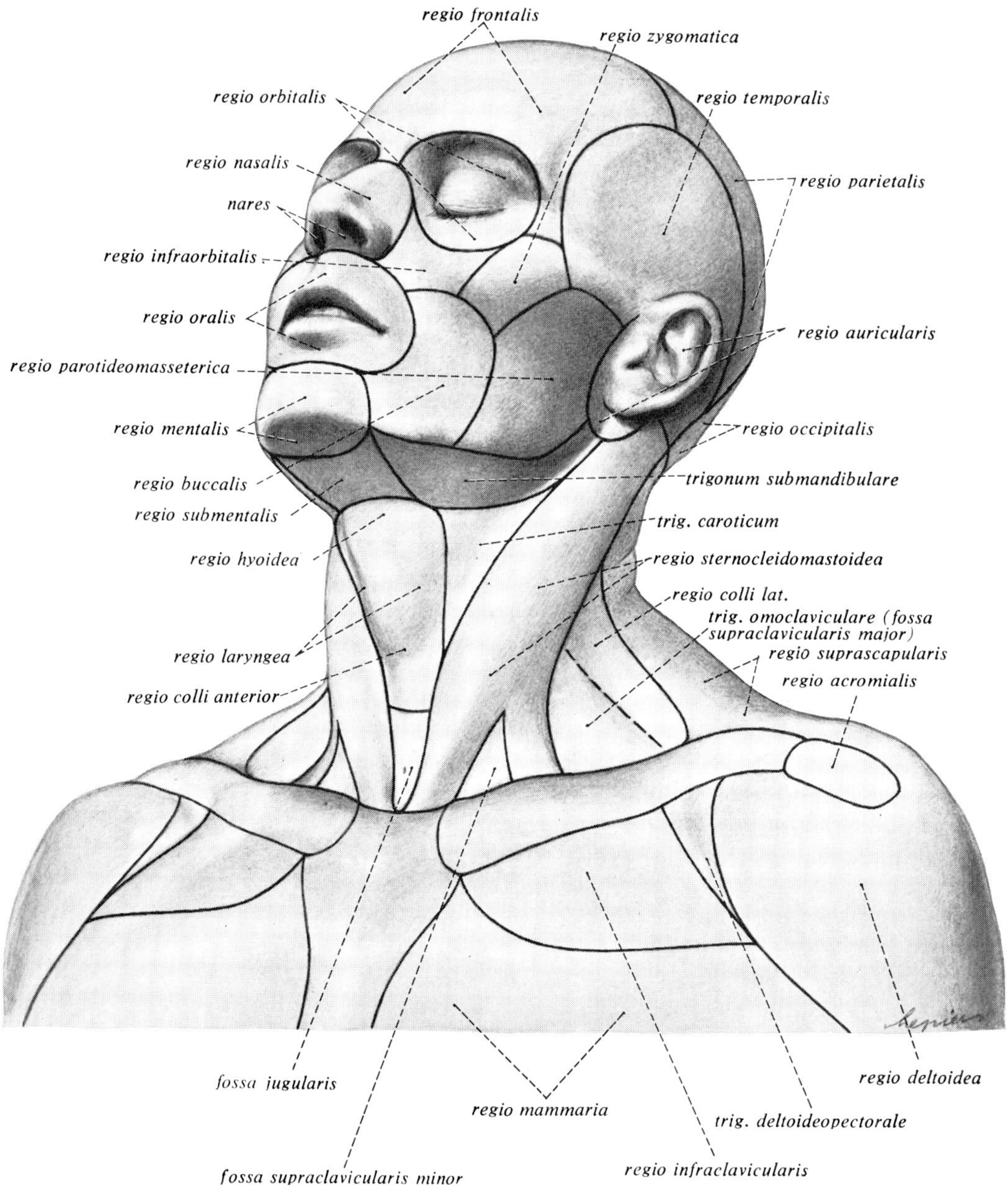

Fig. 3. Regions of the head, neck, and upper body outlined. Ventral view.

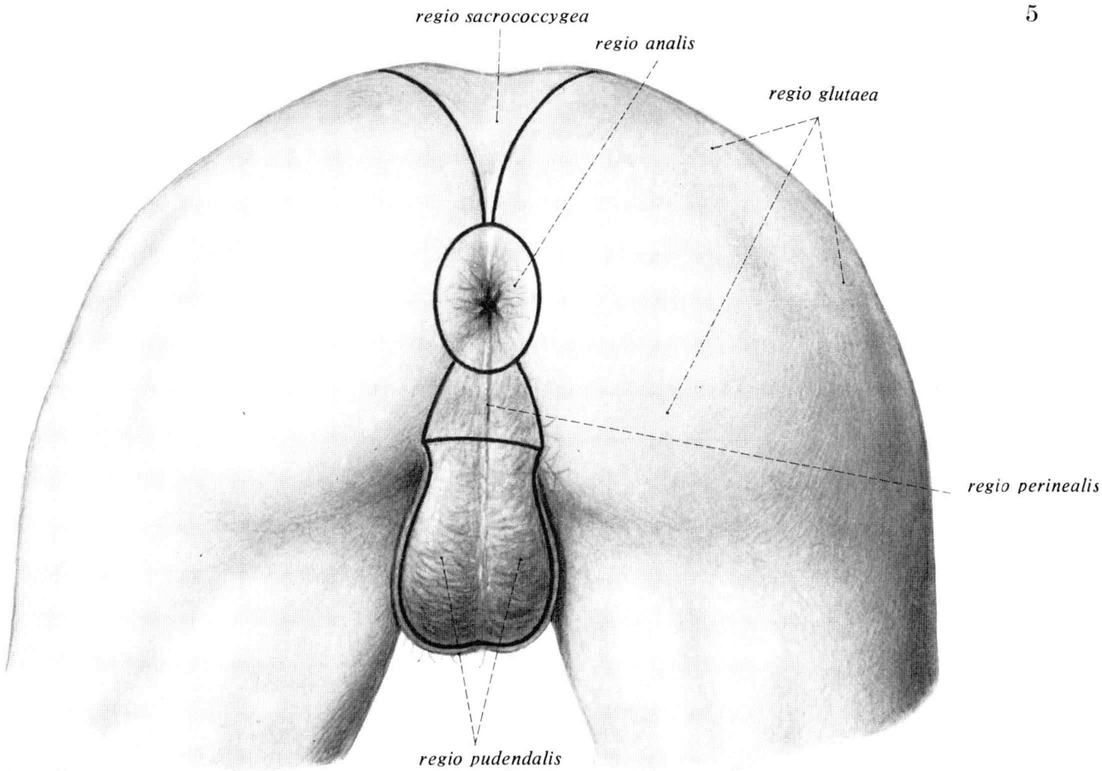

Fig. 4

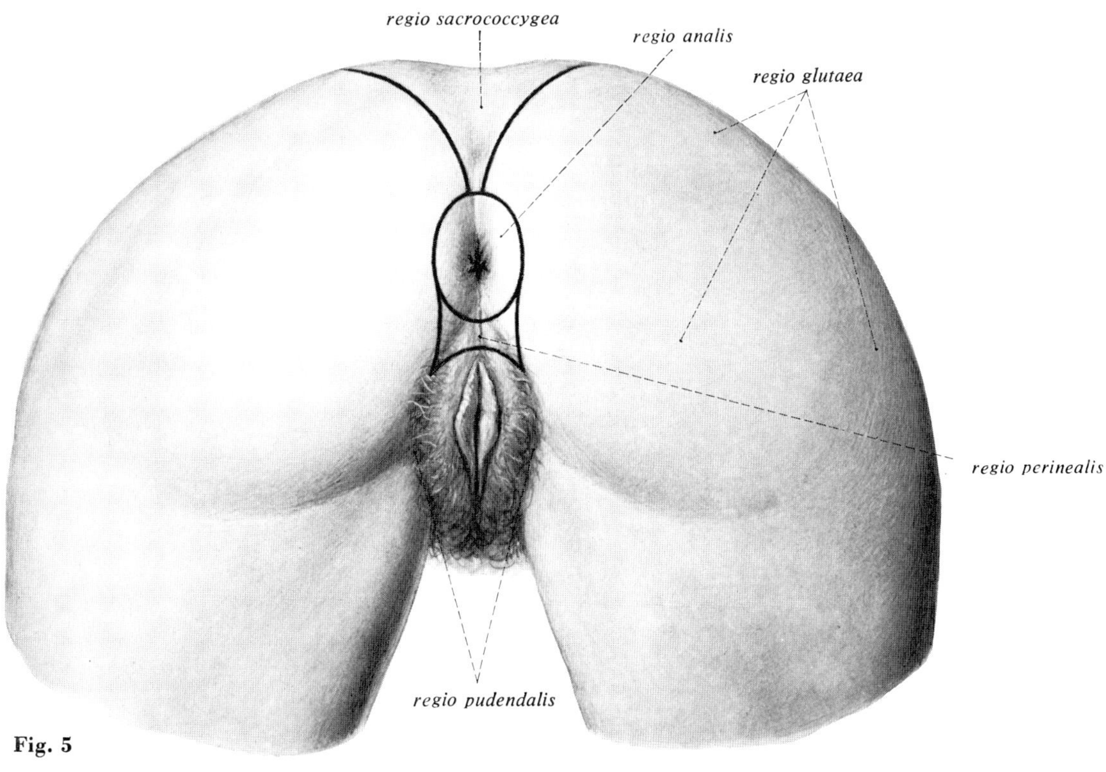

Fig. 5

Figs. 4 and 5. Perineal regions of the body outlined, male and female.

Skeleton

The Bones of the Human Body

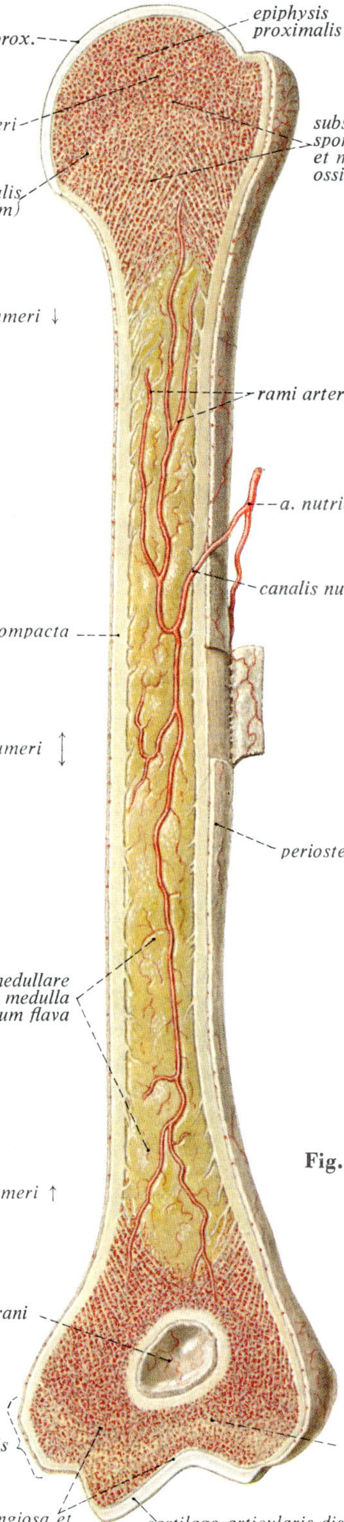

Fig. 6

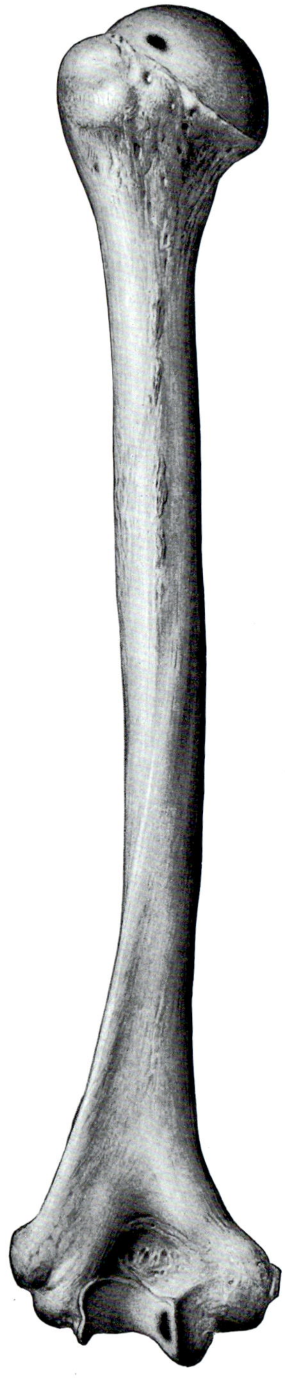

Fig. 7

Figs. 6 and 7. *Humerus*, an example of a long bone. Fig. 6. Longitudinal section to show periosteum, articular cartilage, bone marrow, and blood supply. Epiphyseal lines still discernible. Fig. 7. *Humerus*. Dorsal view.

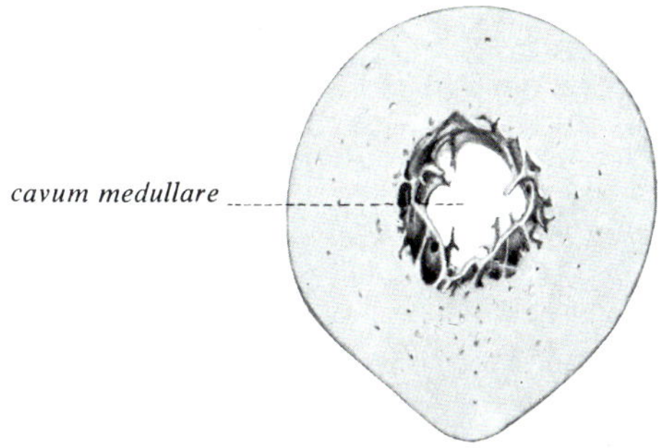

Fig. 8. Cross section of the shaft of a long bone, showing the *cavum medullare*.

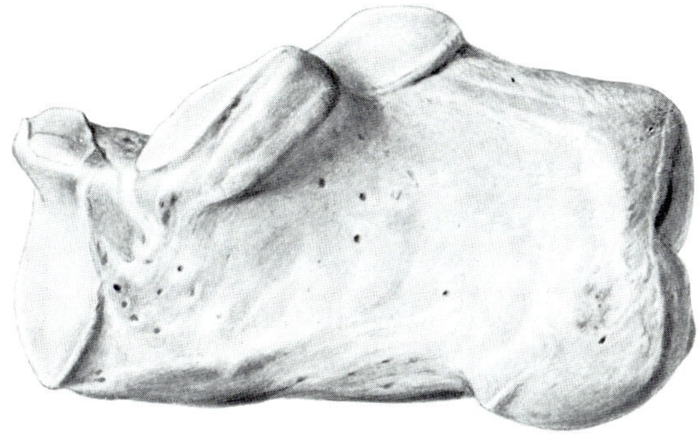

Fig. 9. *Calcaneus,* an example of a short bone.

Fig. 10. *Sternum,* an example of a flat bone.

Fig. 11. *Os temporale.* An example of a pneumatic bone, sectioned to show the *cellulae mastoideae*.

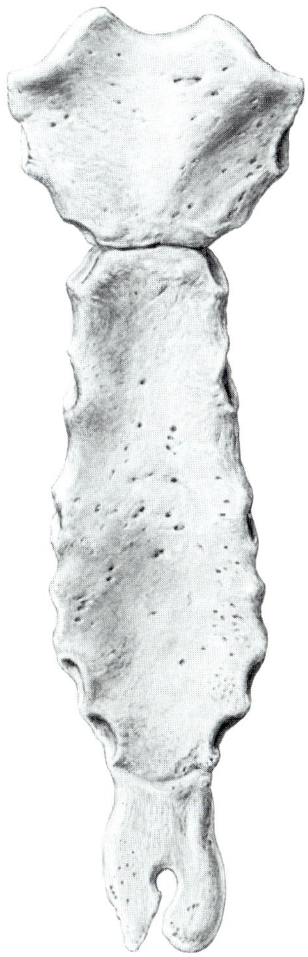

Fig. 10

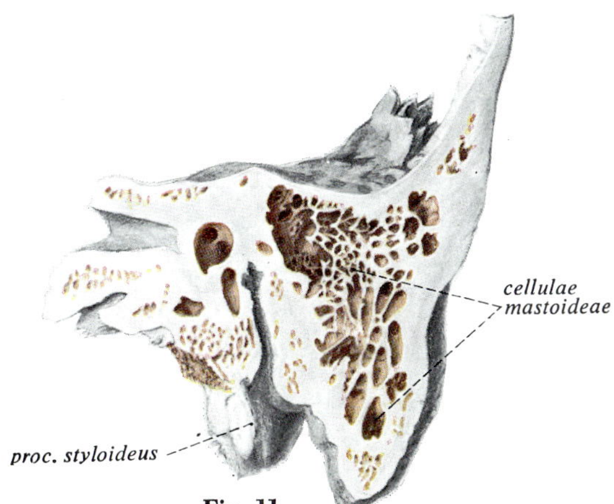

Fig. 11

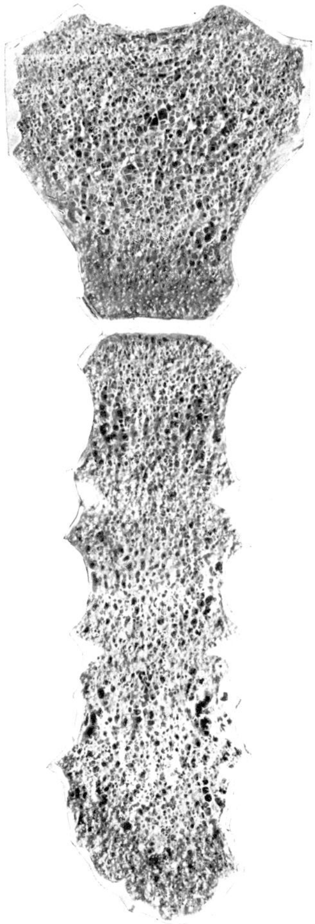

Fig. 12

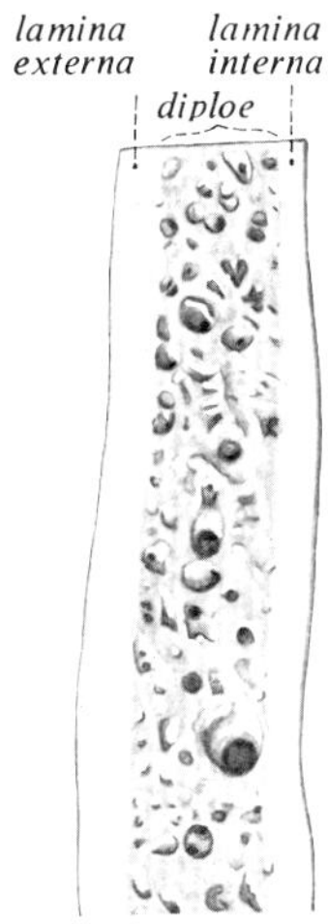

Fig. 13

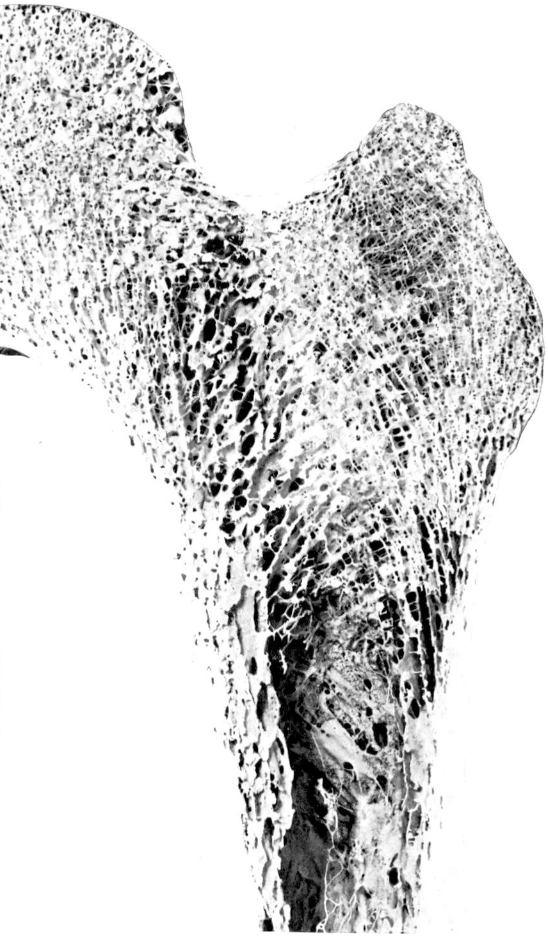

Fig. 14

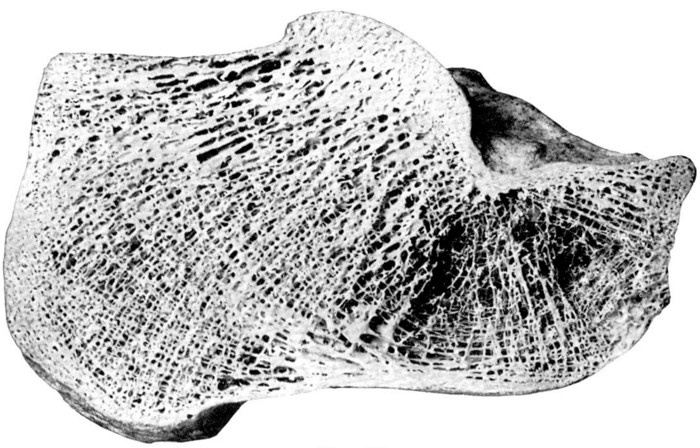

Fig. 15

Fig. 12. Sectioned surface of the *sternum*. The *synchondrosis sternalis* is the fibrocartilage which appears clear between *manubrium* and *corpus sterni*.

Fig. 13. A sectioned flat cranial bone (slightly enlarged).

Fig. 14. Frontal longitudinal section of the proximal end of the *femur*.

Fig. 15. Sagittal longitudinal section of the *calcaneus*. The trabeculae are oriented to give maximum strength and elasticity with minimal weight.

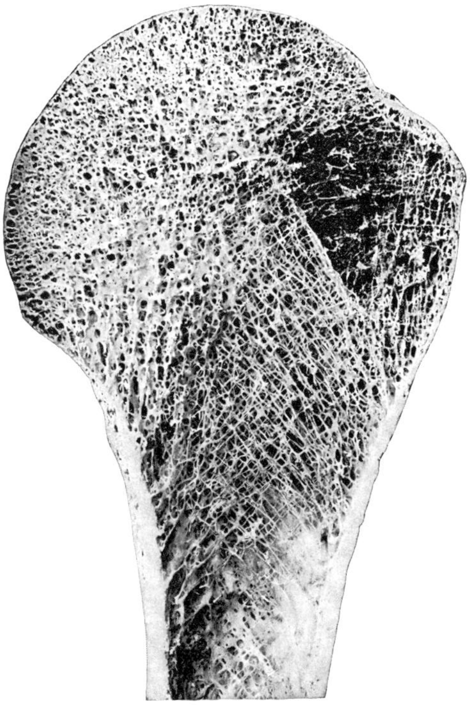

Fig. 16. Frontal longitudinal section through the proximal end of the *humerus*.

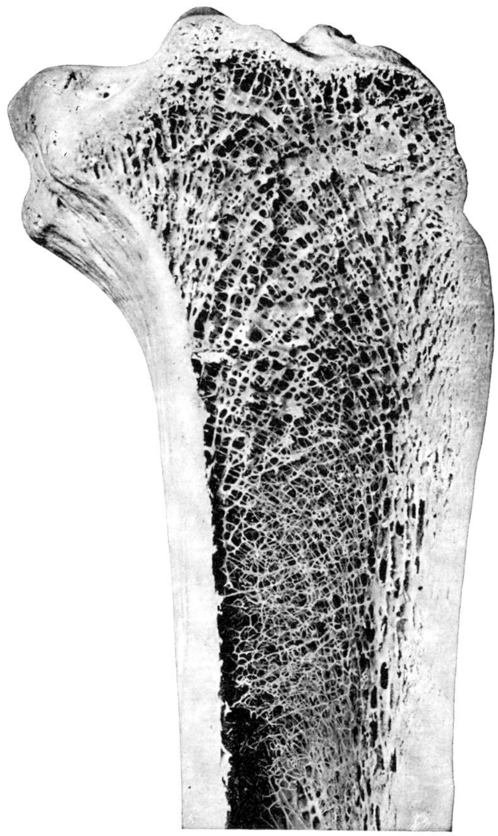

Fig. 17. Sagittal longitudinal section through the proximal end of the *tibia*.

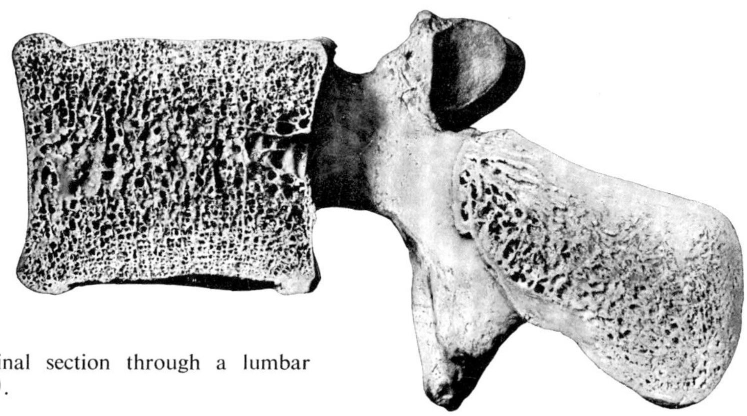

Fig. 18. Sagittal longitudinal section through a lumbar vertebra *(vertebra lumbalis)*.

Note: The structure of the trabeculae in the cancellous bones gives rise to the "trajectorial theory", i.e., the bony trabeculae follow the lines of maximal internal stress. (Figs. 14, 15, 16)

Skeleton

The Trunk

Summary of the Structural Characteristics of the Typical Vertebra

	7 Cervical*	12 Thoracic	5 Lumbar	5 Sacrum Vertebrae
Terminal surfaces of the body of the vertebrae	rectangular small	somewhat triangular	bean-shaped large	fused
Foramen vertebrale	triangular large	round	triangular small	canalis sacralis
Articular surfaces (processus articularis)	oblique, sloping toward dorsal	frontal	sagittal	crista sacralis intermedia
Processus spinosus	processus transversi	club-shaped with foveae costales transversales	processus mamillares et accessorii	crista sacralis lateralis
Spinous processes	horizontal short divided	directed steeply caudalward	horizontal, lateral, large flattened	crista sacralis mediana
Rib rudiments	ventral part of the processus transversus and tuberculum dorsale	none, since the ribs are developed	processus costarii	partes laterales
Characteristic differentiations	foramen transversarium	foveae costales superiores et inferiores	processus mamillares et accessorii	synostosis of the vertebrae

* The first two cervical vertebrae, the *atlas* and *axis*, are not typical cervical vertebrae. They have special characteristics.

Figs. 19-21. Spinal column *(columna vertebralis)*. Fig. 19. Ventral view. Fig. 20. Dorsal view. Fig. 21. Left lateral view. The *fovea costalis transversalis* is missing on the 10th thoracic vertebra.

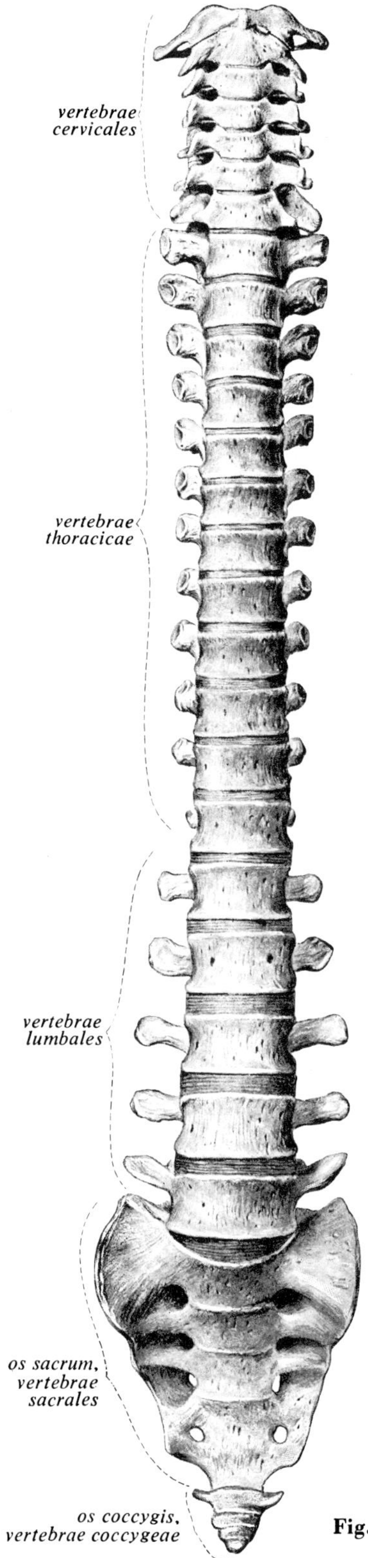
vertebrae cervicales
vertebrae thoracicae
vertebrae lumbales
os sacrum, vertebrae sacrales
os coccygis, vertebrae coccygeae

Fig. 19

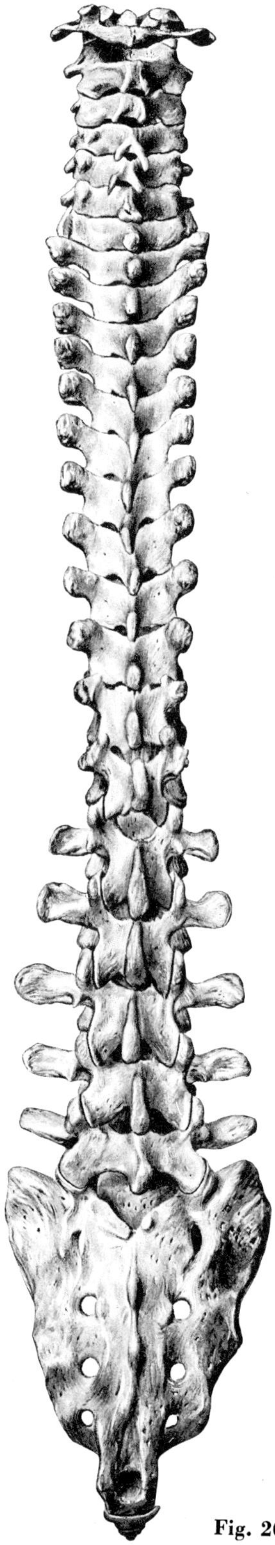

Fig. 20

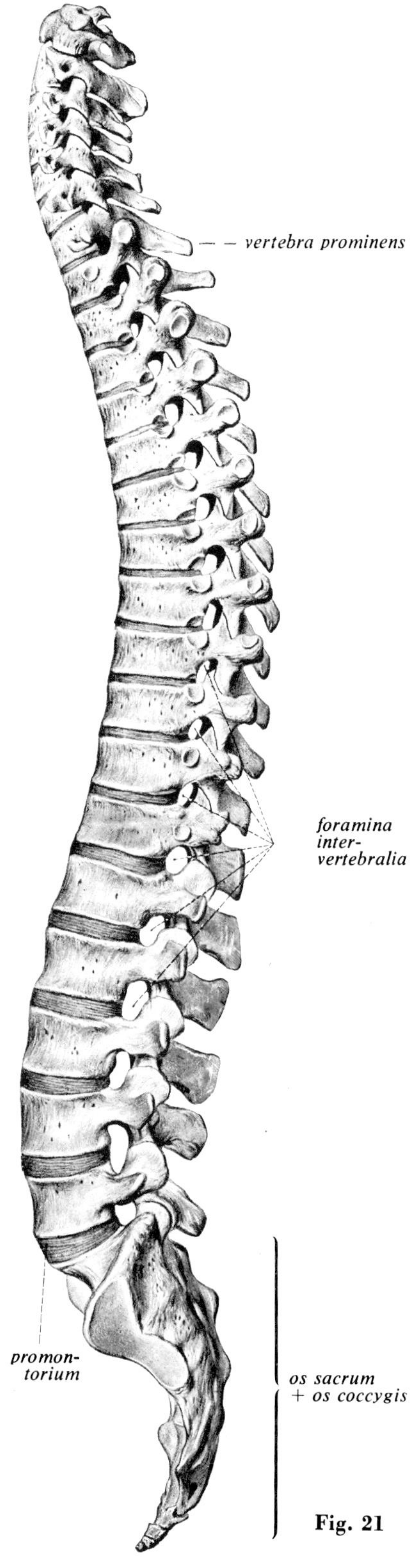
vertebra prominens
foramina inter-vertebralia
promon-torium
os sacrum + os coccygis

Fig. 21

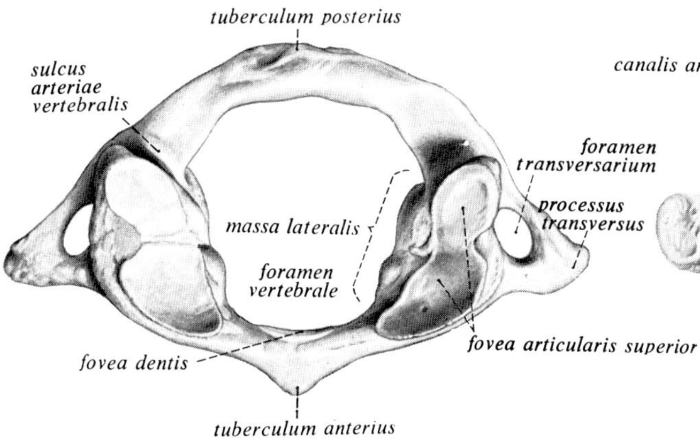

Fig. 22. *Atlas*. Cranial view.

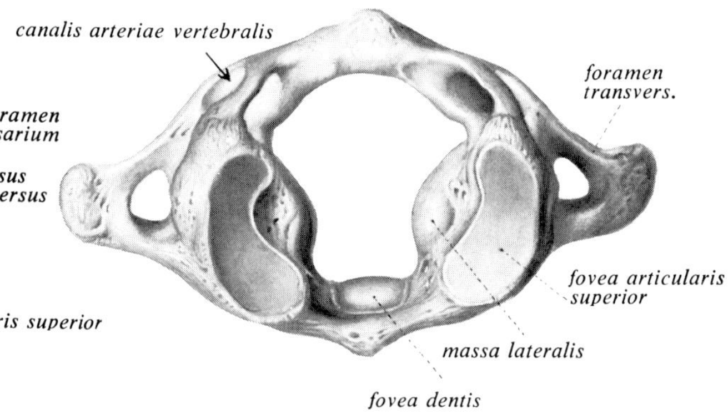

Fig. 23. *Atlas*. Cranial view, with closed *sulcus arteriae vertebralis*.

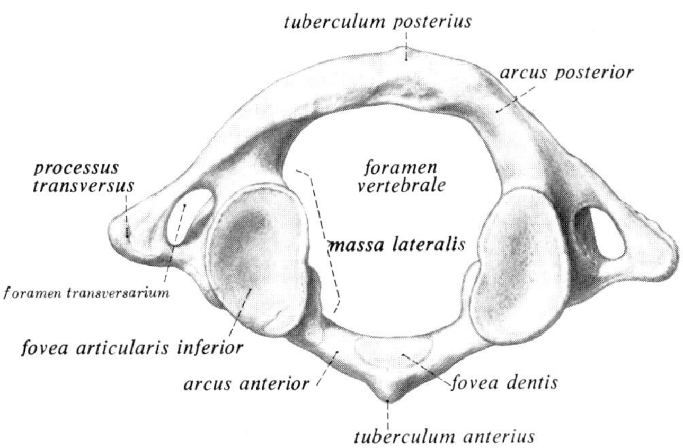

Fig. 24. *Atlas*. Caudal view.

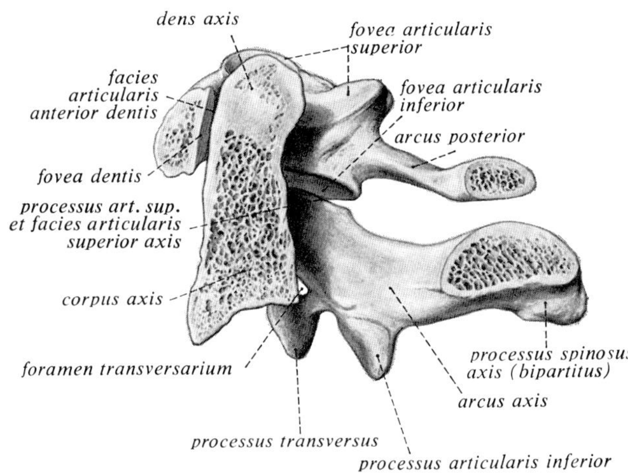

Fig. 25. *Atlas* and *axis*. Median sagittal section.

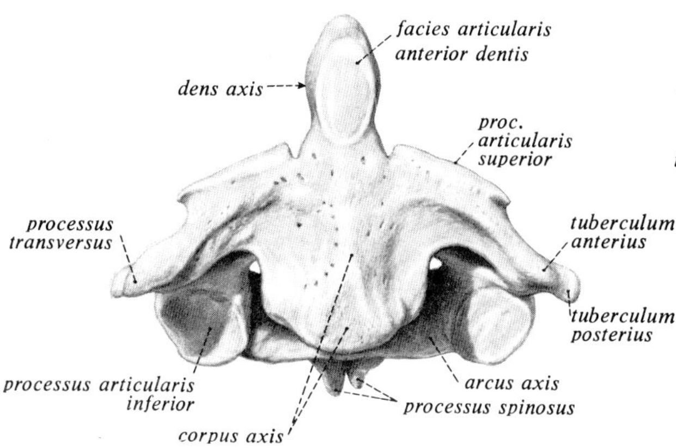

Fig. 26. *Axis*. Ventral view.

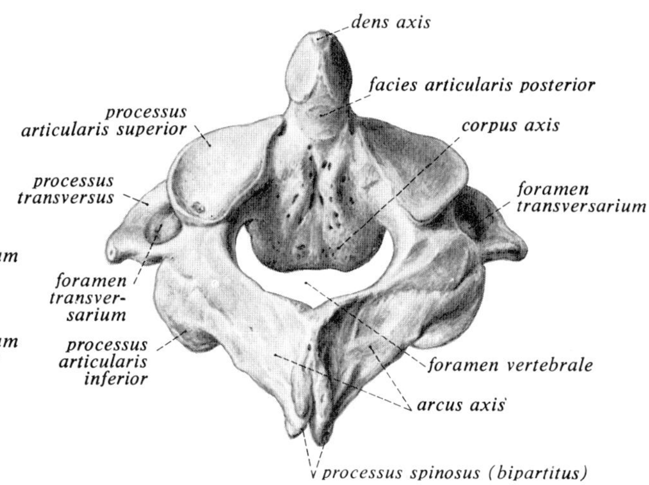

Fig. 27. *Axis*. Dorsal view.

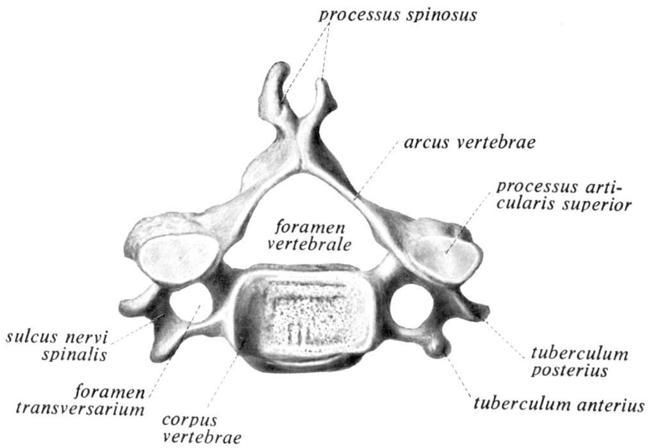

Fig. 28. Fifth *vertebra cervicalis*. Cranial view.

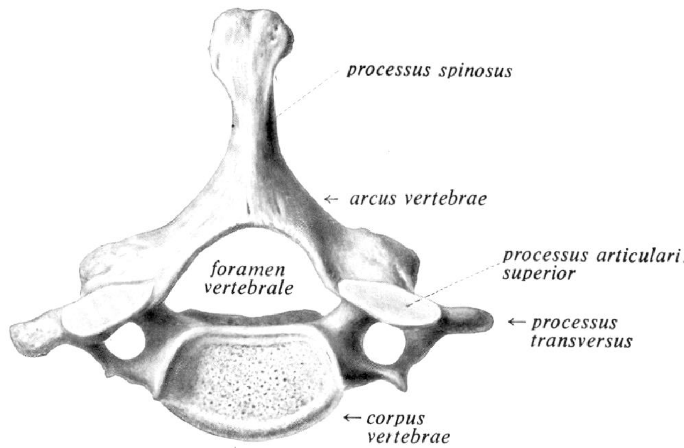

Fig. 29. Seventh cervical vertebra *(vertebra prominens)*. Cranial view.

Fig. 30. Cervical spinal column *(columna cervicalis)*. Dorsal view, somewhat from right side. Roman numerals indicate the number of the cervical vertebra.

Fig. 31. Lower cervical spinal column *(columna cervicalis)*. Ventral view. * Cranial flanges of lateral borders of vertebral bodies.

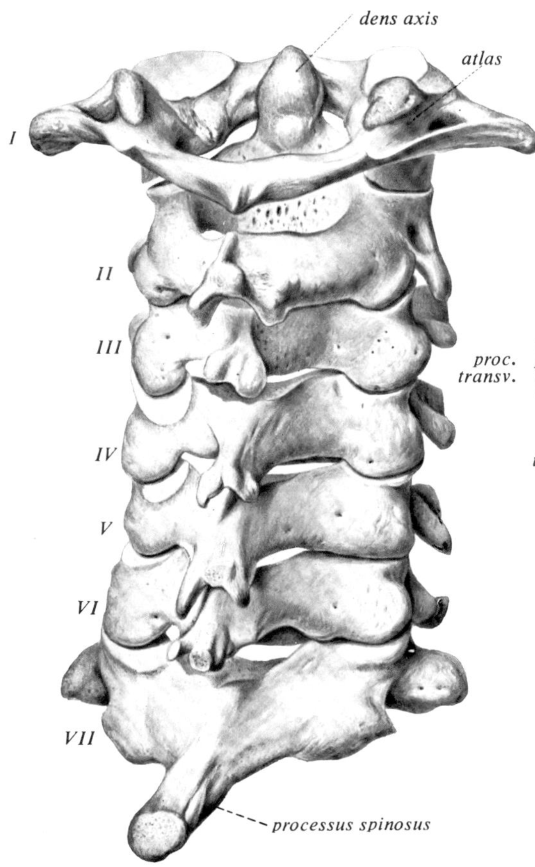

Fig. 30

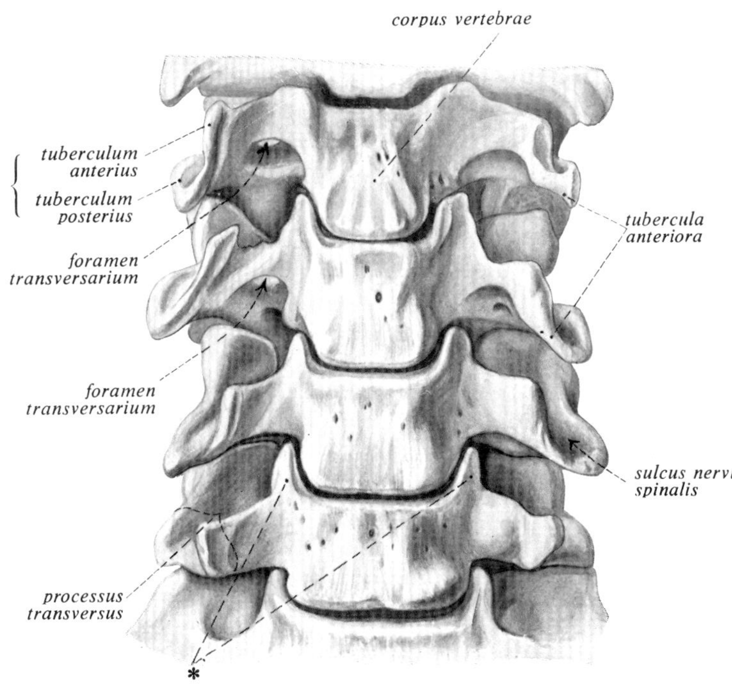

Fig. 31

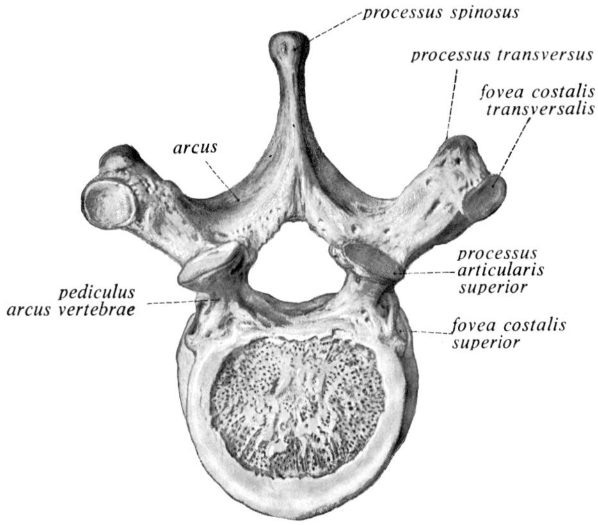

Fig. 32. Sixth *vertebra thoracica*. Cranial view.

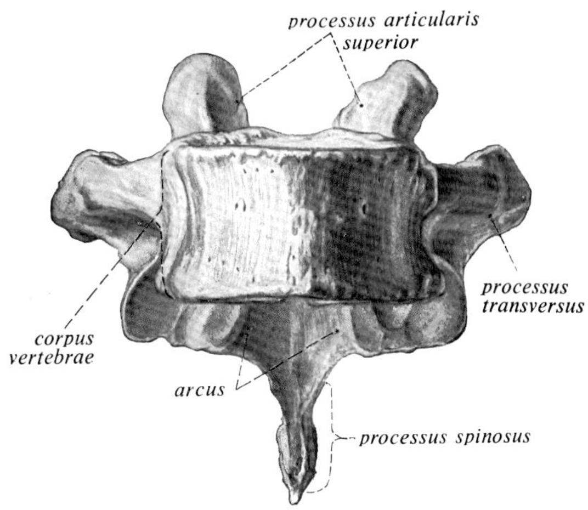

Fig. 33. Tenth *vertebra thoracica*. Ventral view.

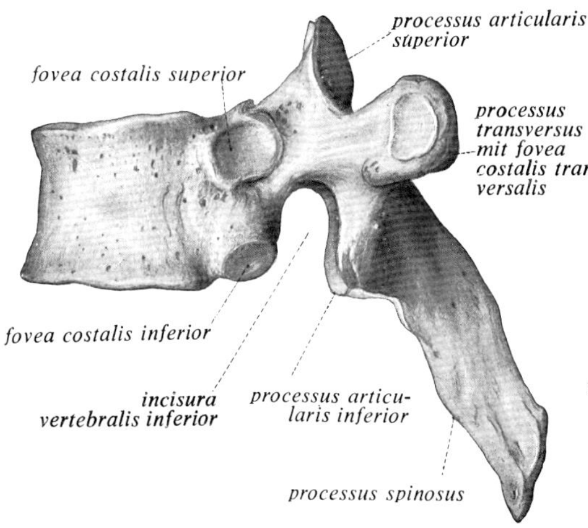

Fig. 34. Sixth *vertebra thoracica*. Left lateral view.

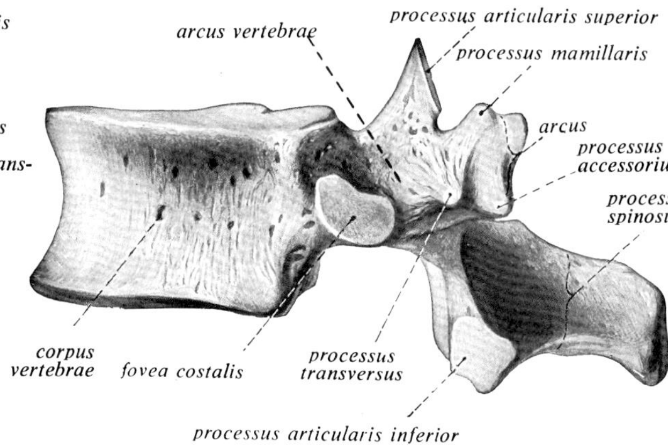

Fig. 35. Twelfth *vertebra thoracica*. Left lateral view.

Note: The sixth thoracic vertebra has three articular surfaces for the ribs: an upper, on the body for the 6th rib; a lower, on the body for the 7th rib; and one on the transverse process for the 6th rib. On the 12th thoracic vertebra, there is only one articular surface present, which is for the 12th rib.

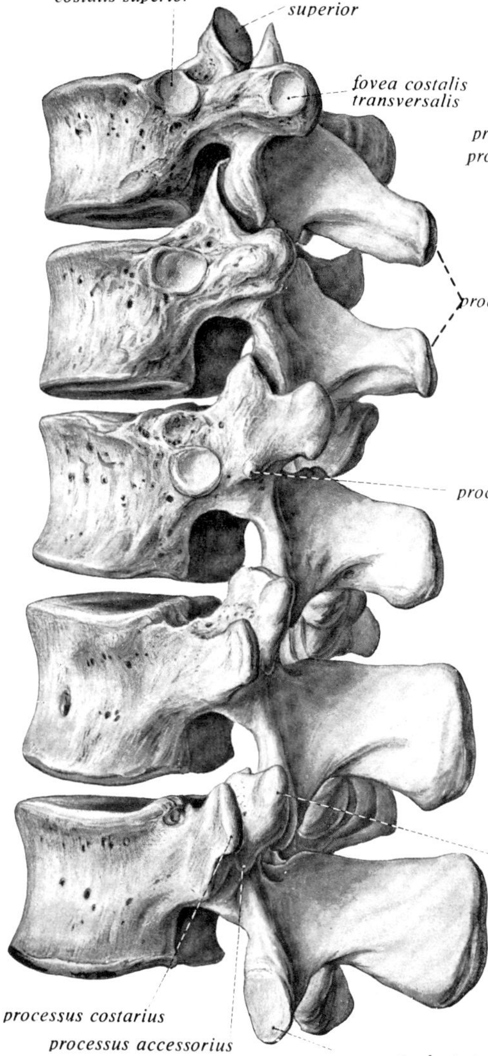

Fig. 36. The last three *vertebrae thoracicae,* X–XII, and the first two *vertebrae lumbales,* I and II. Left lateral view.

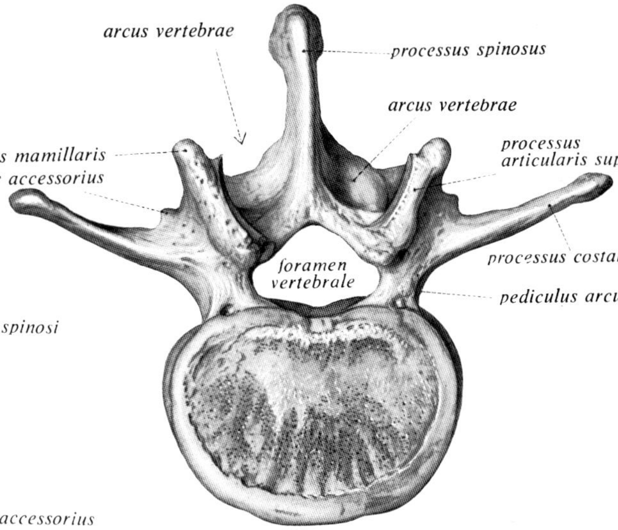

Fig. 37. *Vertebra lumbalis.* Cranial view.

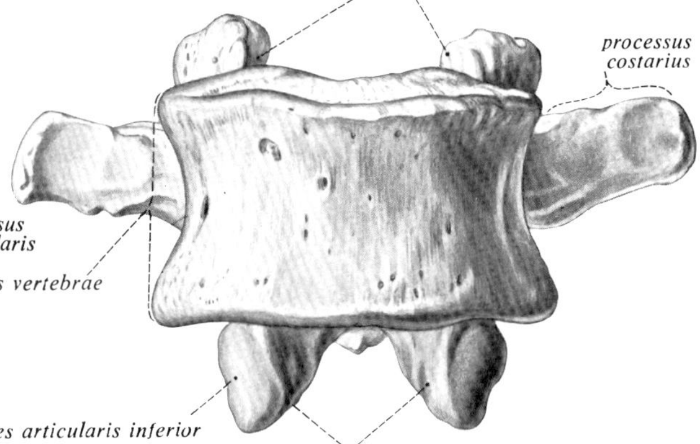

Fig. 38. *Vertebra lumbalis.* Ventral view.

Note: The increase in size of the body of the more caudal vertebrae. The two lower vertebrae of Fig. 36 are lumbar. They have no articular surfaces for ribs, but the rib rudiments, *processus costarii,* are present. The *processus transversus* is divided into an upper *processus mamillaris* and a small lower *processus accessorius.* The articular surfaces of the articular processes are, on the thoracic vertebrae, directed ventrally and dorsally; on the lumbar vertebrae, sagittally (ante- and retroflexion are possible). The *processus spinosi* of the lumbar vertebrae are massive and somewhat quadrilateral and extend more horizontal than those of the thoracic.

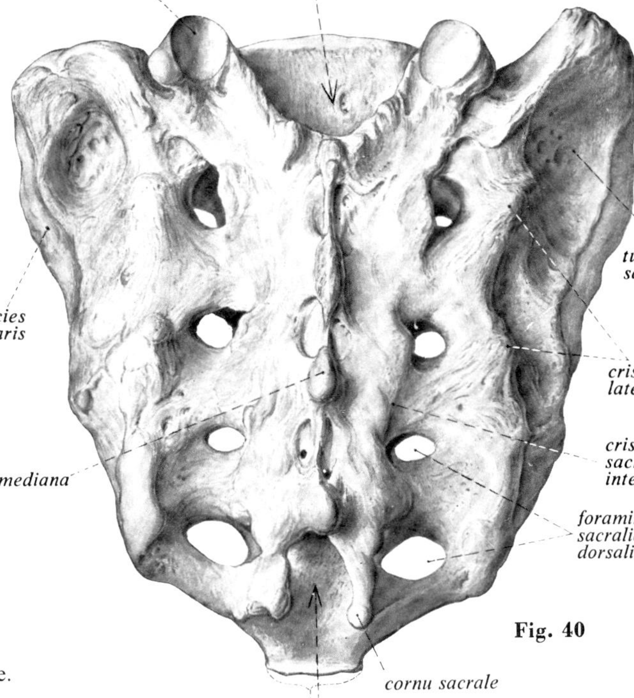

Fig. 40

Fig. 39. *Os sacrum.* Ventral view, pelvic surface.

Fig. 40. *Os sacrum.* Dorsal view.

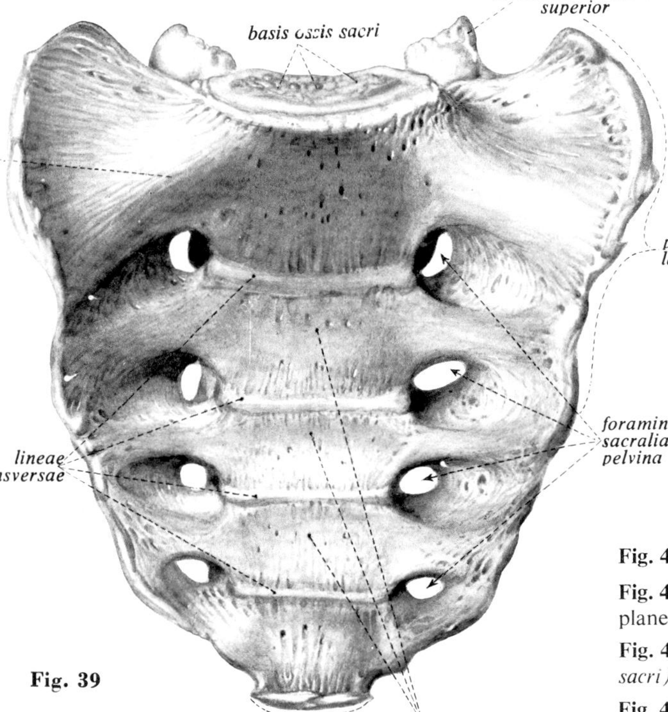

Fig. 39

Fig. 41. *Os sacrum* and *os coccygis.* Right lateral view.

Fig. 42. *Os sacrum* of a young individual. Median sagittal plane.

Fig. 43. *Os sacrum.* Cranial view of the base *(basis ossis sacri).*

Fig. 44. *Os coccygis.* Ventral view.

Fig. 45. *Os coccygis.* Dorsal view.

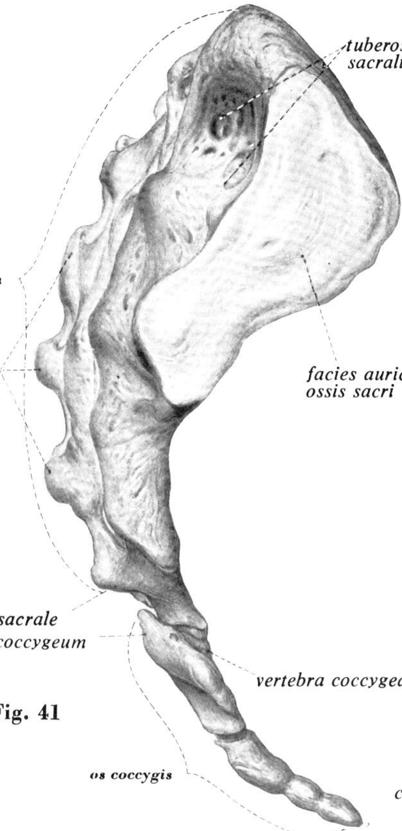
tuberositas sacralis
os sacrum
crista sacralis mediana
facies auricularis ossis sacri
cornu sacrale
cornu coccygeum
vertebra coccygea I
os coccygis

Fig. 41

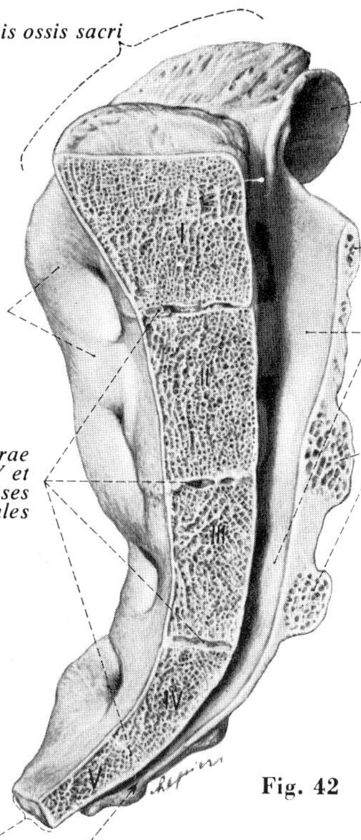
basis ossis sacri
processus articularis superior
crista sacralis mediana
facies pelvina
canalis sacralis
crista sacralis mediana
vertebrae sacrales I–V et synchondroses sacrales
apex ossis sacri
hiatus sacralis

Fig. 42

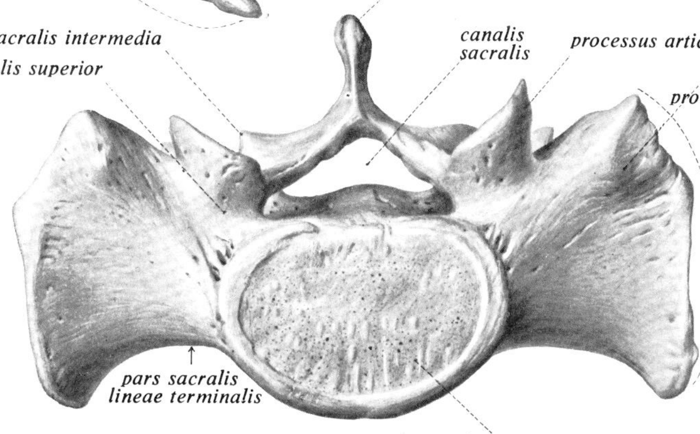
crista sacralis mediana
crista sacralis intermedia
incisura vertebralis superior
canalis sacralis
processus articularis superior
processus costarius vertebrae sacralis I
pars lateralis
pars sacralis lineae terminalis
basis ossis sacri

Fig. 43

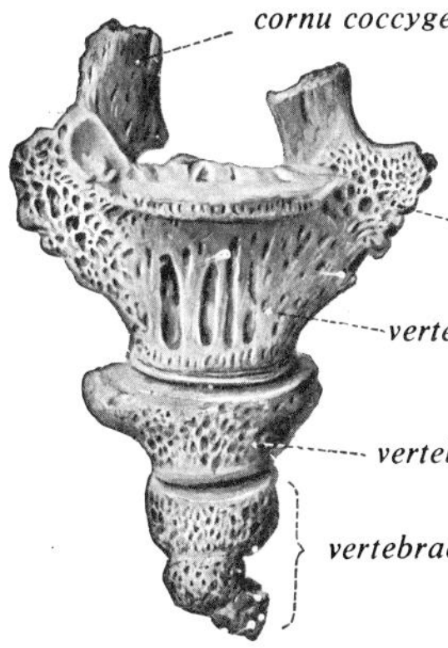
cornu coccygeum
processus transversus
vertebra coccygea I
vertebra coccygea II
vertebrae coccygeae III–V

Fig. 44

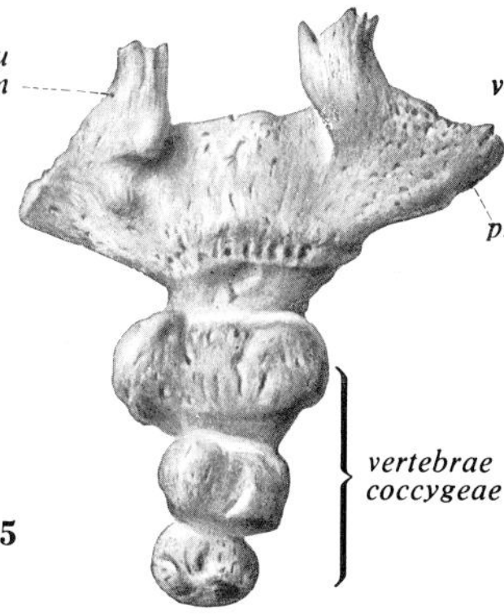
cornu coccygeum
vertebra coccygea I
processus transversus
vertebrae coccygeae II–IV

Fig. 45

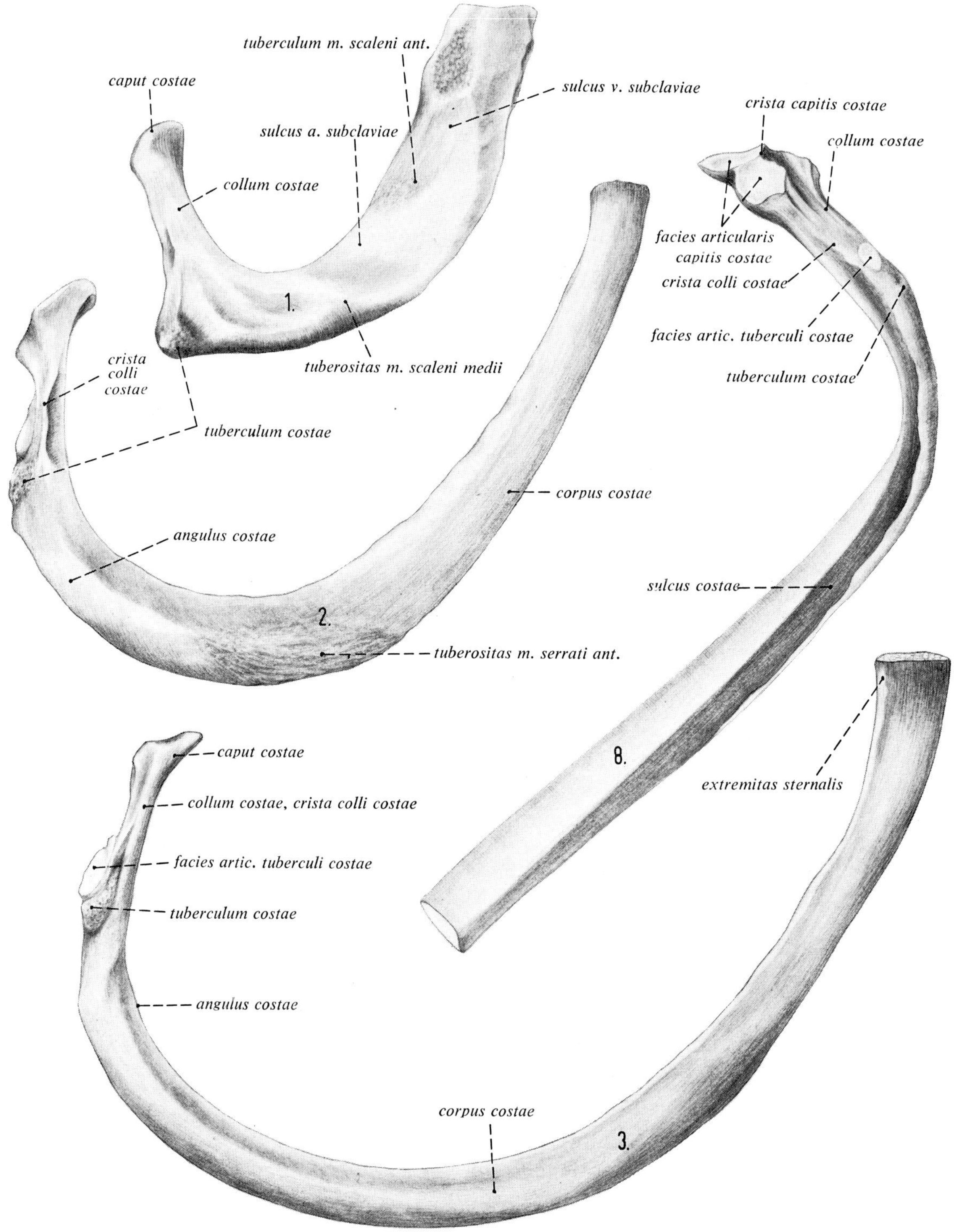

Fig. 46. 1st, 2nd, 3rd, and 8th ribs of the right side of the *thorax,* without *cartilagines costales.* Seen from above. The shortened 8th rib is seen from below.

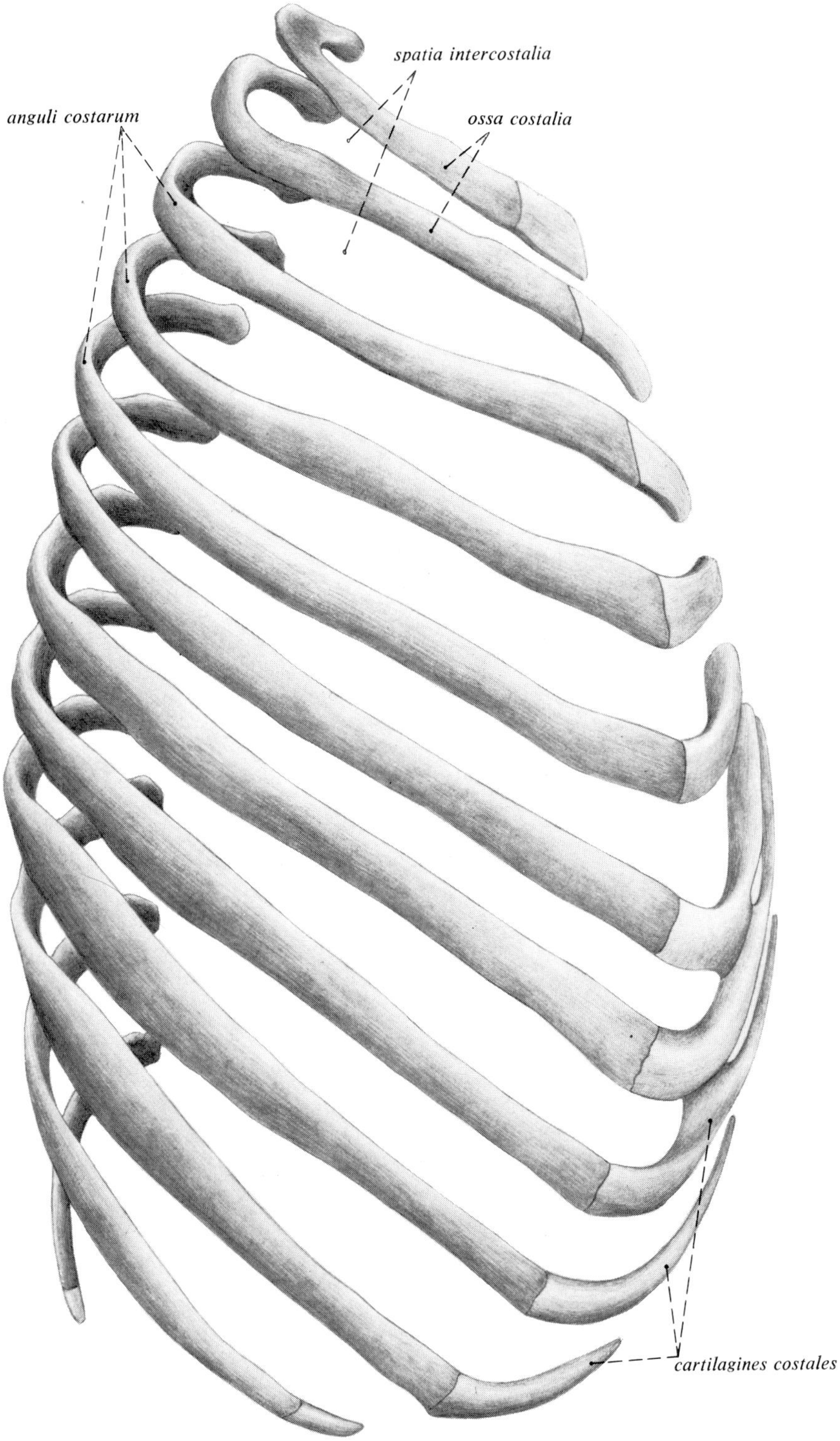

Fig. 47. The ribs of the right side of the *thorax*, in the natural position.

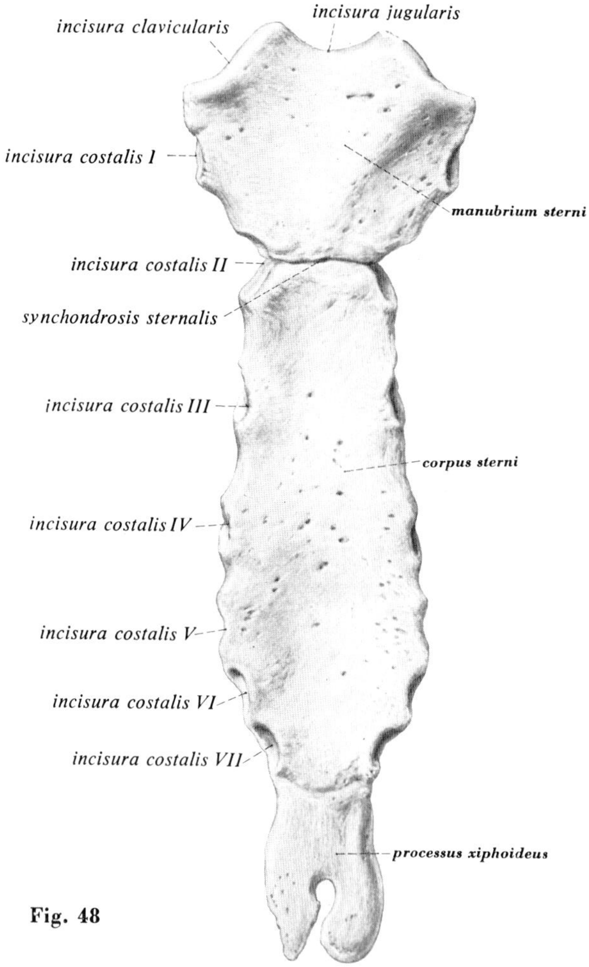

Fig. 48

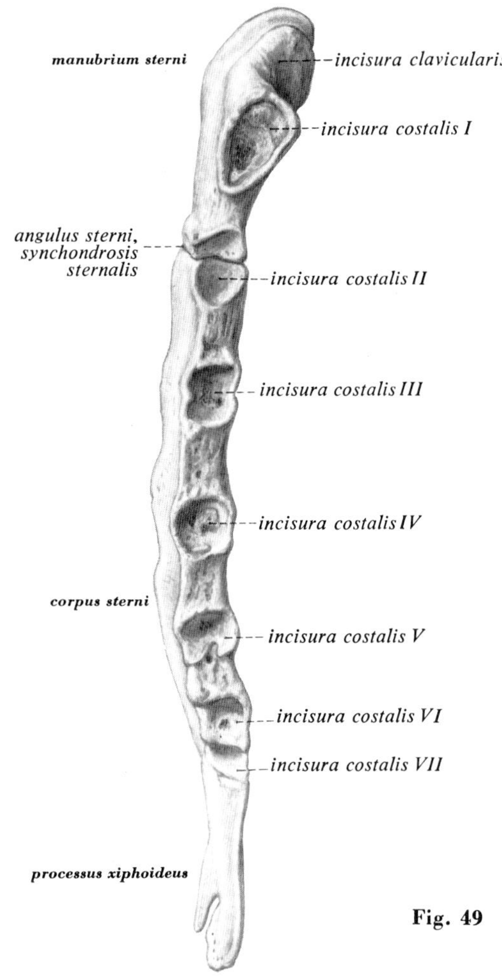

Fig. 49

Figs. 48 and 49. *Sternum* of an adult. Fig. 48. Ventral view. Fig. 49. Lateral view.

Fig. 50. Skeleton of the trunk with shoulder and pelvic girdles and the proximal part of the *femur* in blue. Left median half viewed from the lateral side.

Fig. 51. Skeleton of the trunk, with shoulder and pelvic girdles in blue. Left median half viewed from median aspect.

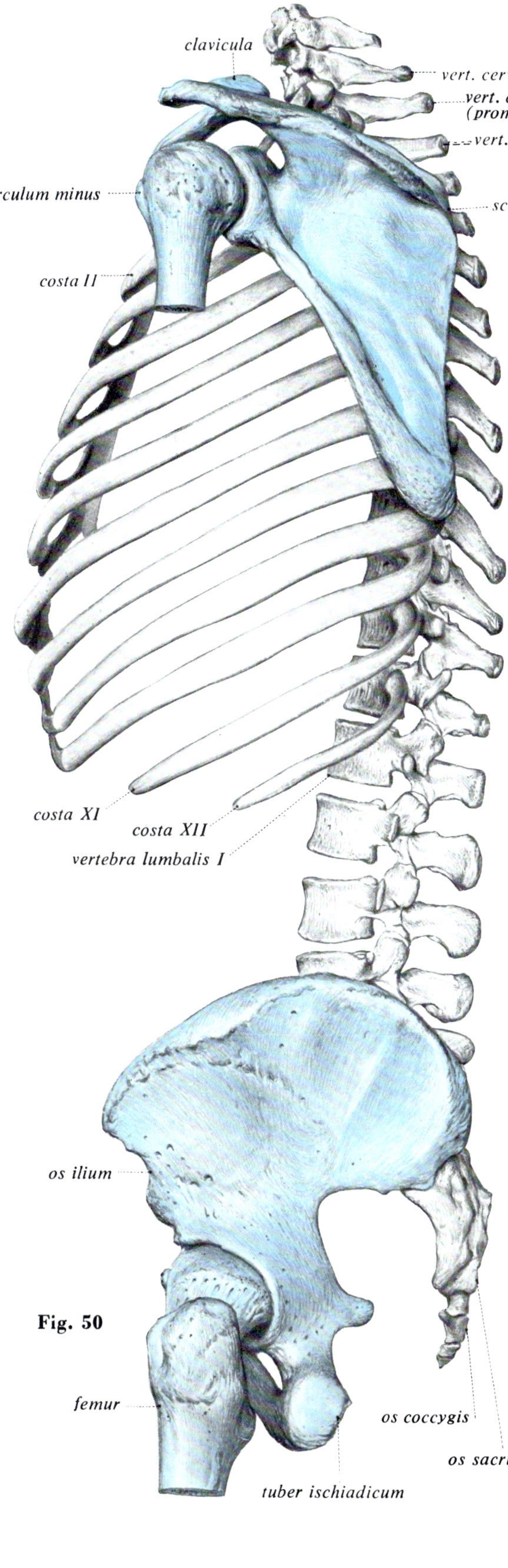
clavicula
vert. cervicalis VI
vert. cervicalis VII
(prominens)
vert. thoracica I
uberculum minus
scapula
costa II
costa XI
costa XII
vertebra lumbalis I
os ilium
femur
os coccygis
os sacrum
tuber ischiadicum

Fig. 50

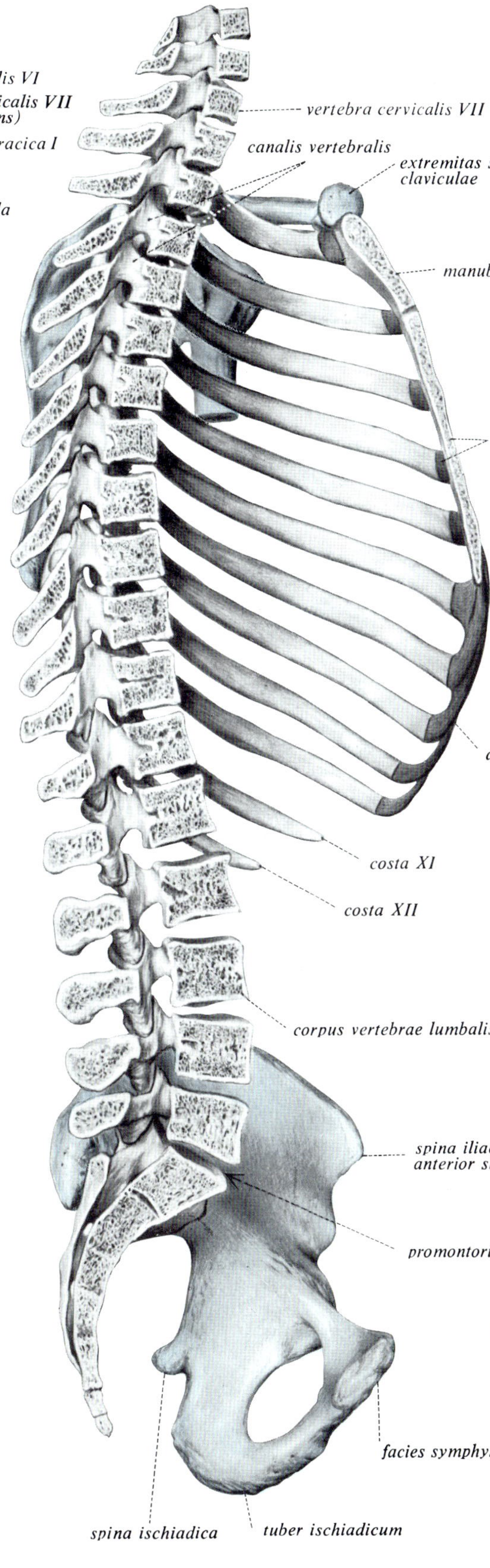
vertebra cervicalis VII
canalis vertebralis
extremitas sternalis
claviculae
manubrium sterni
corpus sterni
arcus costalis
costa XI
costa XII
corpus vertebrae lumbalis III
spina iliaca
anterior superior
promontorium
facies symphysialis
spina ischiadica
tuber ischiadicum

Fig. 51

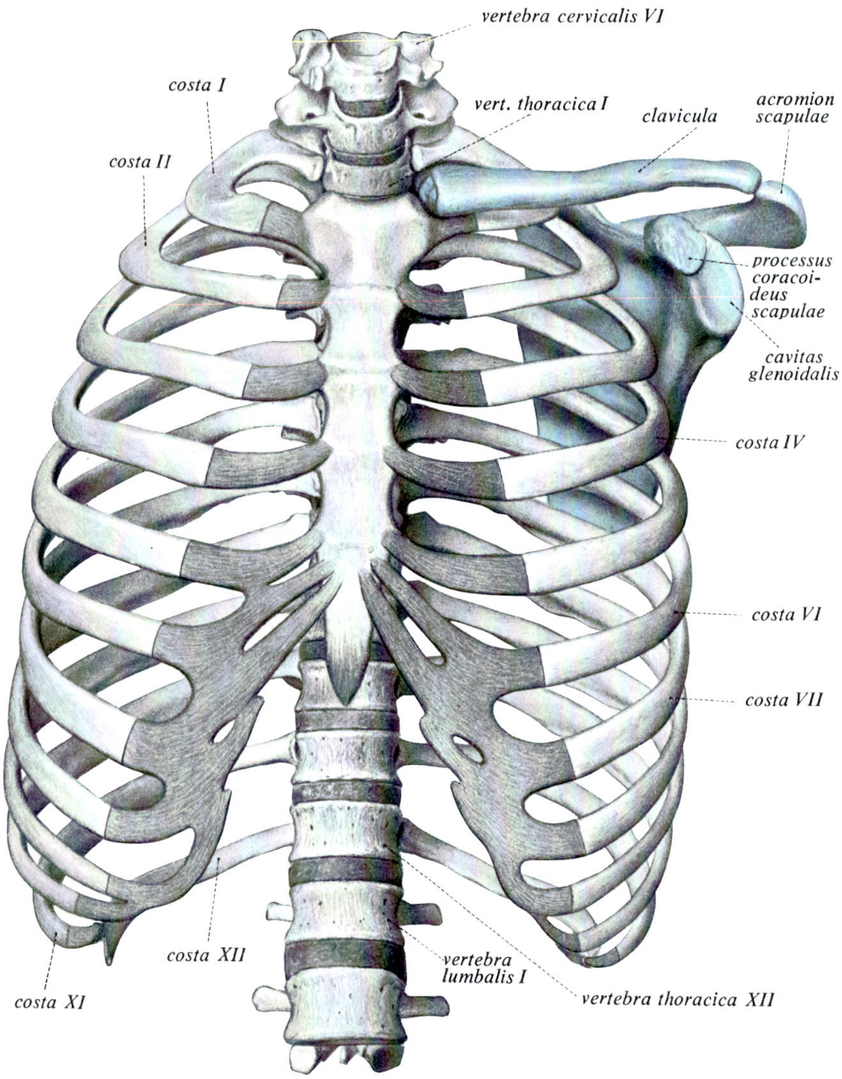

Fig. 52. *Thorax*. Ventral view (moderate inspiration). Left shoulder girdle blue.

Note: The insertion of the second rib meets the *angulus sterni*, i.e., where the *manubrium* meets the body of the *sternum (synchondrosis sternalis)*. This bulge across the *sternum* is always palpable under the skin as an indication of the ending of the second rib.

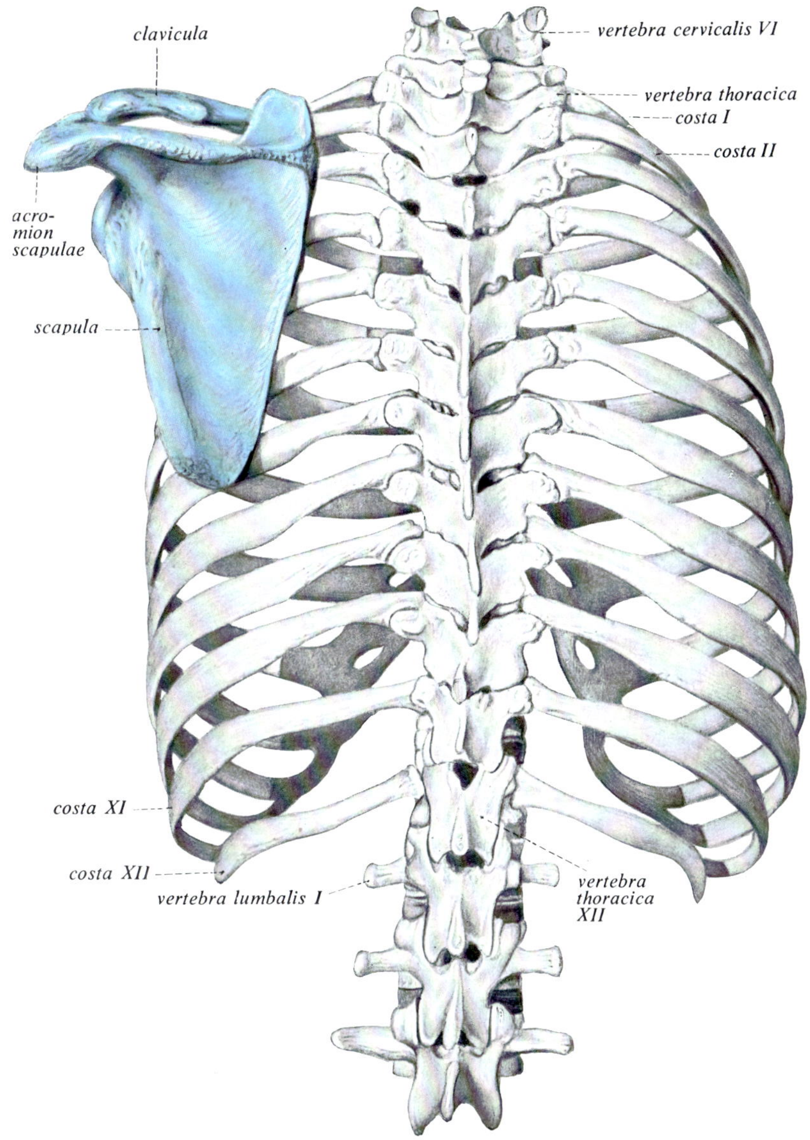

Fig. 53. *Thorax*. Dorsal view (moderate inspiration). Left shoulder girdle blue.

Note: The *apertura thoracis superior* is bounded by the first thoracic vertebra, the first rib, the *manubrium sterni* with its *incisura jugularis*. The *apertura thoracis inferior* is bounded by the 12th thoracic vertebra, the 12th rib, and the cartilaginous *arcus costalis*. The upper seven ribs are called true ribs because they are attached by cartilage to the *sternum*. The remaining 5 are called false ribs because they are not directly attached to the *sternum*. Three of them form the *arcus costalis;* and the 11th and 12th are referred to as floating ribs.

Skeleton

The Skull

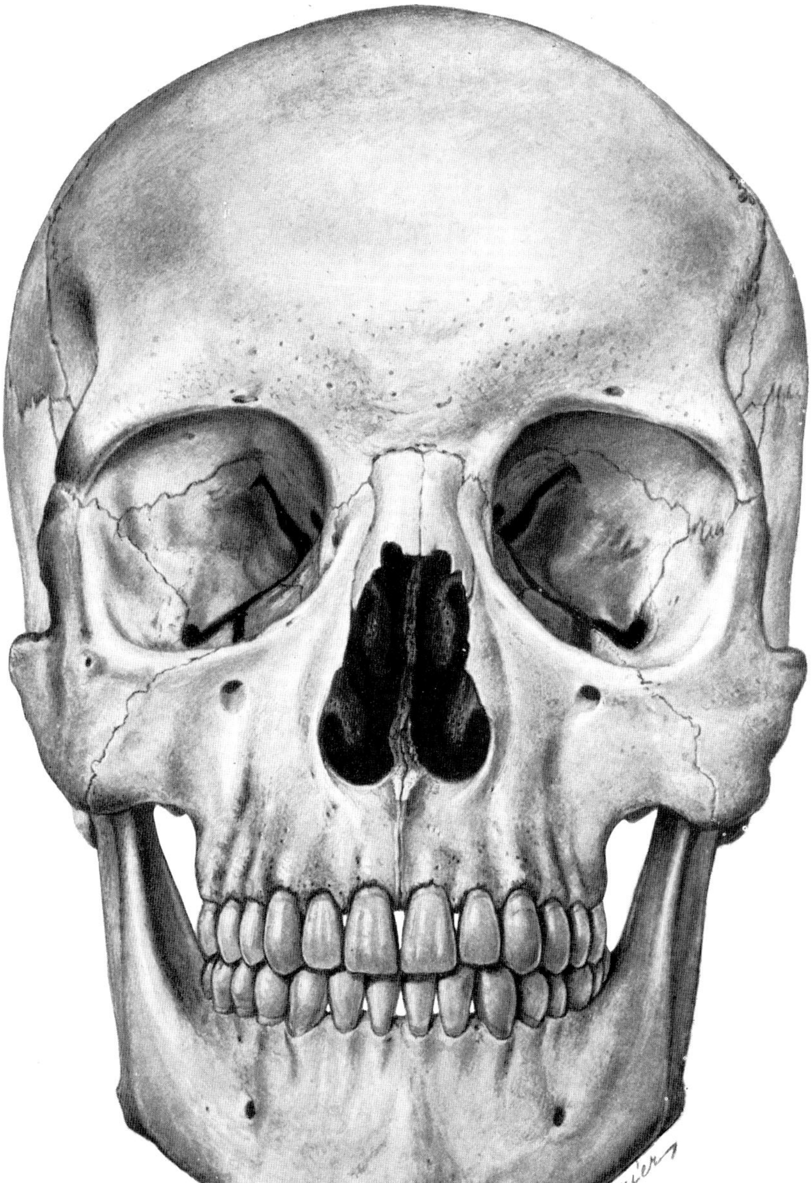

Fig. 54. The skull *(cranium)*. Anterior aspect.

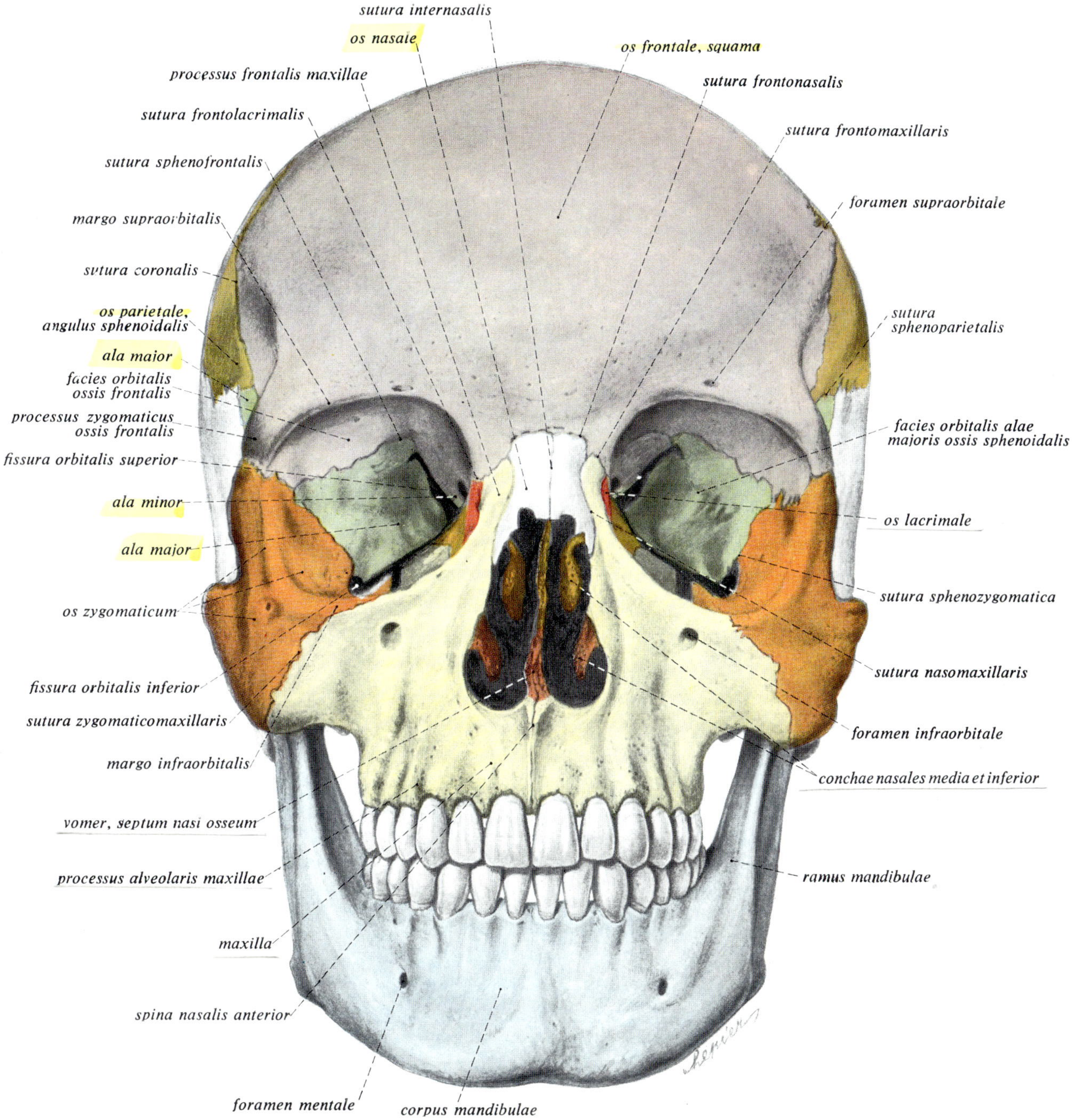

Fig. 55. The skull *(cranium)*. Anterior aspect. The bones are set apart by different colors.

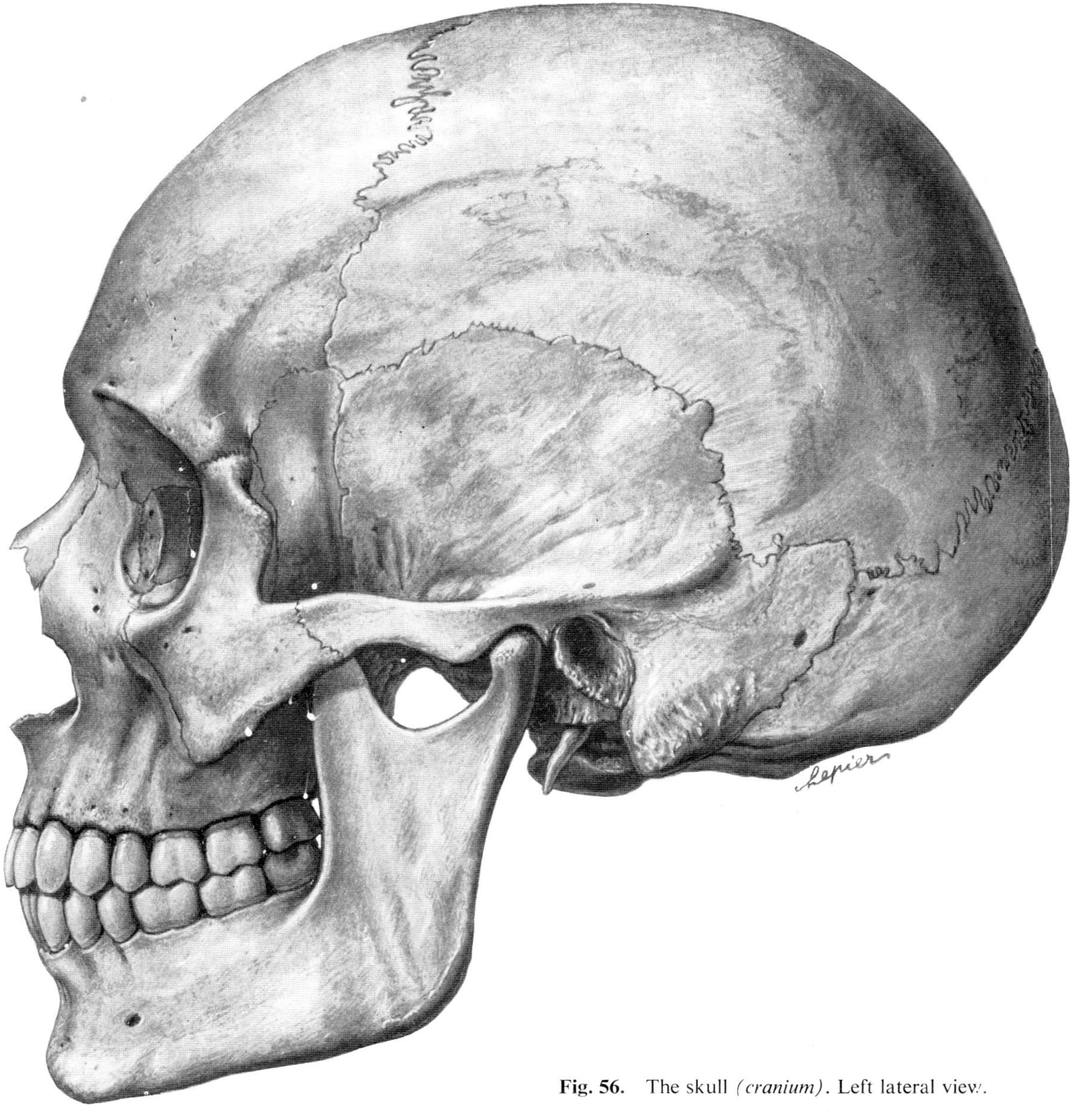

Fig. 56. The skull *(cranium)*. Left lateral view.

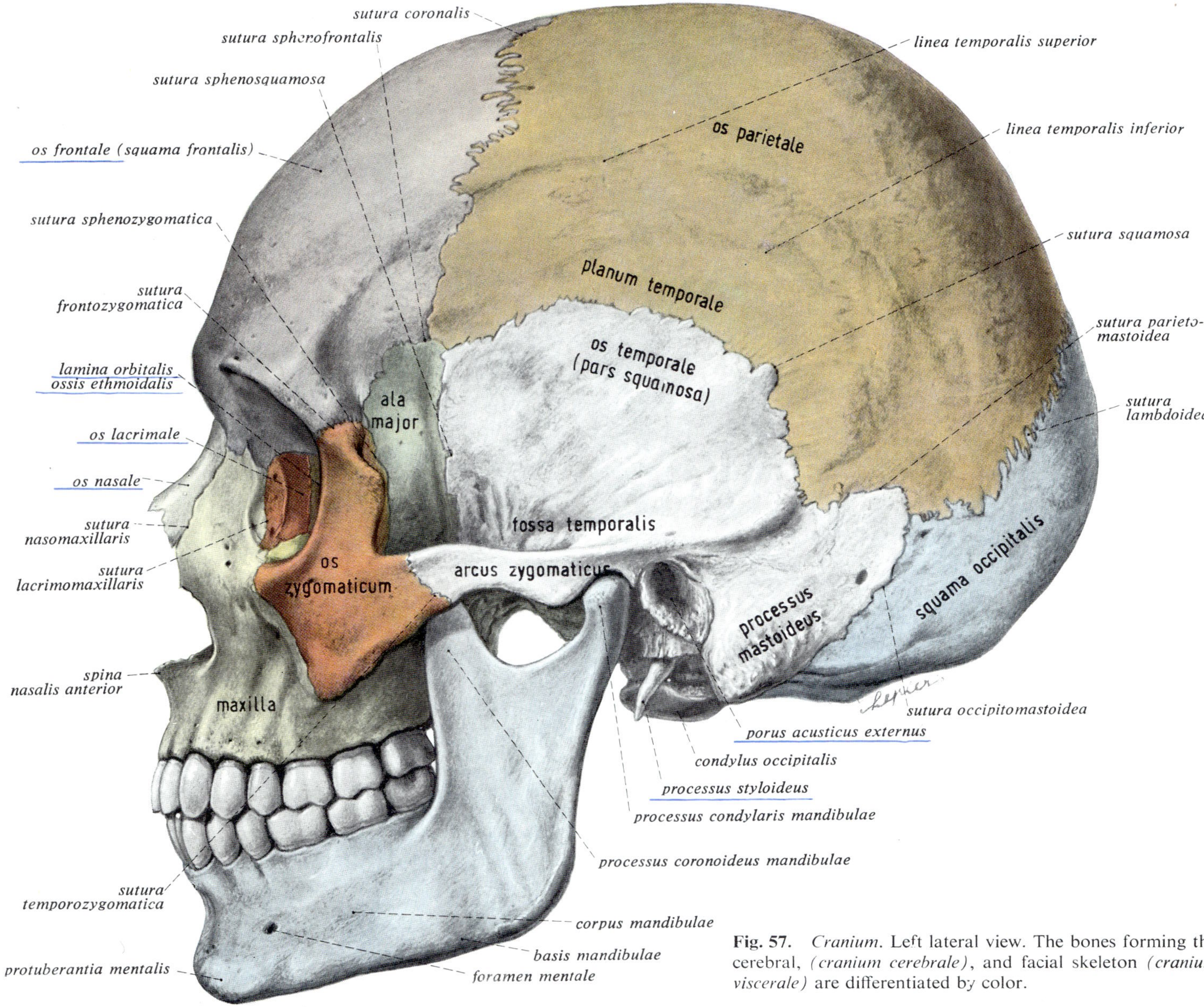

Fig. 57. *Cranium.* Left lateral view. The bones forming the cerebral, *(cranium cerebrale)*, and facial skeleton *(cranium viscerale)* are differentiated by color.

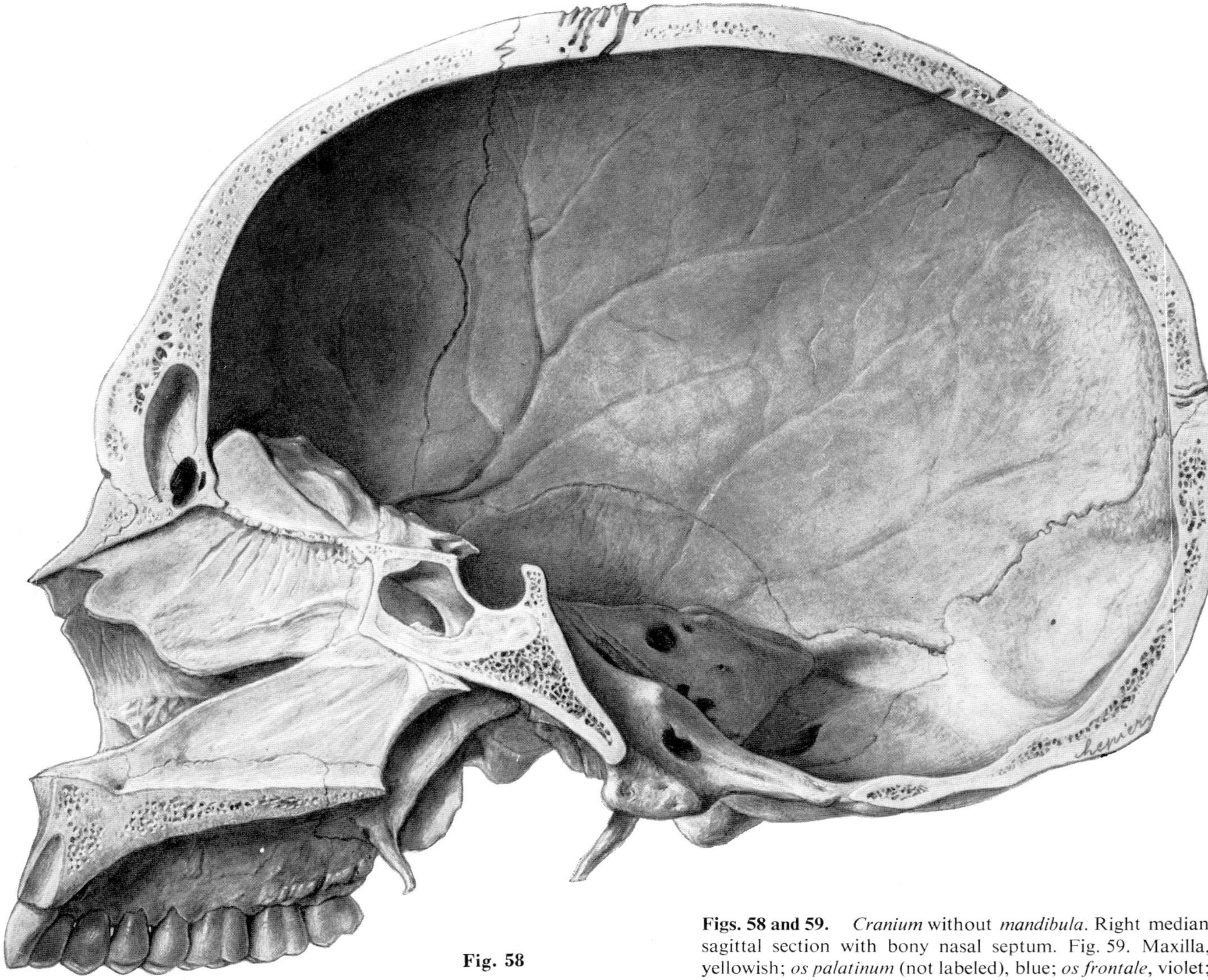

Fig. 58

Figs. 58 and 59. *Cranium* without *mandibula*. Right median sagittal section with bony nasal septum. Fig. 59. Maxilla, yellowish; *os palatinum* (not labeled), blue; *os frontale*, violet; *os sphenoidale*, greenish; *os temporale*, not colored; vomer, brick-red; *os occipitale*, blue; *os ethmoidale*, orange; *os parietale*, brownish.

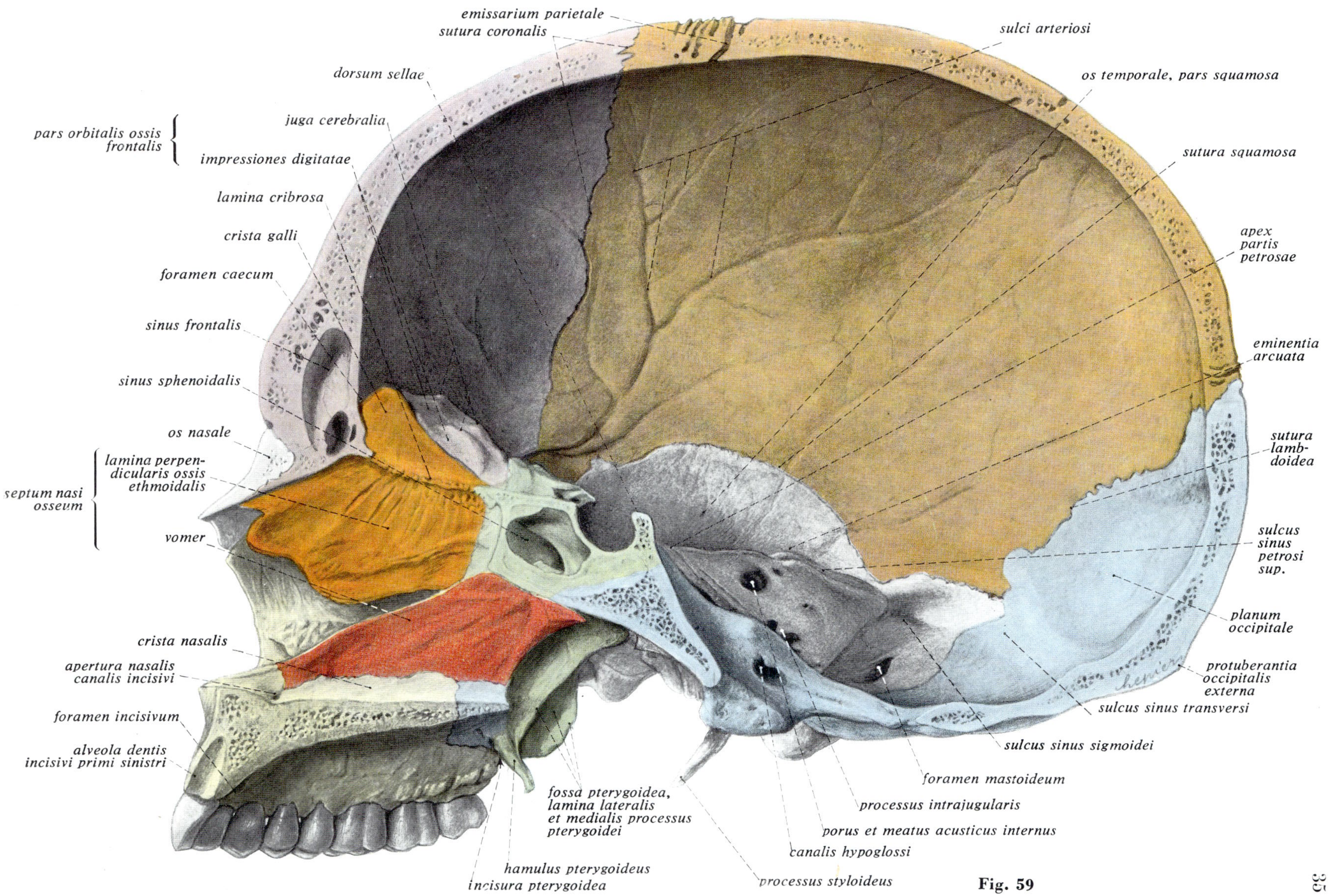
emissarium parietale
sutura coronalis
dorsum sellae
pars orbitalis ossis frontalis
juga cerebralia
impressiones digitatae
lamina cribrosa
crista galli
foramen caecum
sinus frontalis
sinus sphenoidalis
os nasale
septum nasi osseum
lamina perpendicularis ossis ethmoidalis
vomer
crista nasalis
apertura nasalis canalis incisivi
foramen incisivum
alveola dentis incisivi primi sinistri
fossa pterygoidea, lamina lateralis et medialis processus pterygoidei
hamulus pterygoideus
incisura pterygoidea
processus styloideus
canalis hypoglossi
porus et meatus acusticus internus
processus intrajugularis
foramen mastoideum
sulcus sinus sigmoidei
sulcus sinus transversi
protuberantia occipitalis externa
planum occipitale
sulcus sinus petrosi sup.
sutura lambdoidea
eminentia arcuata
apex partis petrosae
sutura squamosa
os temporale, pars squamosa
sulci arteriosi

Fig. 59

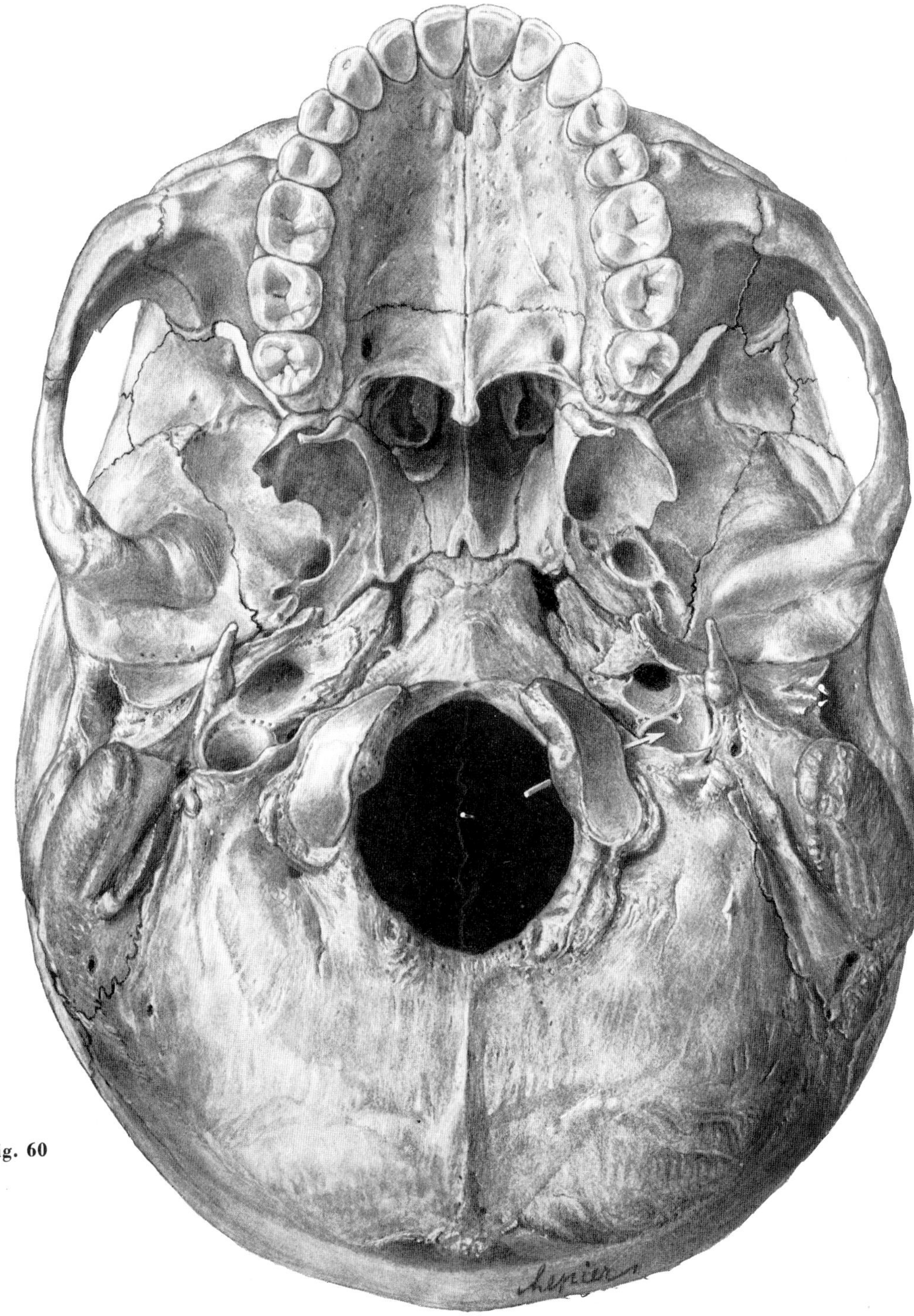

Fig. 60

Figs. 60 and 61. The base of the skull *(basis cranii externa)*, without *mandibula*, from below. Arrow in the *canalis hypoglossi* in Fig. 61.

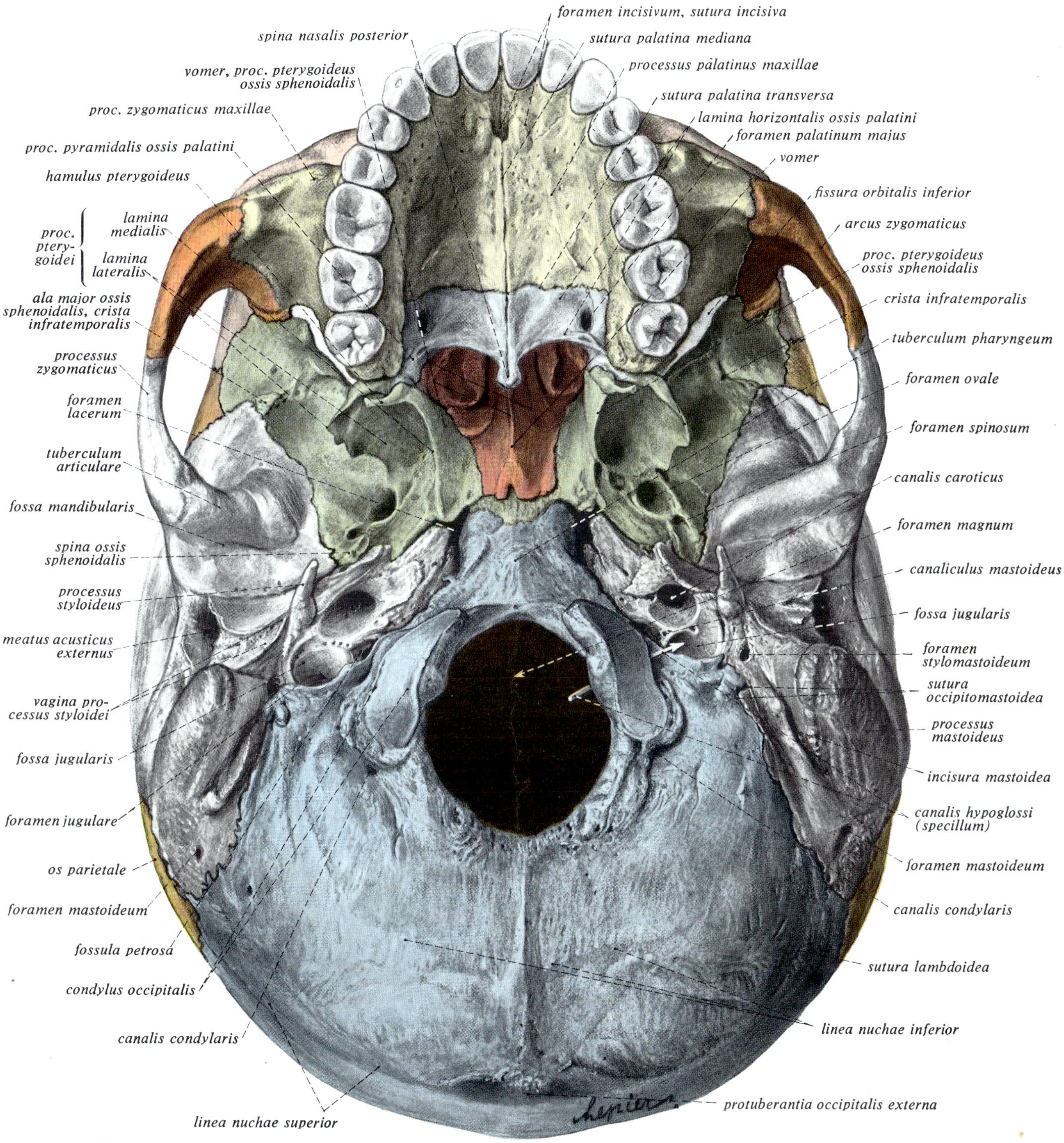
foramen incisivum, sutura incisiva
spina nasalis posterior
sutura palatina mediana
vomer, proc. pterygoideus ossis sphenoidalis
processus palatinus maxillae
proc. zygomaticus maxillae
sutura palatina transversa
lamina horizontalis ossis palatini
proc. pyramidalis ossis palatini
foramen palatinum majus
vomer
hamulus pterygoideus
fissura orbitalis inferior
proc. pterygoidei
lamina medialis
lamina lateralis
arcus zygomaticus
proc. pterygoideus ossis sphenoidalis
ala major ossis sphenoidalis, crista infratemporalis
crista infratemporalis
tuberculum pharyngeum
processus zygomaticus
foramen ovale
foramen lacerum
foramen spinosum
tuberculum articulare
canalis caroticus
fossa mandibularis
foramen magnum
spina ossis sphenoidalis
canaliculus mastoideus
processus styloideus
fossa jugularis
meatus acusticus externus
foramen stylomastoideum
vagina processus styloidei
sutura occipitomastoidea
processus mastoideus
fossa jugularis
incisura mastoidea
foramen jugulare
canalis hypoglossi (specillum)
os parietale
foramen mastoideum
foramen mastoideum
canalis condylaris
fossula petrosa
sutura lambdoidea
condylus occipitalis
linea nuchae inferior
canalis condylaris
protuberantia occipitalis externa
linea nuchae superior

Fig. 61

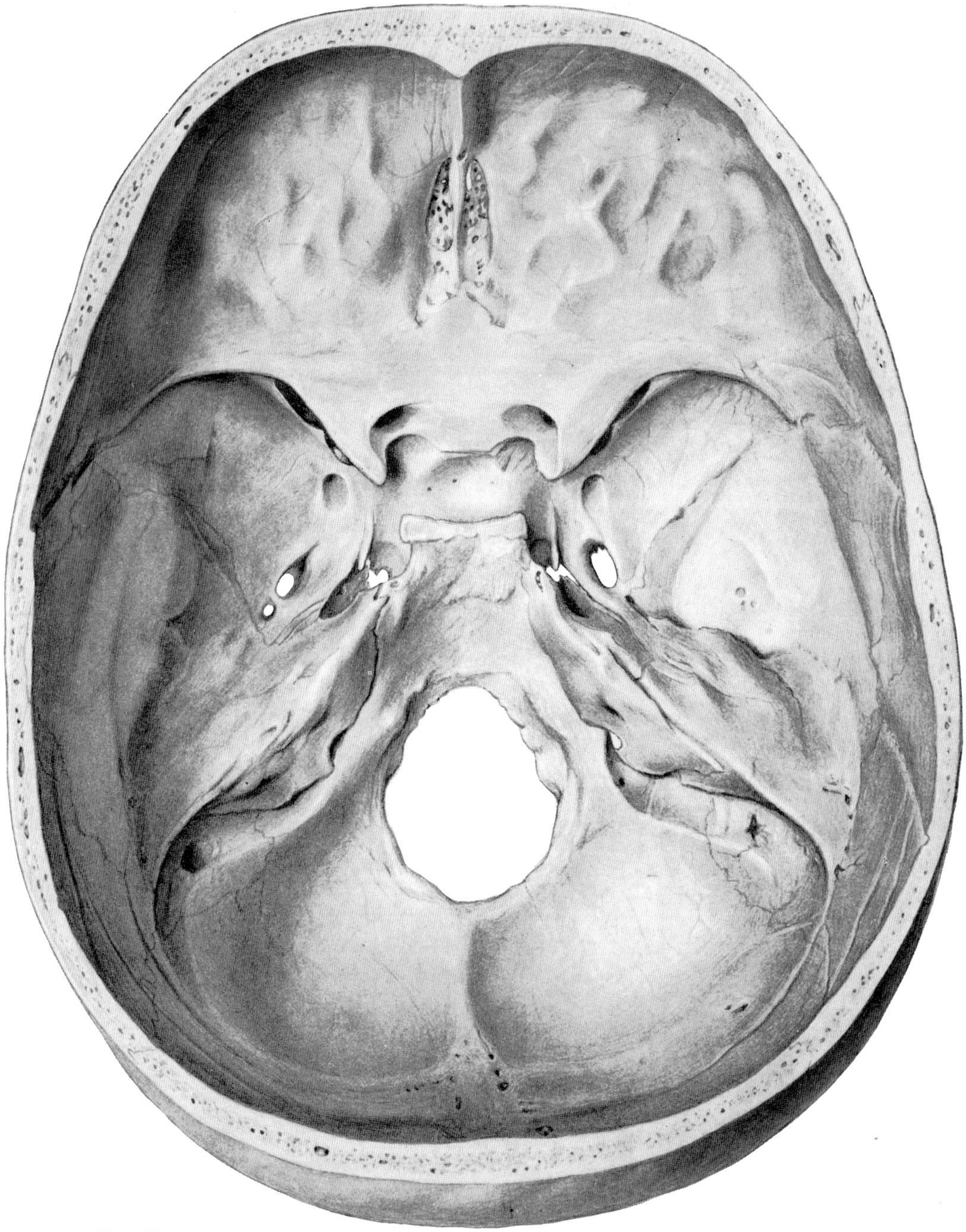

Fig. 62

Figs. 62 and 63. The base of the skull, *(basis cranii interna)*. Interior surfaces. Eight bones form the *cranium;* two are paired, so there are only six names to remember.

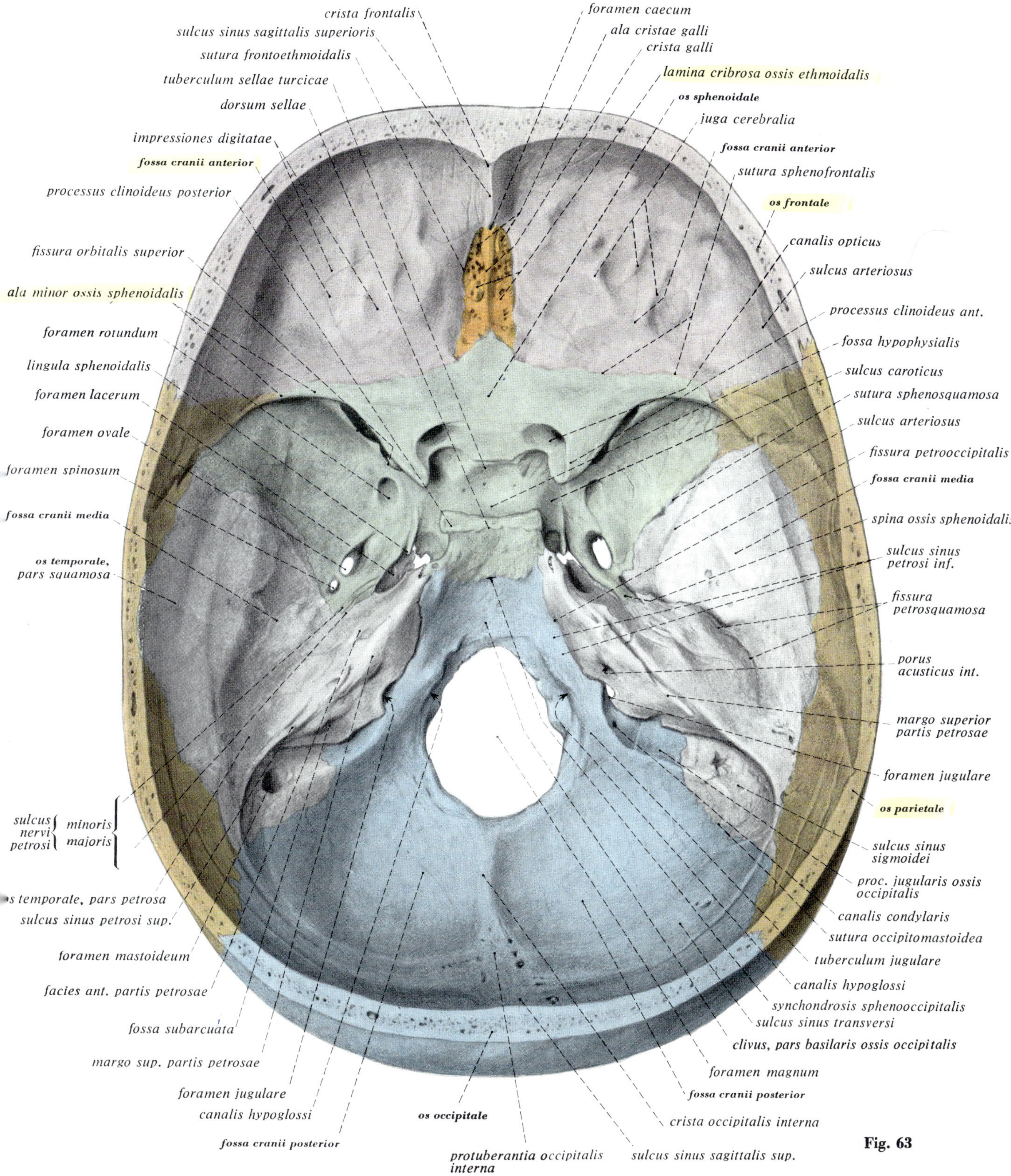
crista frontalis
sulcus sinus sagittalis superioris
sutura frontoethmoidalis
tuberculum sellae turcicae
dorsum sellae
impressiones digitatae
fossa cranii anterior
processus clinoideus posterior
fissura orbitalis superior
ala minor ossis sphenoidalis
foramen rotundum
lingula sphenoidalis
foramen lacerum
foramen ovale
foramen spinosum
fossa cranii media
os temporale, pars squamosa
sulcus nervi petrosi minoris
sulcus nervi petrosi majoris
os temporale, pars petrosa
sulcus sinus petrosi sup.
foramen mastoideum
facies ant. partis petrosae
fossa subarcuata
margo sup. partis petrosae
foramen jugulare
canalis hypoglossi
fossa cranii posterior
os occipitale
protuberantia occipitalis interna
sulcus sinus sagittalis sup.
crista occipitalis interna
fossa cranii posterior
foramen magnum
clivus, pars basilaris ossis occipitalis
sulcus sinus transversi
synchondrosis sphenooccipitalis
canalis hypoglossi
tuberculum jugulare
sutura occipitomastoidea
canalis condylaris
proc. jugularis ossis occipitalis
sulcus sinus sigmoidei
os parietale
foramen jugulare
margo superior partis petrosae
porus acusticus int.
fissura petrosquamosa
sulcus sinus petrosi inf.
spina ossis sphenoidalis
fossa cranii media
fissura petrooccipitalis
sulcus arteriosus
sutura sphenosquamosa
sulcus caroticus
fossa hypophysialis
processus clinoideus ant.
sulcus arteriosus
canalis opticus
os frontale
sutura sphenofrontalis
fossa cranii anterior
juga cerebralia
os sphenoidale
lamina cribrosa ossis ethmoidalis
crista galli
ala cristae galli
foramen caecum

Fig. 63

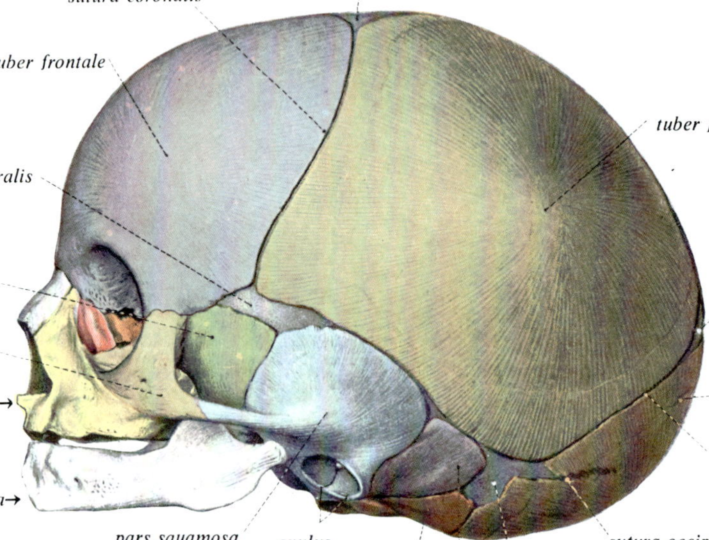

Fig. 64

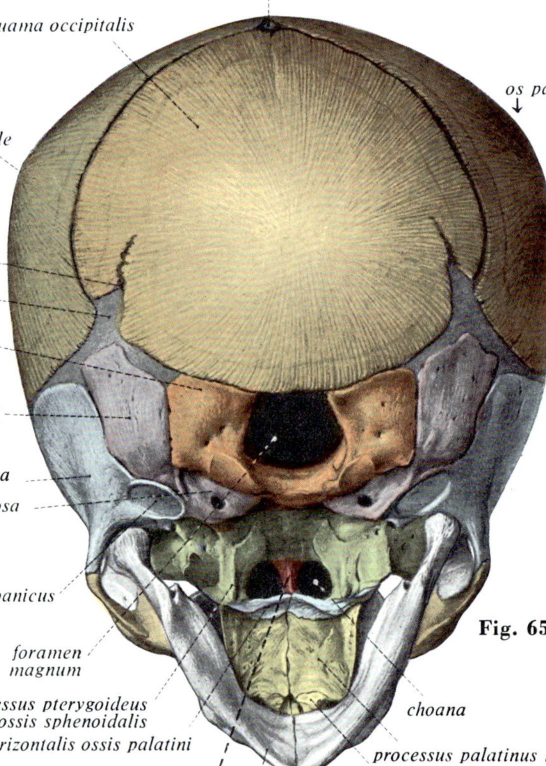

Fig. 65

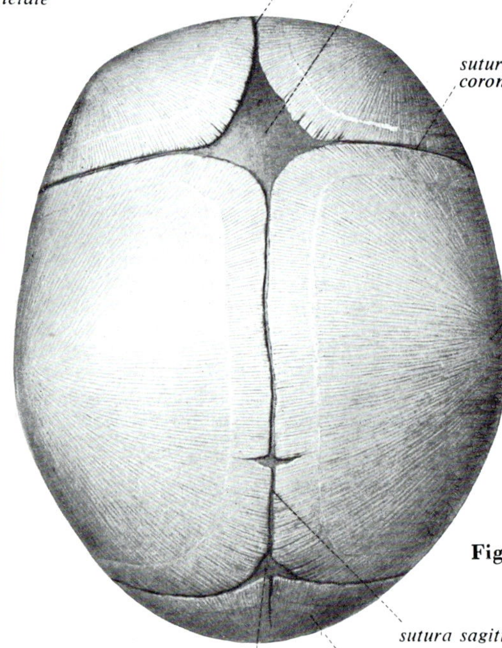

Fig. 66

Figs. 64–66. The skull, *(cranium)*, at birth. Fig. 64. Lateral view. Fig. 65. View from below and dorsally. Fig. 66. View from above.

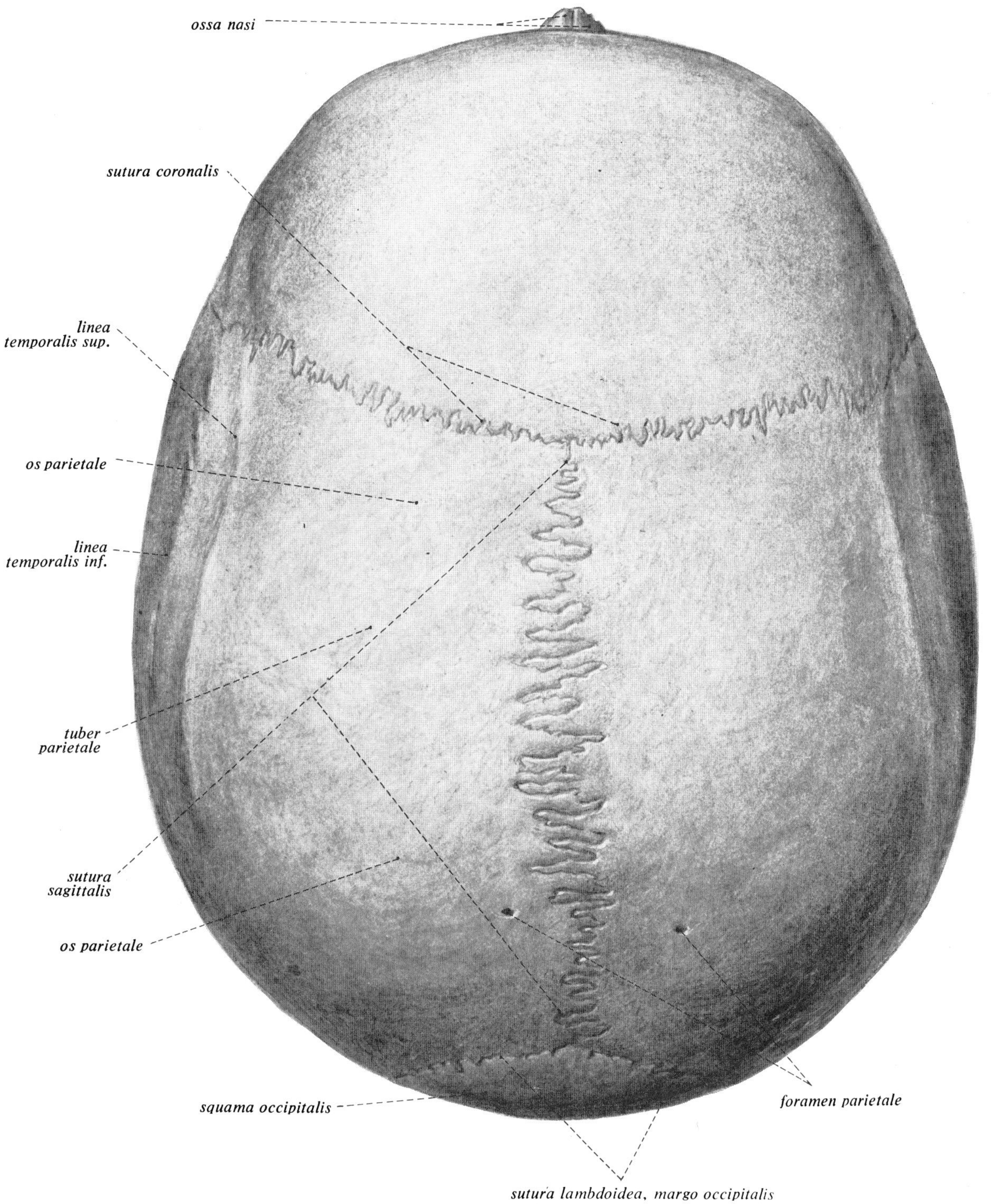

Fig. 67. *Calvaria.* Sutures of the neurocranium from above.

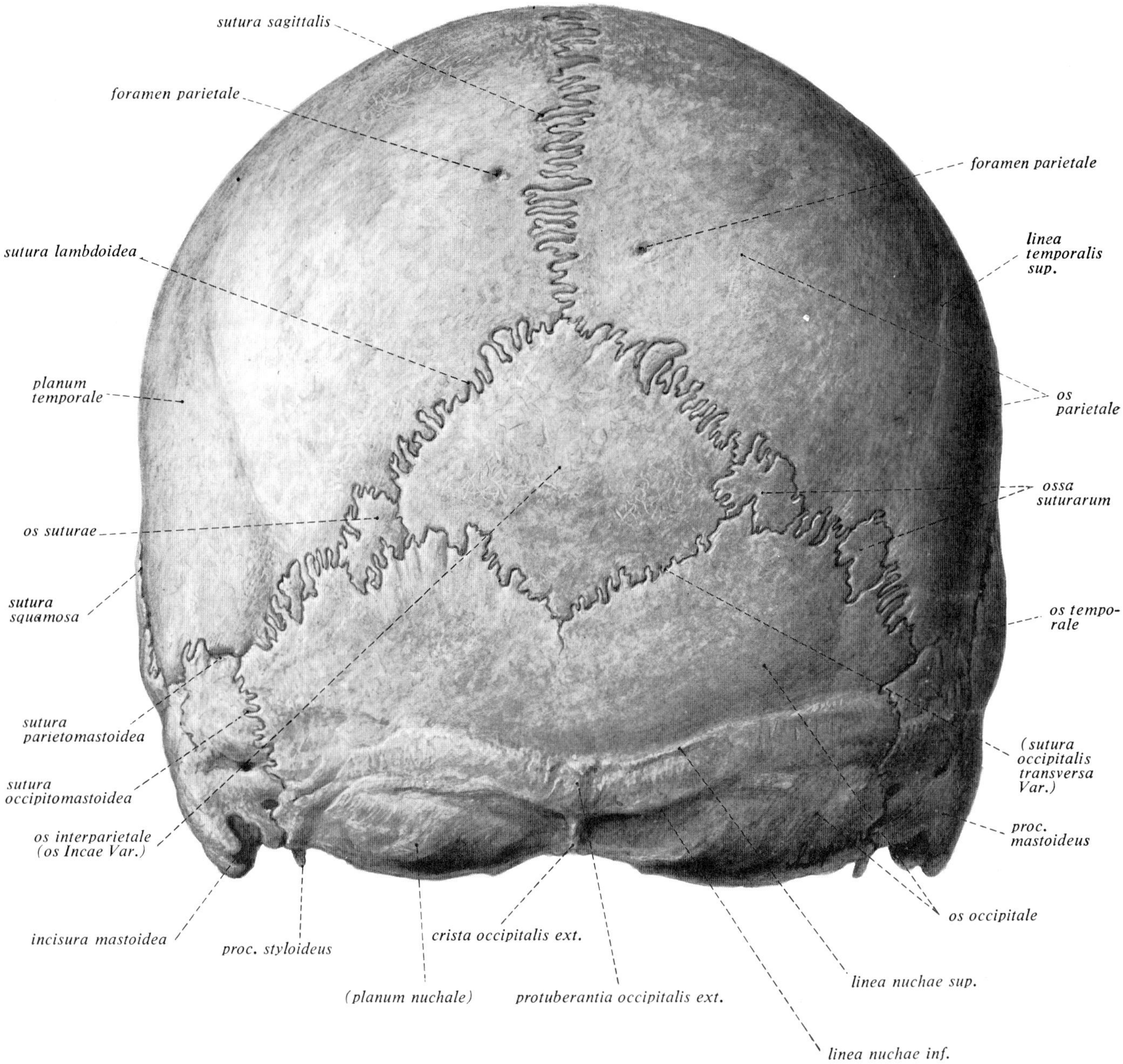

Fig. 68. Sutures of the *cranium.* Dorsal view. Sutural bones (Wormian) and *os interparietale* formerly called the Inca bone.

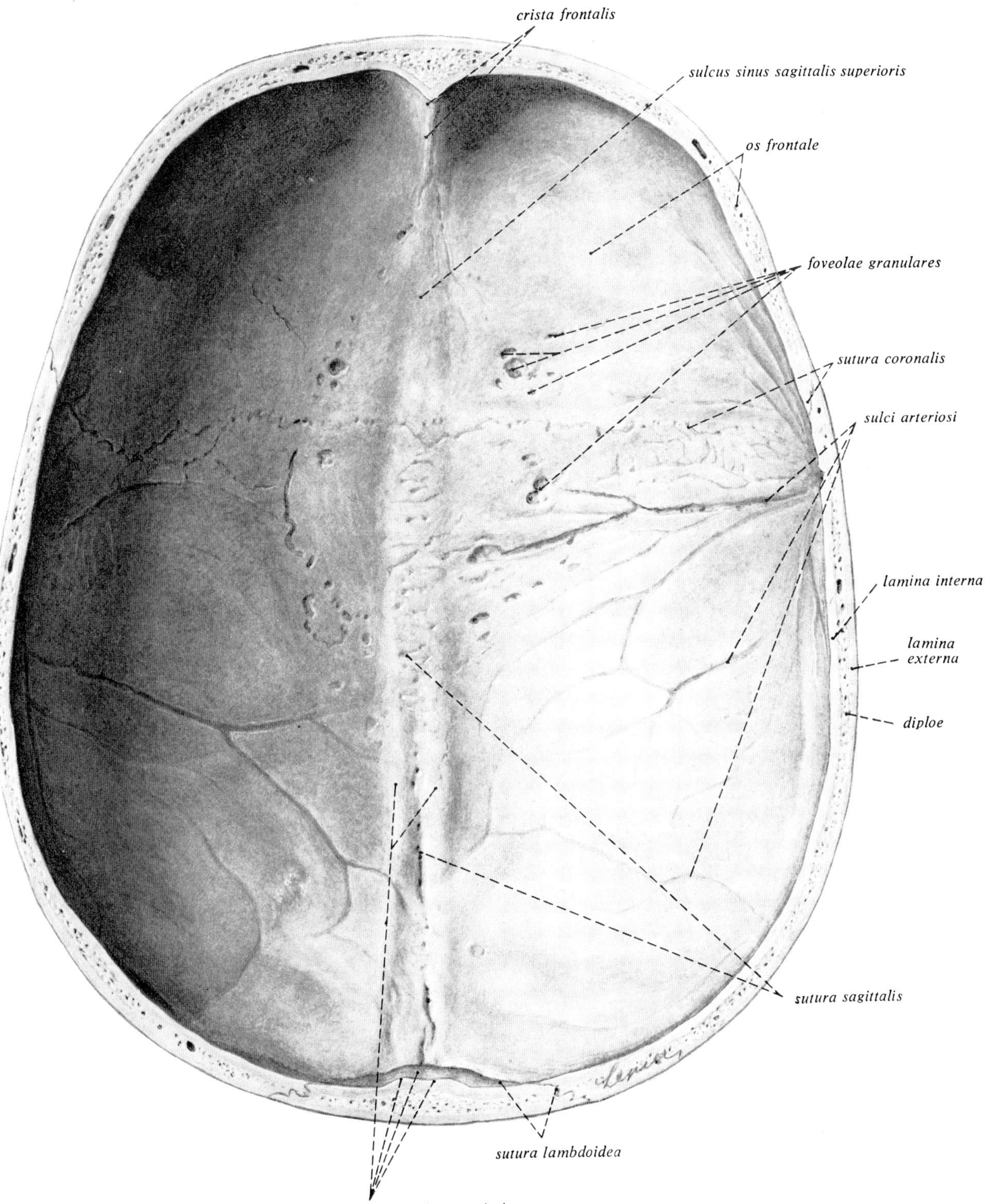

Fig. 69. *Calvaria*, the neurocranial roof. Inner or cerebral surface.

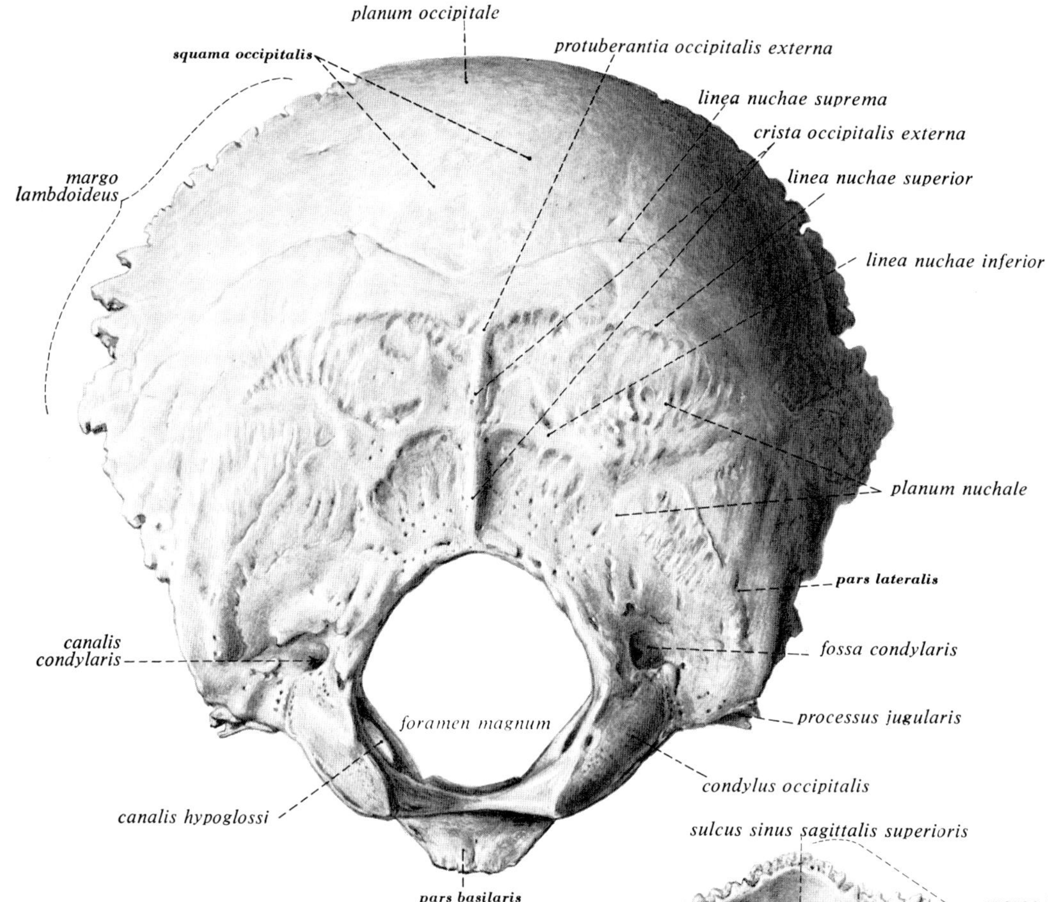

Fig. 70. *Os occipitale*. Dorsal, outer surface.

Fig. 71. *Os occipitale*. Ventral, inner surface. Centre: *Squama occipitalis* and *foramen occipitale magnum.*

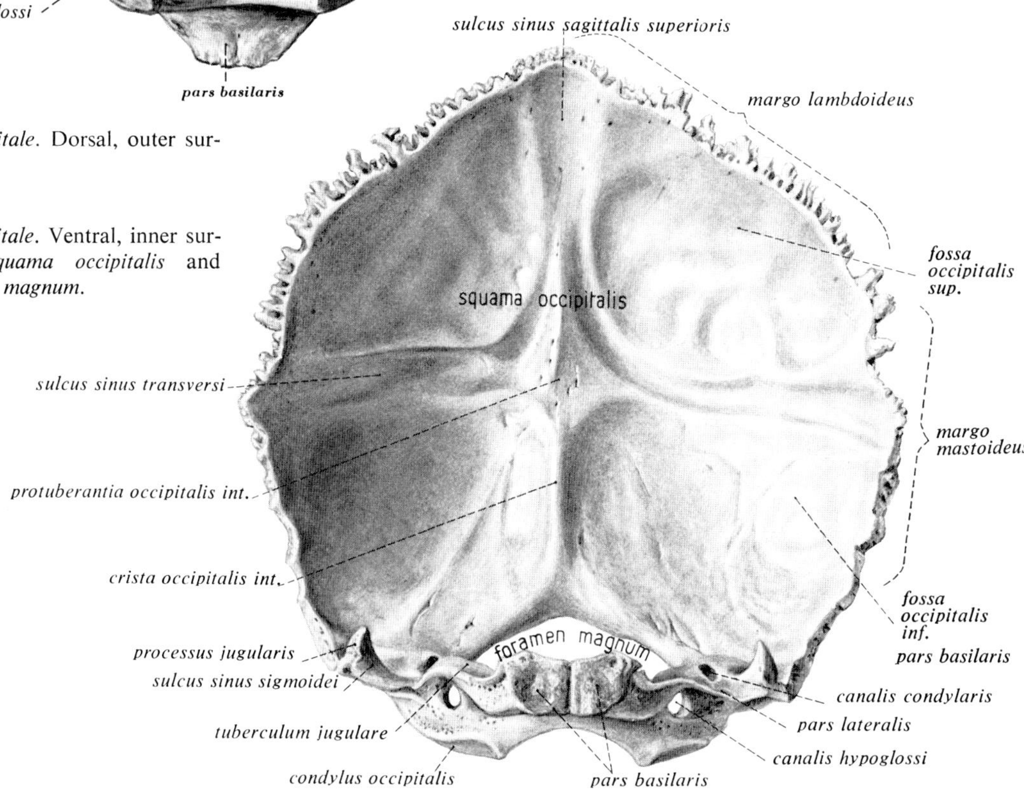

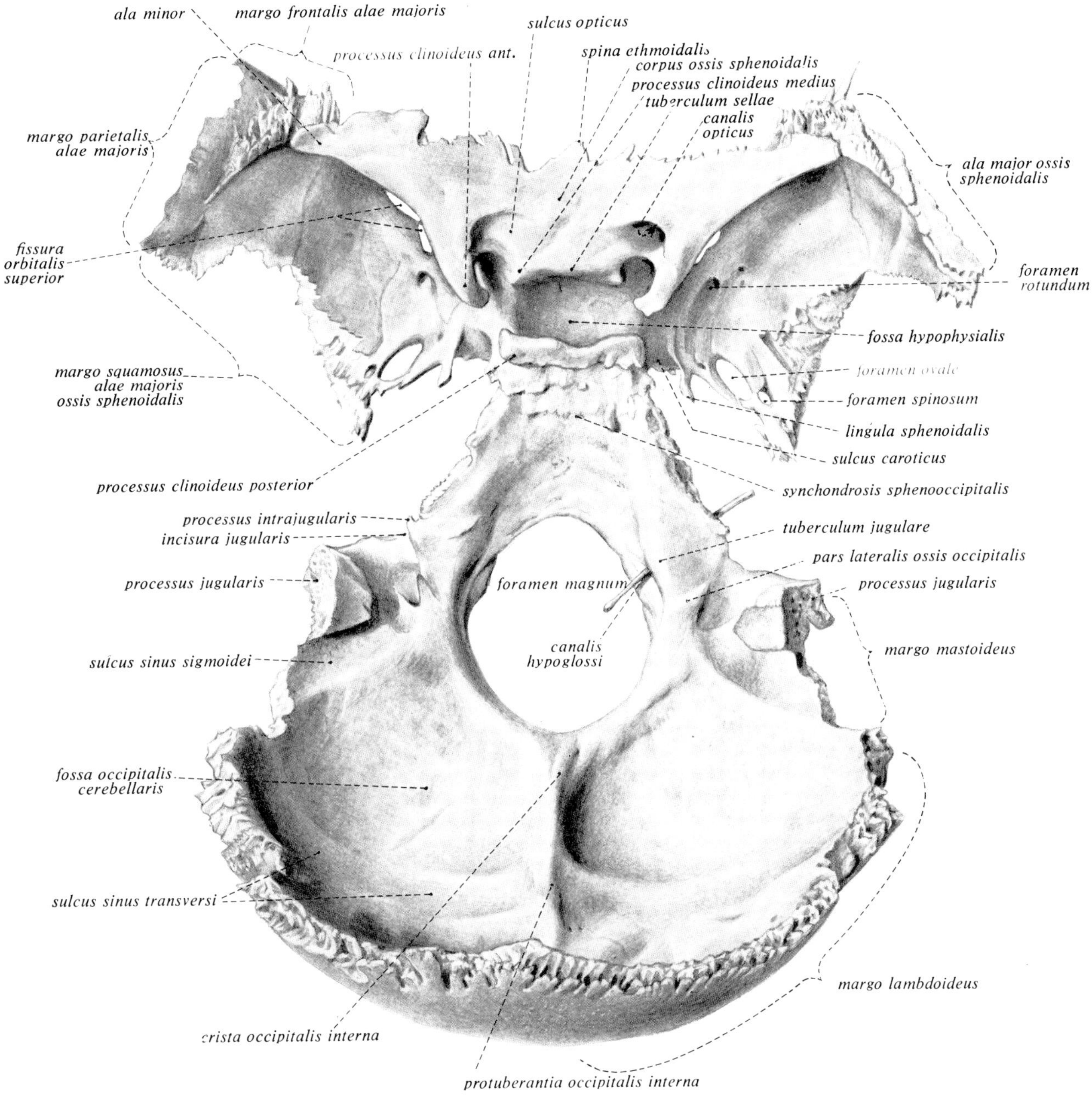

Fig. 72. *Os occipitale* and *os sphenoidale*. Seen from inside the skull. These are the bones of a growing youth, so the *synchondrosis sphenooccipitalis* is still present. The *pars petrosa* of the *os temporale* in the space between *os occipitale* and *os sphenoidale* is not shown.

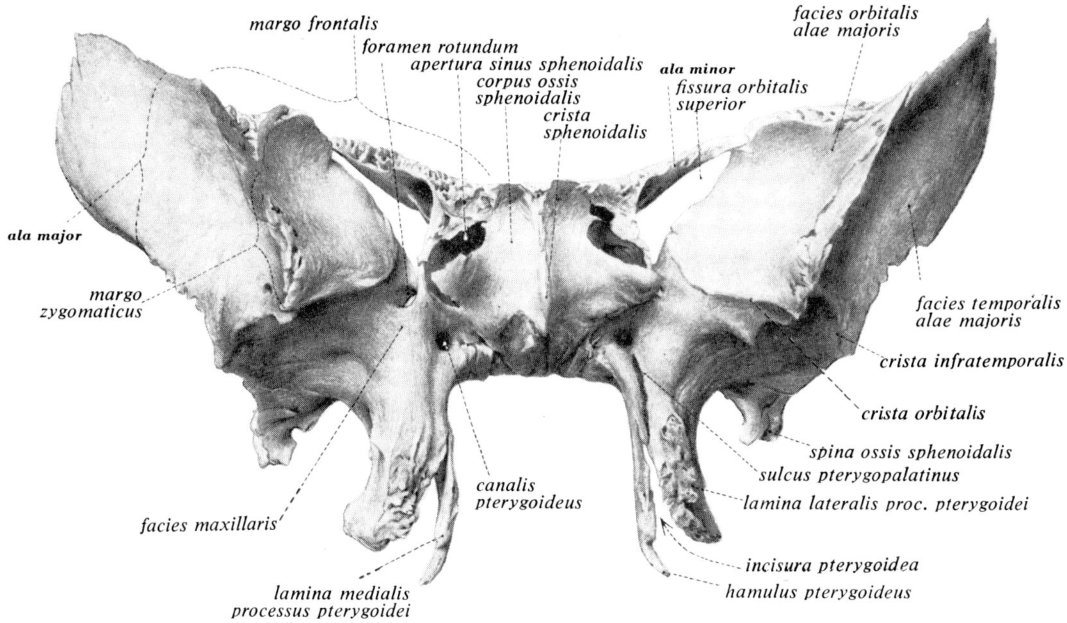

Fig. 73. *Os sphenoidale.* Ventral view.

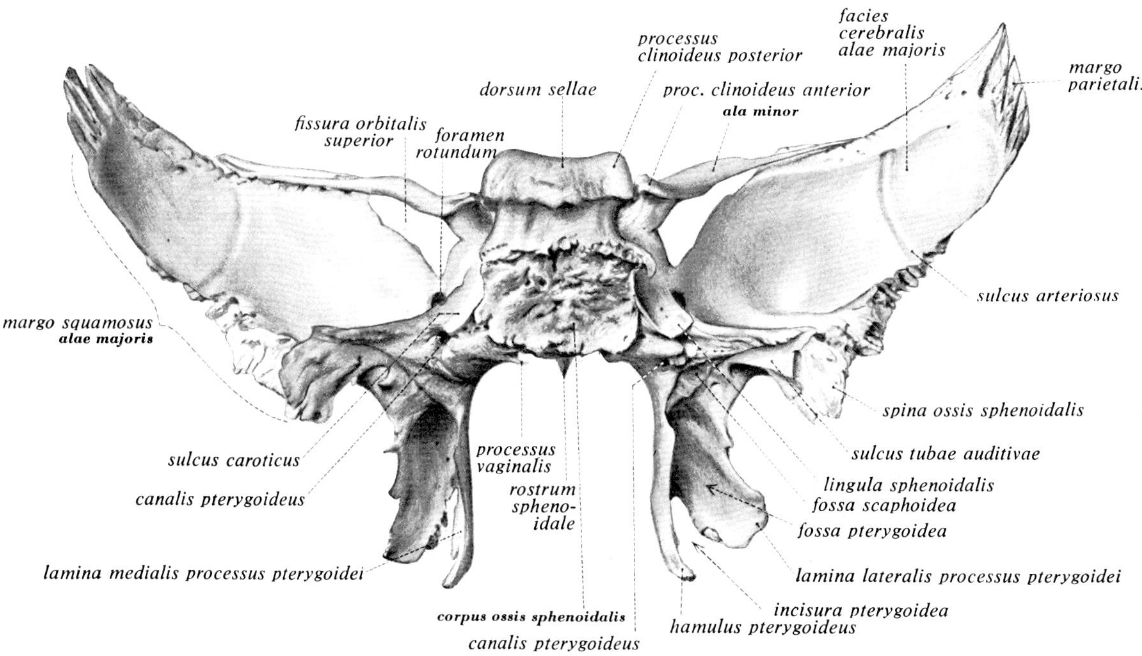

Fig. 74. *Os sphenoidale.* Dorsal view. A young person with an unossified *synchondrosis sphenooccipitalis.*

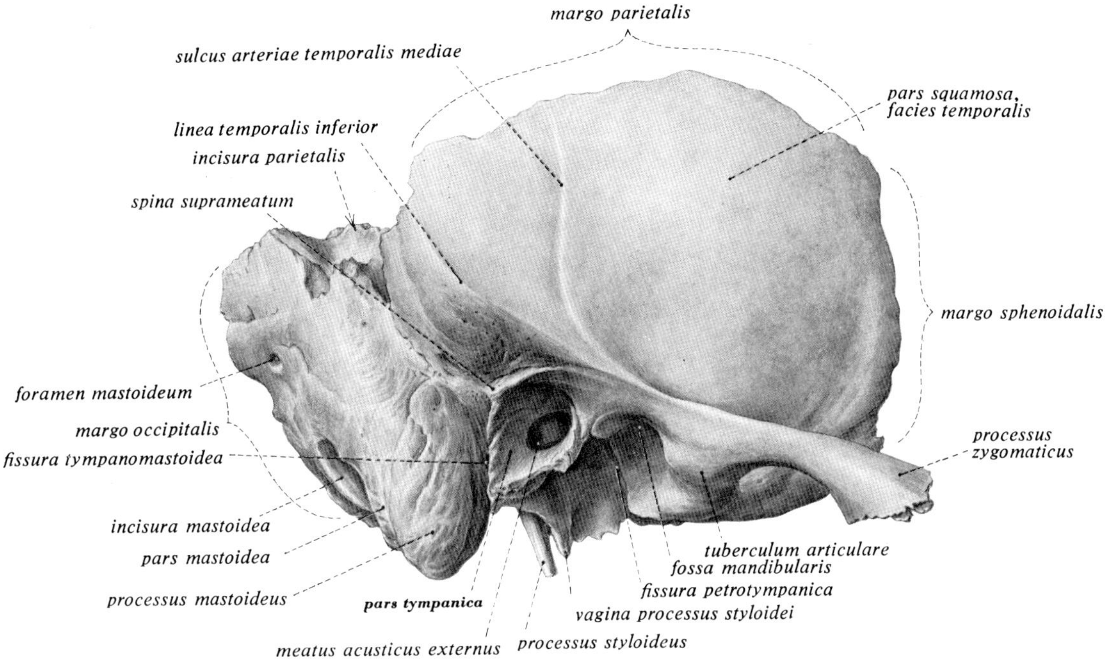

Fig. 75

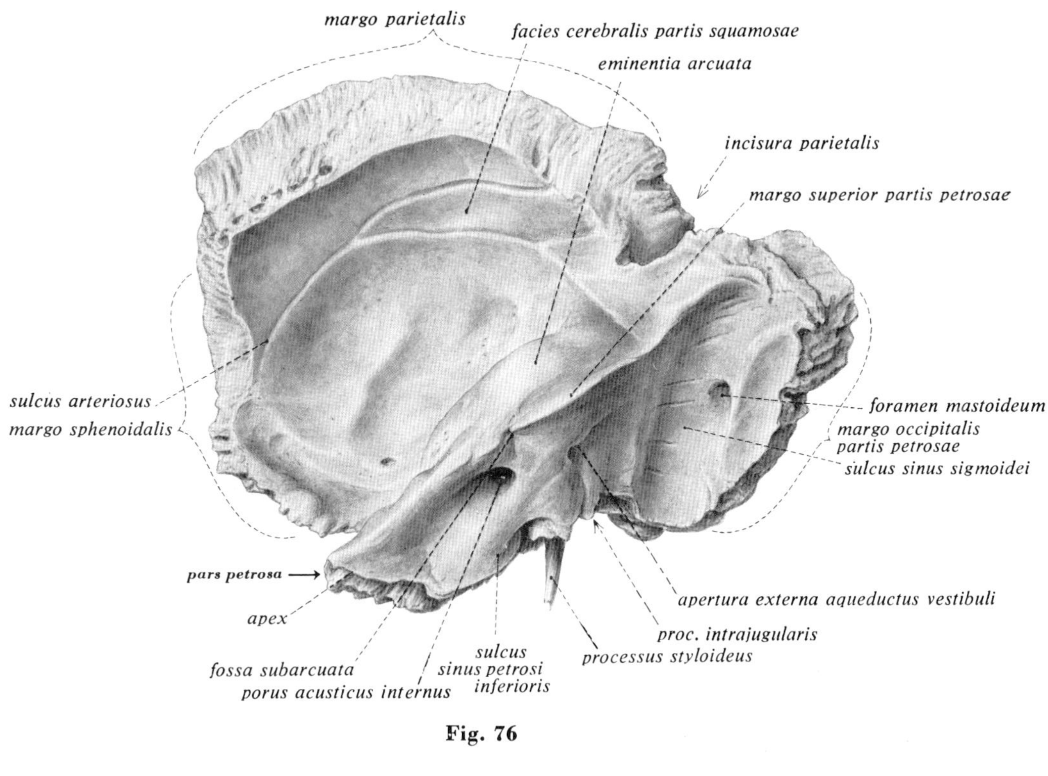

Fig. 76

Figs. 75 and 76. Right *os temporale*. Fig. 75. Lateral view. Fig. 76. Medial view.

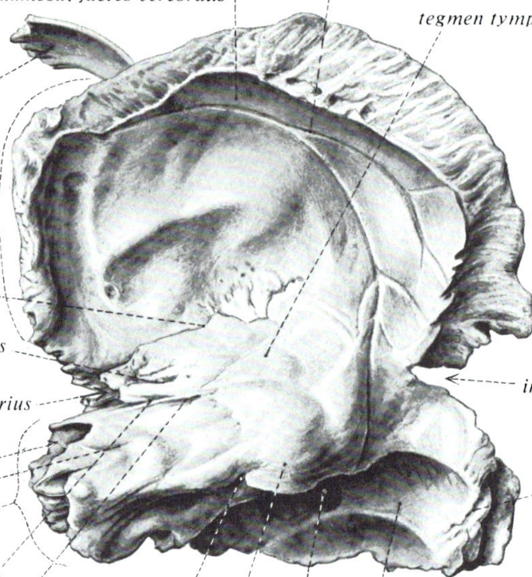

Fig. 77

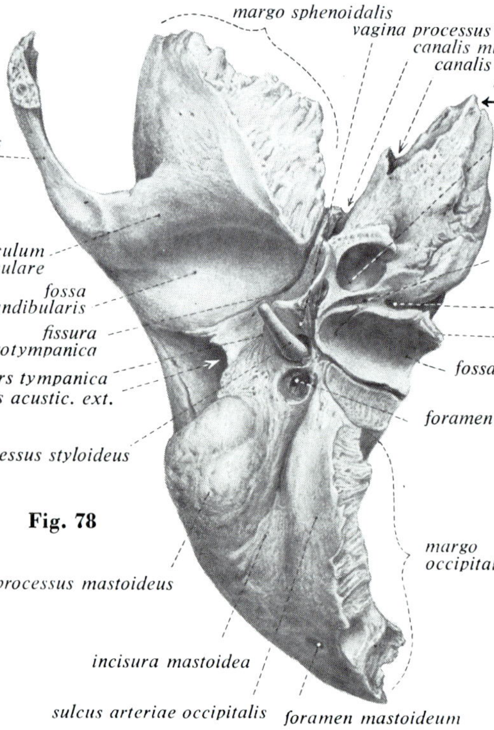

Fig. 78

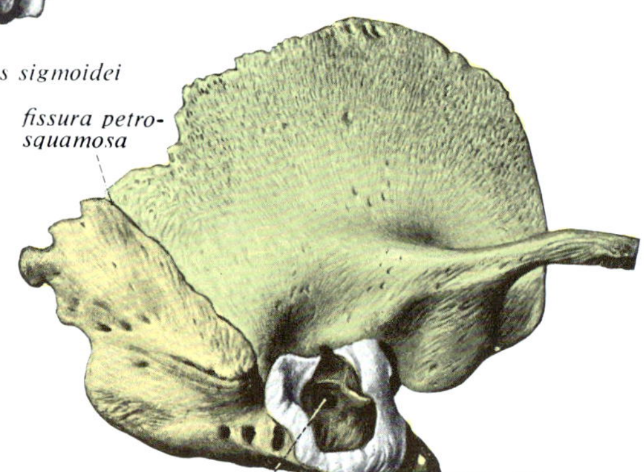

Fig. 79

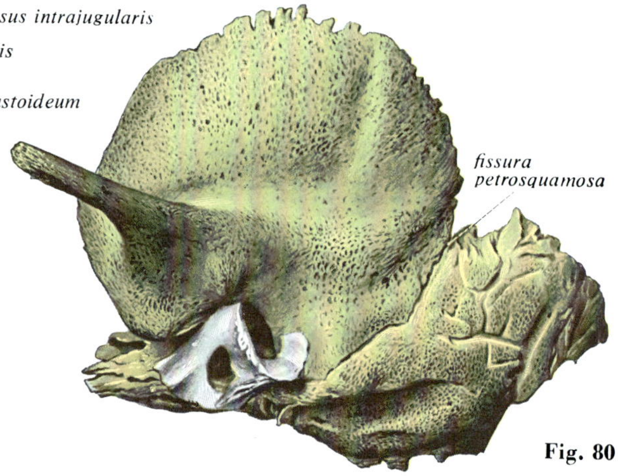

Fig. 80

Fig. 77. Right *os temporale*. Inner cranial surface, displaying apex of petrous portion.
Fig. 78. Right *os temporale*. Caudal view, from below.
Figs. 79 and 80. Right and left *ossa temporalia* of newborn. *Pars squamosa*, green; *pars petrosa*, yellow; *pars tympanica*, not colored.

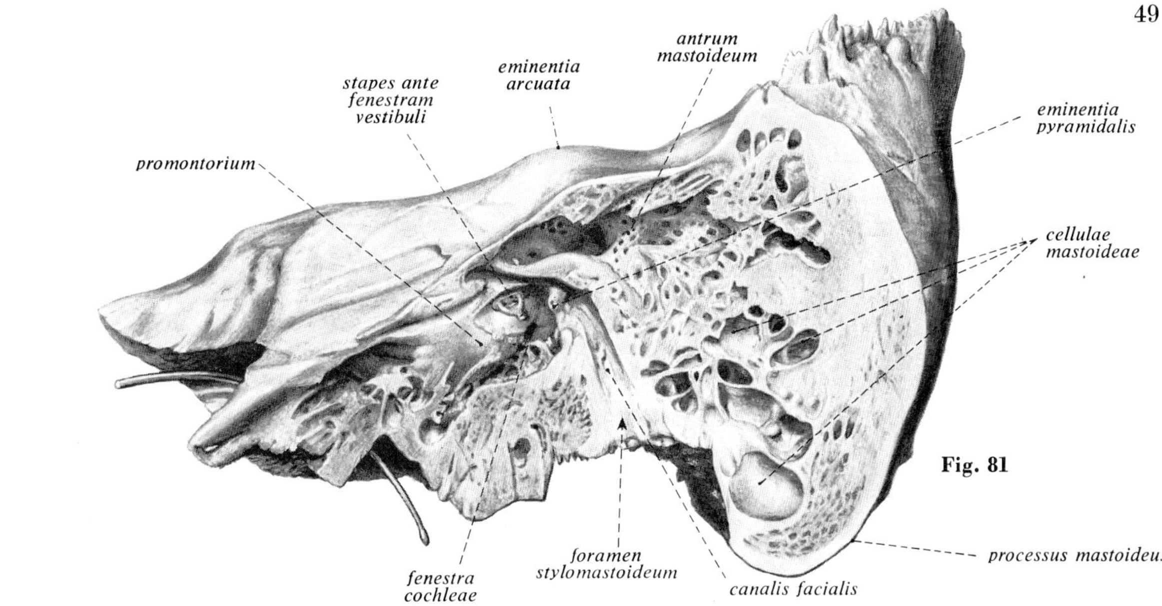

Fig. 81

Figs. 81–84. Sawcuts through the *os temporale*. Fig. 81. Left medial half, with probe in the *canalis caroticus*. Fig. 82. Lateral half.

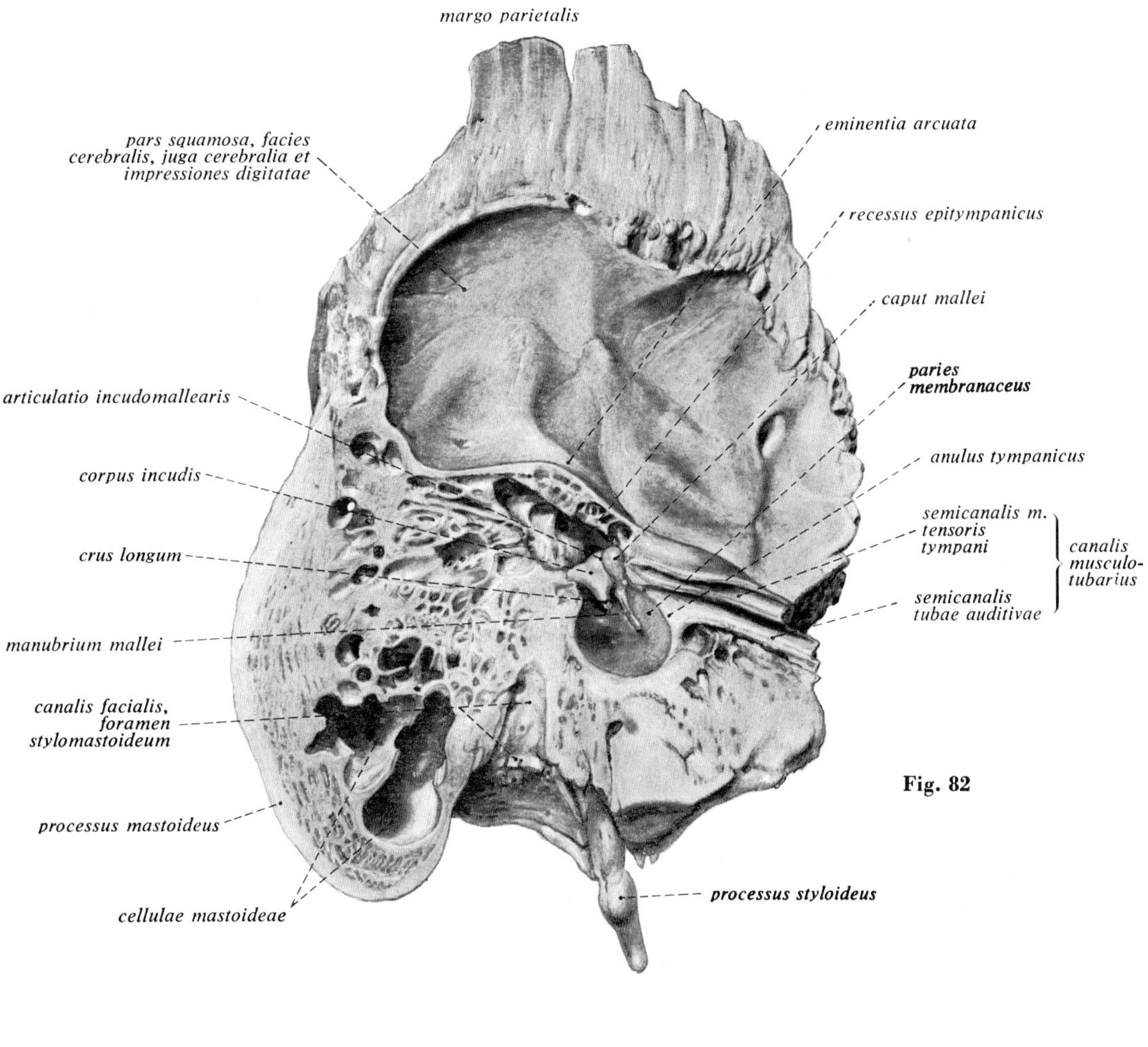

Fig. 82

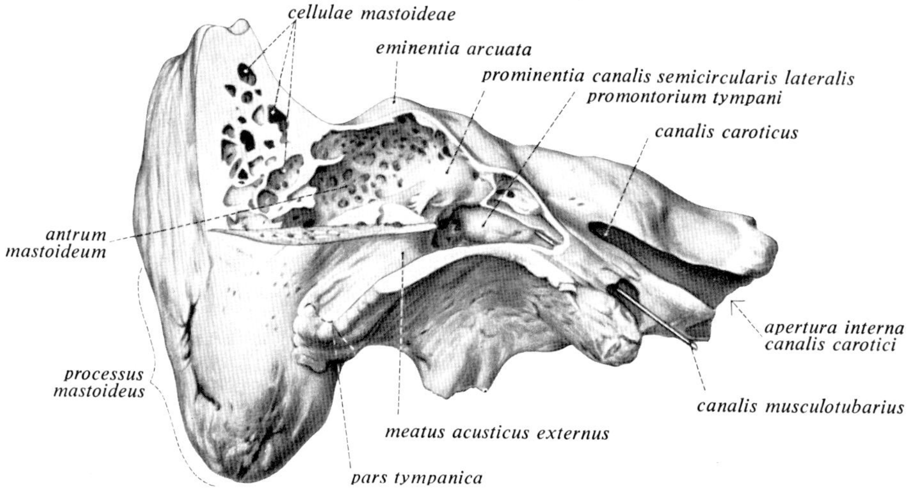

Fig. 83. Right *os temporale,* from ventral. *Cellulae mastoideae, antrum, cavum tympani and meatus acusticus externus,* as well as a part of the *canalis musculotubarius* (with probe) were exposed by a sawcut.

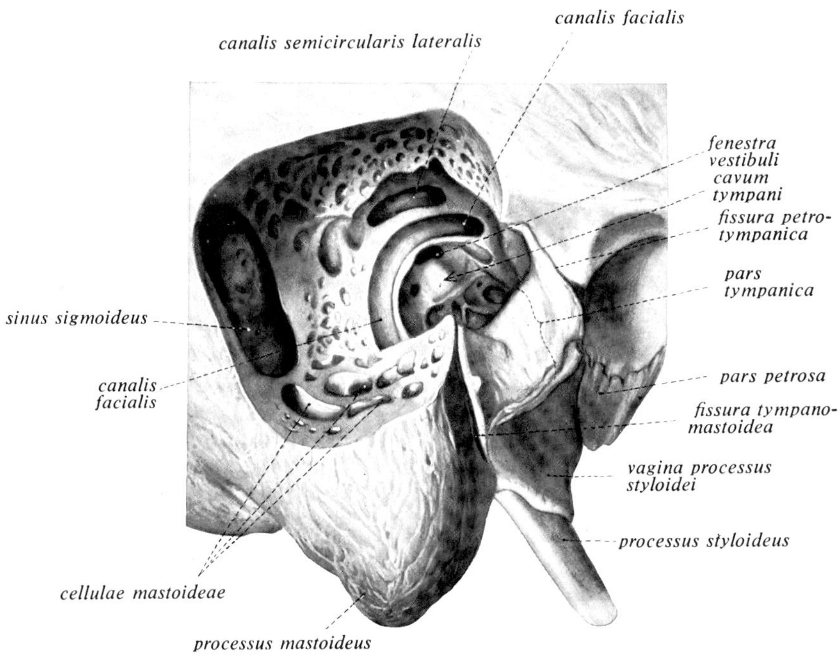

Fig. 84. Right *os temporale*. Opened and dissected from lateral side, revealing the inner space with the relative positions between *sinus sigmoideus, canalis facialis*, and bony configuration of the organs of equilibrium and hearing.

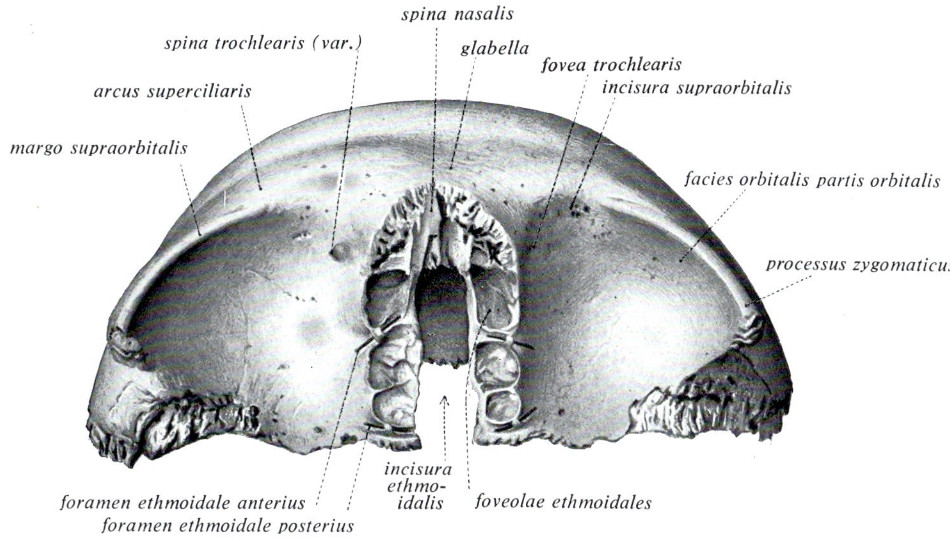

Fig. 85. *Os frontale*. Seen from below.

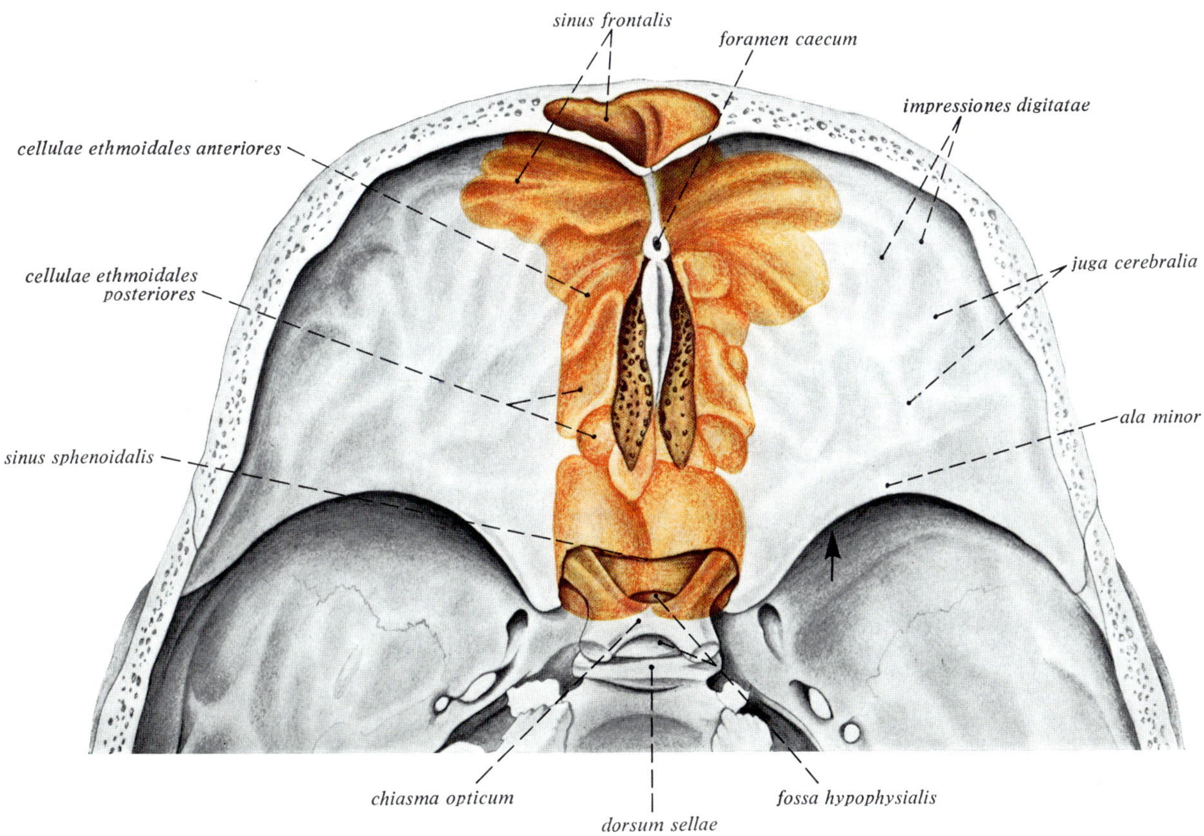

Fig. 86. *Sinus paranasales* and their projection on the *fossa cranii anterior* from which they are separated by only thin bony plates. The arrow points to the entrance of the *fissura orbitalis superior*.

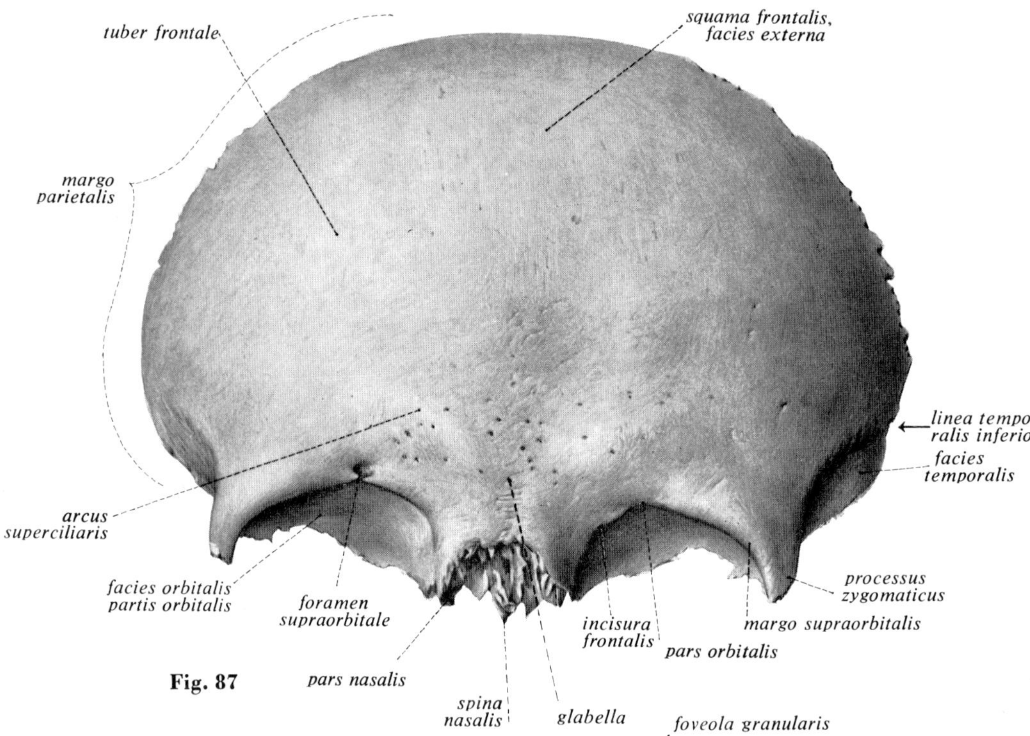

Fig. 87

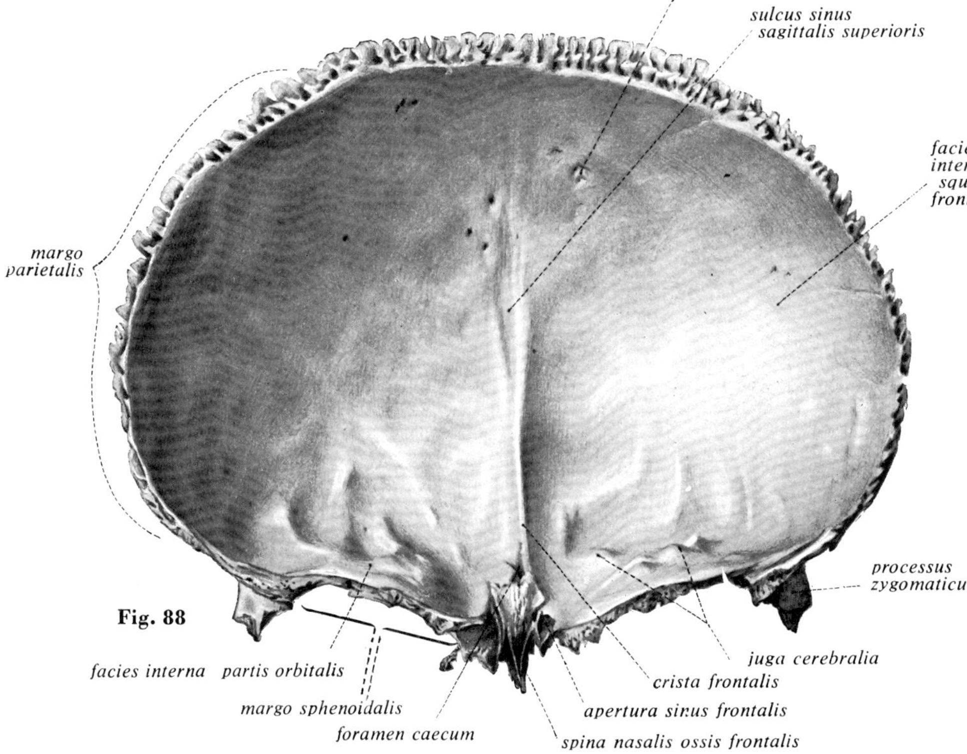

Fig. 88

Figs. 87 and 88. *Os frontale*. Fig. 87. Ventral or external view. Fig. 88. Dorsal or internal view.

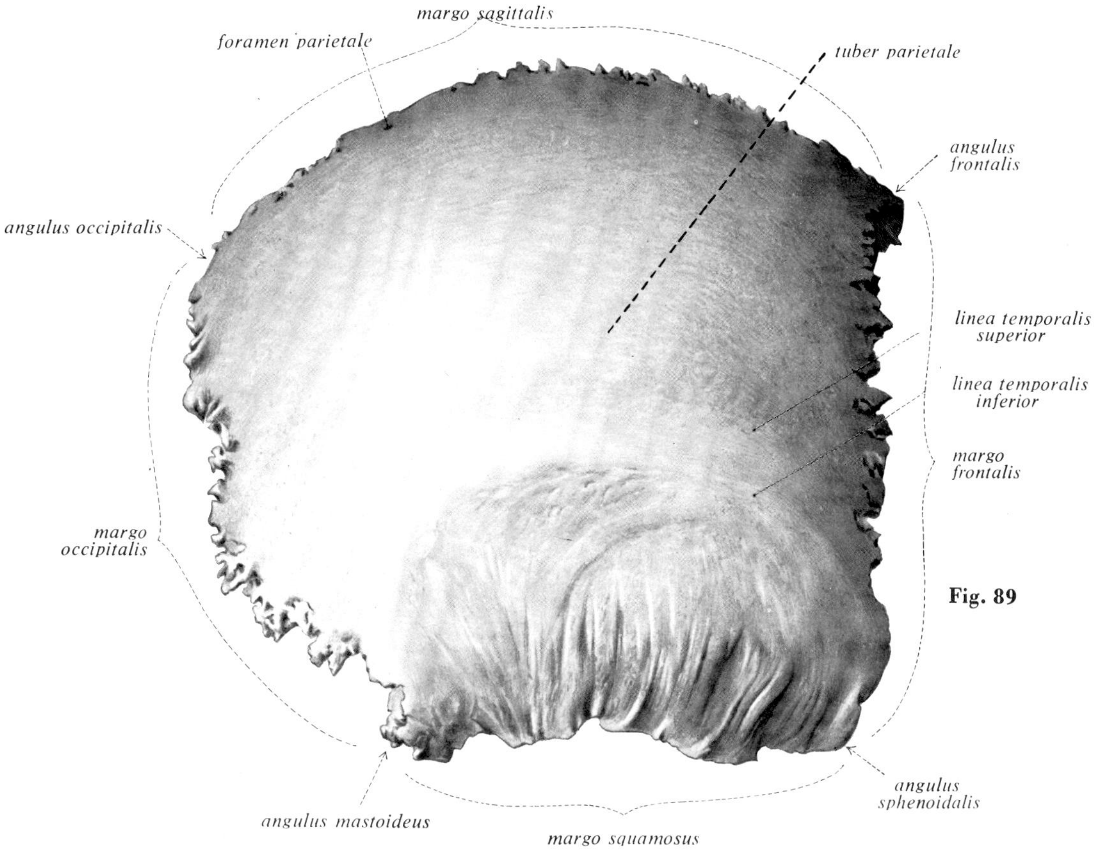

Fig. 89

Figs. 89 and 90. Right *os parietale*. Fig. 89. External view. Fig. 90. Internal view.

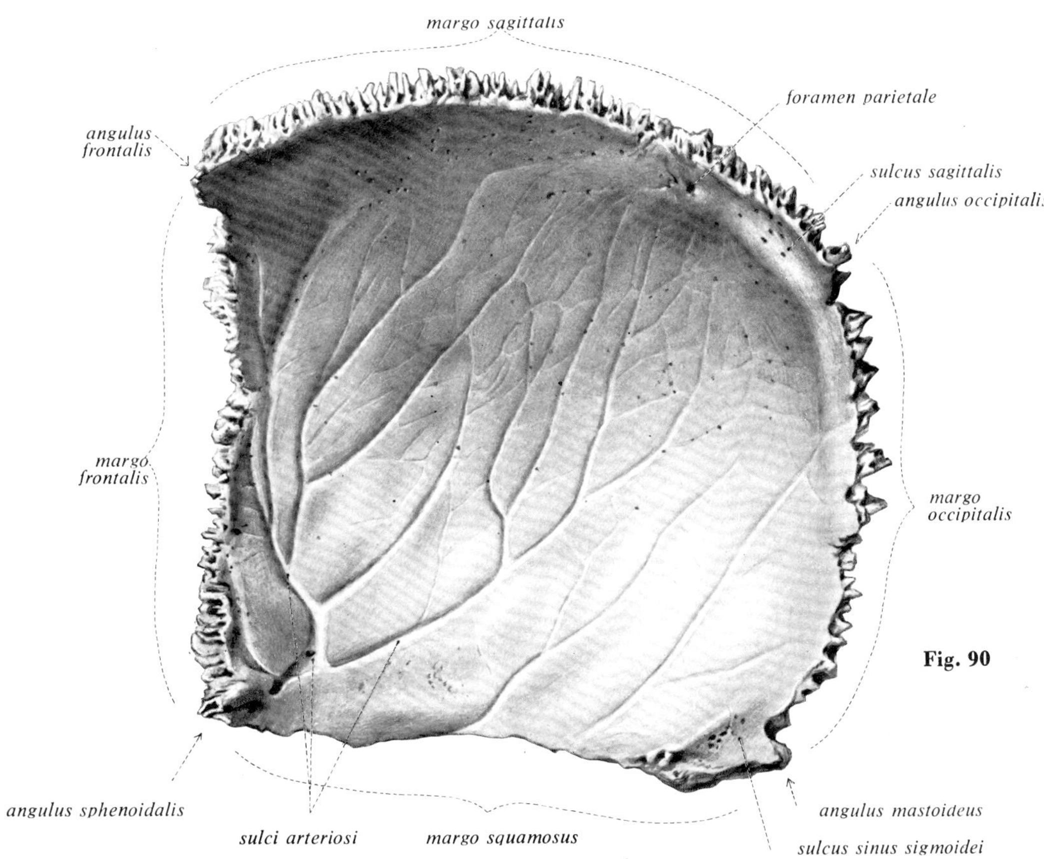

Fig. 90

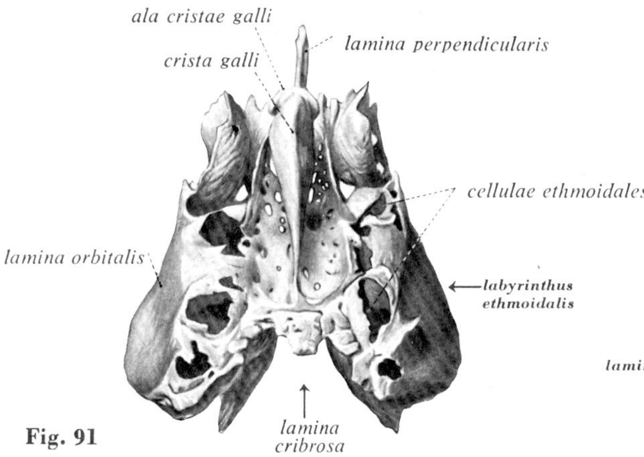

Fig. 91

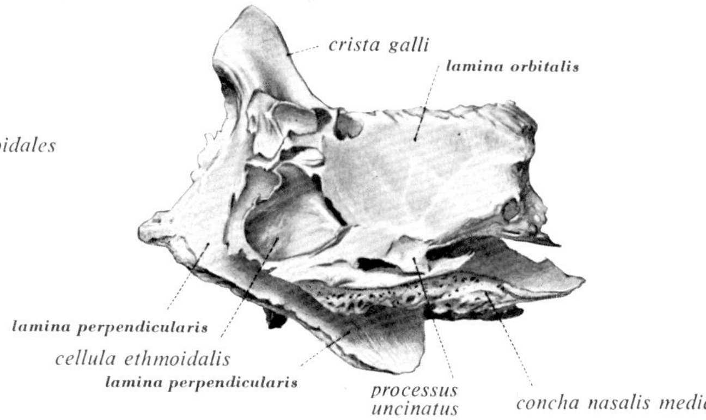

Fig. 92

Figs. 91 and 92. *Os ethmoidale.*
Fig. 91. Cranial view, from above. Fig. 92. Left lateral view.

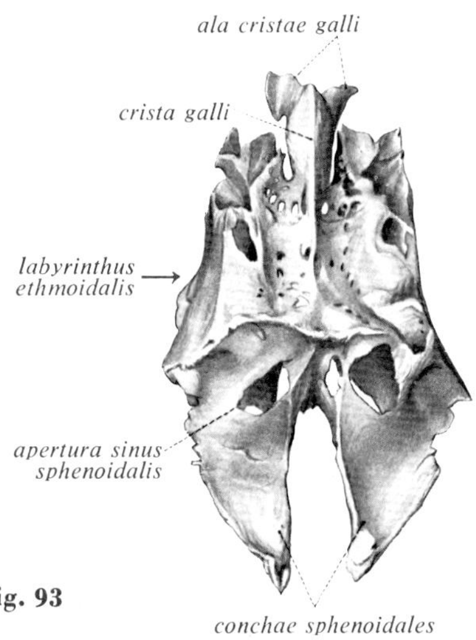

Fig. 93

Fig. 93. *Os ethmoidale* and *conchae sphenoidales.* From above and dorsal.

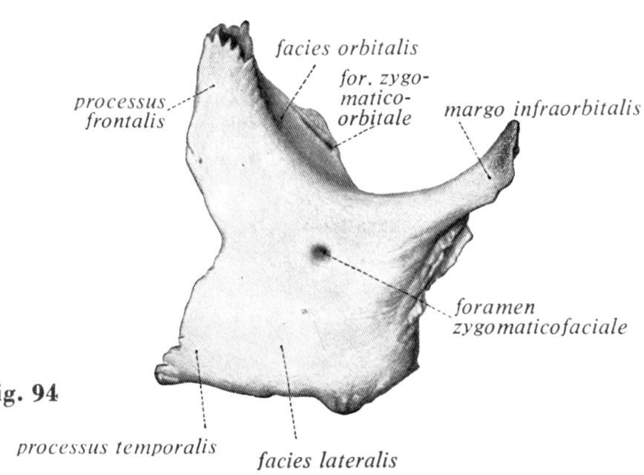

Fig. 94

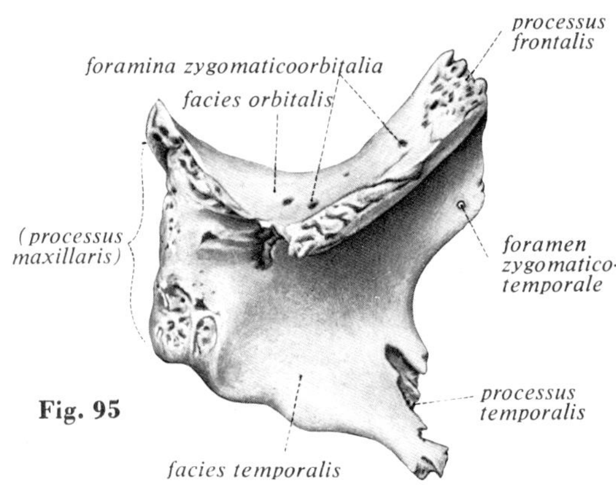

Fig. 95

Figs. 94 and 95. Right *os zygomaticum.* Fig. 94. Lateral, external surface. Fig. 95. Temporal surface.

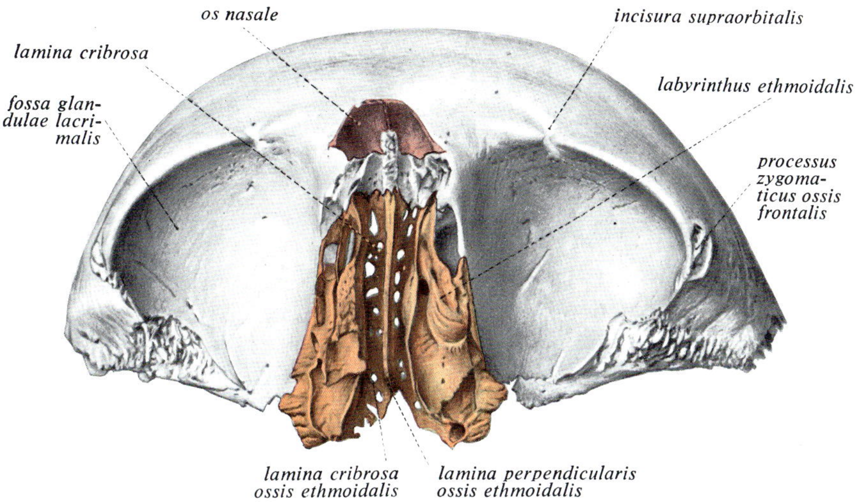

Fig. 96. *Os frontale* with a large part of the *os ethmoidale,* and *ossa nasalia* attached. Caudal view: *os frontale,* not colored; *os ethmoidale*, orange; *os nasale,* reddish.

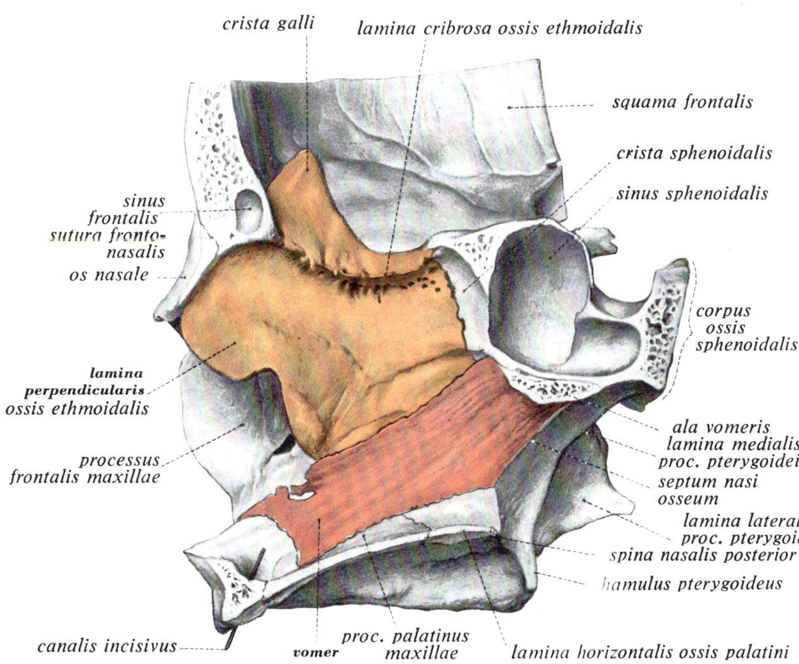

Fig. 97. Bony portion of the nasal septum *(septum nasi osseum).* Seen from the left side. *Os ethmoidale,* orange; vomer, reddish.

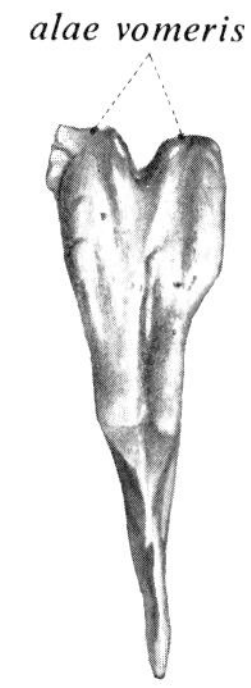

Fig. 98

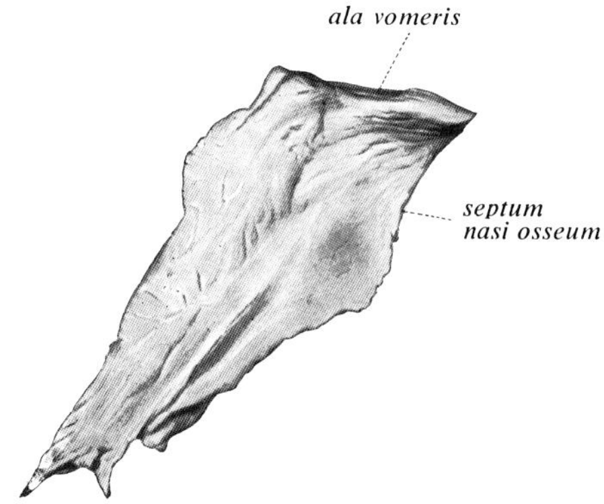

Fig. 99

Fig. 98. *Vomer*. Dorsal view.
Fig. 99. *Vomer*. Left lateral view.

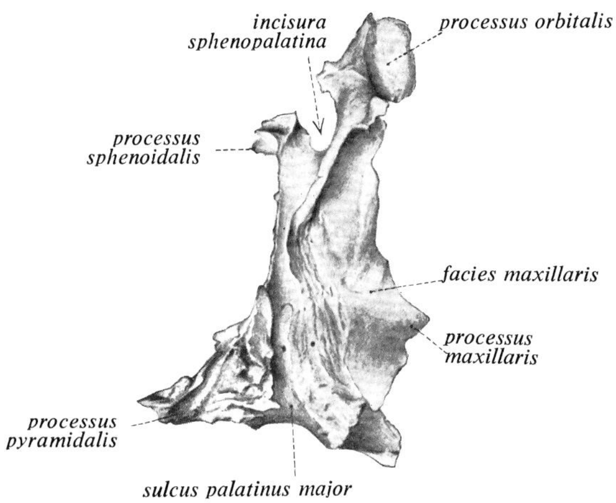

Fig. 100

Figs. 100–102. Right *os palatinum*.
Fig. 100. Lateral. Fig. 101. Dorsal. Fig. 102. Medial views.

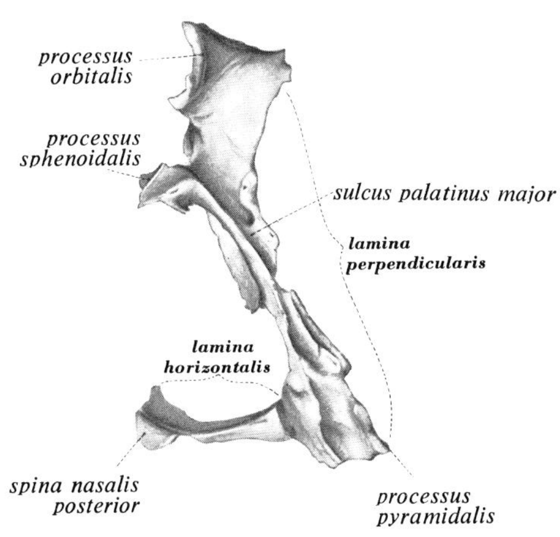

Fig. 101

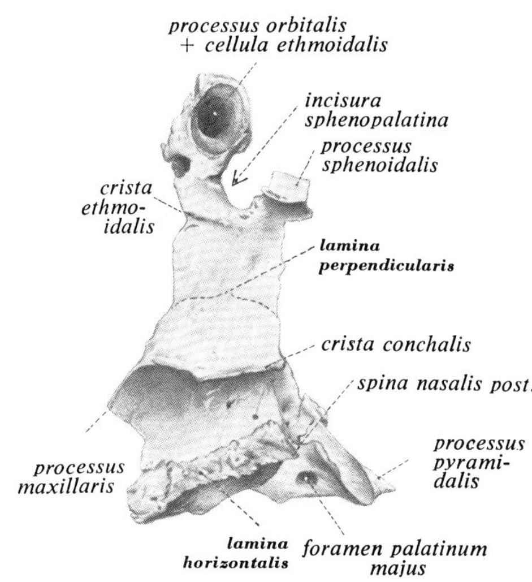

Fig. 102

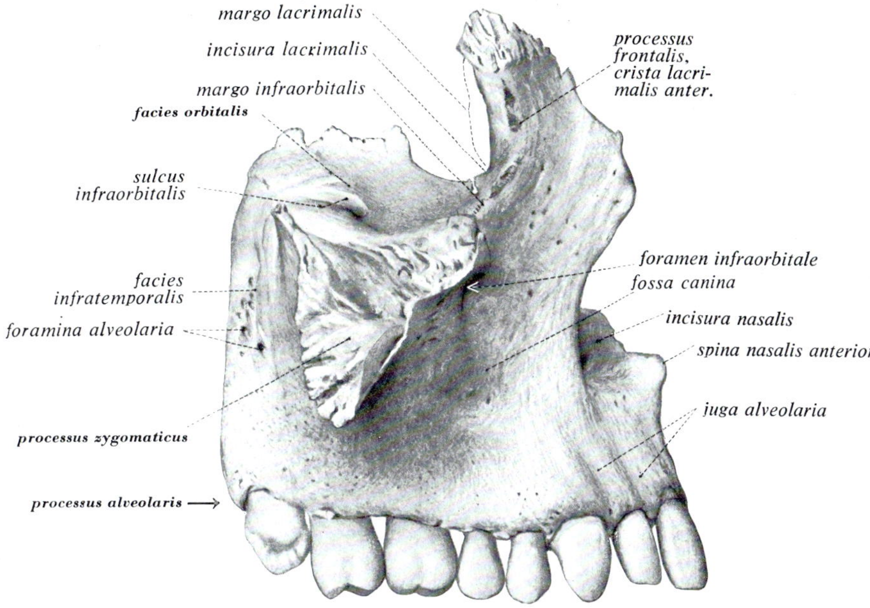

Fig. 103. Right *maxilla.* Lateral view.

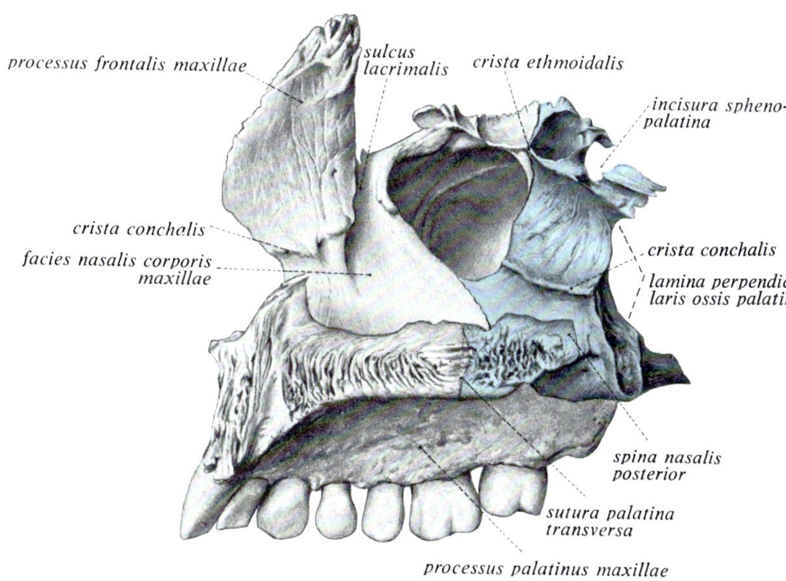

Fig. 104. Right *maxilla* and *os palatinum. Os palatinum*, blue.

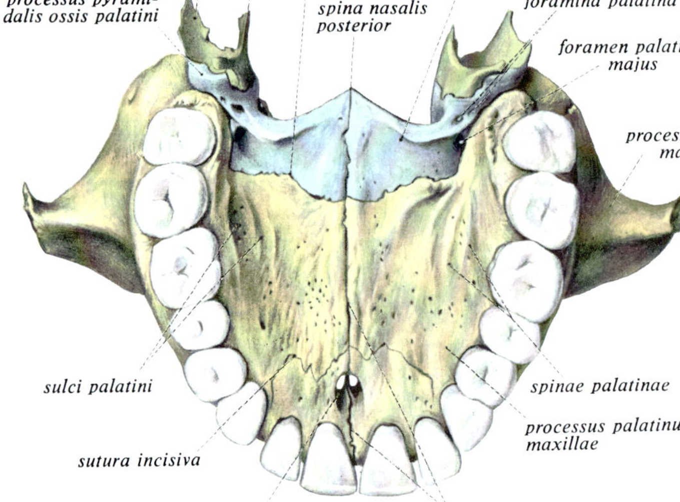

Fig. 105

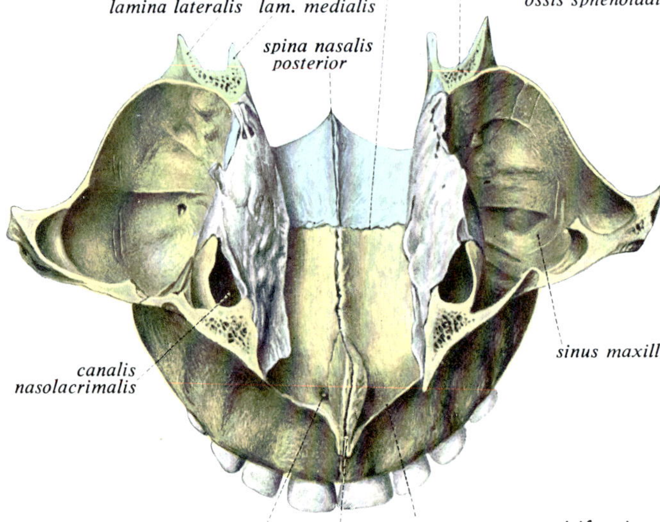

Fig. 106

Figs. 105 and 106. Hard palate *(Os palatinum)*. Fig. 105. Oral view, from below. Fig. 106. With *concha nasalis inferior* (not labeled nor colored) and *sinus maxillaris*, from above. *Maxilla,* yellow; *os palatinum*, blue; *os sphenoidale,* green.

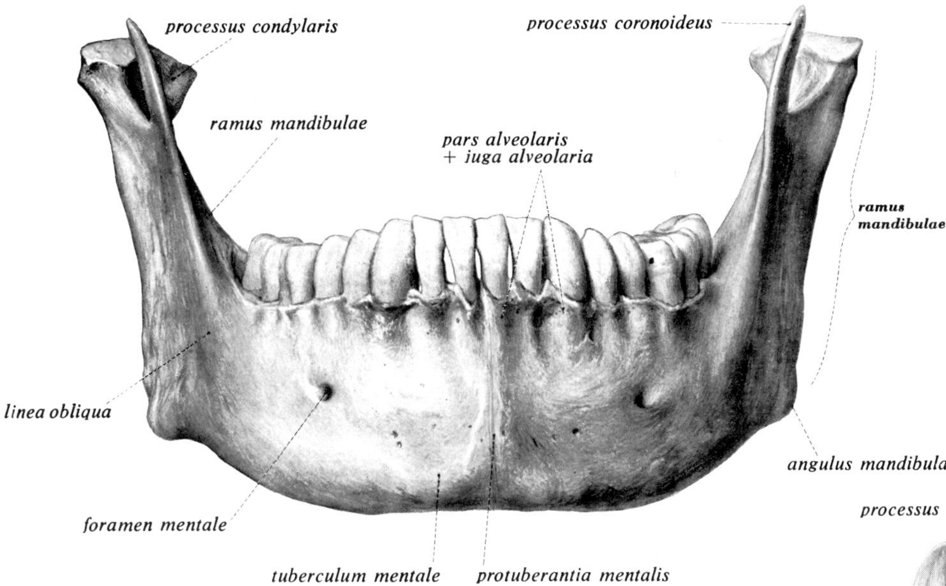

Fig. 107. *Mandibula.* Seen from in front.

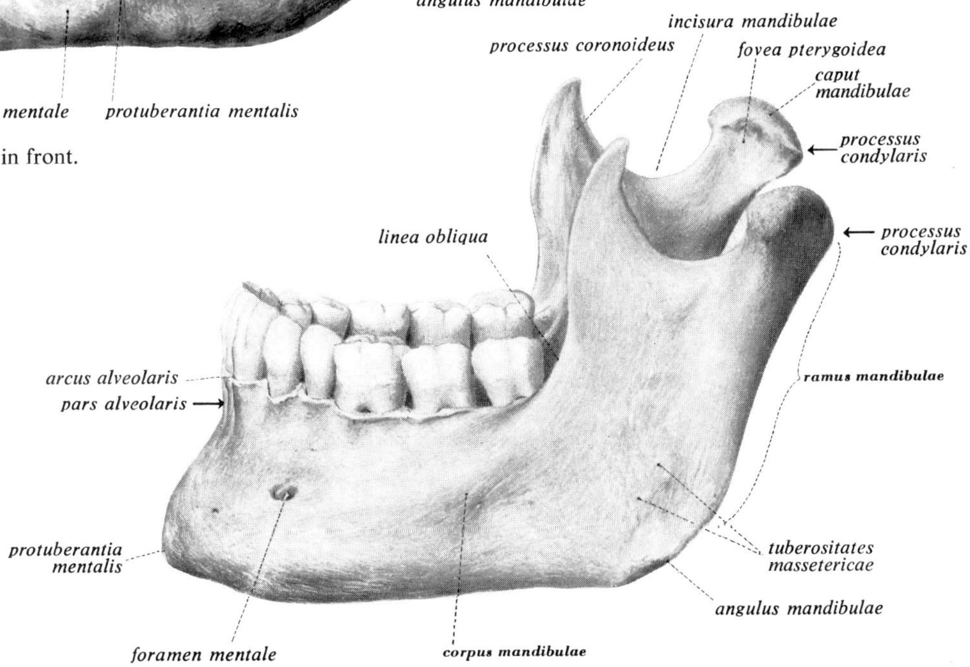

Fig. 108. *Mandibula.* Seen from left lateral side.

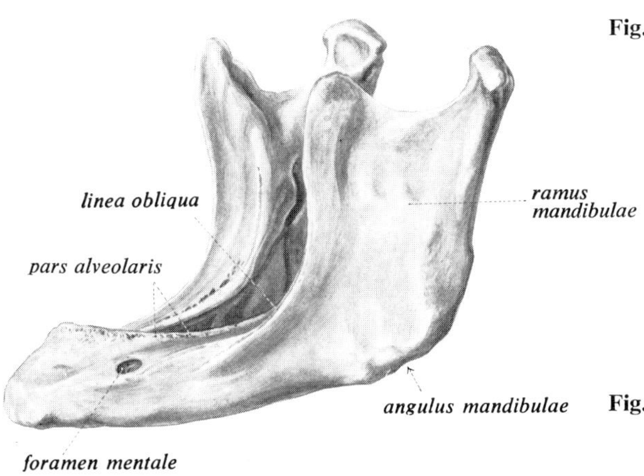

Fig. 109. *Mandibula* of an aged woman.

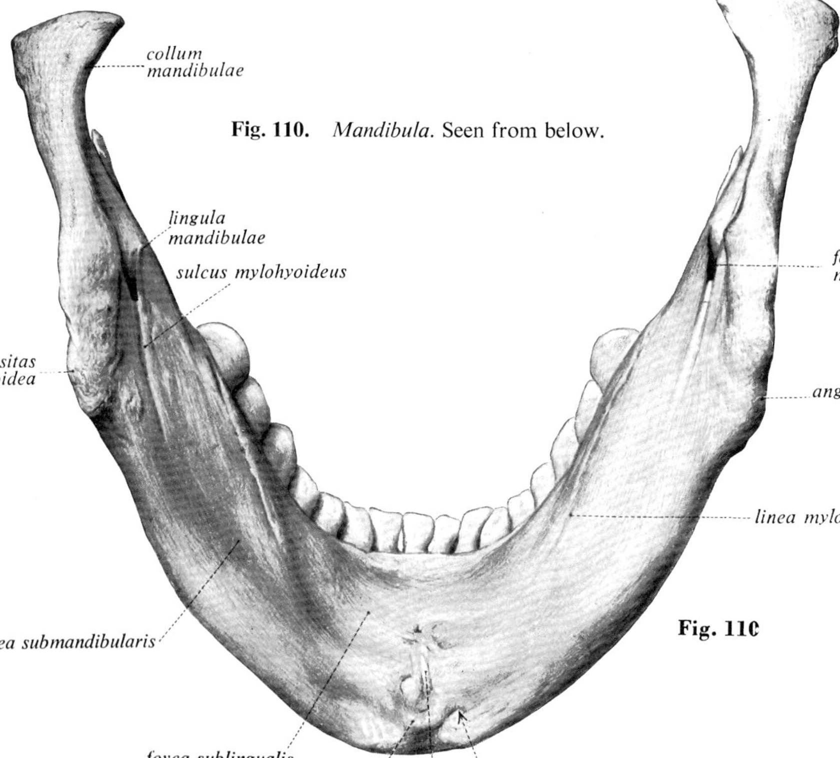

Fig. 110. *Mandibula*. Seen from below.

Fig. 110

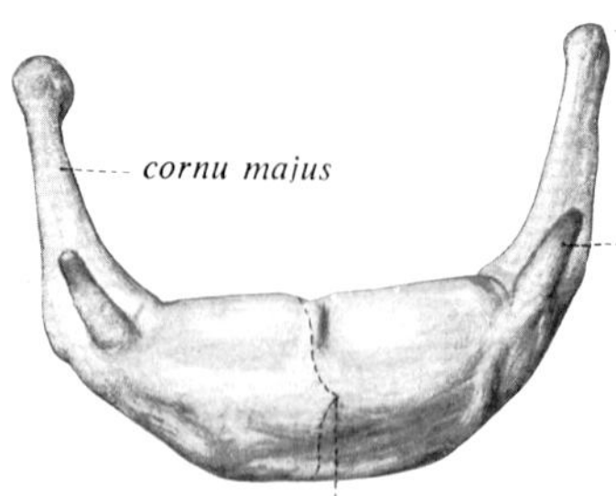

Fig. 112

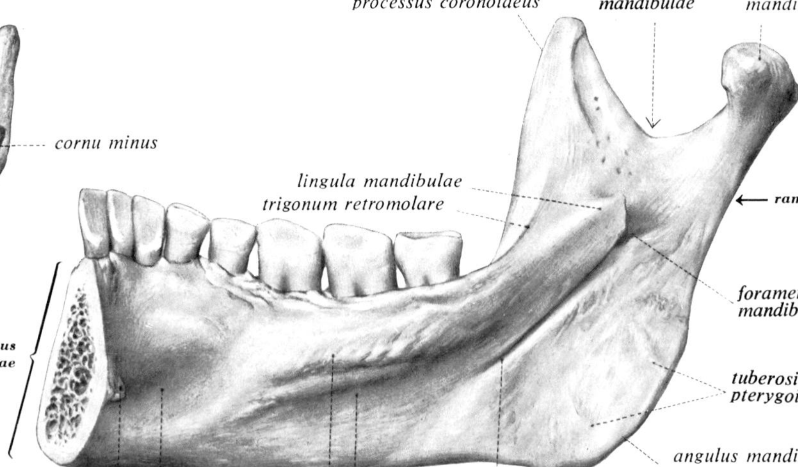

Fig. 111

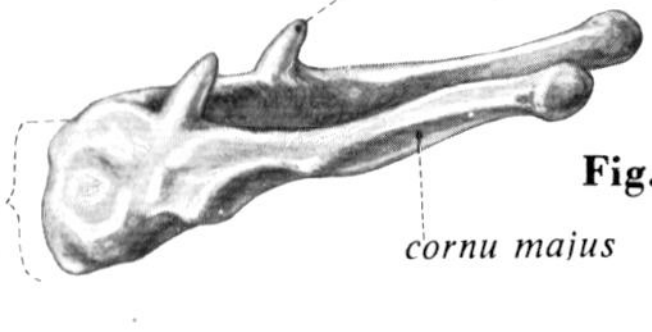

Fig. 113

Fig. 111. Right half of *mandibula*. Medial view.
Fig. 112. *Os hyoideum*. Cranial and frontal view.
Fig. 113. *Os hyoideum*. Seen from left lateral side.

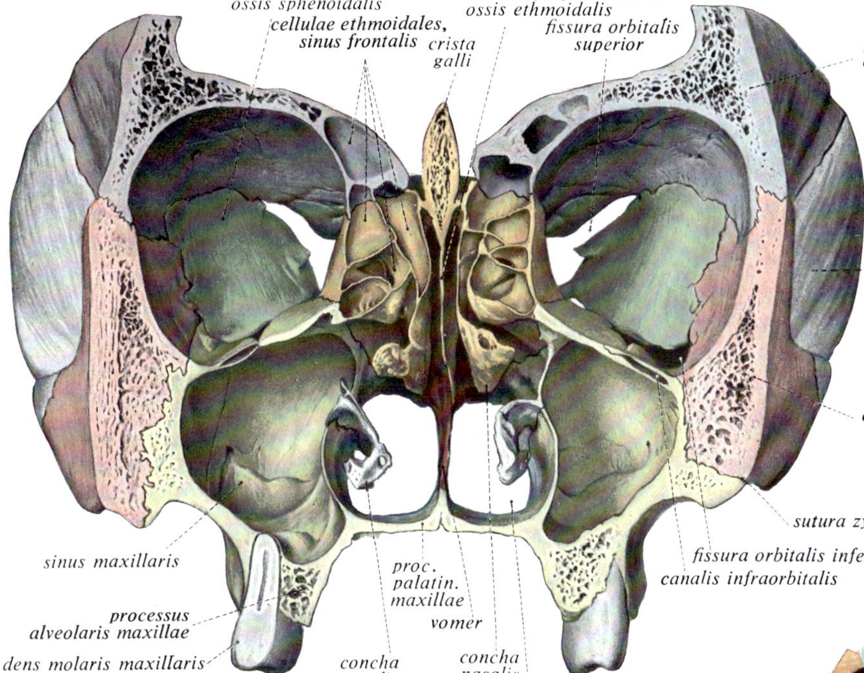

Fig. 114

Figs. 114–116. *Os frontale,* pink-violet; *os ethmoidale,* orange; *maxilla,* yellow; *os sphenoidale,* pale green; *os palatinum,* pale blue; *vomer* and *os lacrimale,* reddish; *concha nasalis inferior* and *os temporale,* uncolored; *os zygomaticum* in Fig. 114, pinkish-red.

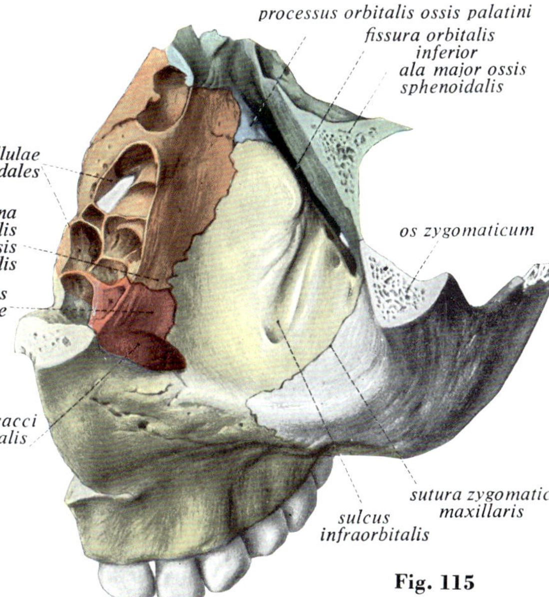

Fig. 115

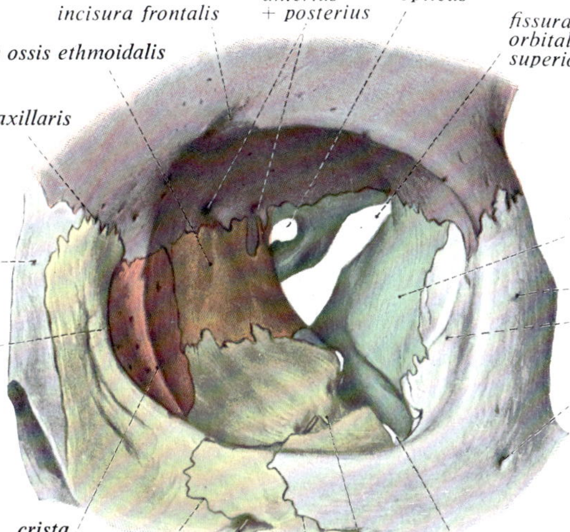

Fig. 116

Fig. 114. Frontal section of the *cranium. Orbita* and *cavum nasi, sinus maxillaris* and *labyrinthus ethmoidalis.*
Fig. 115. Floor of left orbital cavity.
Fig. 116. Left *orbita.* Seen from in front.
* Sound in the *canalis infraorbitalis.*

Fig. 117. Medial wall of the left *orbita* and *fossa pterygopalatina.* Explanation of coloring below.

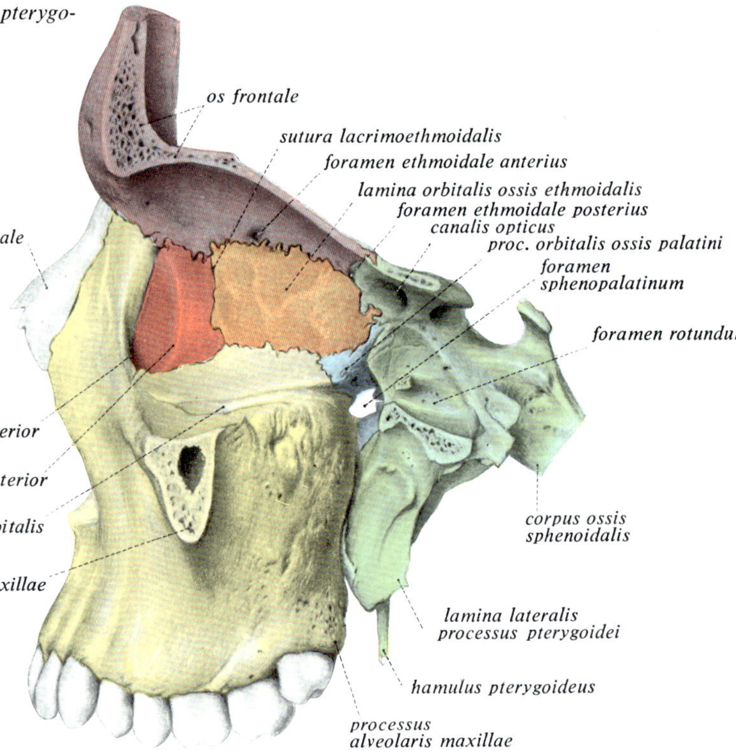

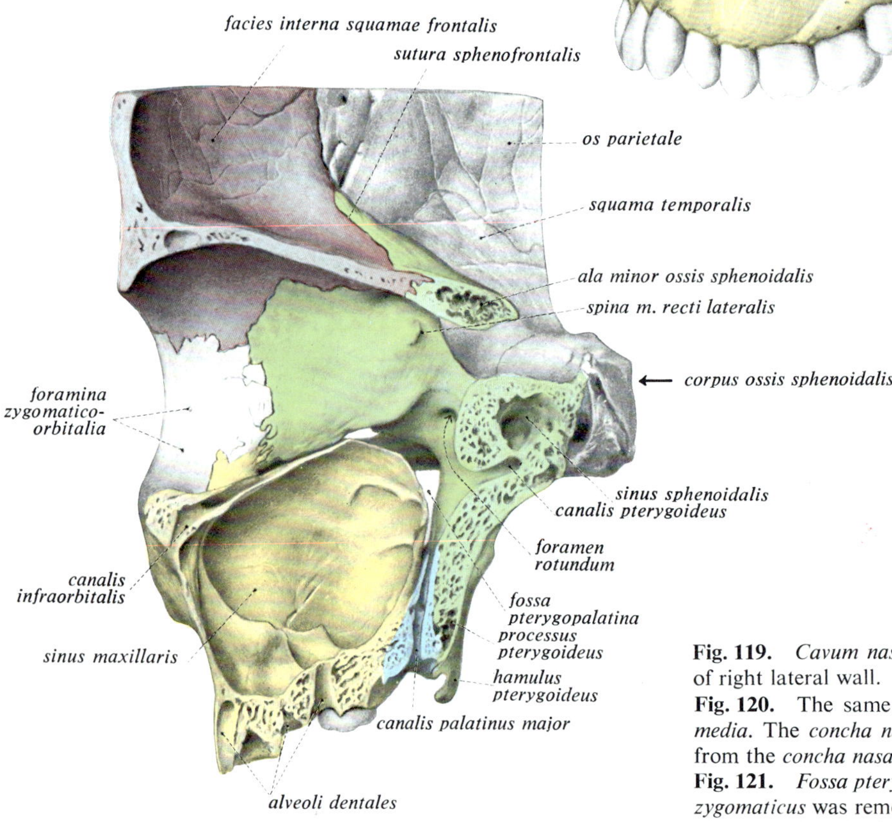

Fig. 118. Lateral wall of right orbital cavity, maxillary sinus, and the pterygopalatine fossa.

Fig. 119. *Cavum nasi. Septum nasi* removed to view bones of right lateral wall.

Fig. 120. The same view after resection of *concha nasalis media.* The *concha nasalis superior* is not sharply delimited from the *concha nasalis media.*

Fig. 121. *Fossa pterygopalatina.* Left lateral view. The *arcus zygomaticus* was removed.

Figs. 119–121. *Os frontale*, pale violet; *os lacrimale*, reddish; *os ethmoidale*, peach-orange; *maxilla*, yellow; *os palatinum*, pale blue; *os sphenoidale*, pale green.

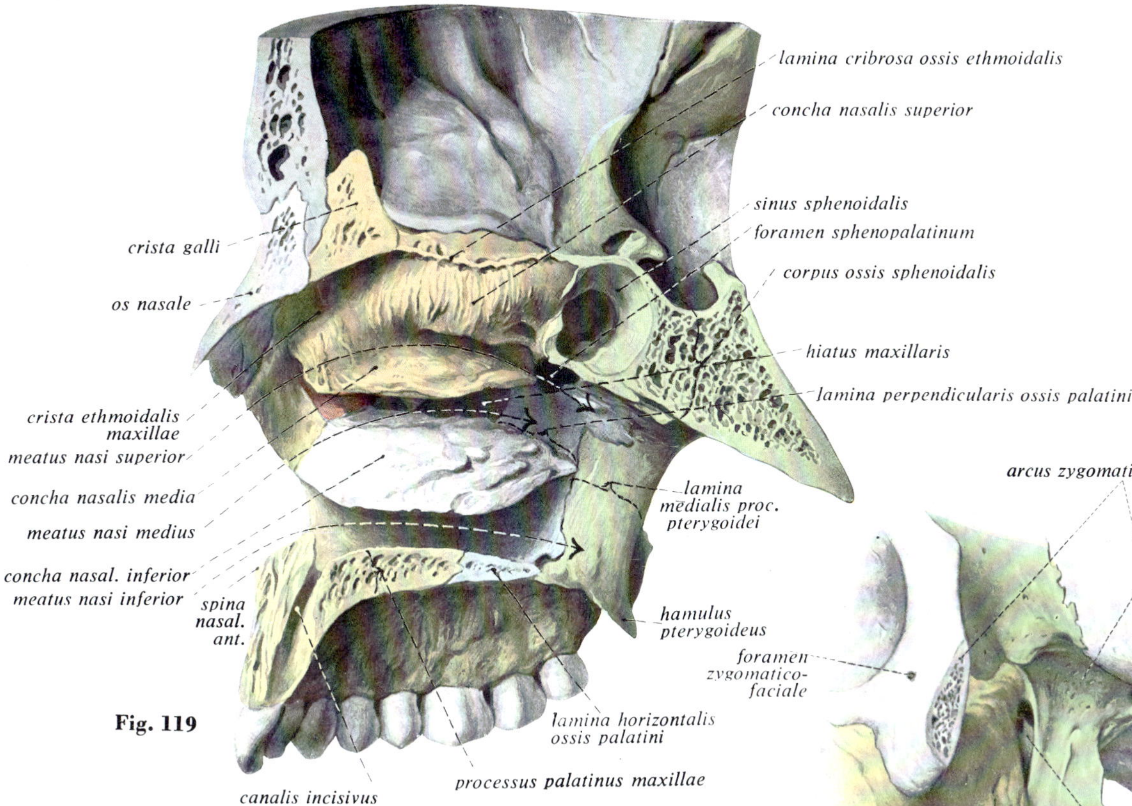
lamina cribrosa ossis ethmoidalis
concha nasalis superior
sinus sphenoidalis
foramen sphenopalatinum
corpus ossis sphenoidalis
hiatus maxillaris
lamina perpendicularis ossis palatini
crista galli
os nasale
crista ethmoidalis maxillae
meatus nasi superior
concha nasalis media
meatus nasi medius
concha nasal. inferior
meatus nasi inferior
spina nasal. ant.
lamina medialis proc. pterygoidei
hamulus pterygoideus
lamina horizontalis ossis palatini
processus palatinus maxillae
canalis incisivus

Fig. 119

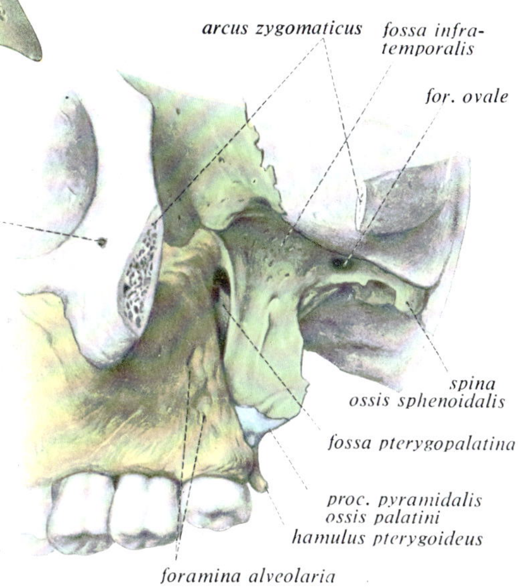
arcus zygomaticus
fossa infratemporalis
for. ovale
foramen zygomaticofaciale
spina ossis sphenoidalis
fossa pterygopalatina
proc. pyramidalis ossis palatini
hamulus pterygoideus
foramina alveolaria

Fig. 121

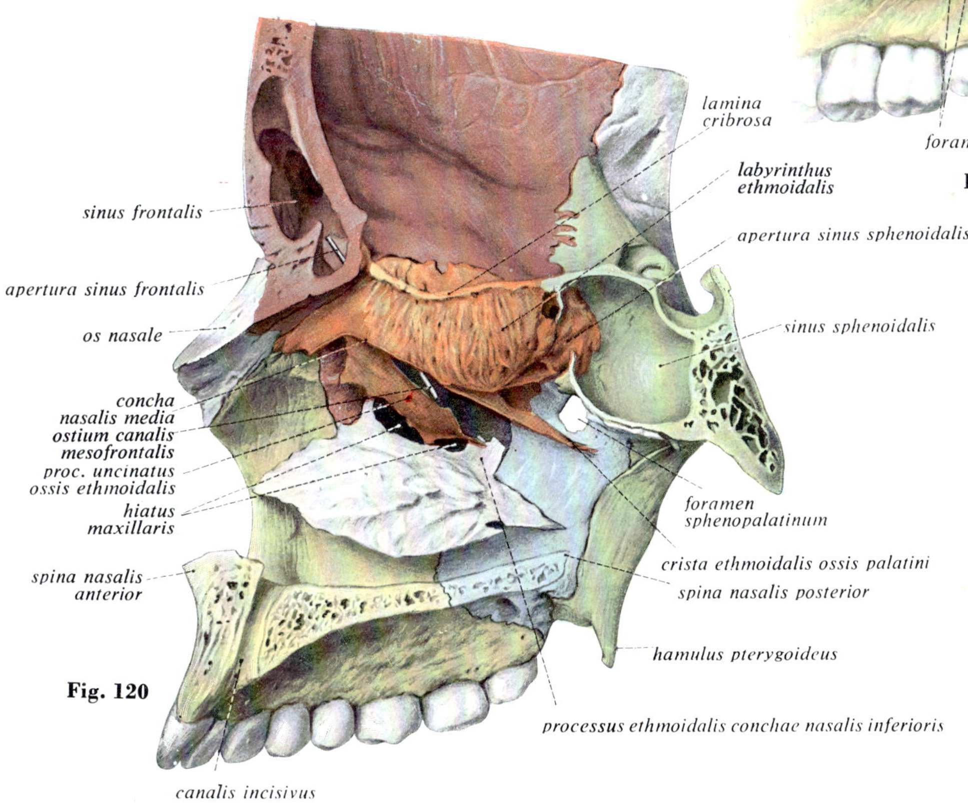
lamina cribrosa
labyrinthus ethmoidalis
apertura sinus sphenoidalis
sinus frontalis
apertura sinus frontalis
os nasale
sinus sphenoidalis
concha nasalis media
ostium canalis mesofrontalis
proc. uncinatus ossis ethmoidalis
hiatus maxillaris
foramen sphenopalatinum
crista ethmoidalis ossis palatini
spina nasalis anterior
spina nasalis posterior
hamulus pterygoideus
processus ethmoidalis conchae nasalis inferioris
canalis incisivus

Fig. 120

Skeleton

The Shoulder Girdle and Upper Limb

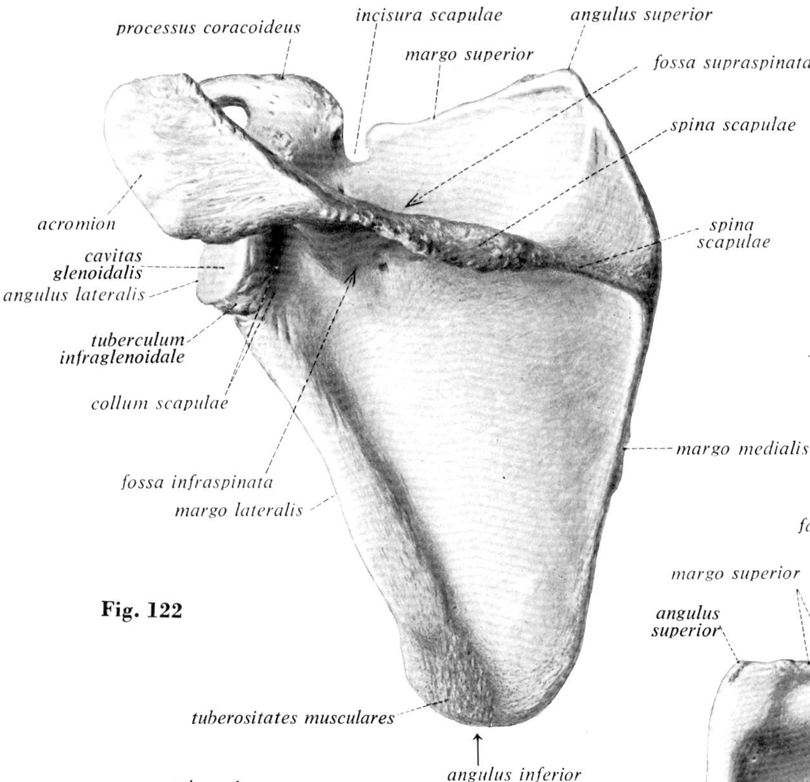

Fig. 122

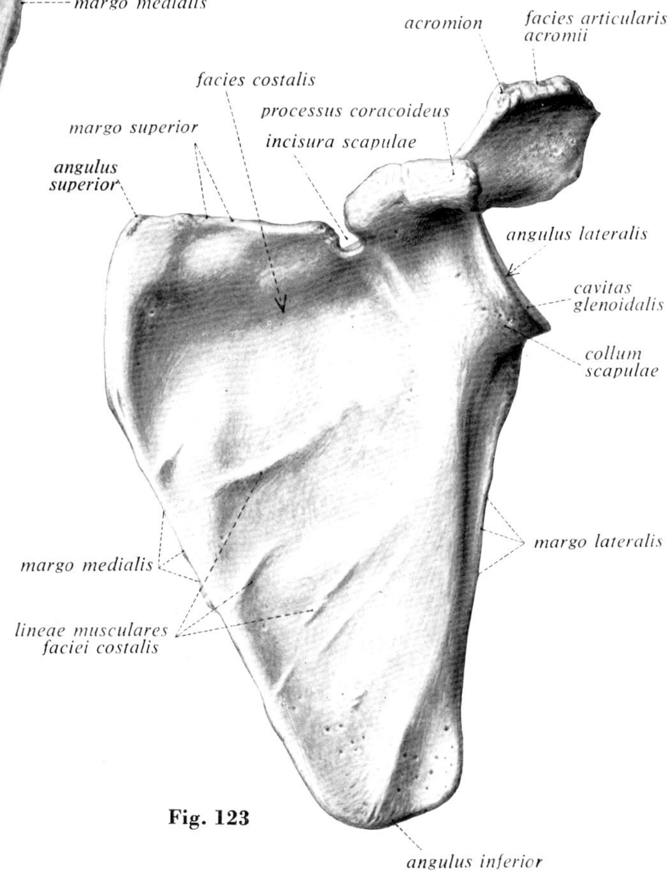

Fig. 123

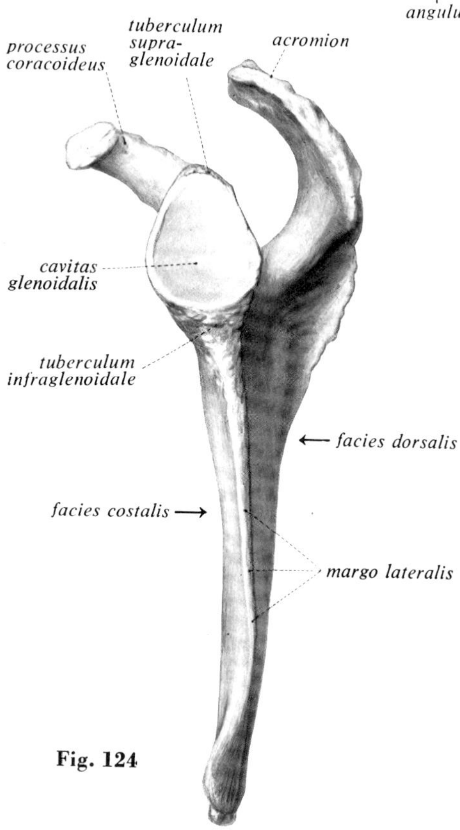

Fig. 124

Figs. 122–124. The left *scapula*. Fig. 122. Dorsal view. Fig. 123. Ventral view. Fig. 124. Lateral view.

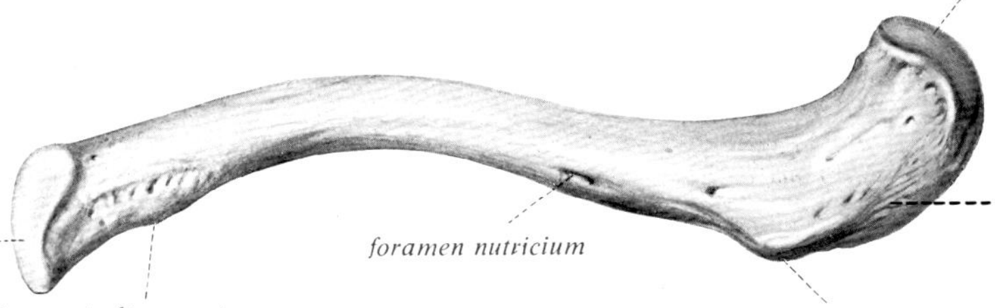

Fig. 125

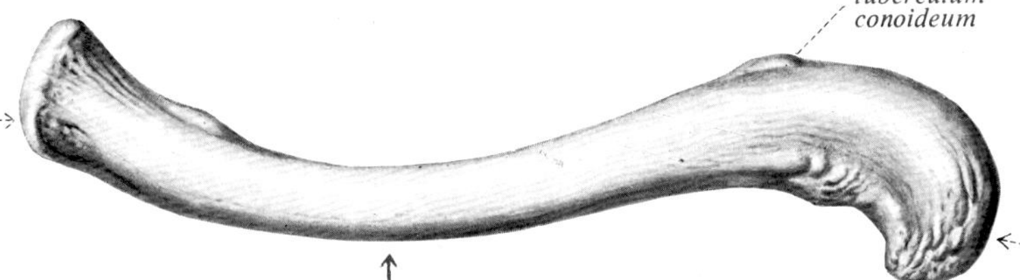

Fig. 126

Figs. 125 and 126. The left *clavicula*.
Fig. 125. Caudal view. Fig. 126. Cranial view.

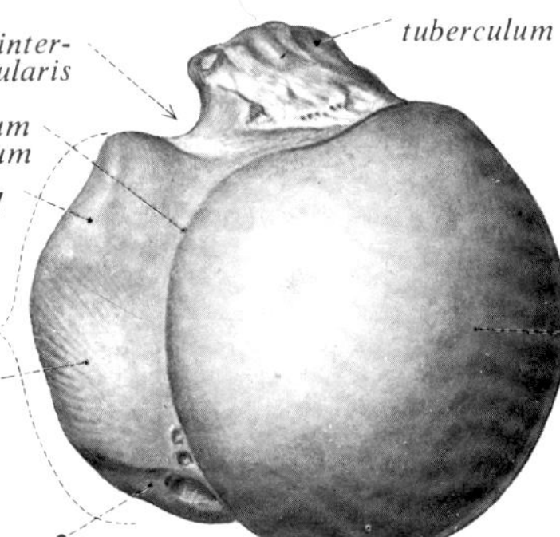

Fig. 127. Head of left *humerus (caput humeri)*. Proximal view. Facets for:
1. *M. supraspinatus*. 2. *M. infraspinatus*. 3. *M. teres minor*.

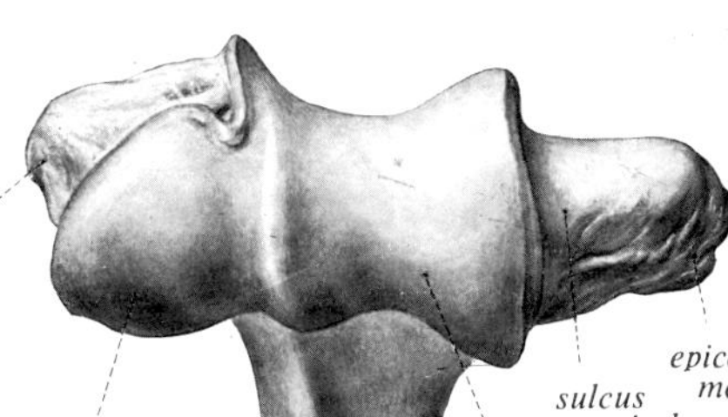

Fig. 128. Distal end of the left *humerus*.

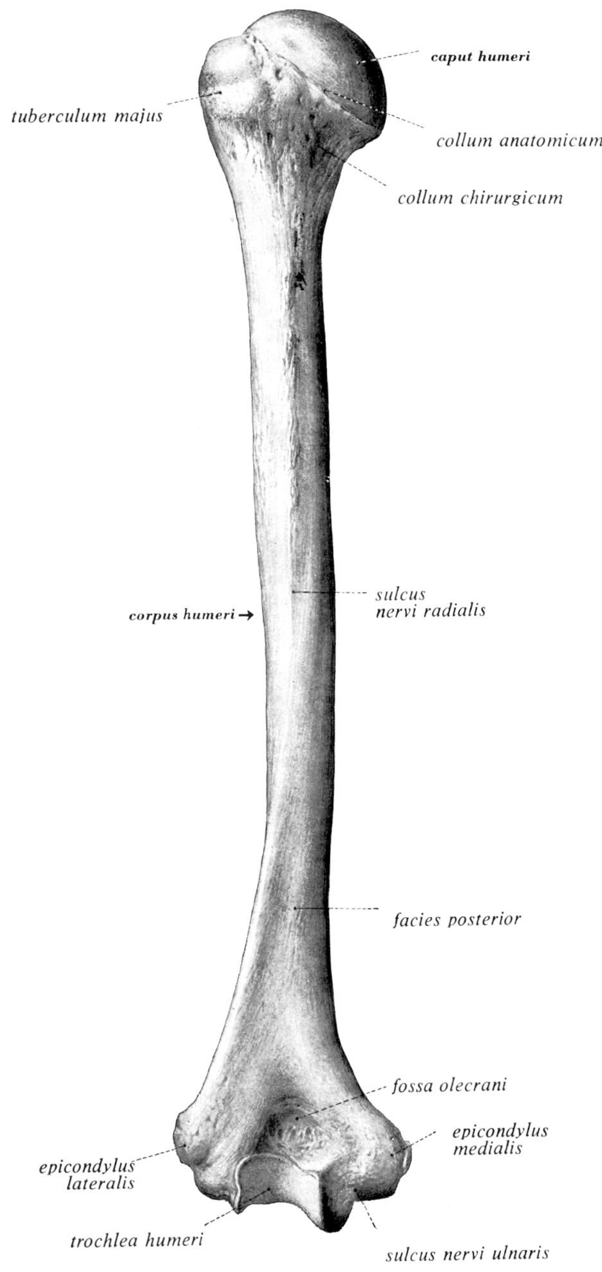

Fig. 129

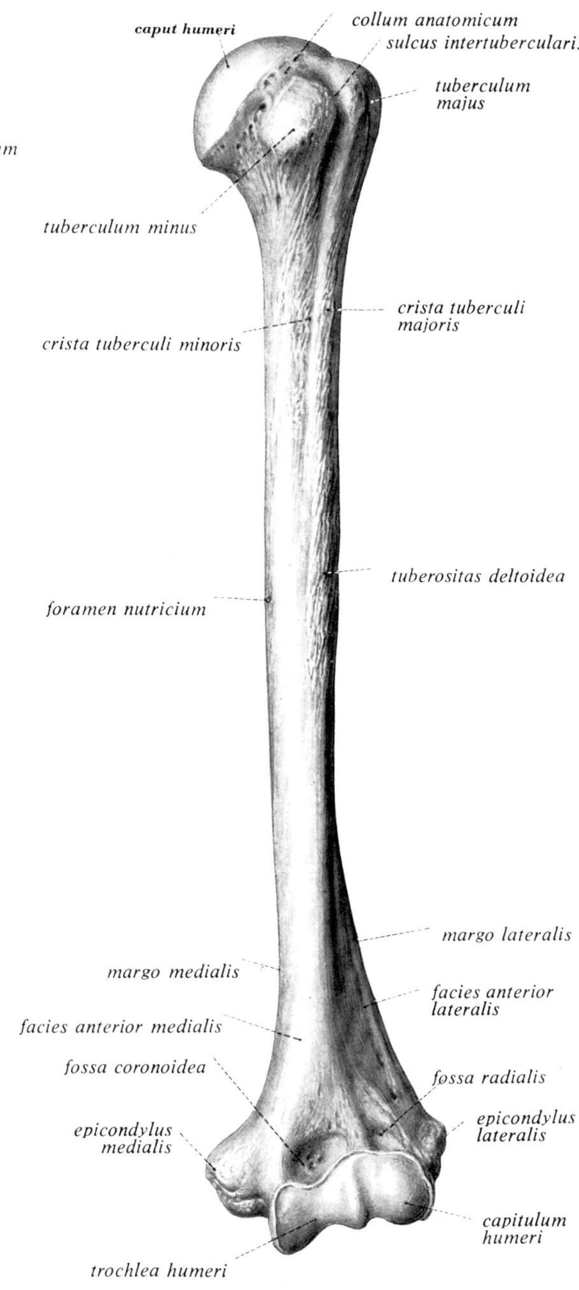

Fig. 130

Figs. 129 and 130. Left *humerus*. Fig. 129. Dorsal view. Fig. 130. Ventral view.

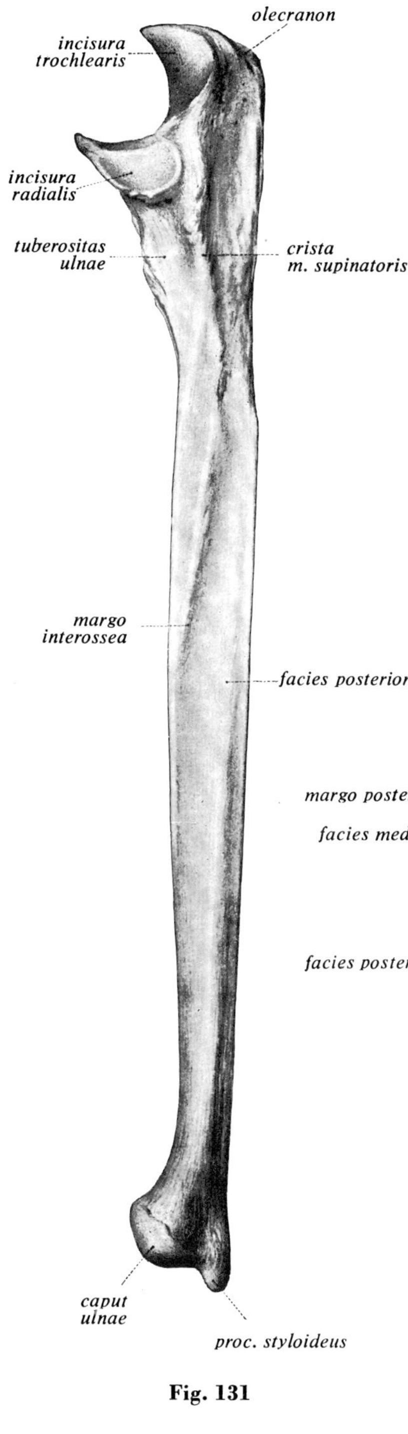

Fig. 131

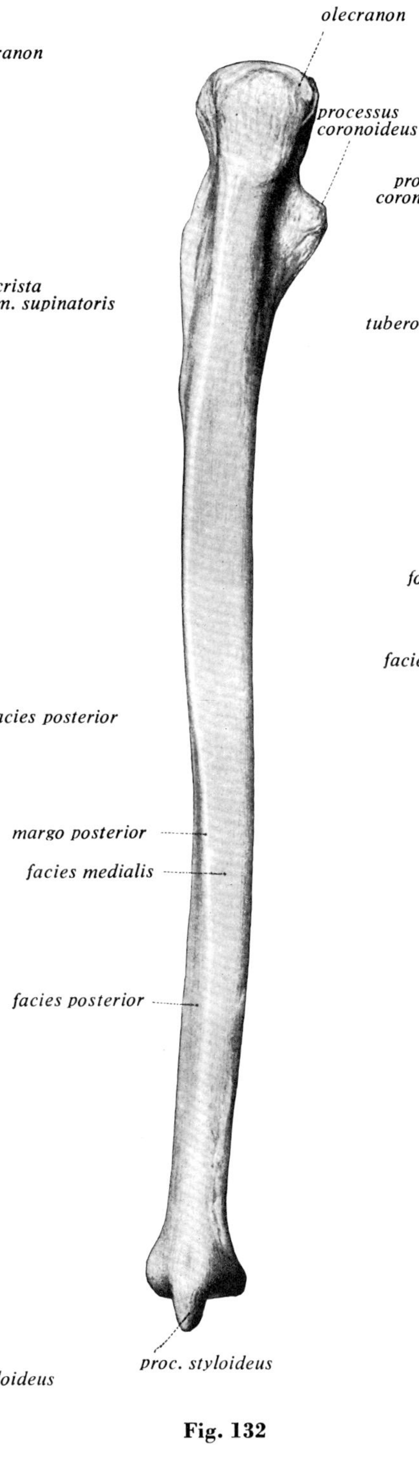

Fig. 132

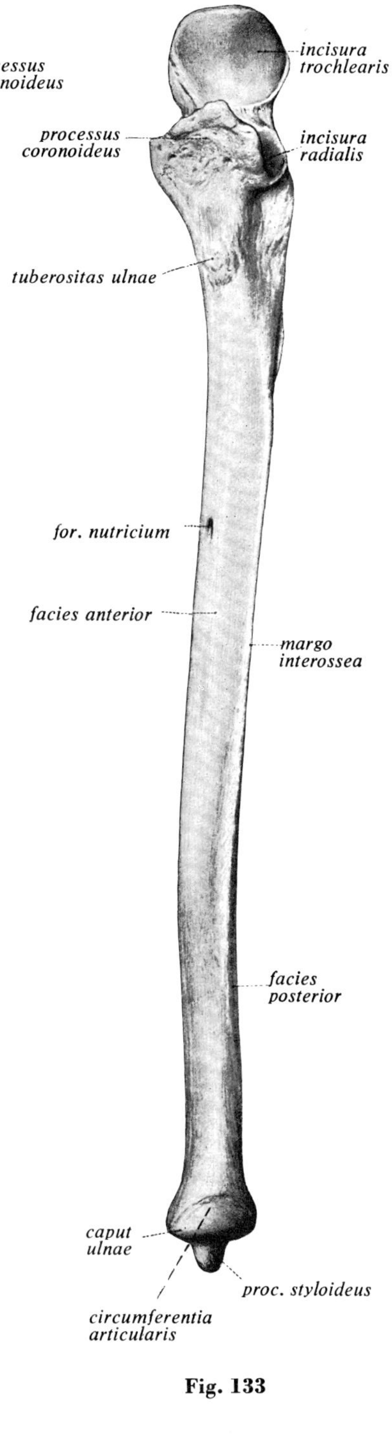

Fig. 133

Figs. 131–133. The left *ulna*. Fig. 131. Lateral (radial) aspect. Fig. 132. Dorsal aspect. Fig. 133. Palmar or anterior aspect.

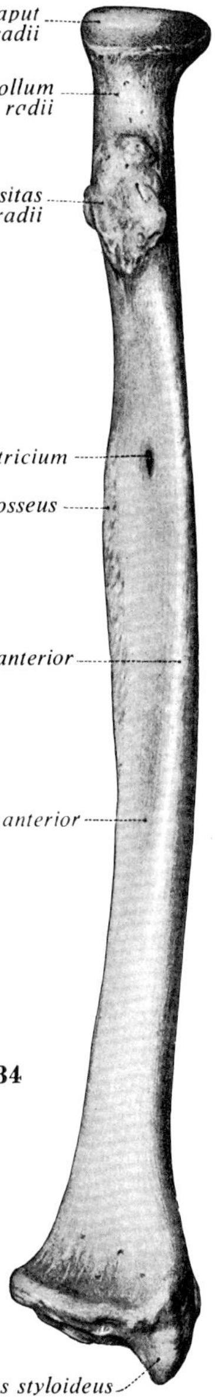

Fig. 134

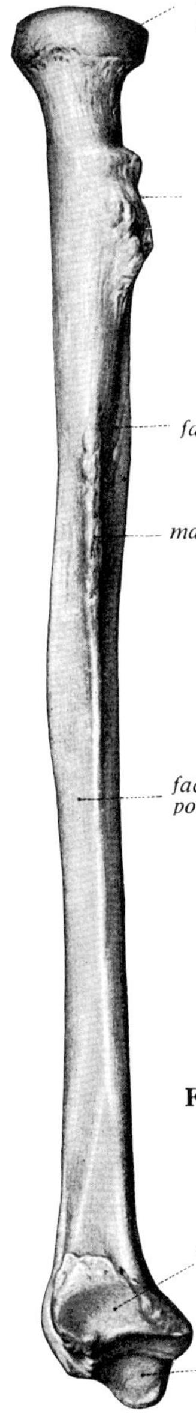

Fig. 135

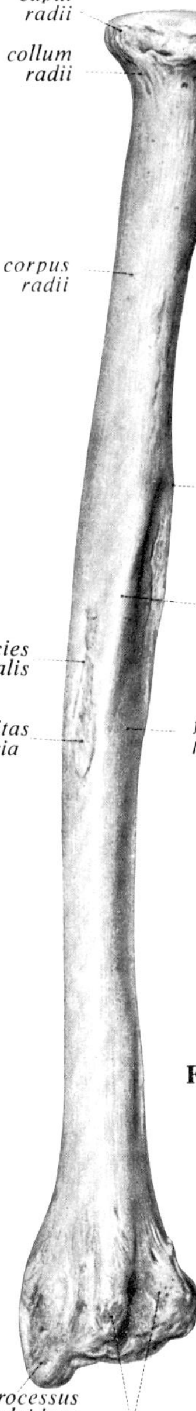

Fig. 136

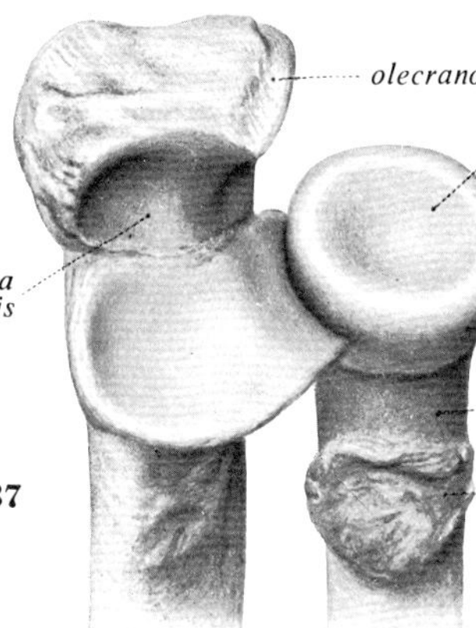

Fig. 137

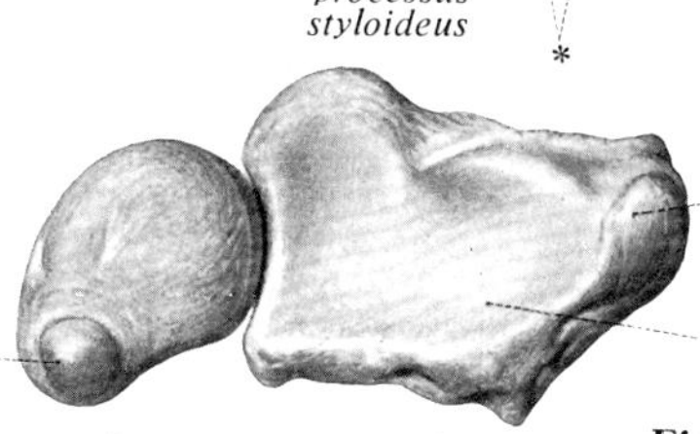

Fig. 138

Fig. 134. Left *radius*. Anterior view.
Fig. 135. Left *radius*. Medial view.
Fig. 136. Left *radius*. Posterior view.
Fig. 137. Proximal ends of *radius* and *ulna*.
Fig. 138. Distal ends of *radius* and *ulna*. Distal view.
* Grooves and crests for extensor tendons.

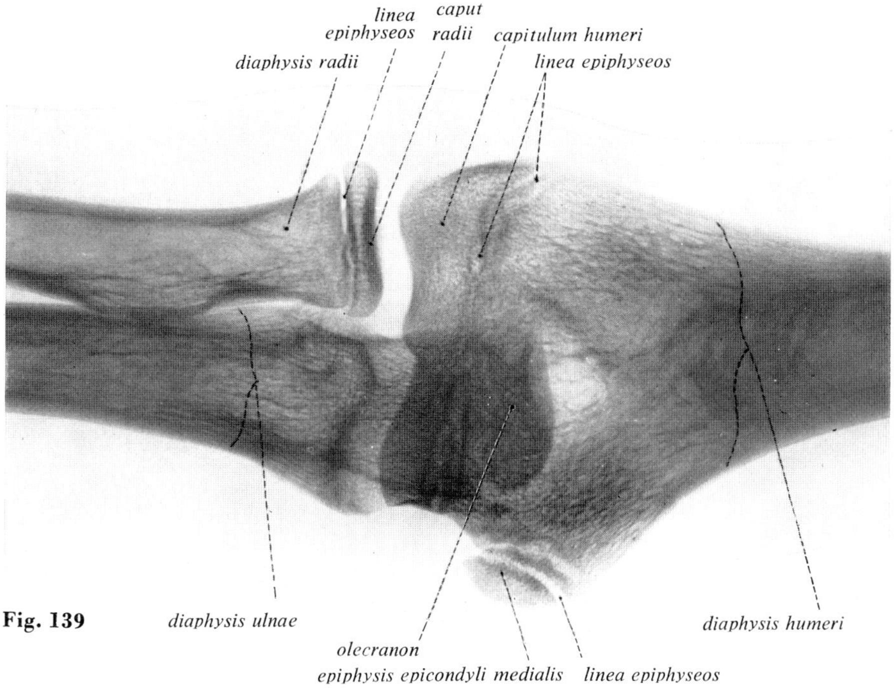

Fig. 139

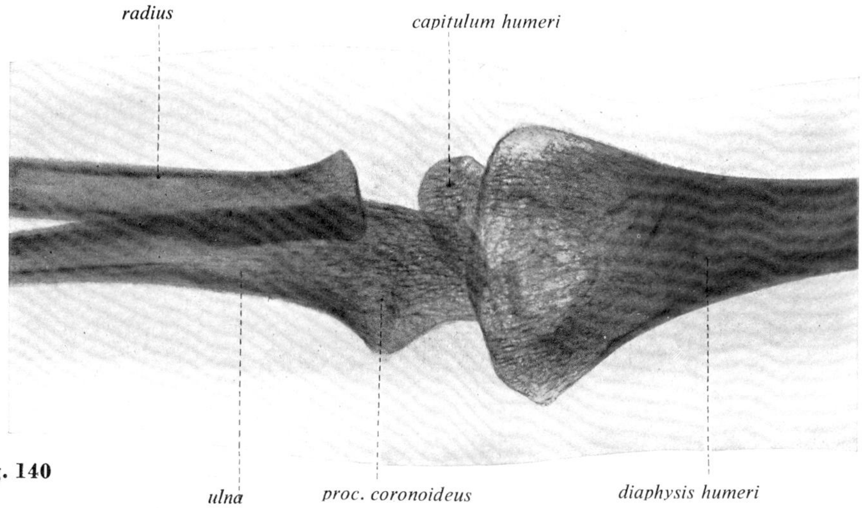

Fig. 140

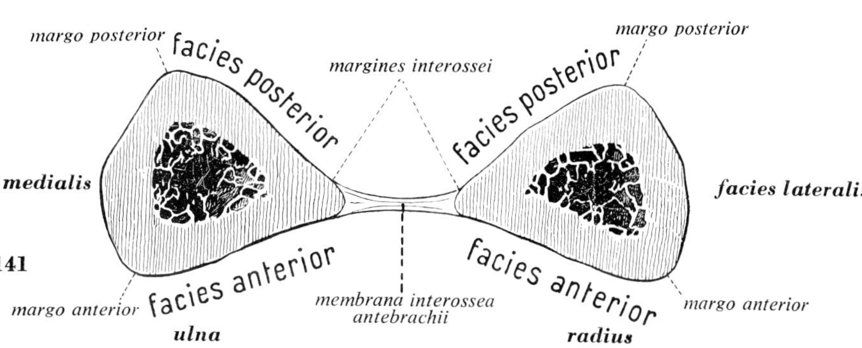

Fig. 141

Fig. 139. X-ray picture of the elbow *(regio cubiti)* of a 17 year old boy.
Fig. 140. X-ray picture of the elbow *(regio cubiti)* of a 5½ year old boy.
Fig. 141. Surfaces and borders of the bones of the left forearm. Diagrammatic section near the middle of its length. *Facies anterior* = Anterior surface; *facies posterior* = Posterior surface.

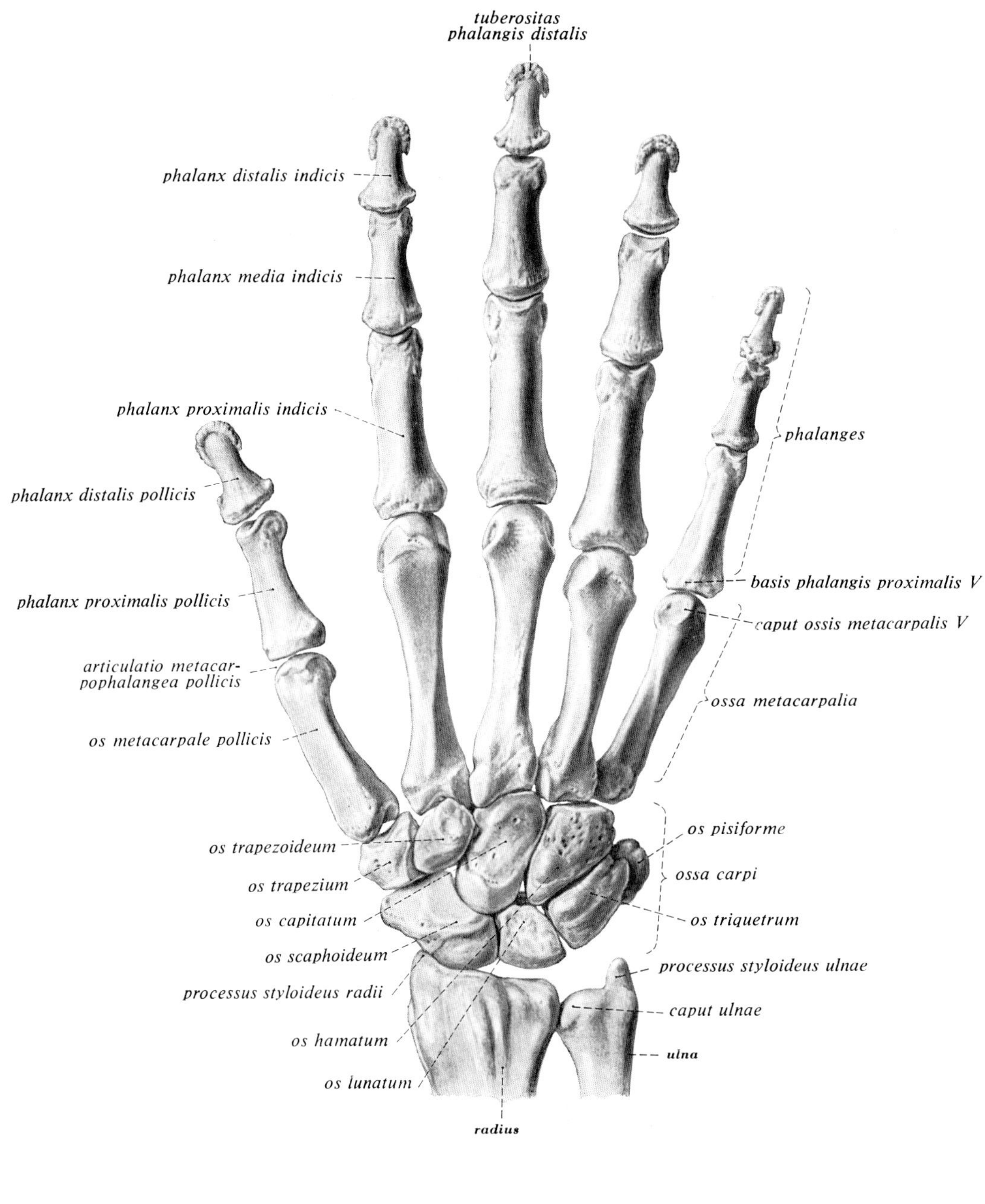

Fig. 142. Skeleton of right hand with extended, slightly spread fingers, and the distal end of the forearm with bones in their natural position. Dorsal view.

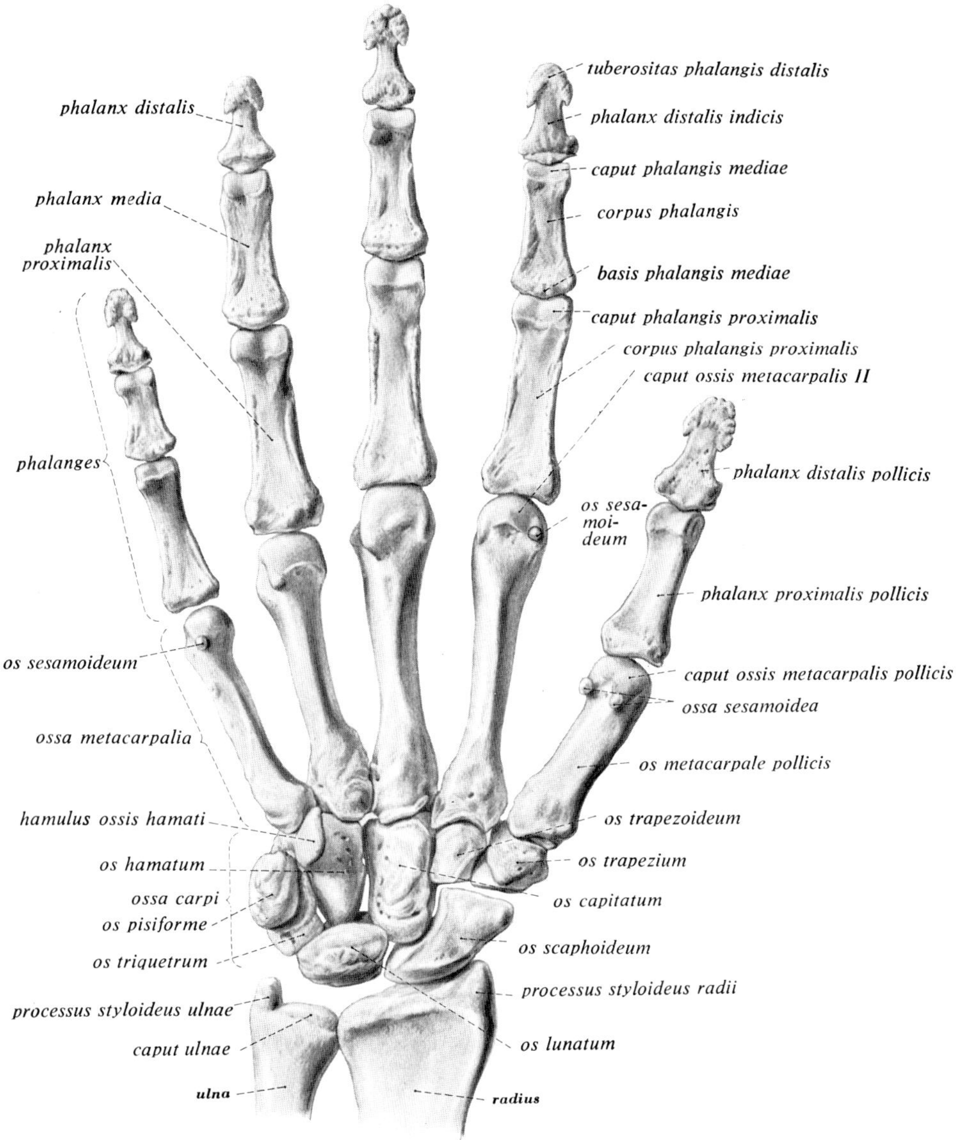

Fig. 143. Skeleton of the right hand (same object as in Fig. 142). Palmar view.

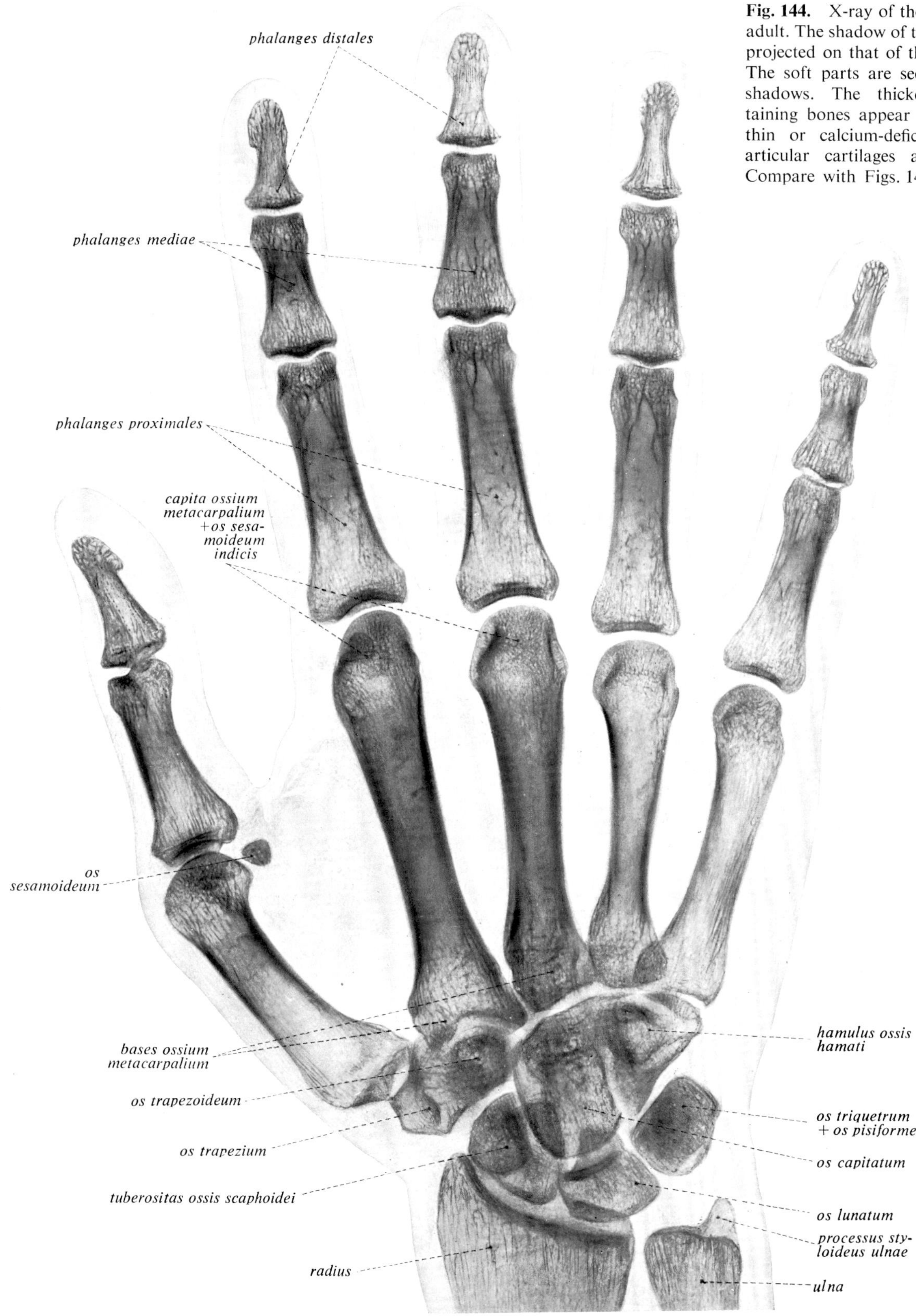

Fig. 144. X-ray of the left hand of an adult. The shadow of the *os pisiforme* is projected on that of the *os triquetrum*. The soft parts are seen only as faint shadows. The thicker calcium-containing bones appear darker than the thin or calcium-deficient ones. The articular cartilages are not visible. Compare with Figs. 145 and 146.

Fig. 145. X-ray picture of the left hand of a 15½ year old. The distal epiphyses of the *radius* and *ulna*, as well as the distal resp. proximal epiphyses of the metacarpals and phalanges, are not yet united with their respective diaphyses. Note the definite epiphyseal lines.

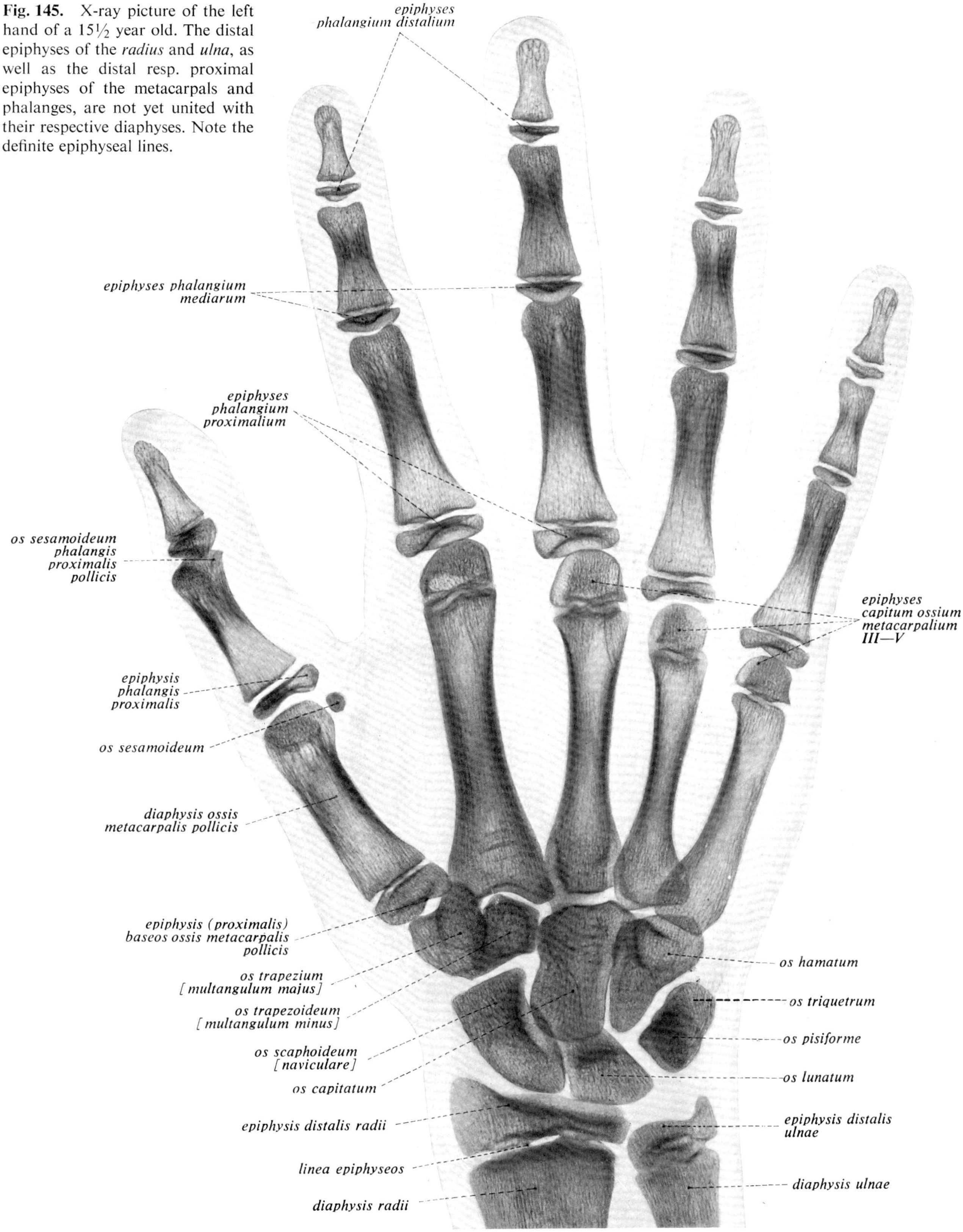

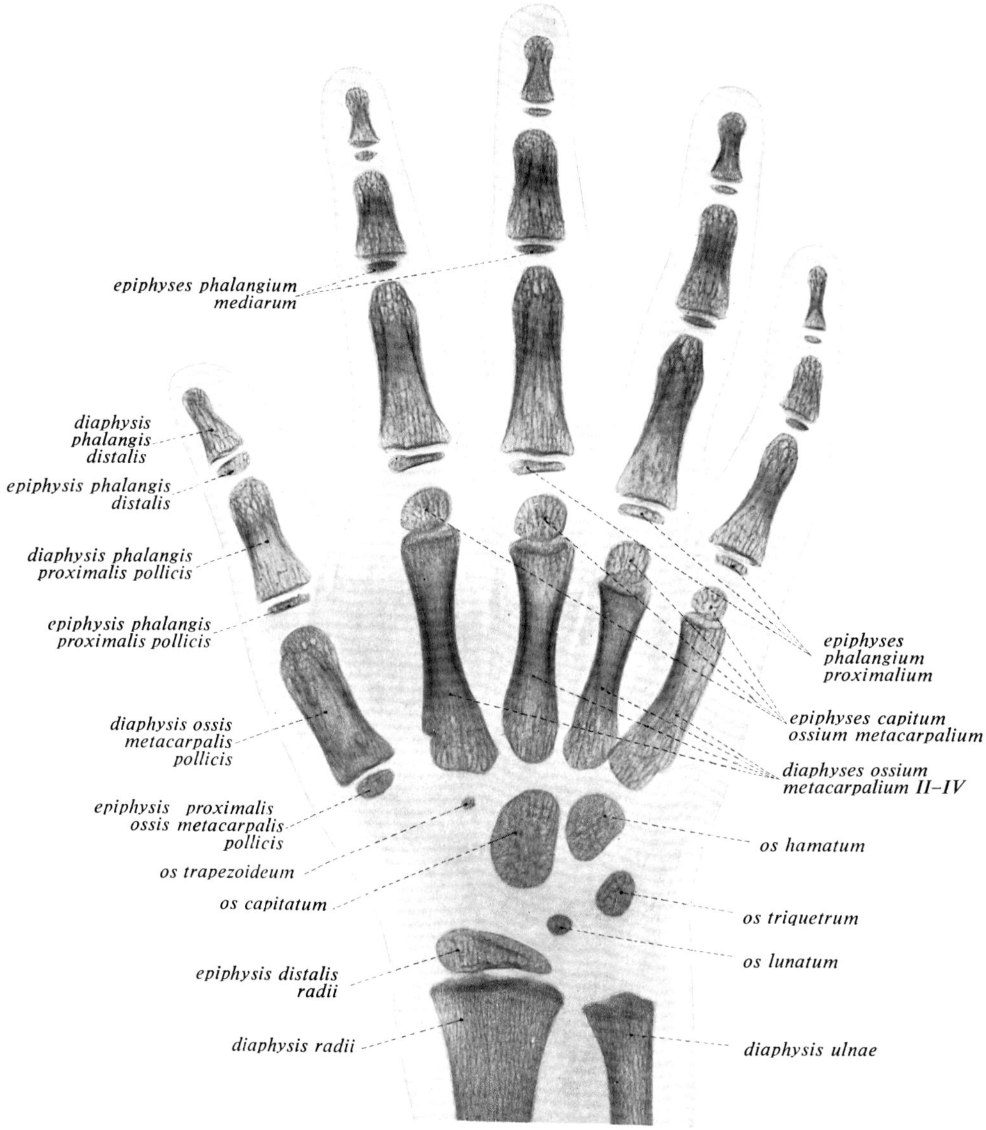

Fig. 146. X-ray picture of the hand of a $5\frac{1}{2}$ year old boy. The phalanges of the fingers have only one proximal epiphysis; the *ossa metacarpalia* II–V have only one distal. From this, one can see the *os metacarpale pollicis* as the proximal phalanx of the thumb. The center of ossification of the *os trapezoideum* and *os lunatum* are still very small; that of the *os scaphoideum* is absent. It is, therefore, possible to determine the age of children through investigation of the ossification. (Compare with Fig. 184.)

Skeleton

The Pelvic Girdle and Lower Limb

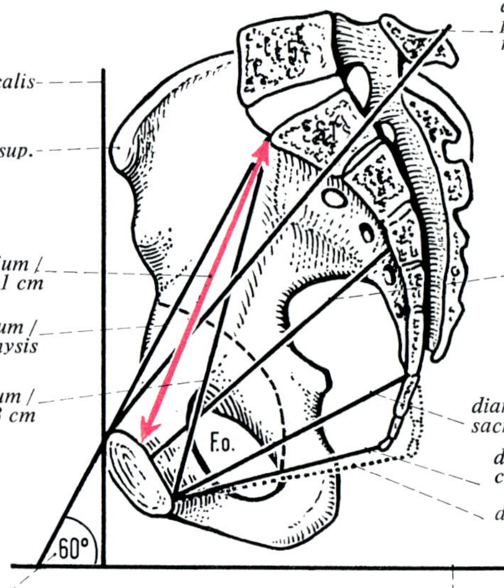

Fig. 147. Median sagittal section through the *pelvis* of an adult female, showing important obstetrical diameters and axes. *Conjugata "anatomica":* Diameter from the *promontorium* to the superior margin of the *symphysis pubica. Conjugata "vera"* = *"gynaecologica":* Diameter connects the *promontorium* with the middle of the most prominent part of the posterior aspect of the *symphysis pubica.* The dotted line indicates the *axis pelvis.*

♂

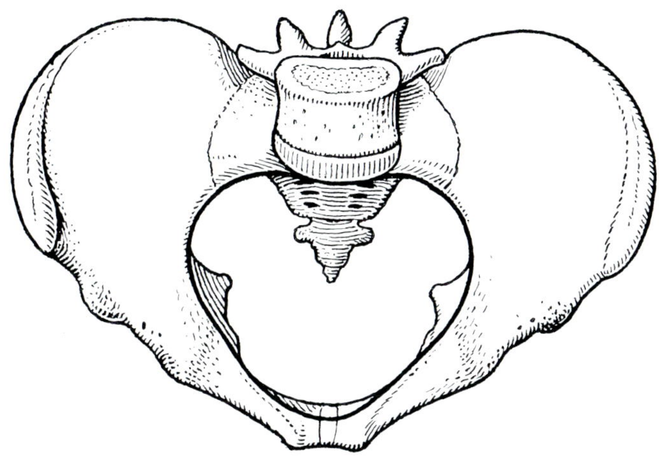

Fig. 148a. Male *pelvis:* Heartshaped pelvic aperture; true pelvis becomes narrower toward the outlet, hence funnel-shaped, subpubic angle.

♀

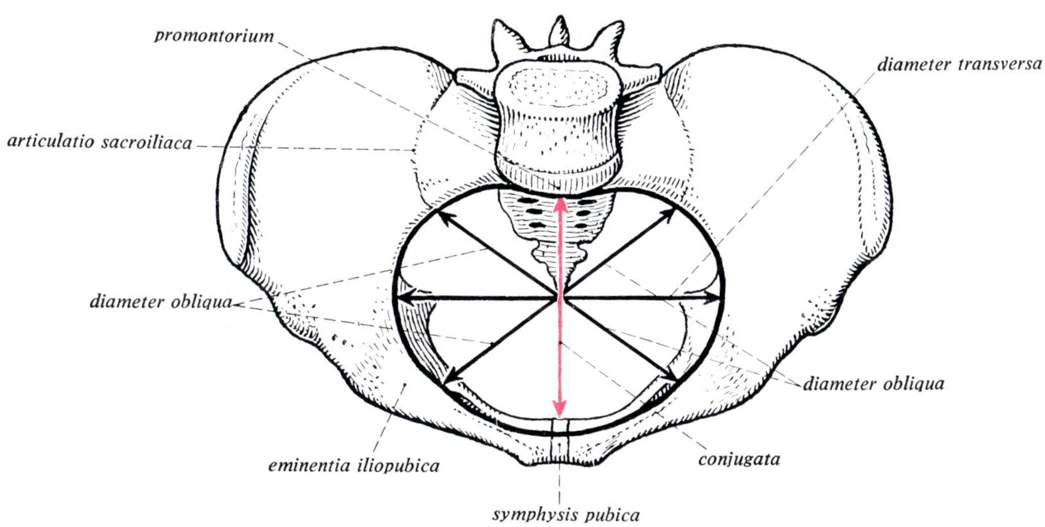

Fig. 148b. Female *pelvis:* Slanting oval of the pelvic aperture; cylindrical true *pelvis* not narrowed toward outlet, *arcus pubis.*

Note: The sex differences, especially in the shape, size, and diameter of the superior aperture of the *pelvis,* also as to the *sacrum* and position of the *fossa iliaca.* The left *diameter obliqua I* (12.5 cm.) from the left *eminentia ileopubica* to the right *articulatio sacroiliaca;* the right *diameter obliqua II* (12.5 cm.) from the right *eminentia ileopectinea* to the left *articulatio sacroiliaca; conjugata* (11 cm.) from the *promontorium* to the most prominent part of the posterior aspect of the symphysis of the pubis (red arrow).

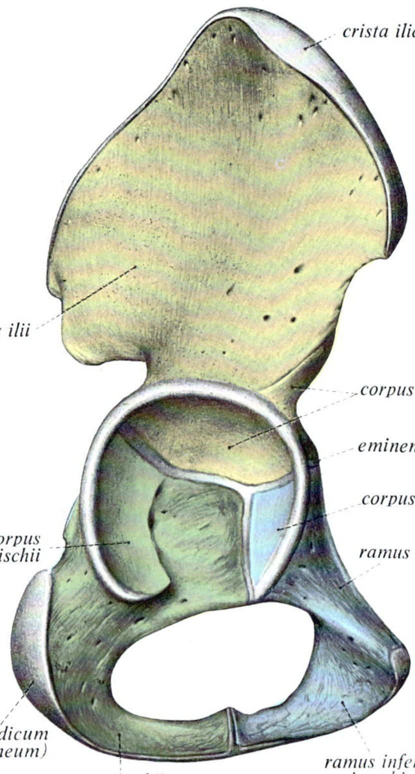

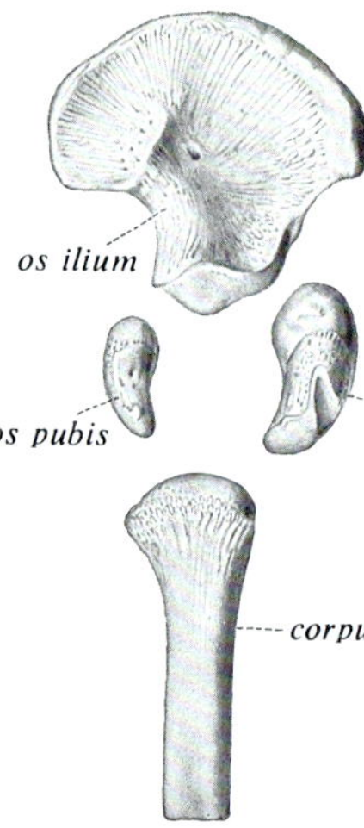

Fig. 150. Right hip bone *(os coxae)* and proximal part of the *femur* at birth. The 3 parts of the hip bone *(os ischium, os ilium* and *os pubis)* are not united at this stage, and the head *(caput)* and neck *(collum)* of the *femur* are cartilaginous.

Fig. 149. Hip bone *(os coxae)* of a child about 5 to 6 years old. Seen from lateral. *Os ilium*, yellow; *os ischium*, green; *os pubis*, blue. The three parts first form a starlike synchondrosis. The separating cartilaginous lines are present only in the young. Later synostosis takes place when they fuse to form the *os coxae* in the area of the *acetabulum*.

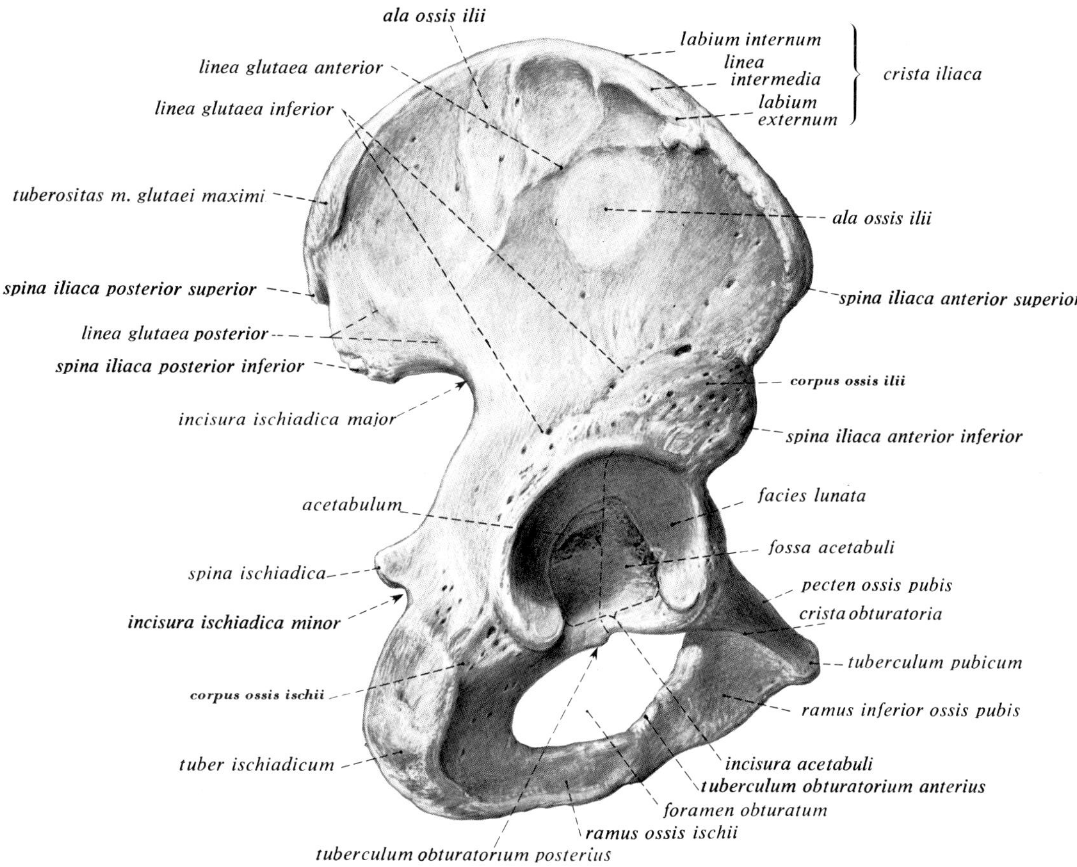
ala ossis ilii
linea glutaea anterior
linea glutaea inferior
labium internum
linea intermedia
labium externum
crista iliaca
tuberositas m. glutaei maximi
ala ossis ilii
spina iliaca posterior superior
spina iliaca anterior superior
linea glutaea posterior
spina iliaca posterior inferior
corpus ossis ilii
incisura ischiadica major
spina iliaca anterior inferior
acetabulum
facies lunata
fossa acetabuli
spina ischiadica
pecten ossis pubis
incisura ischiadica minor
crista obturatoria
tuberculum pubicum
corpus ossis ischii
ramus inferior ossis pubis
tuber ischiadicum
incisura acetabuli
tuberculum obturatorium anterius
foramen obturatum
ramus ossis ischii
tuberculum obturatorium posterius

Fig. 151. Right hip bone *(os coxae)*. Lateral view.

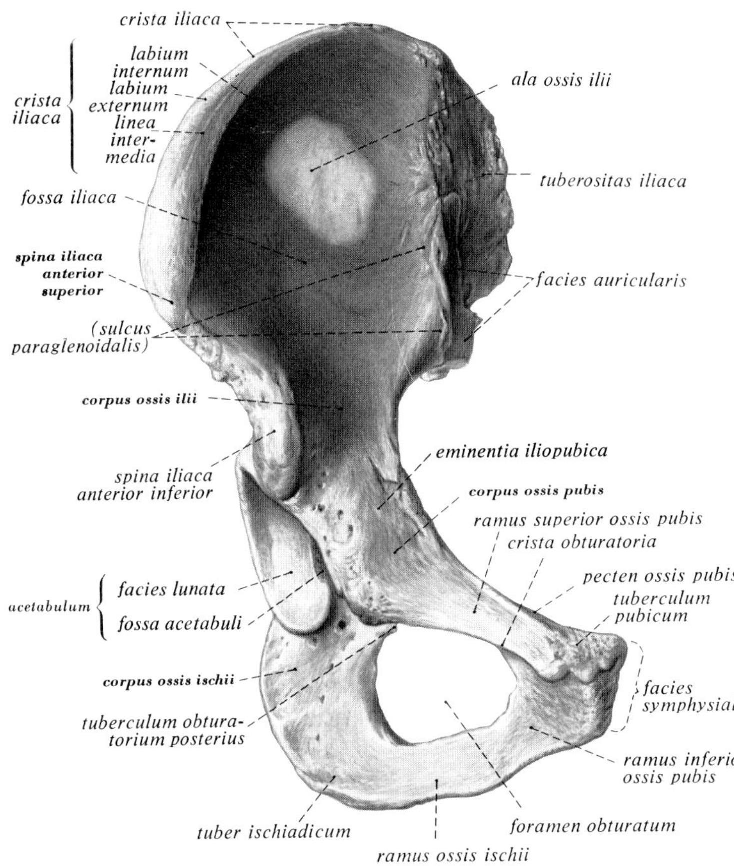
crista iliaca
crista iliaca
labium internum
labium externum
linea intermedia
ala ossis ilii
tuberositas iliaca
fossa iliaca
spina iliaca anterior superior
facies auricularis
(sulcus paraglenoidalis)
corpus ossis ilii
eminentia iliopubica
spina iliaca anterior inferior
corpus ossis pubis
ramus superior ossis pubis
crista obturatoria
pecten ossis pubis
acetabulum
facies lunata
fossa acetabuli
tuberculum pubicum
corpus ossis ischii
facies symphysialis
tuberculum obturatorium posterius
ramus inferior ossis pubis
tuber ischiadicum
foramen obturatum
ramus ossis ischii

Fig. 152. Right hip bone *(os coxae)*. Ventral view.

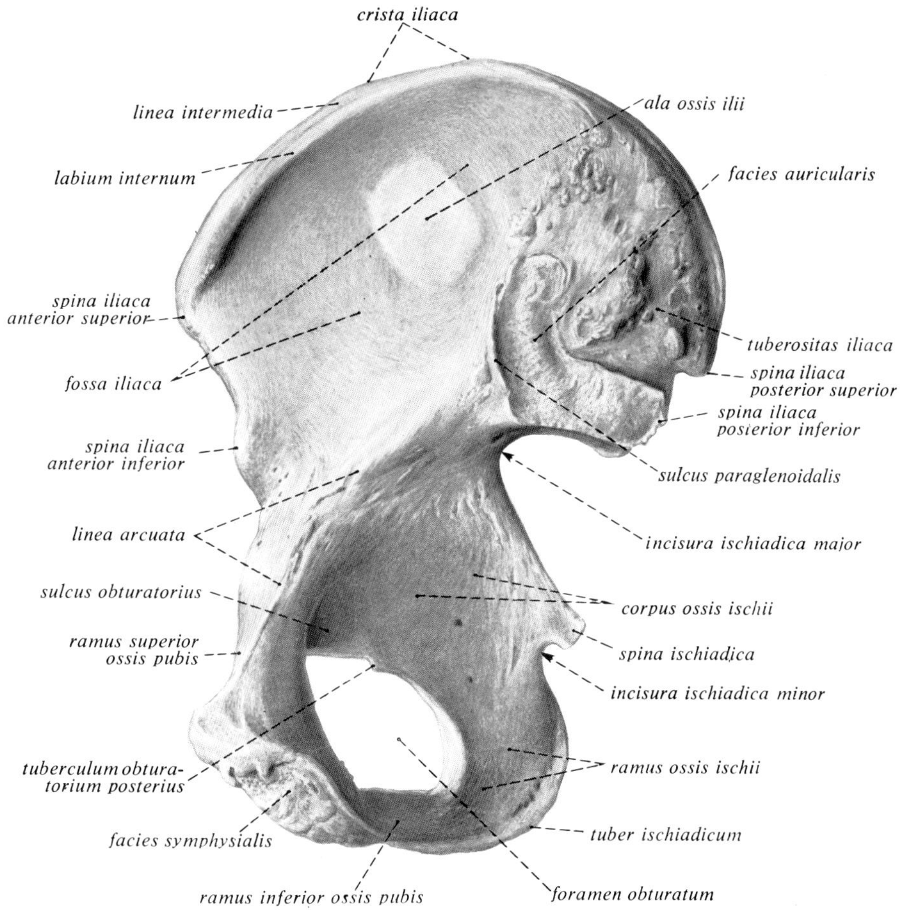
crista iliaca
linea intermedia
ala ossis ilii
labium internum
facies auricularis
spina iliaca anterior superior
tuberositas iliaca
spina iliaca posterior superior
fossa iliaca
spina iliaca posterior inferior
spina iliaca anterior inferior
sulcus paraglenoidalis
incisura ischiadica major
linea arcuata
sulcus obturatorius
corpus ossis ischii
ramus superior ossis pubis
spina ischiadica
incisura ischiadica minor
tuberculum obturatorium posterius
ramus ossis ischii
facies symphysialis
tuber ischiadicum
ramus inferior ossis pubis
foramen obturatum

Fig. 153. Right hip bone *(os coxae)*. Medial view.

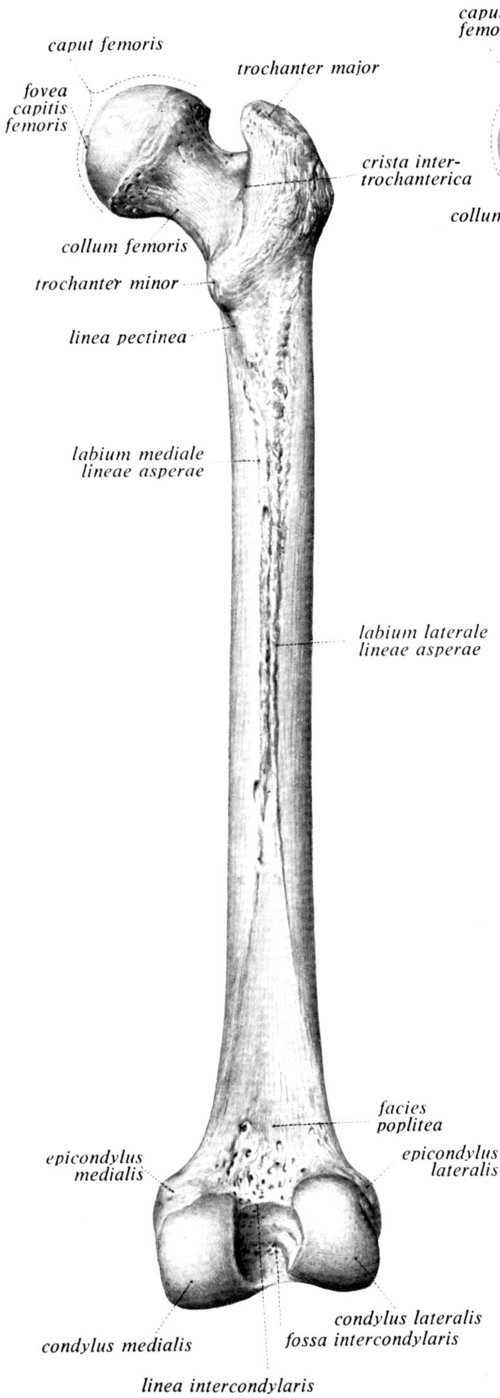

Fig. 154

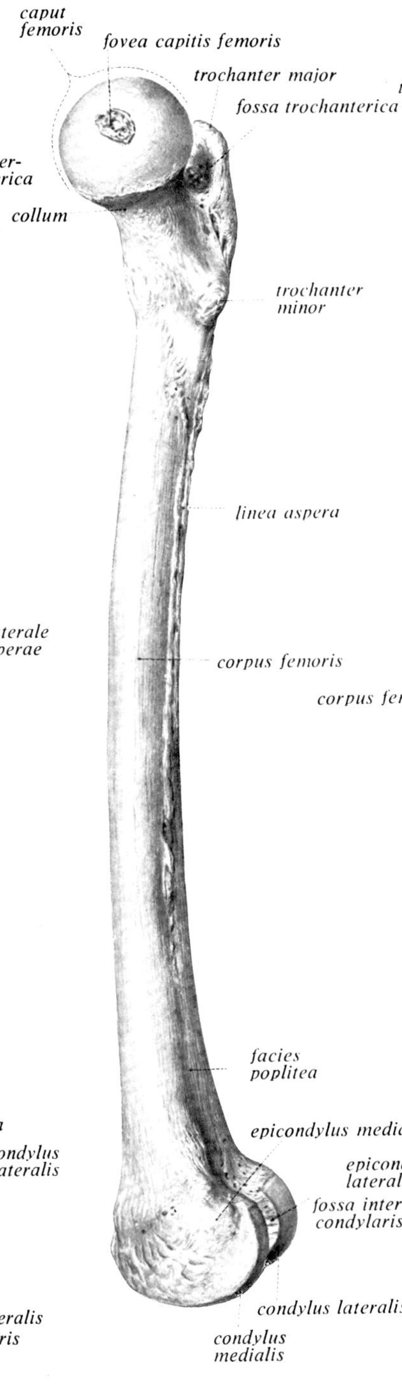

Fig. 155

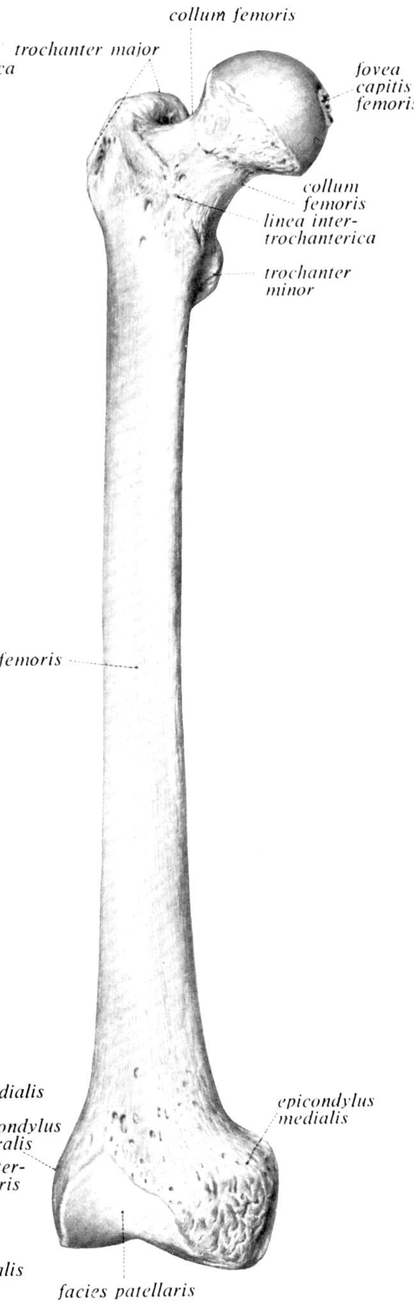

Fig. 156

Figs. 154–156. Right *femur*. Fig. 154. Dorsal; Fig. 155. medial; and Fig. 156. ventral views.

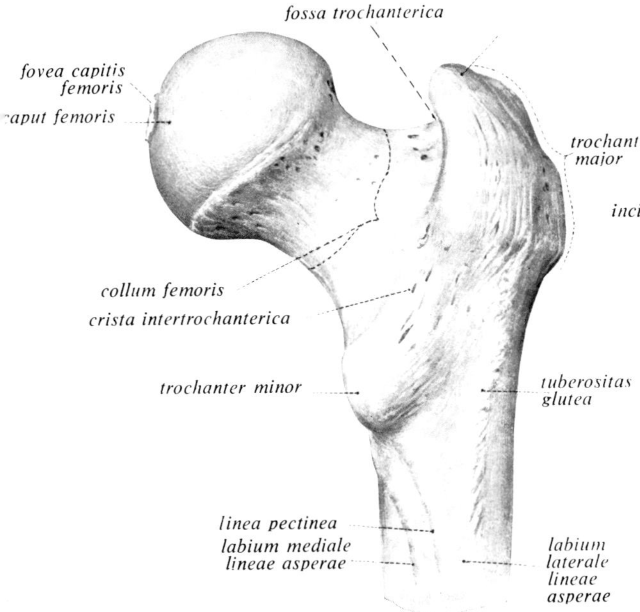

Fig. 157. Proximal end of right *femur*. Dorsal view.

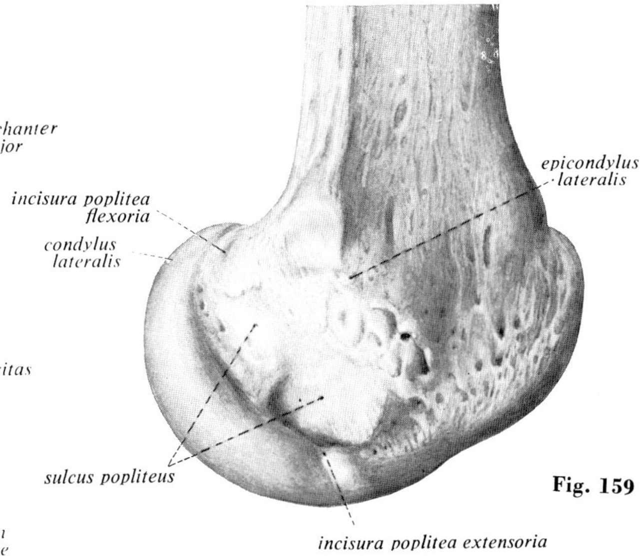

Fig. 159

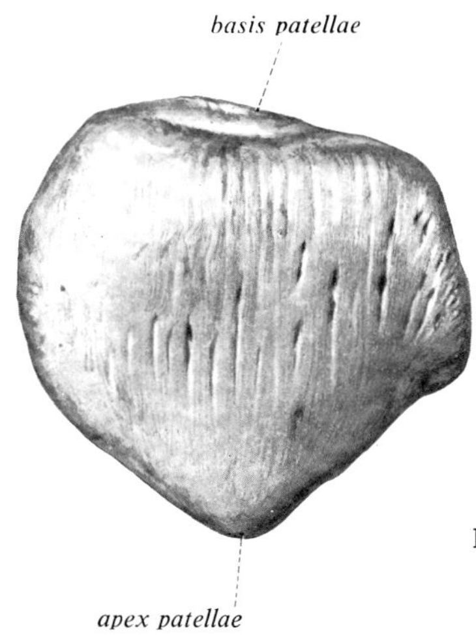

Fig. 160

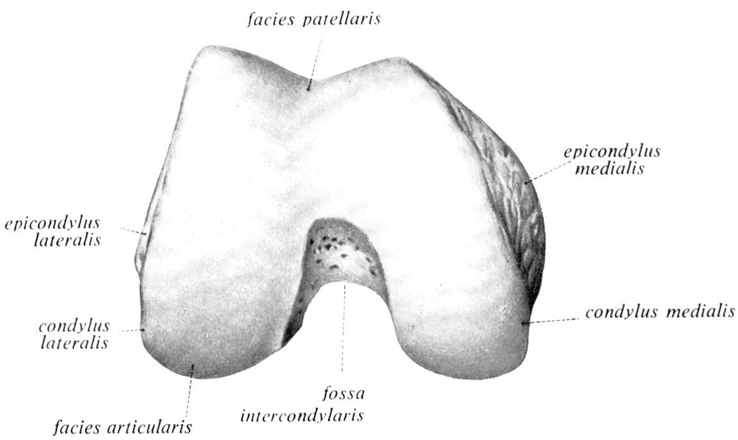

Fig. 158. Distal end of right *femur*. Seen from below.

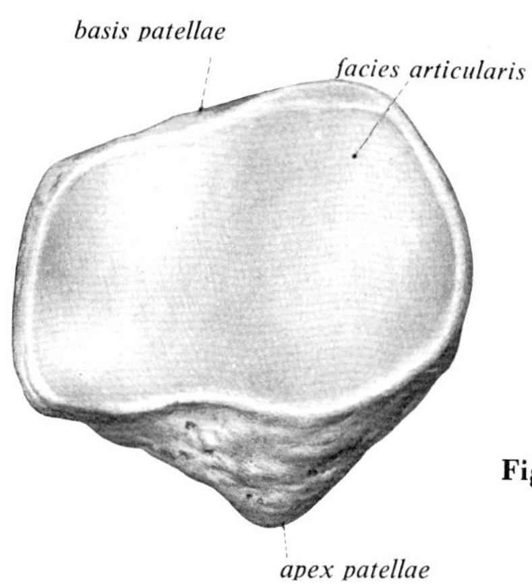

Fig. 161

Fig. 159. Distal end of right *femur*. Lateral view.
Fig. 160. *Patella*. Ventral view.
Fig. 161. *Patella*. Dorsal view.

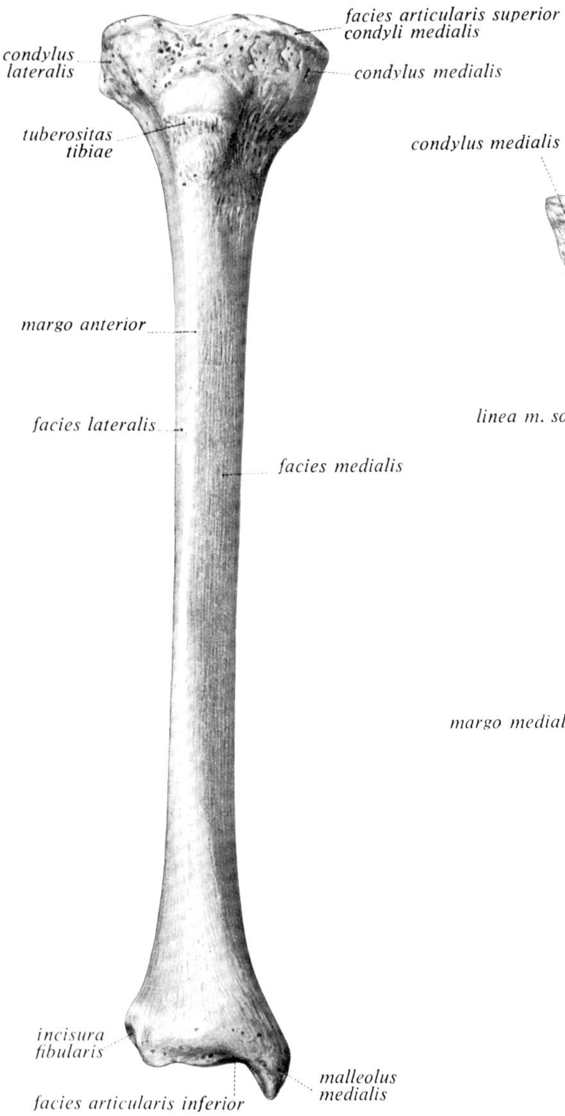

Fig. 162

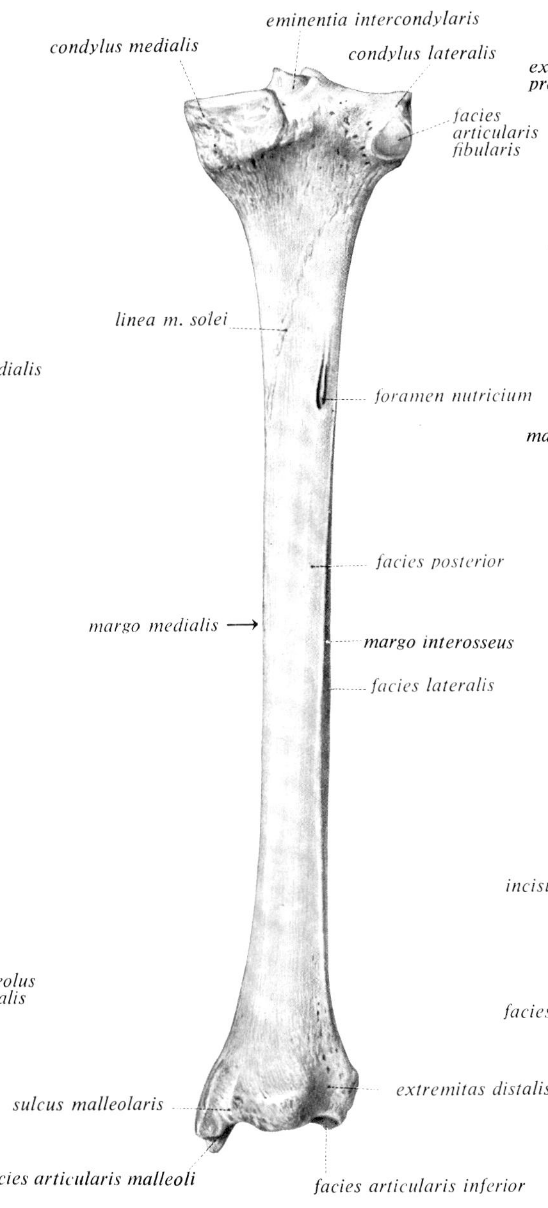

Fig. 163

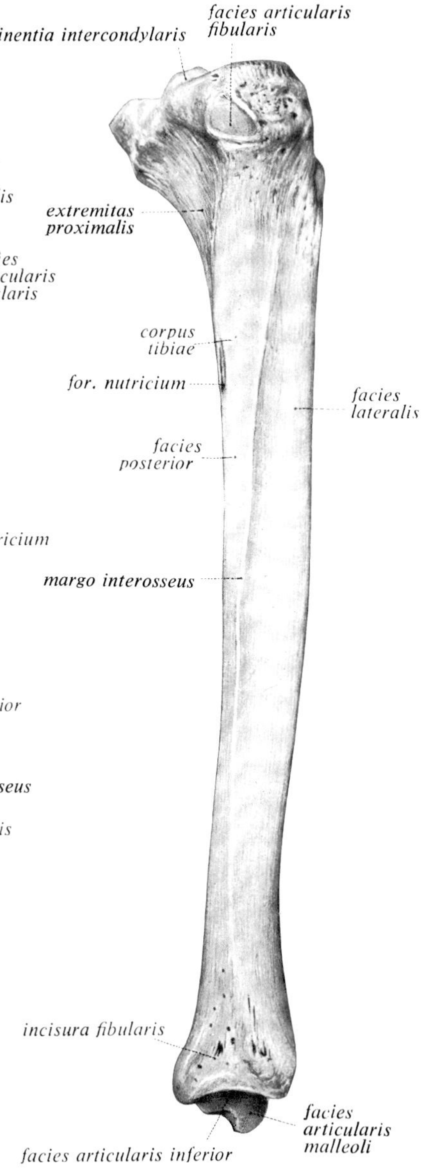

Fig. 164

Figs. 162–164. Right *tibia*. Fig. 162. Ventral; Fig. 163. Dorsal; Fig. 164. Lateral views.

Figs. 165 and 166. Right *fibula*. Fig. 165. Medial; Fig. 166. Lateral views.
Fig. 167. Right *tibia* and *fibula*. Dorsal view.
Fig. 168. Proximal ends of the right *tibia* and *fibula*. Proximal view.
Fig. 169. Distal ends of right *tibia* and *fibula*. Distal view.

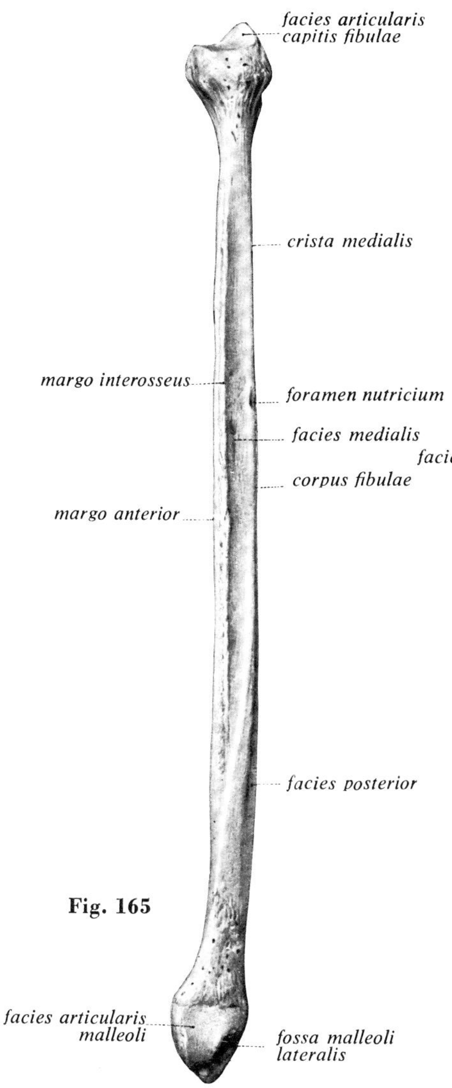
facies articularis capitis fibulae
crista medialis
margo interosseus
foramen nutricium
facies medialis
corpus fibulae
margo anterior
facies posterior
facies articularis malleoli
fossa malleoli lateralis

Fig. 165

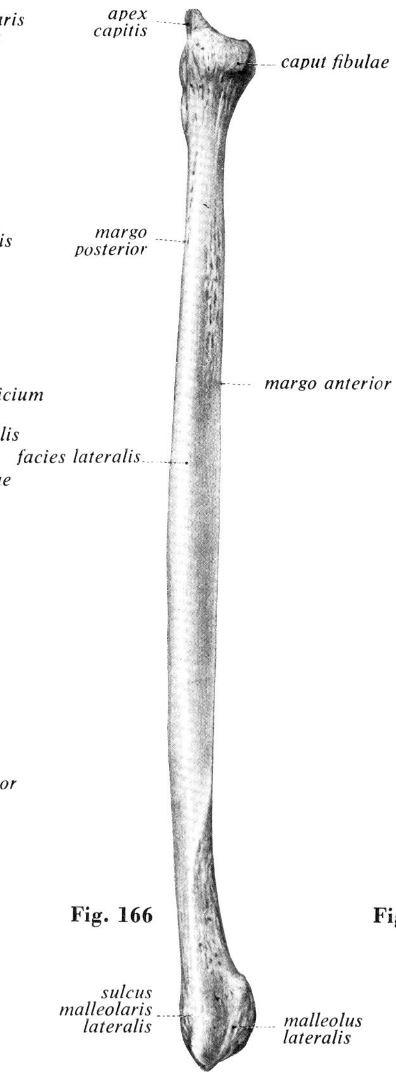
apex capitis
caput fibulae
margo posterior
margo anterior
facies lateralis
sulcus malleolaris lateralis
malleolus lateralis

Fig. 166

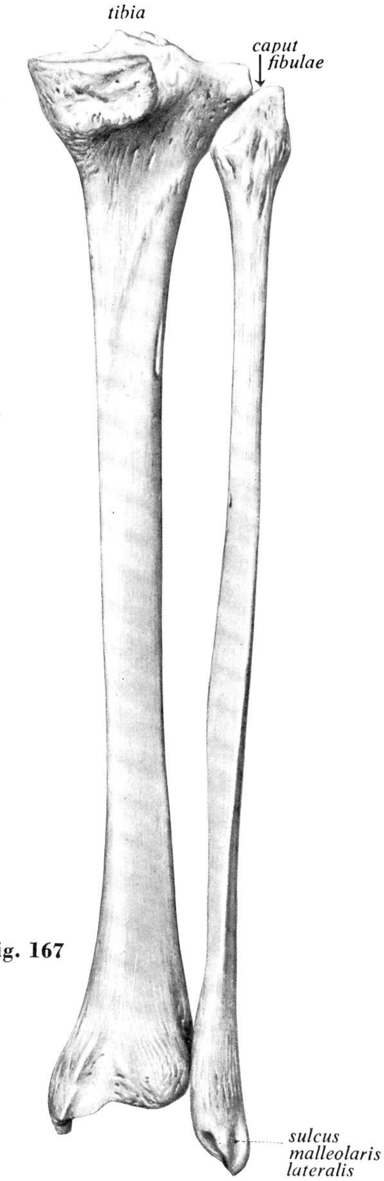
tibia
caput fibulae
sulcus malleolaris lateralis

Fig. 167

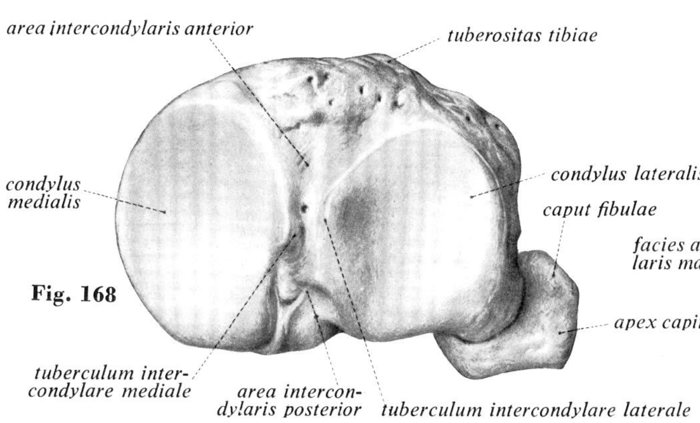
area intercondylaris anterior
tuberositas tibiae
condylus medialis
condylus lateralis
caput fibulae
apex capitis fibulae
tuberculum intercondylare mediale
area intercondylaris posterior
tuberculum intercondylare laterale

Fig. 168

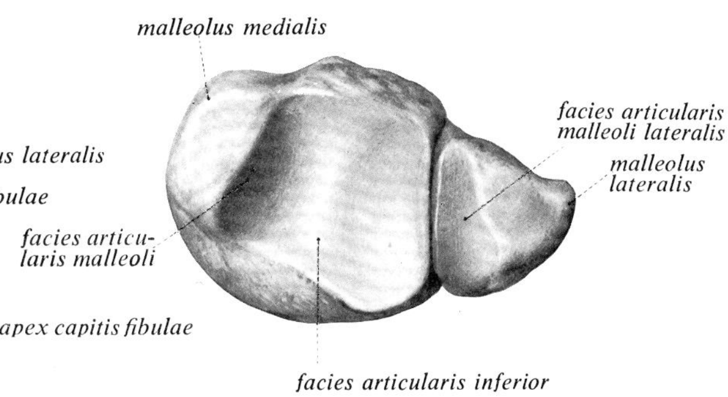
malleolus medialis
facies articularis malleoli lateralis
malleolus lateralis
facies articularis malleoli
facies articularis inferior

Fig. 169

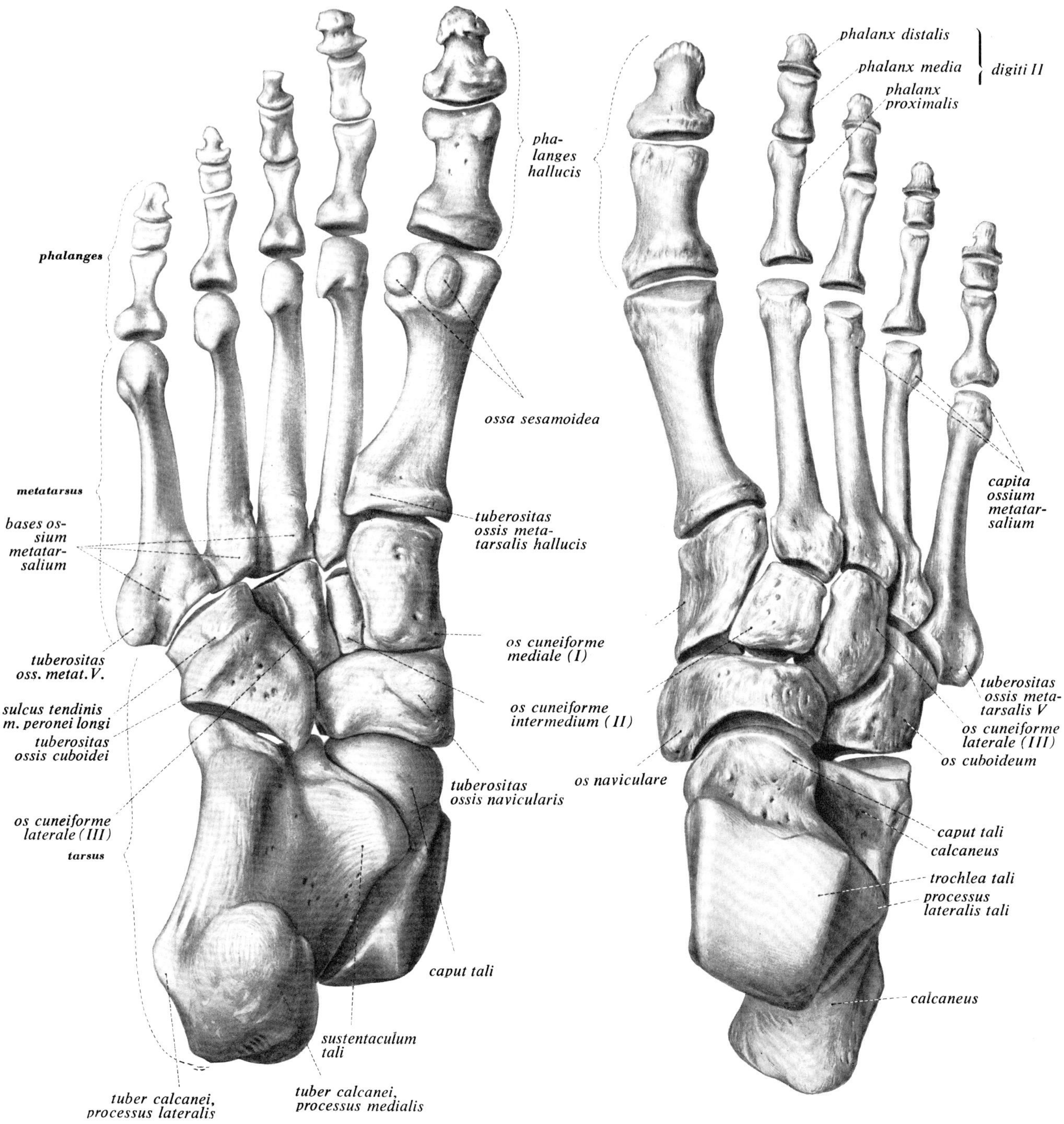

Figs. 170 and 171. The foot and ankle bones *(ossa pedis)* in their natural position. Fig. 170. Plantar view. Fig. 171. Dorsal view.

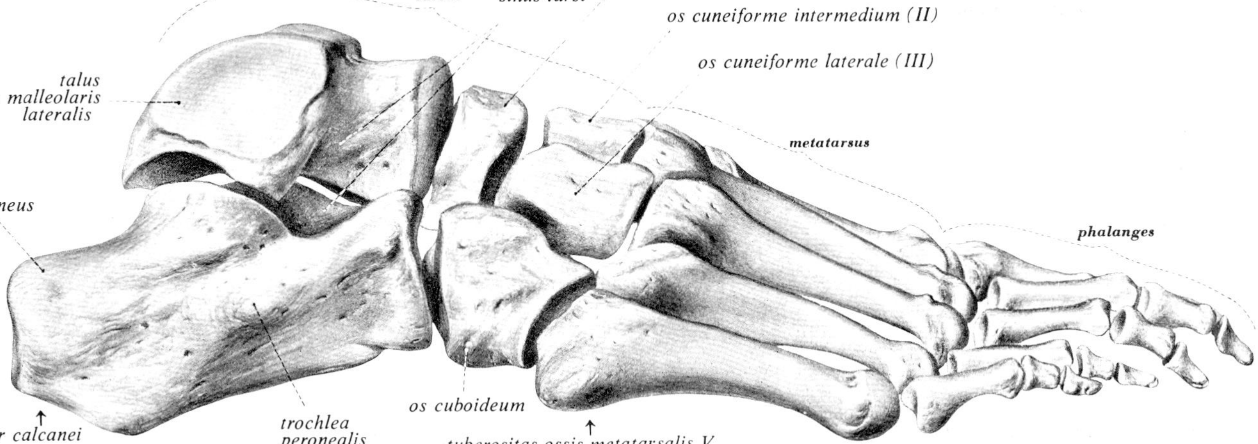

Fig. 172. Skeleton of the right foot. Lateral view.

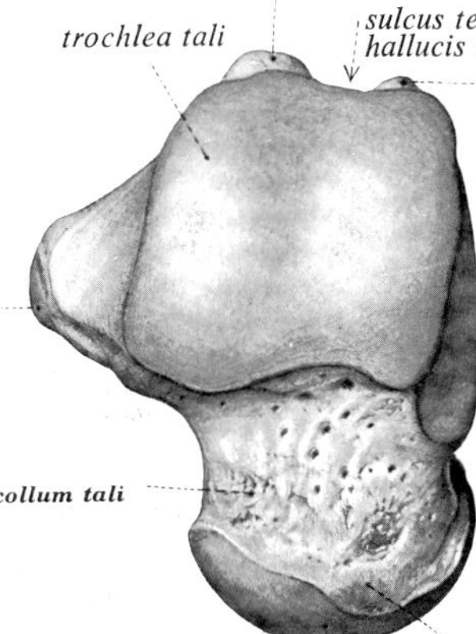

Fig. 173. The right *talus*. Proximal or dorsal view.

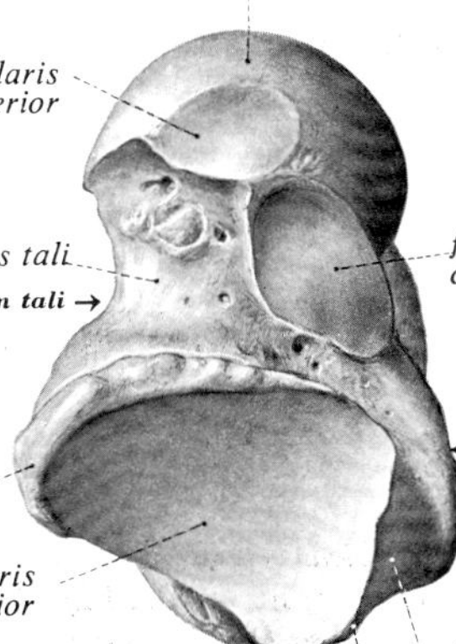

Fig. 174. The right *talus*. Plantar view.

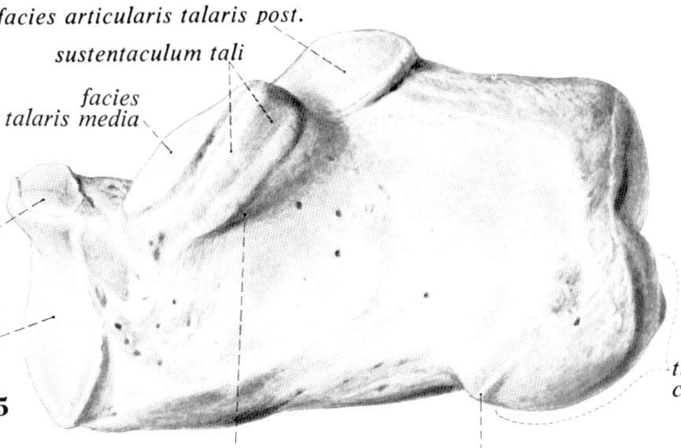

Fig. 175

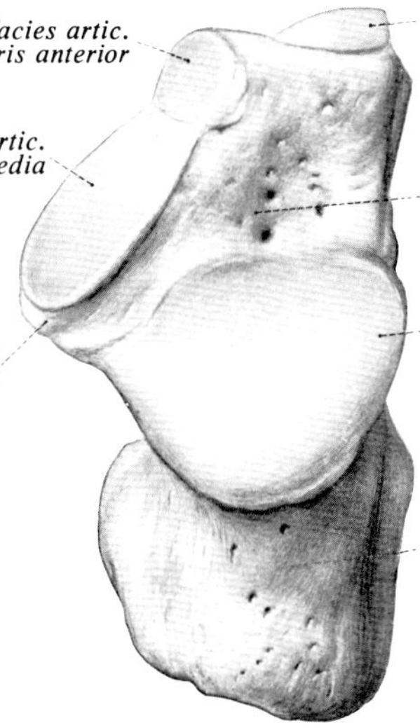

Fig. 177

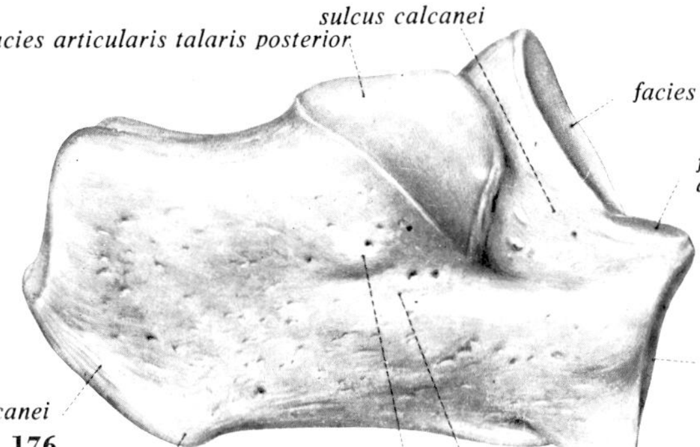

Fig. 176

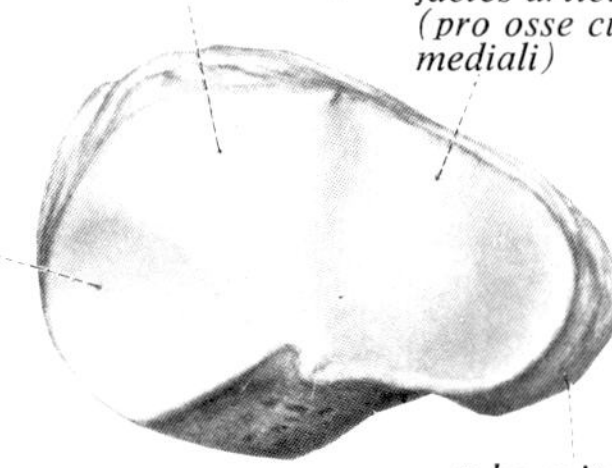

Fig. 178

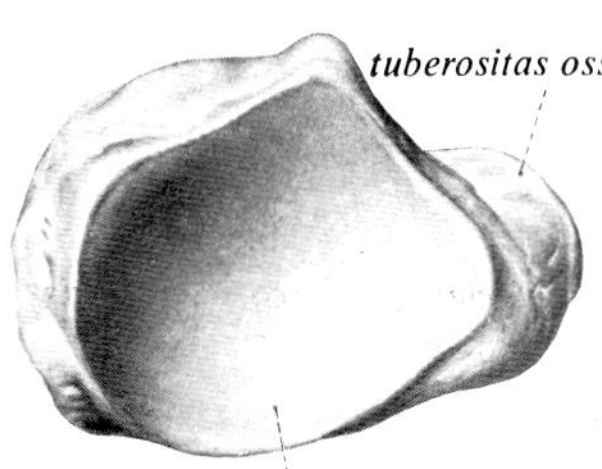

Fig. 179

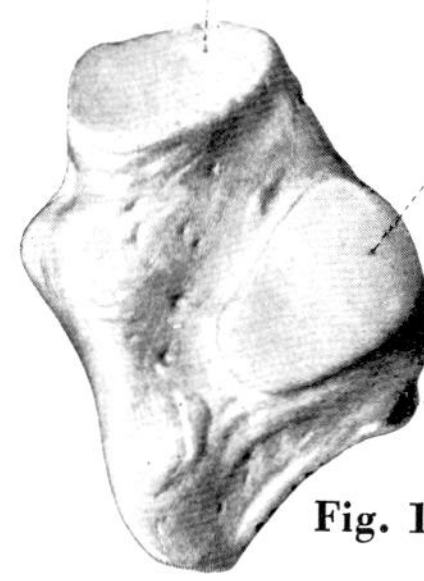

Fig. 180

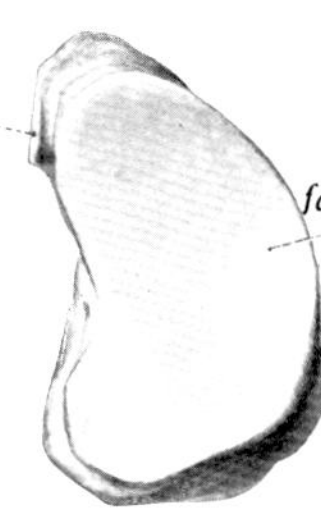

Fig. 181

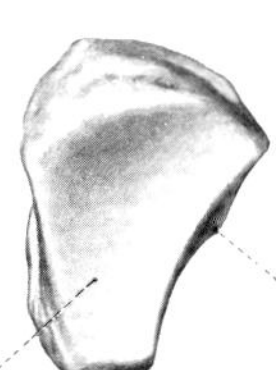

Fig. 182

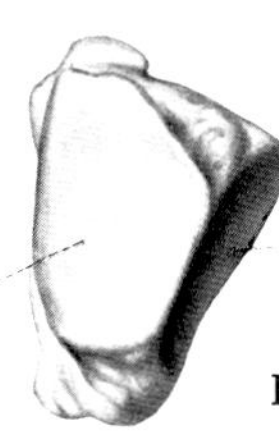

Fig. 183

Figs. 175–177. Right *calcaneus*. Fig. 175. Medial view. Fig. 176. Lateral view. Fig. 177. Proximal or dorsal view.
Figs. 178 and 179. Right *os naviculare*. Fig. 178. Distal view. Fig. 179. Proximal view.
Fig. 180. Right *os cuboideum*. Medial view. (See also Fig. 172.)
Figs. 181–183. Right *ossa cuneiformia*. Fig. 181. *Os cuneiforme mediale*, distal aspect. Fig. 182 *Os cuneiforme intermedium*, proximal aspect. Fig. 183. *Os cuneiforme laterale*, proximal aspect.

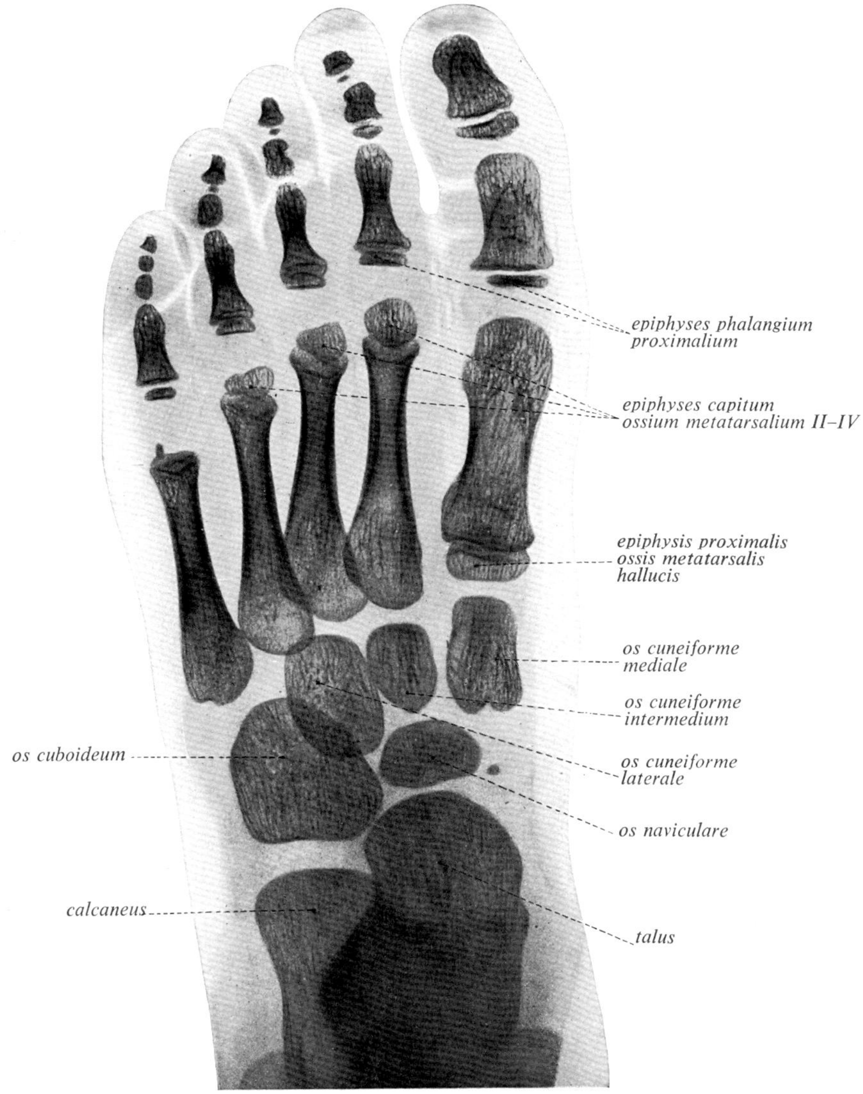

Fig. 184. X-ray of the left foot of a 5½ year old boy.

Note: The development of the distal-formed epiphyses, the *ossa metatarsalia* II–IV, as well as the proximal epiphyses of the phalanges and that of *os metatarsale* I (compare with Fig. 146). The x-ray picture distinctly shows the epiphyseal "gaps" which make up the cartilaginous epiphyseal juncture, the zone for growth and length.

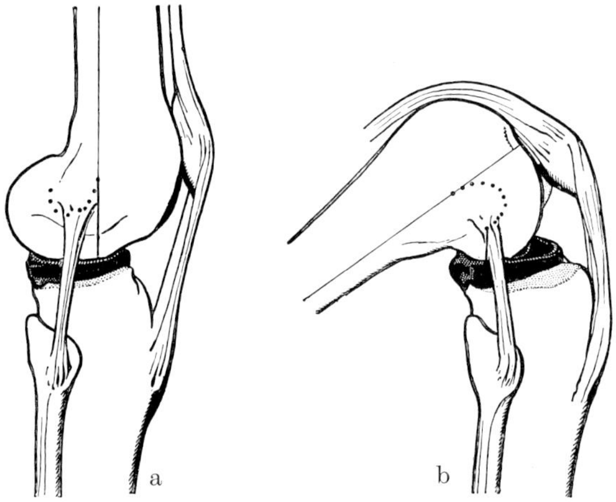

Fig. 185. Right knee joint *(articulatio genus)*, lateral view. a Extended. b Flexed. With stronger flexion, the *meniscus*, especially the lateral on the cartilaginous plate of the *tibia* (stippling) will be pushed backward.

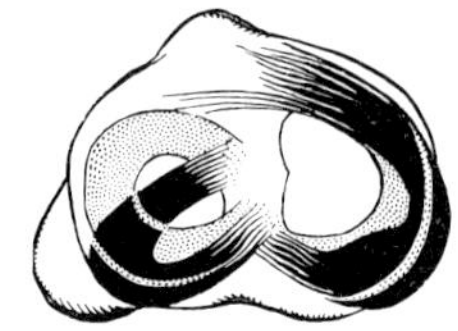

Fig. 186. View of the head of the left *tibia, (facies articularis superior tibiae)*. Position of *meniscus* in extension of knee joint, stippled; in flexion, black. Note the greater movement of the lateral meniscus. (Figs. 185 and 186 after H. Virchow from Benninghoff-Goerttler: Lehrbuch der Anatomie des Menschen Vol. I: 10, Urban & Schwarzenberg, Munich–Berlin–Vienna 1968.)

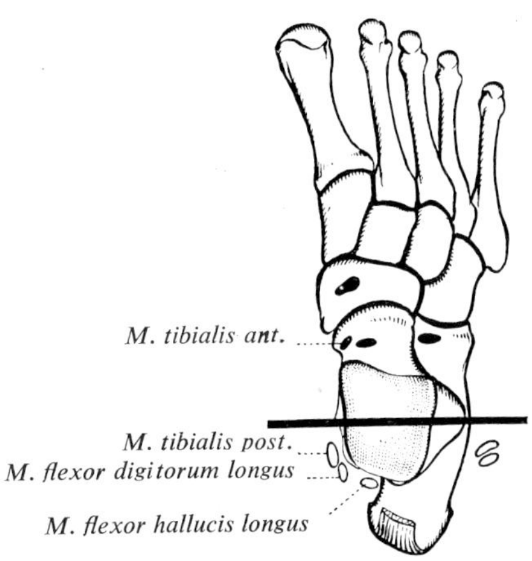

Fig. 187. Axis of the upper ankle joint, *(articulatio talocruralis)*, with the tendons of the muscles for this joint. Tendons of the extensors, black; tendons of the flexors, white. Compare with Fig. 188.

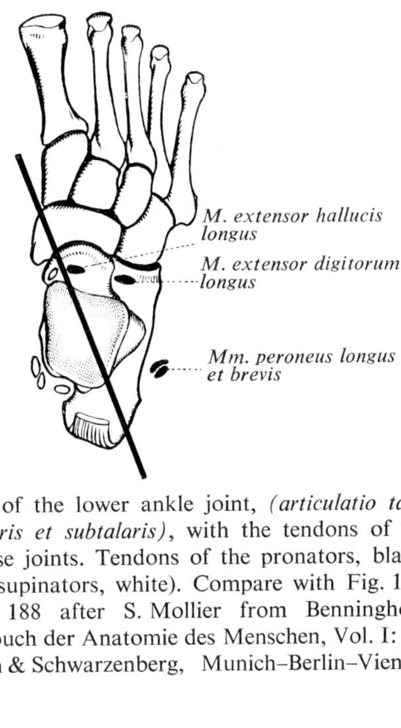

Fig. 188. Axis of the lower ankle joint, *(articulatio talocalcaneonavicularis et subtalaris)*, with the tendons of the muscles for these joints. Tendons of the pronators, black; tendons of the supinators, white). Compare with Fig. 187. (Figs. 187 and 188 after S. Mollier from Benninghoff-Goerttler: Lehrbuch der Anatomie des Menschen, Vol. I: 10, pub. by Urban & Schwarzenberg, Munich–Berlin–Vienna, 1968.)

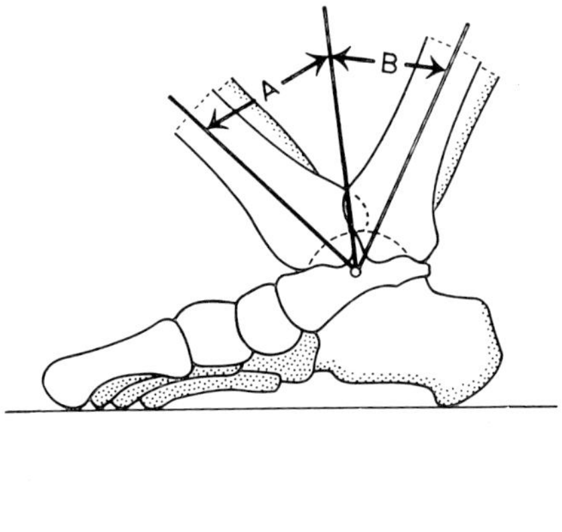

Fig. 189. Flexion and extension in the upper ankle joint, *(articulatio talocruralis)*, when the foot is solidly planted and the leg below the knee is moved back and forth. (From S. Mollier: Plastische Anatomie, 2. pub. by Bergmann, Munich, 1938.)

Joints and Ligaments

Vertebral Column, Thorax, Skull

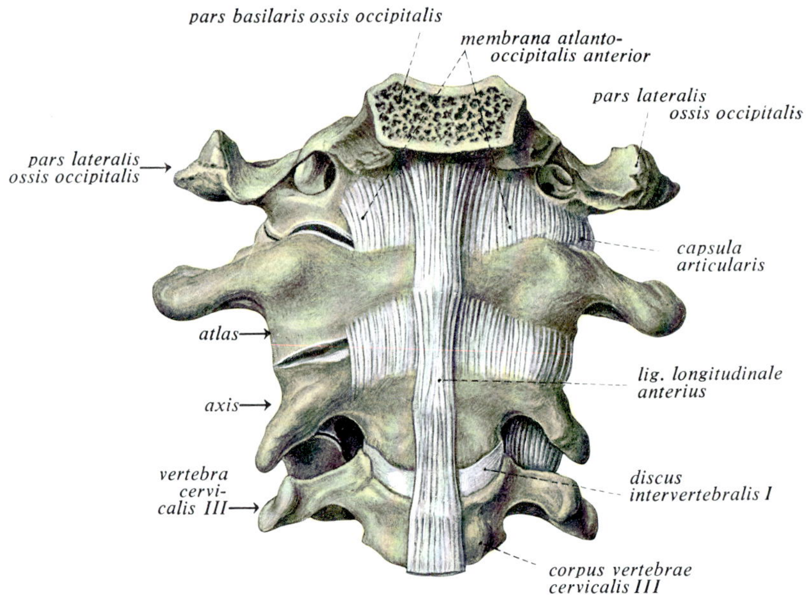

Fig. 190. Part of the *os occipitale*, the first three vertebrae, *membrana atlantooccipitalis anterior*, and the cranial end of the *ligamentum longitudinale anterius*. Articular capsules are removed on the right. Ventral view.

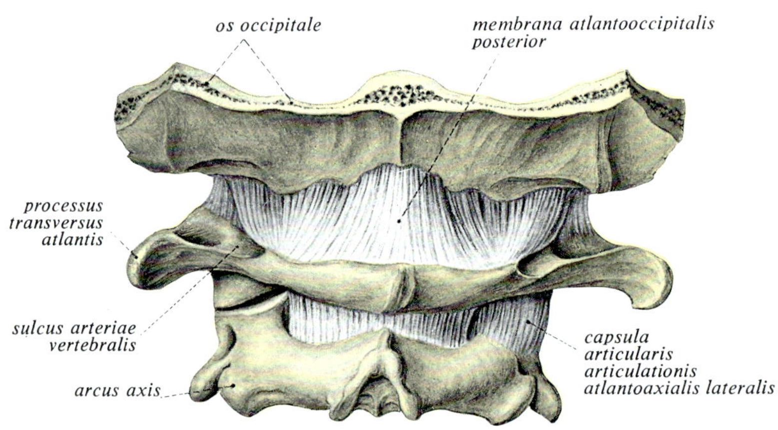

Fig. 191. Part of the *os occipitale*, *atlas*, and *axis* with their ligaments, and *membrana atlantooccipitalis anterior*. The articular capsule of the *articulatio atlantoaxialis laterales* removed on left. Dorsal view.

Note: The *articulationes atlantooccipitales, atlantoaxiales laterales*, and the *articulatio atlantoaxialis mediana* form a functional unit with the effect of a ball and socket joint. Dissection of the articular portions demonstrates the safeguard against dislocation.

Fig. 192. *Membrana tectoria.* Dorsal view. The dorsal section of the occipital bone and the arches of the three cranial cervical vertebrae are sawed off. The articular capsules of the intervertebral joints are removed on the right.

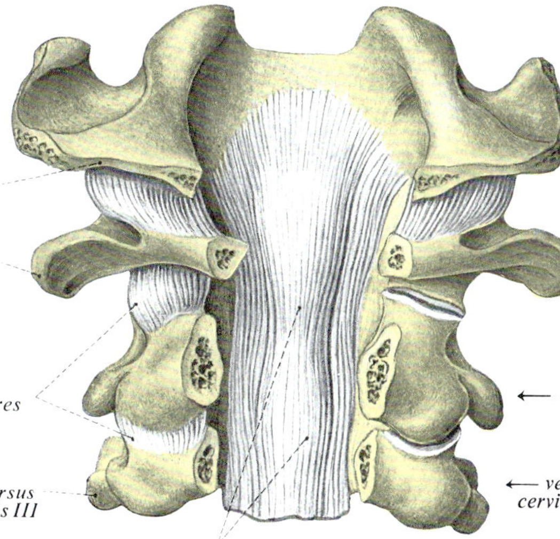

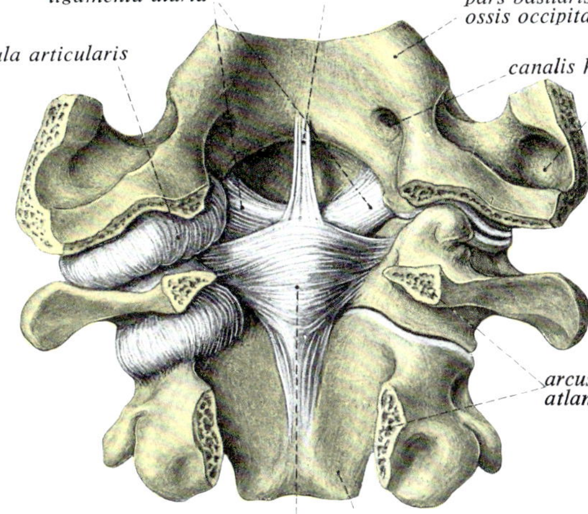

Fig. 193. *Ligamentum cruciforme atlantis* after removal of the *membrana tectoria.* Seen from dorsal. Prepared as in Fig. 192.

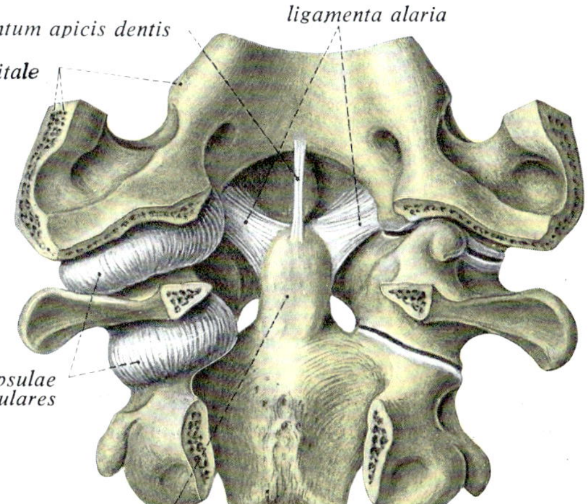

Fig. 194. *Ligamenta alaria* and *ligamentum apicis dentis* after removal of the *ligamentum cruciforme atlantis.* Seen from dorsal. Prepared as in Fig. 192.

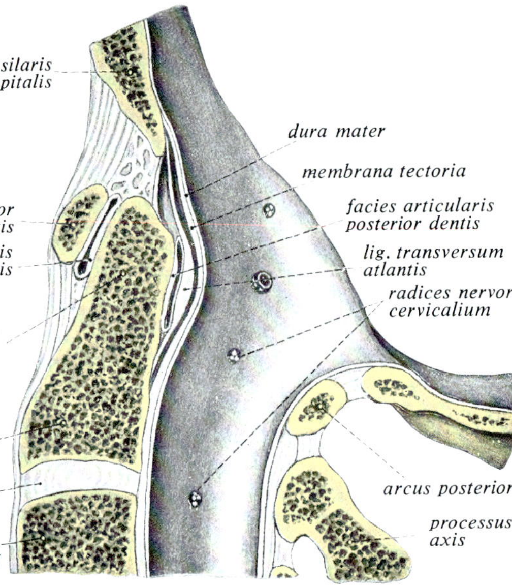

Fig. 195. *Articulationes atlantoaxiales*. Median longitudinal section.

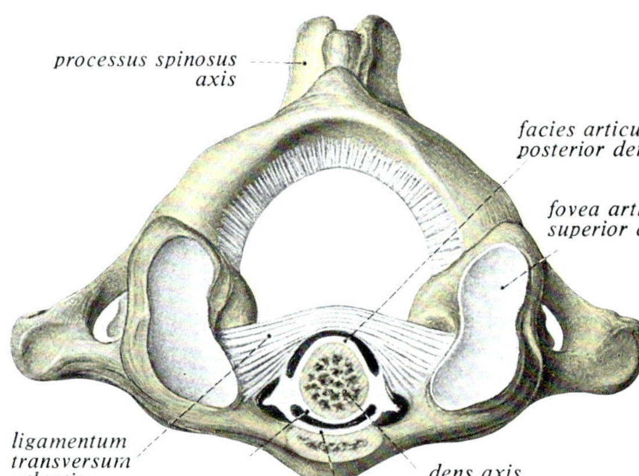

Fig. 196. *Articulatio atlantoaxialis mediana*. The atlas is removed from the atlantooccipital articulation. *Dens axis* and the ventral arch of the *atlas* are sawed through horizontally. Cranial view.

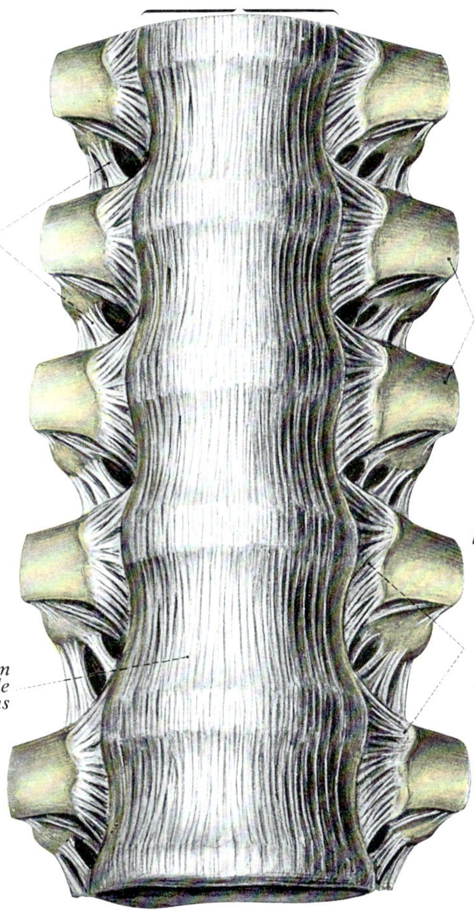

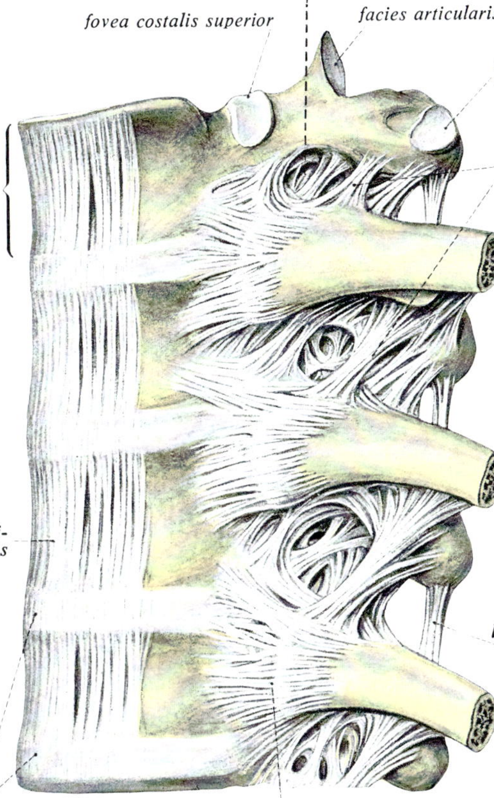

Fig. 197. Preparation of the *ligamentum longitudinale anterius* of the caudal section of the thoracic vertebral column with the costovertebral articulations. Ventral view.

Fig. 198. Preparation of the middle and caudal thoracic vertebrae and ribs. The most cranial rib was disarticulated and removed. Left lateral view.

Note: The heads of the ribs articulate with the (12) vertebrae and the (10) *discus intervertebrales* forming the *articulationes costovertebrales*. These are gliding joints between the heads of the ribs and the demifacet of two adjacent vertebrae. Only the 11th and 12th thoracic vertebrae have a whole *fovea costalis* on the upper lateral surface of the vertebrae.

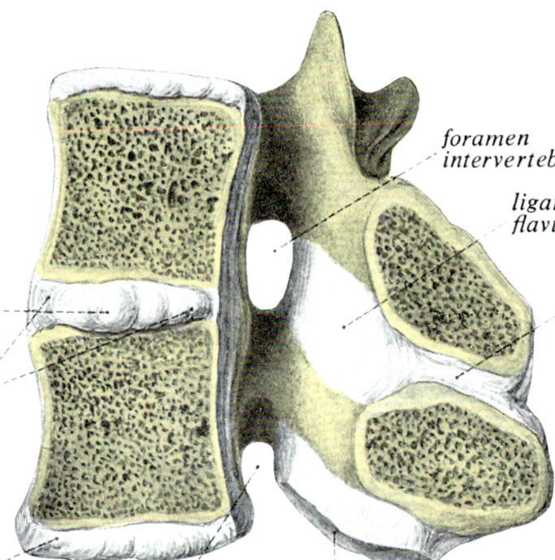

Fig. 199. Two thoracic vertebrae with their ligaments *(ligamenta flava)*. Cut through the median sagittal plane.

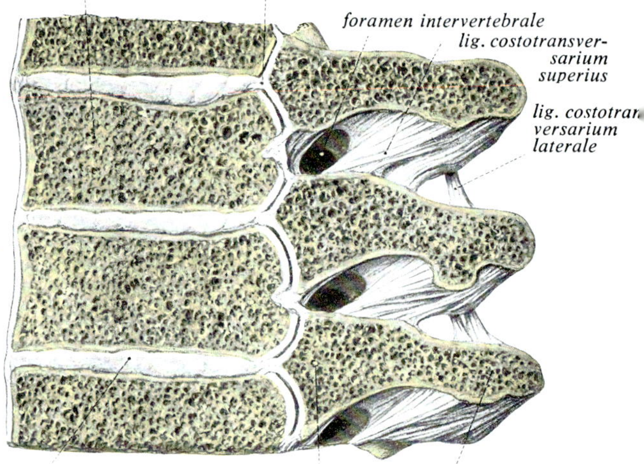

Fig. 200. Sawcut through the vertebral bodies, the *articulationes costovertebrales* and the vertebral ends of the ribs. The cut is at the 45° angle to the median plane. The *crista capitis costae* is closely bound up with the *discus intervertebralis* through the *ligamentum intraarticulare*. The rib belongs to the body of the vertebra below.

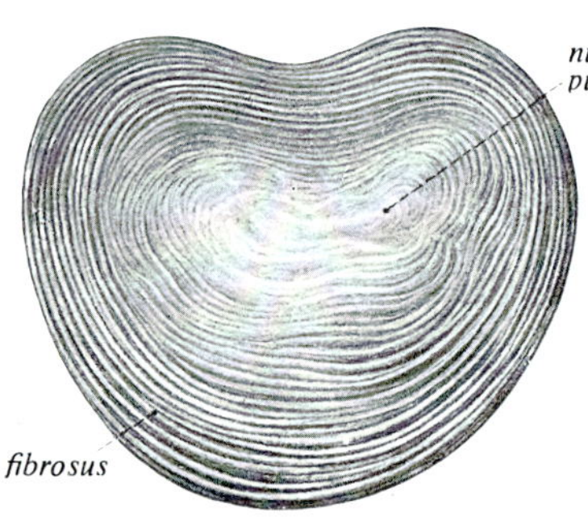

Fig. 201. Articulating surface view of an isolated *discus intervertebralis. (Lumbar vertebra.)*

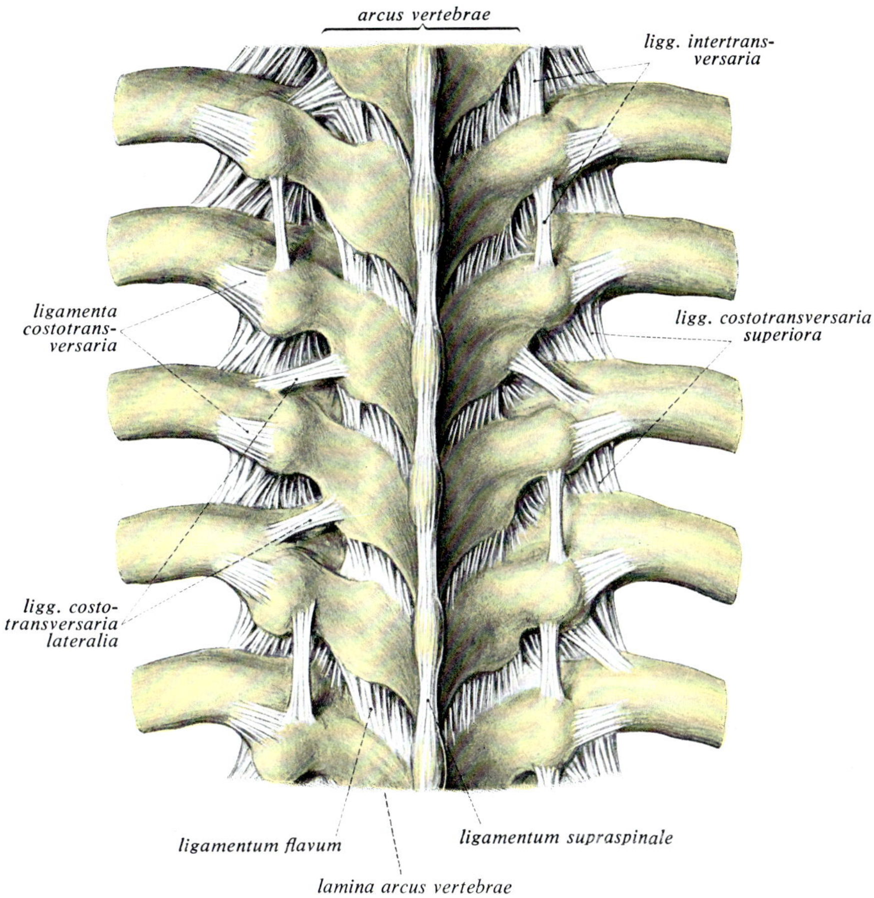

Fig. 202. Preparation of the ligaments of the middle and caudal thoracic vertebrae and ribs. *Articulationes vertebrarum.* Dorsal view.

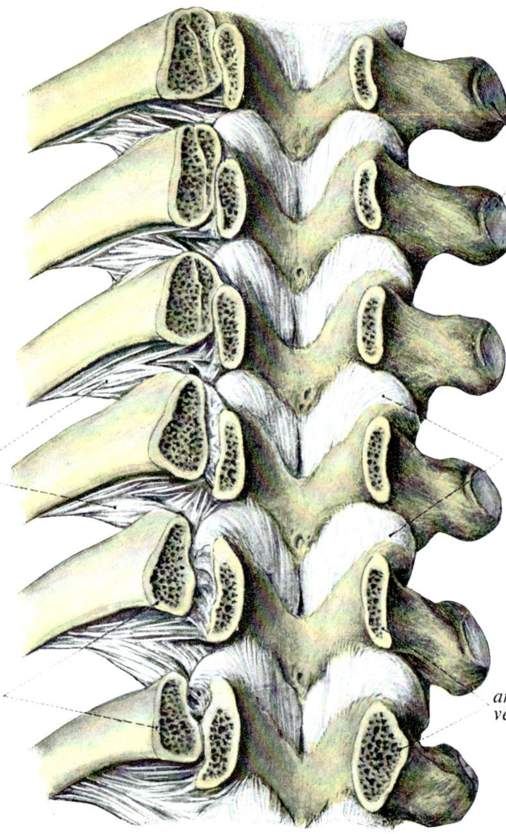

Fig. 203. *Ligamenta flava* of the thoracic vertebrae. (Seen from inside the *canalis vertebralis.*) The vertebral bodies are sawed off to display the lamina. The ribs on the left are disarticulate and removed; on the right, they are in their natural position.

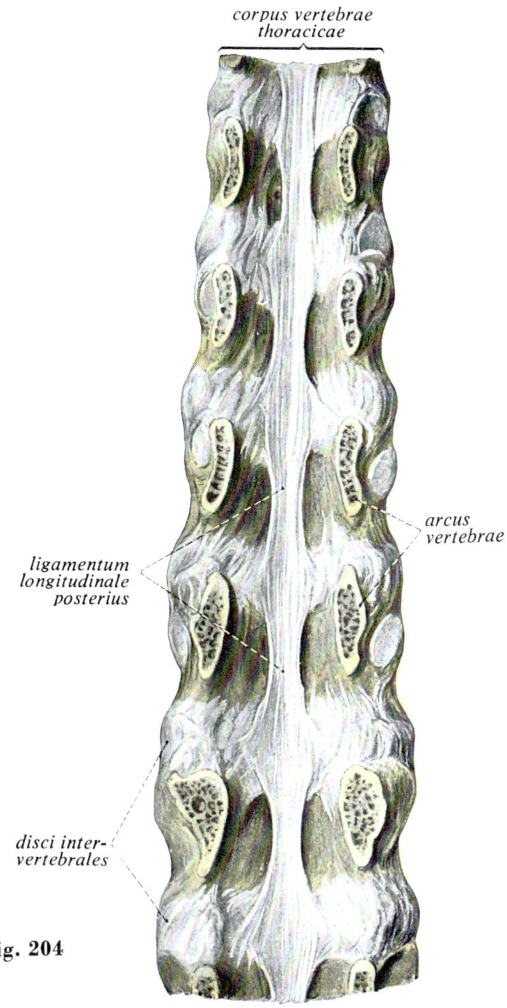

Fig. 204

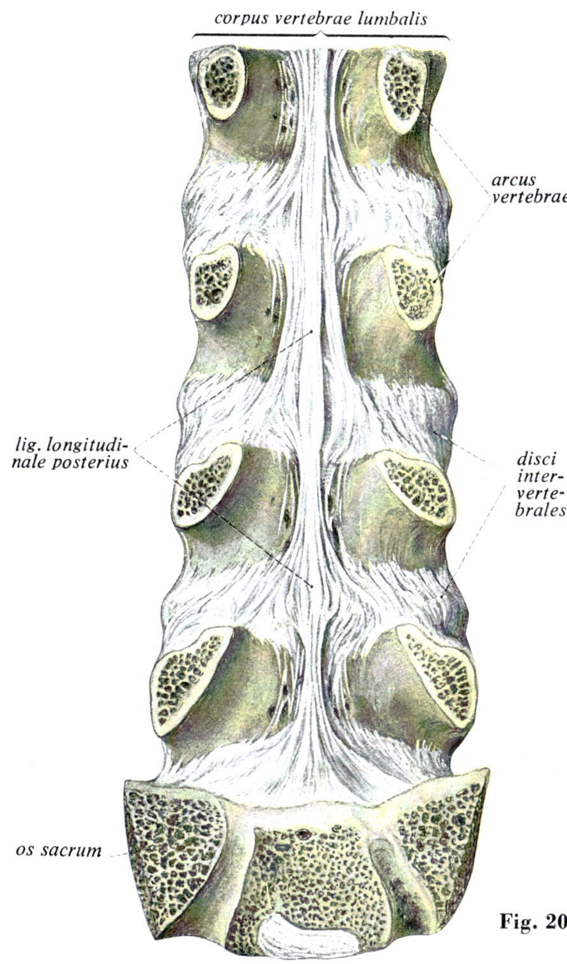

Fig. 205

Figs. 204 and 205. *Ligamentum longitudinale posterius* and *disci intervertebrales*. Vertebral canal opened by removing the vertebral arches from the dorsal side. Fig. 204. Caudal region of the thoracic vertebrae. Fig. 205. Region of the lumbar portion of the spine and the sacrum.

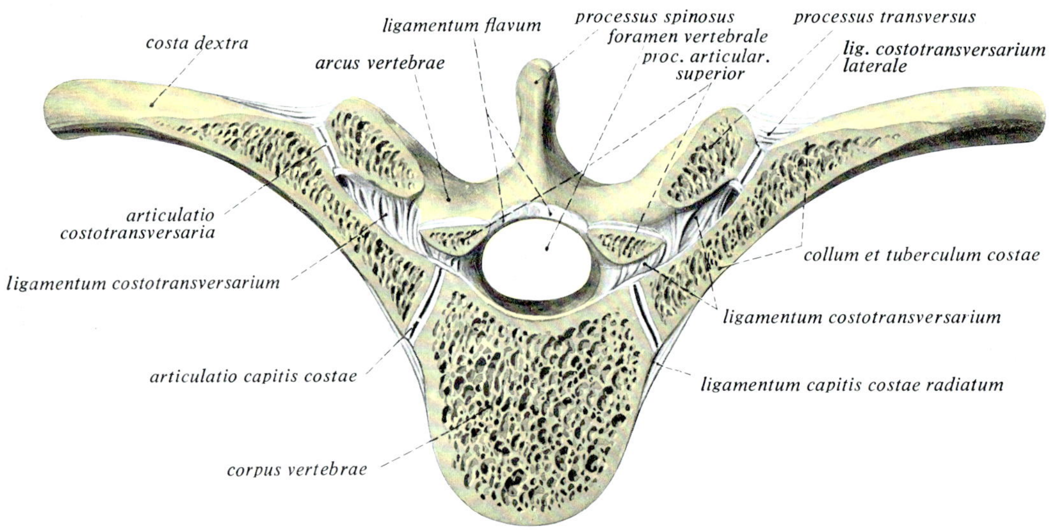

Fig. 206. Horizontal section through a thoracic vertebra, with the *articulationes costovertebrales*.

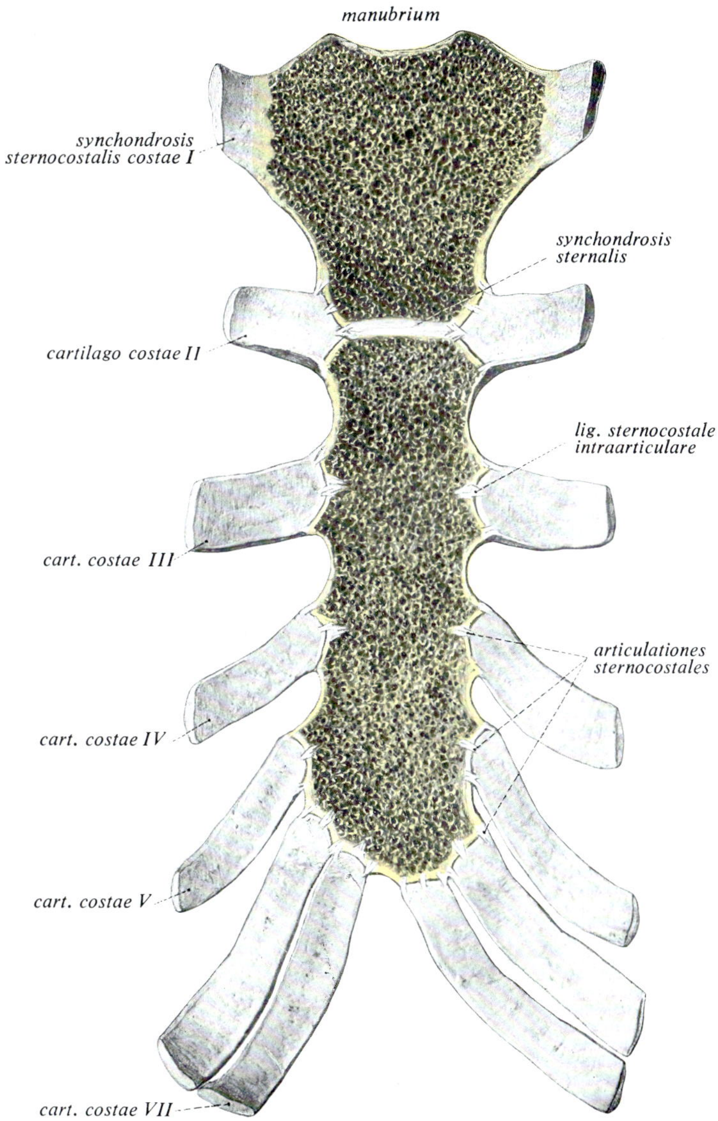

Fig. 207. The *sternum* with costal cartilages. *Articulationes sternocostales* sawed lengthwise in the frontal plane.

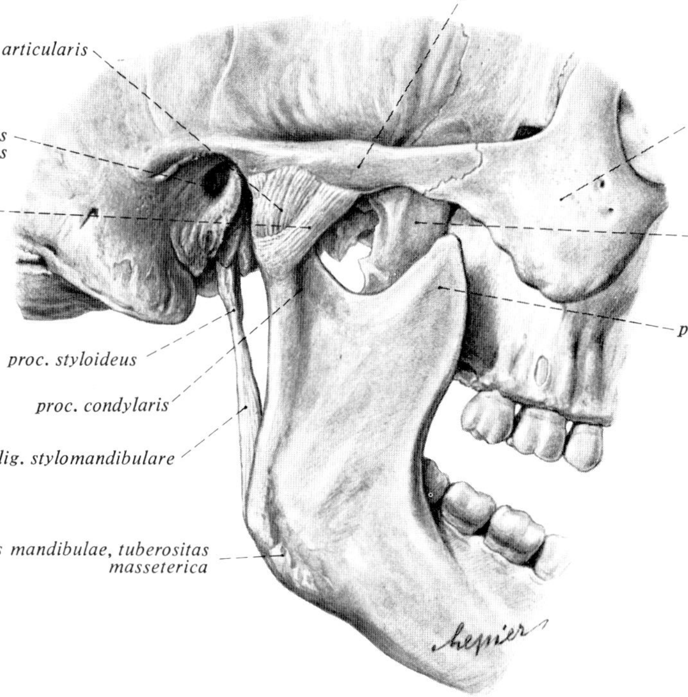

Fig. 208. The right *articulatio temporomandibularis* with ligaments. Lateral view.

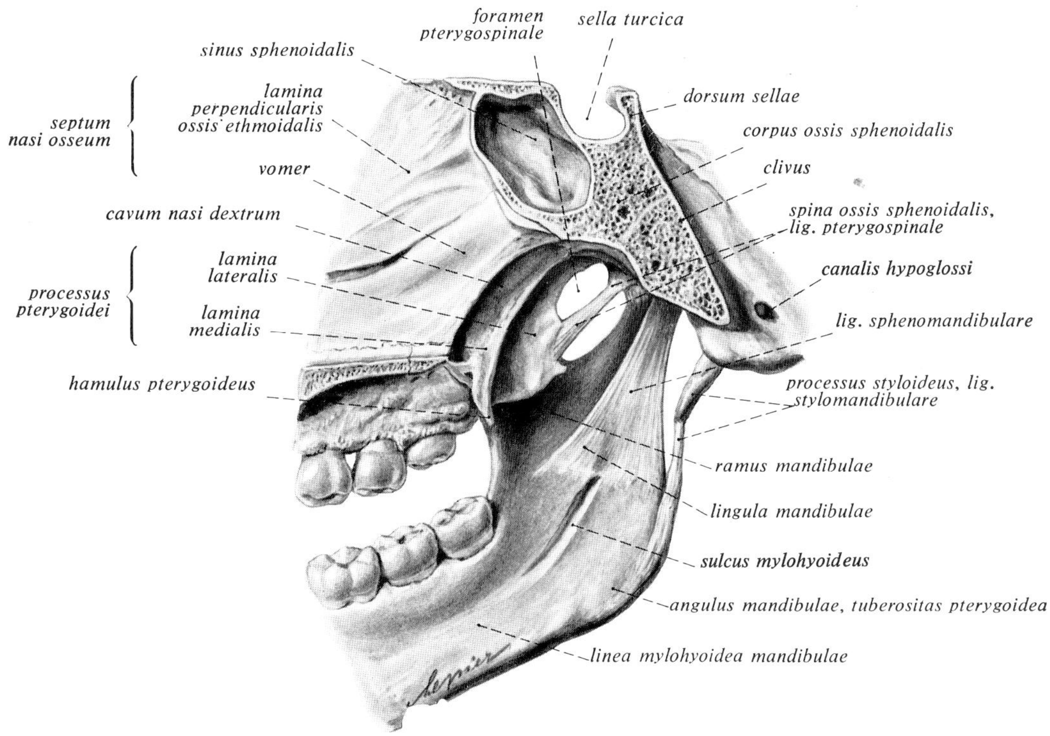

Fig. 209. The right *articulatio temporomandibularis* with ligaments. Medial view.

Joints and Ligaments

Shoulder Girdle and Upper Limb

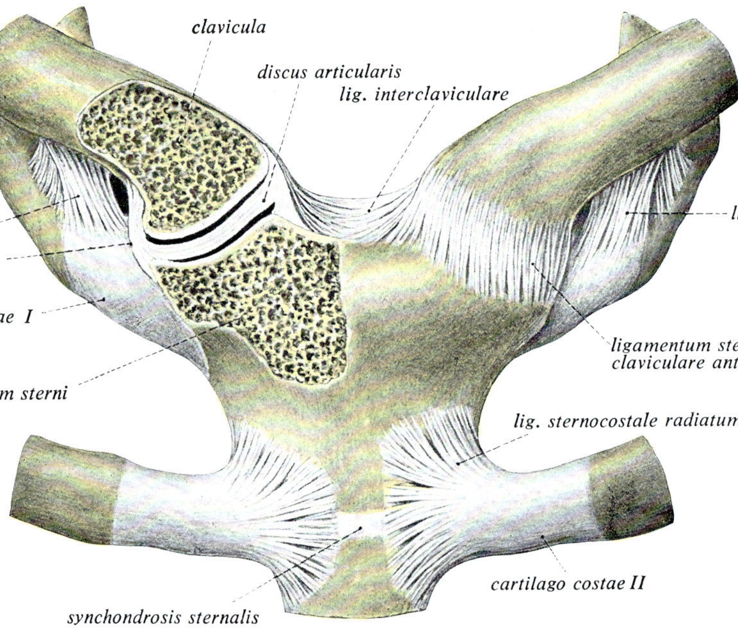

Fig. 210. Both sternoclavicular joints *(articulationes sternoclaviculares)* and the articulations of the cranial ribs with the sternum. Ventral view. The right sternoclavicular joint was opened by a frontal sawcut.

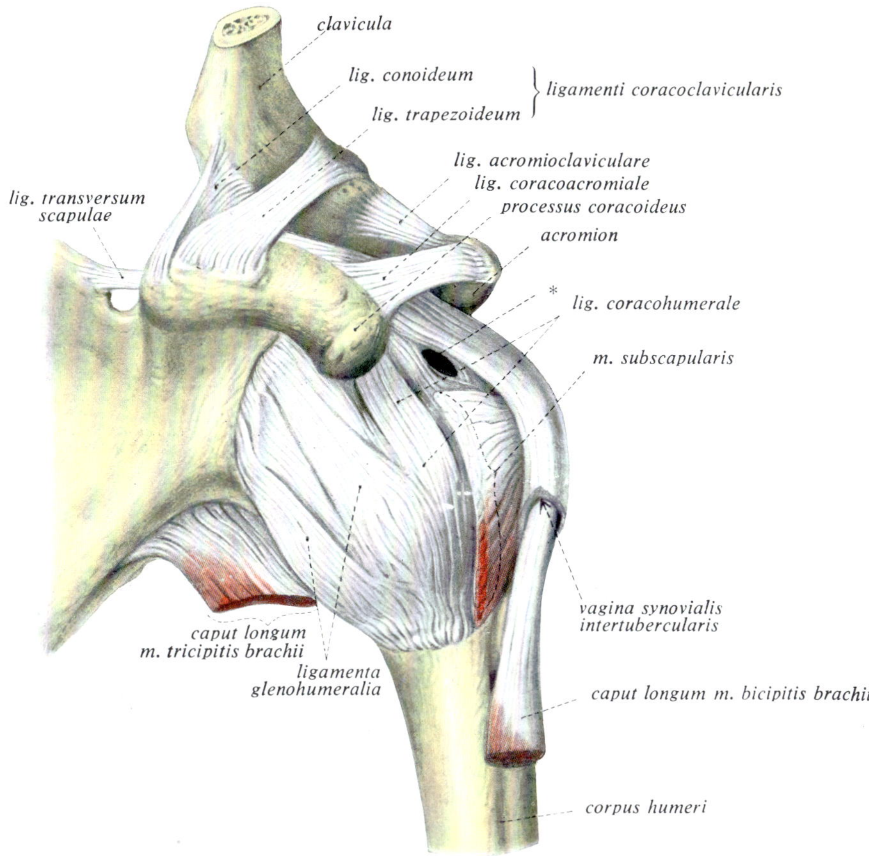

Fig. 211. Left shoulder joint *(articulatio humeri)* and acromioclavicular joint *(articulatio acromioclavicularis)*. Ventral view. * Communication point with the subacromial bursa *(bursa subacromialis)*.

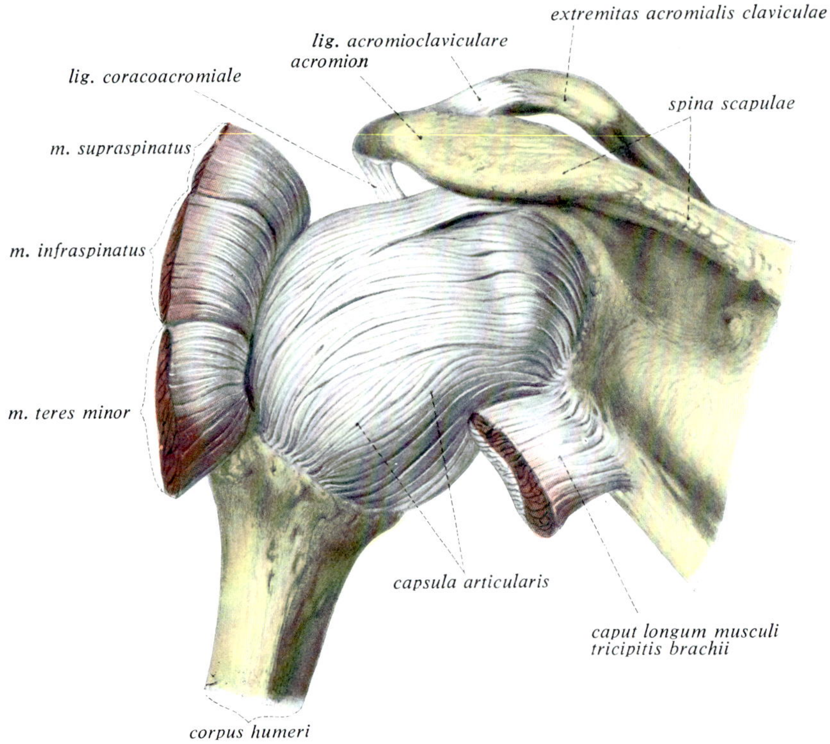

Fig. 212. Left shoulder joint *(articulatio humeri)*. Dorsal view. The muscle attachments of the *mm. supraspinatus, infraspinatus, teres minor* and *caput longum musculi tricipitis* show the relationship to the joint capsule.

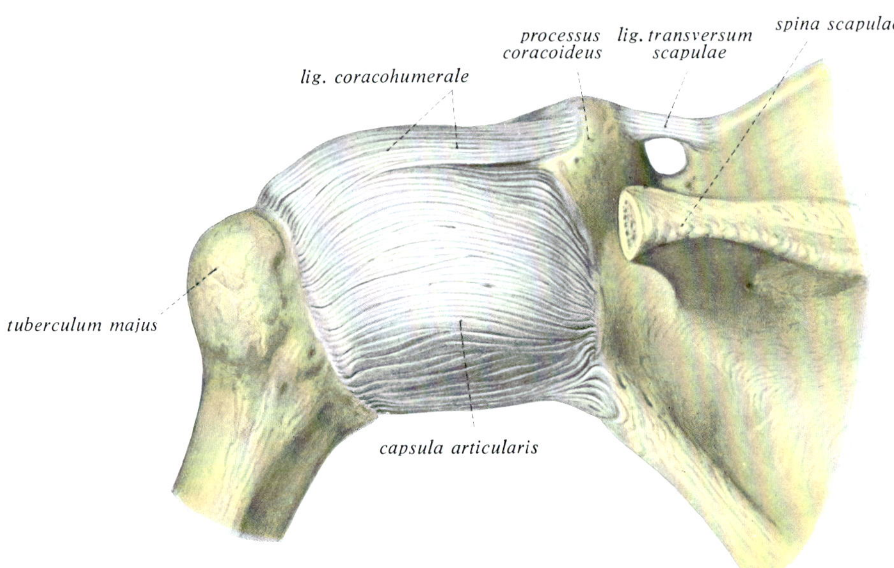

Fig. 213. Left shoulder joint *(articulatio humeri)* without muscle attachments. Dorsocranial view. The *acromiom scapulae* is cut off with a saw.

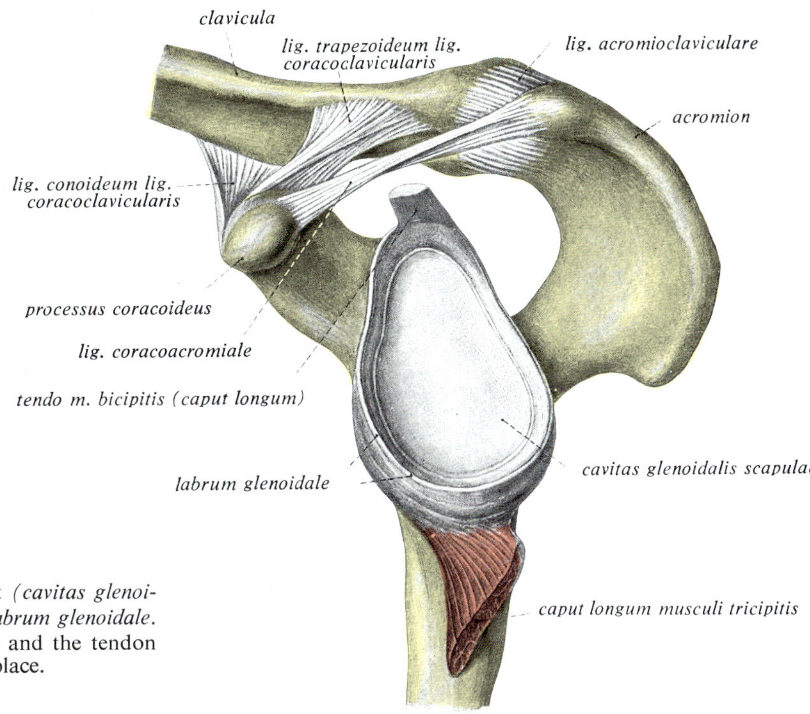

Fig. 214. Socket of the left shoulder joint *(cavitas glenoidalis)*. The joint capsule is cut off at the *labrum glenoidale*. The origin of the *caput longum m. tricipitis* and the tendon of the ***caput longum m. bicipitis*** is kept in place.

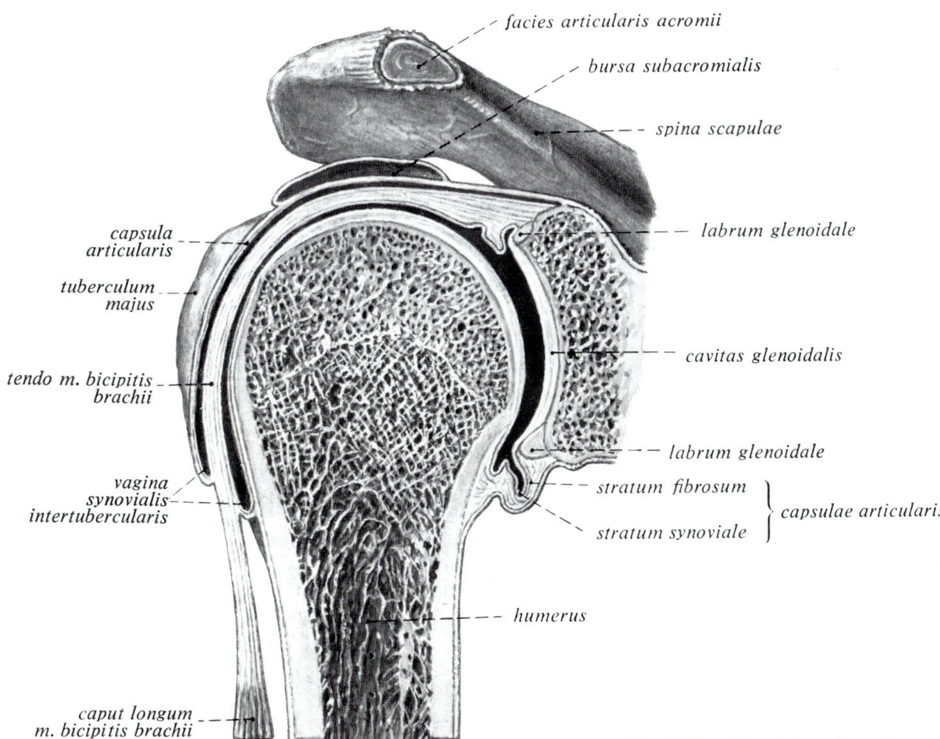

Fig. 215. Frontal section through the right shoulder joint *(articulatio humeri)*. Dorsal half.

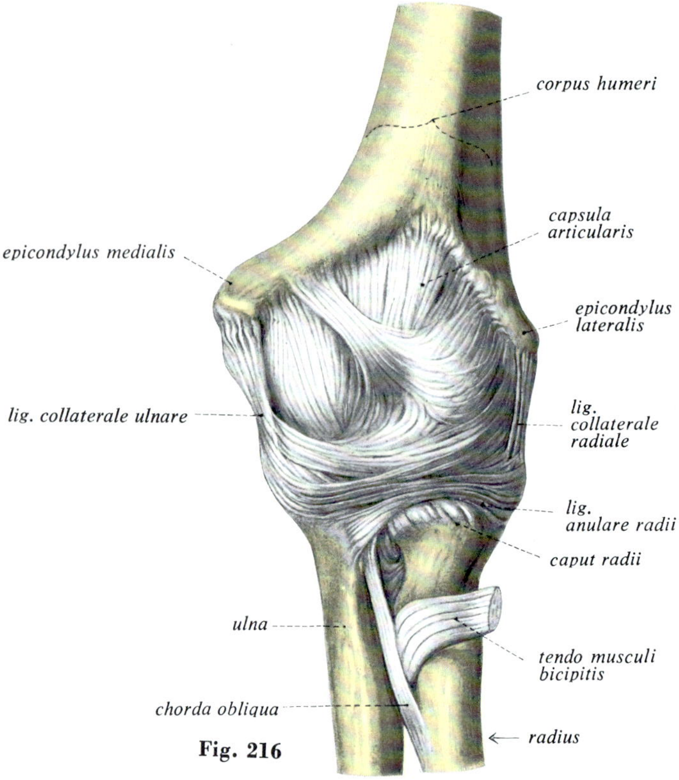

Fig. 216

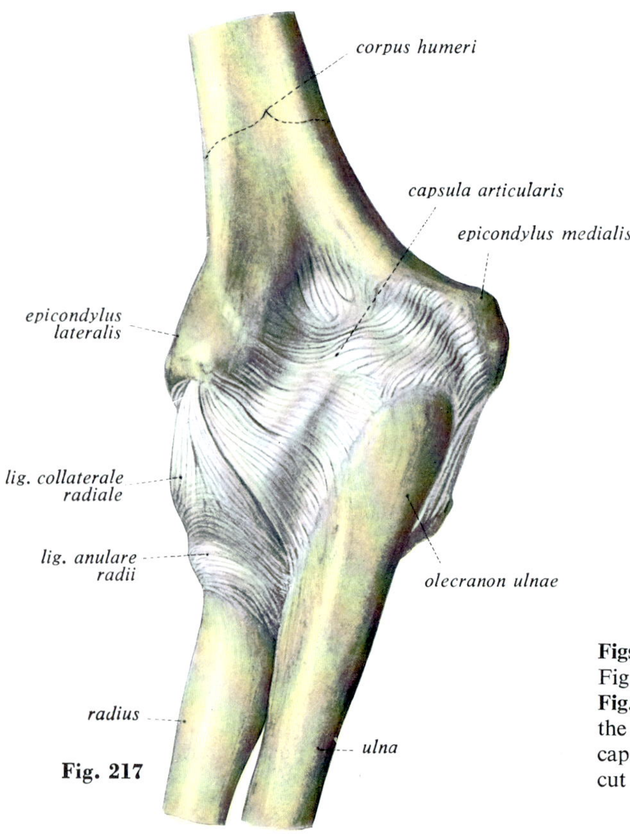

Fig. 217

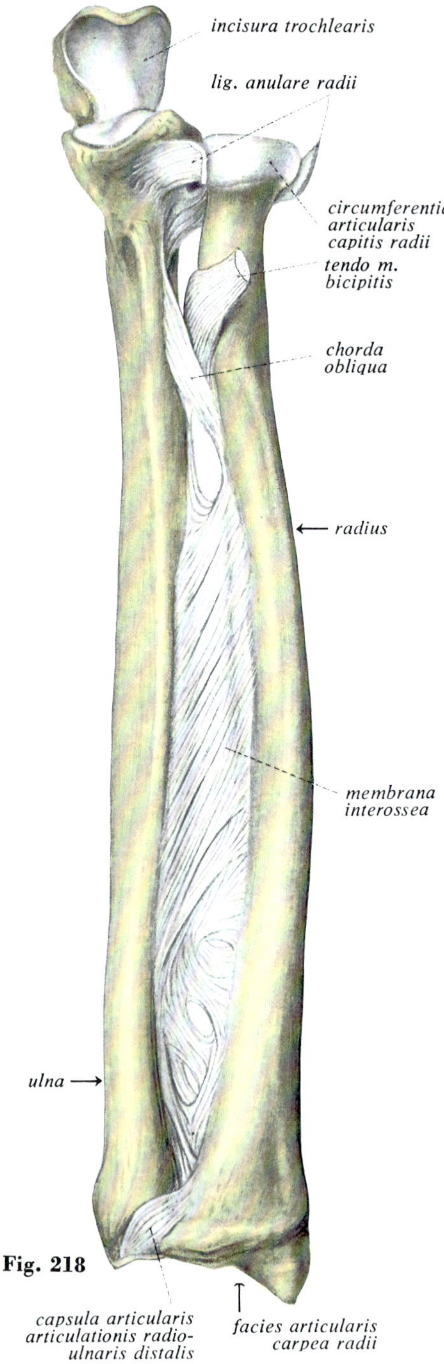

Fig. 218

Figs. 216 and 217. Left elbow joint *(articulatio cubiti)*. Fig. 216. Palmar view. Fig. 217. Dorsoradial view.

Fig. 218. Both left forearm bones, the *radius* and *ulna*, and the *membrana interossea*. The elbow joint was opened, the capsule removed; the *ligamentum anulare radii* has been cut to expose the cylindrical head of the *radius*.

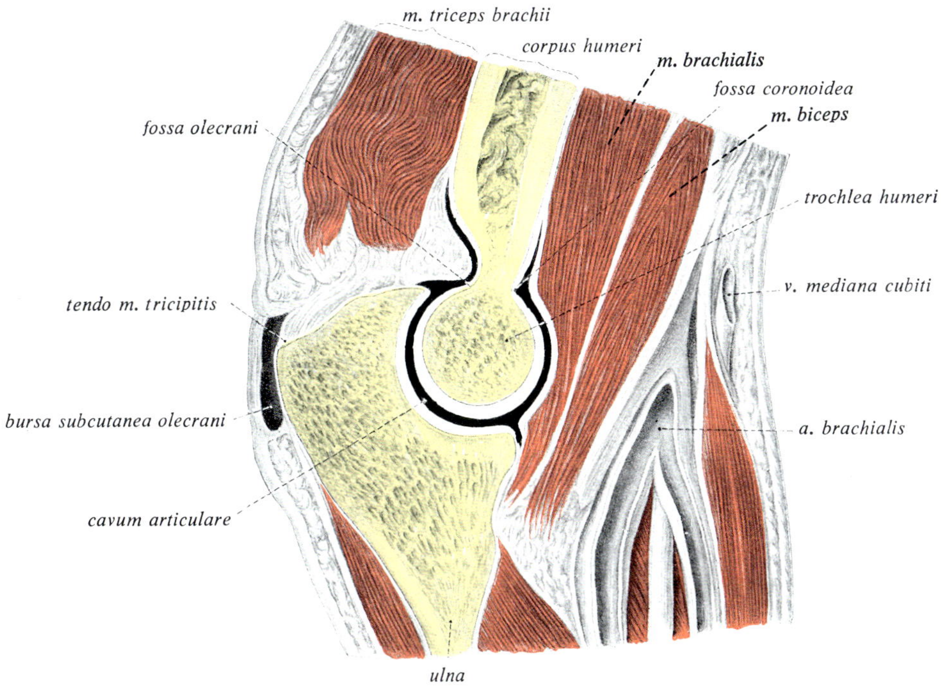

Fig. 219. Sagittal section (frozen) of the left elbow joint *(articulatio humeroulnaris)*.

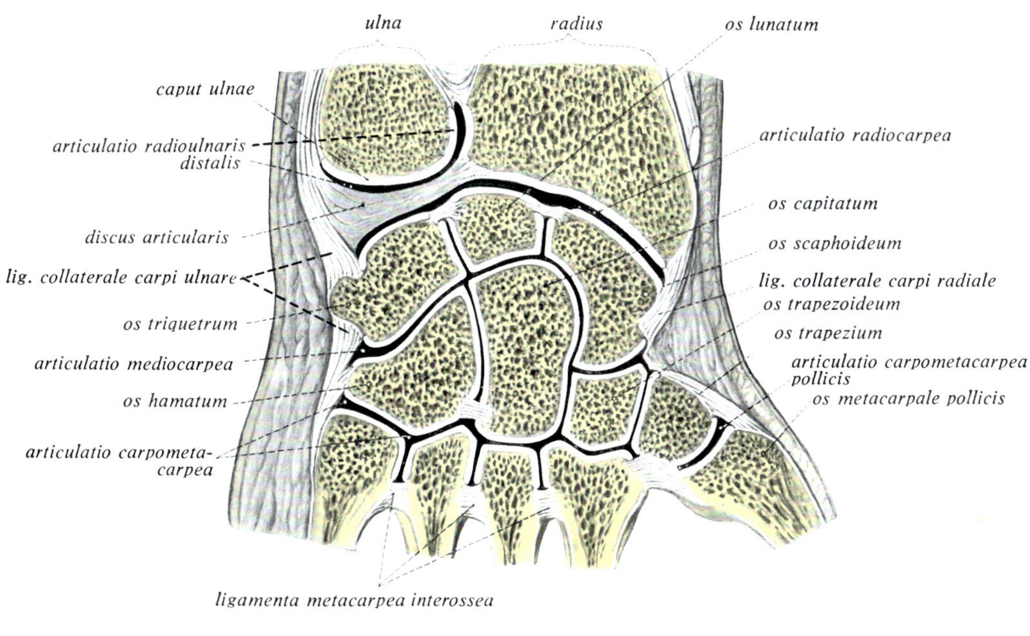

Fig. 220. Section through the wrist joints, cut parallel to the dorsal surface of the hand *(dorsum manus)*.

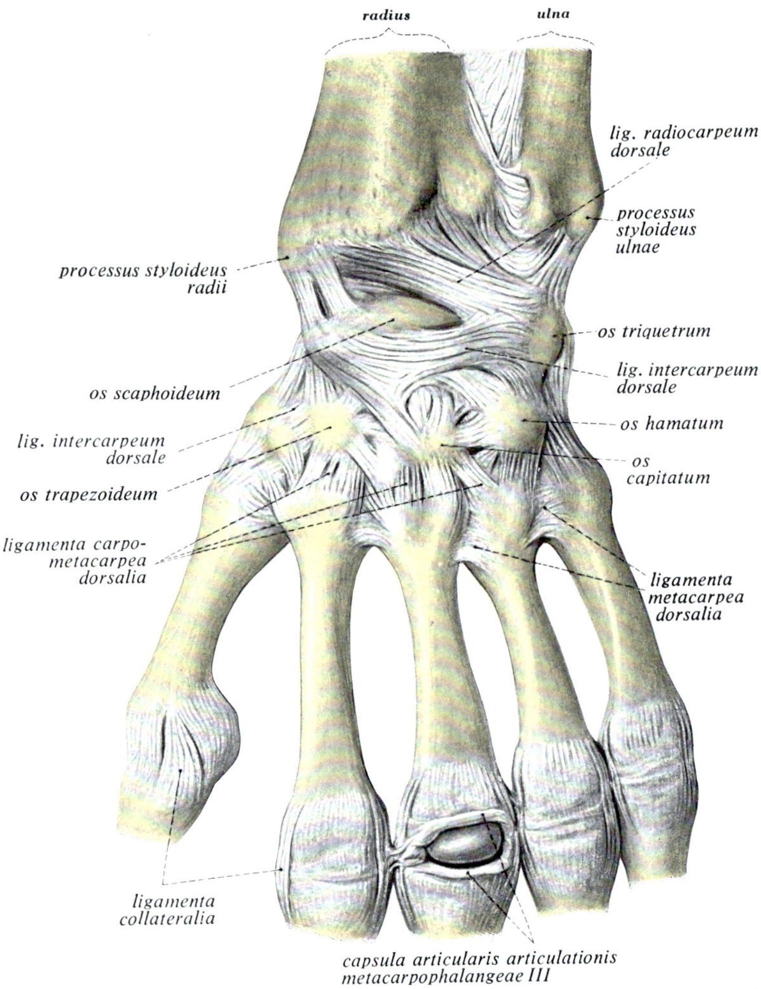

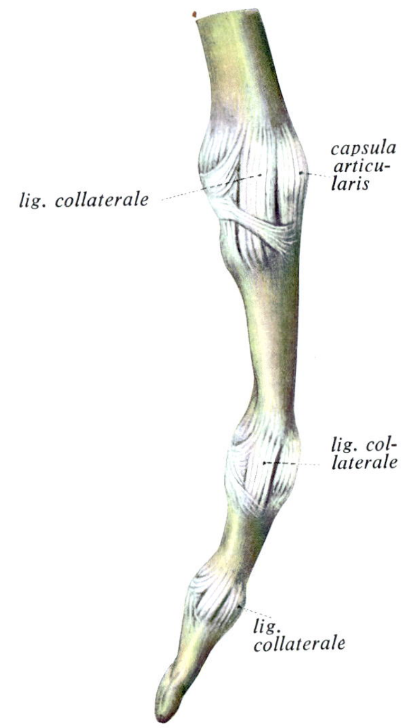

Fig. 221. Articulations and ligaments of the hand and wrist *(articulationes et ligamenta manus)*. Dorsal view.

Fig. 222. Articulations of the middle finger *(articulationes digiti medii)*. Lateral view.

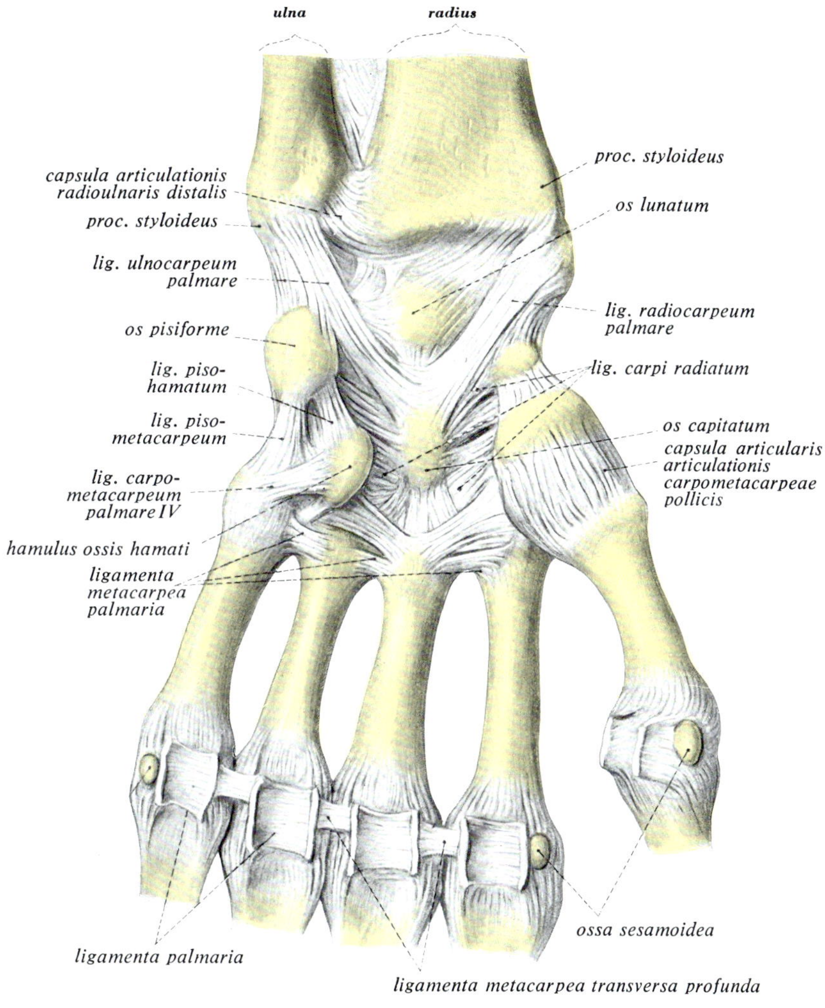

Fig. 223. Articulations and ligaments of the hand and wrist *(articulationes et ligamenta manus)*. Palmar view. The flexor retinaculum *(ligamentum carpi transversum)* was removed. The sesamoid bones of the thumb, index and little finger were exposed.

Joints and Ligaments

Pelvic Girdle and Lower Limb

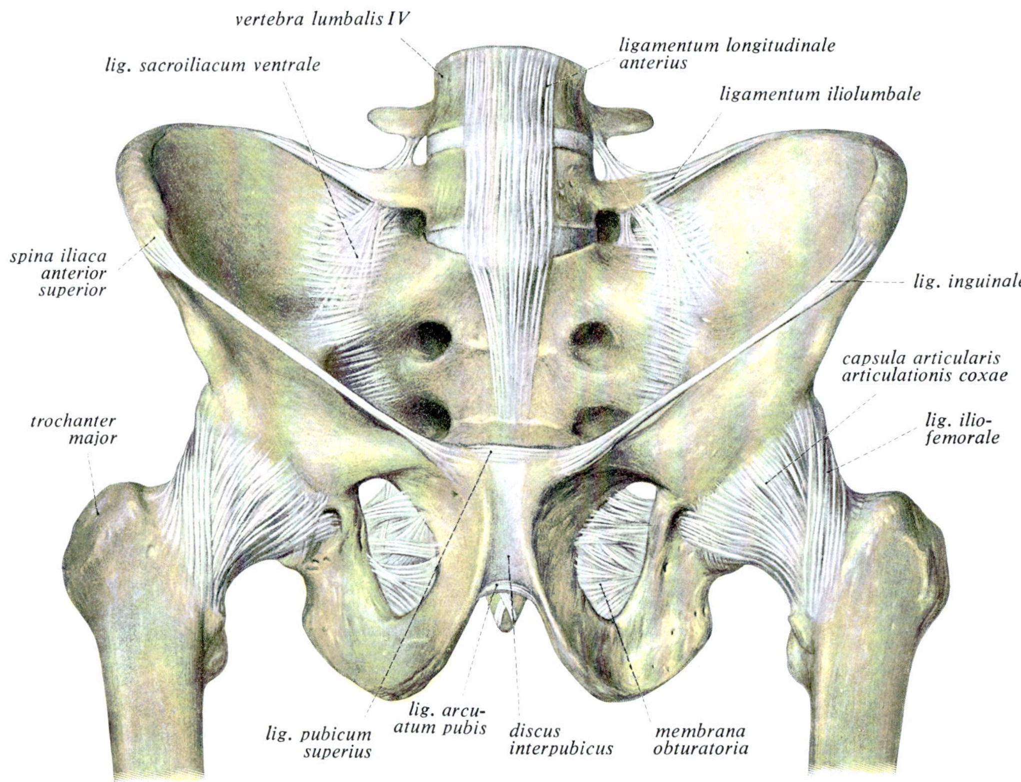

Fig. 224. Male pelvis with its ligaments *(ligamenta pelvis)*. Ventral view. Compare with Fig. 225.

Note: 1. The differences between the male and female pelves are primarily related to an enlarged pelvic outlet in the female to facilitate the function of childbearing.

The Chief Differences between Male and Female Pelves:

(1) The *angulus or arcus pubicus* is wider and more rounded in the female pelvis than in the male.
(2) The *tuberositates ischiadici* are more widely separated and everted in the female pelvis than in the male.
(3) The *symphysis pubica* is more shallow in the female. The distance between the *ligamentum arcuatum pubis* and the *ligamentum pubicum superius* is greater in the male pelvis.
(4) The *ossa ilia* have more flare in the female pelvis. This results in a shallow, wide, *pelvis major* in the female; and a narrower, deeper *pelvis major* in the male.
(5) The *os sacrum* is broader and less curved in the female.
(6) The *foramen obturatorium* is smaller and somewhat triangular in shape in the female.

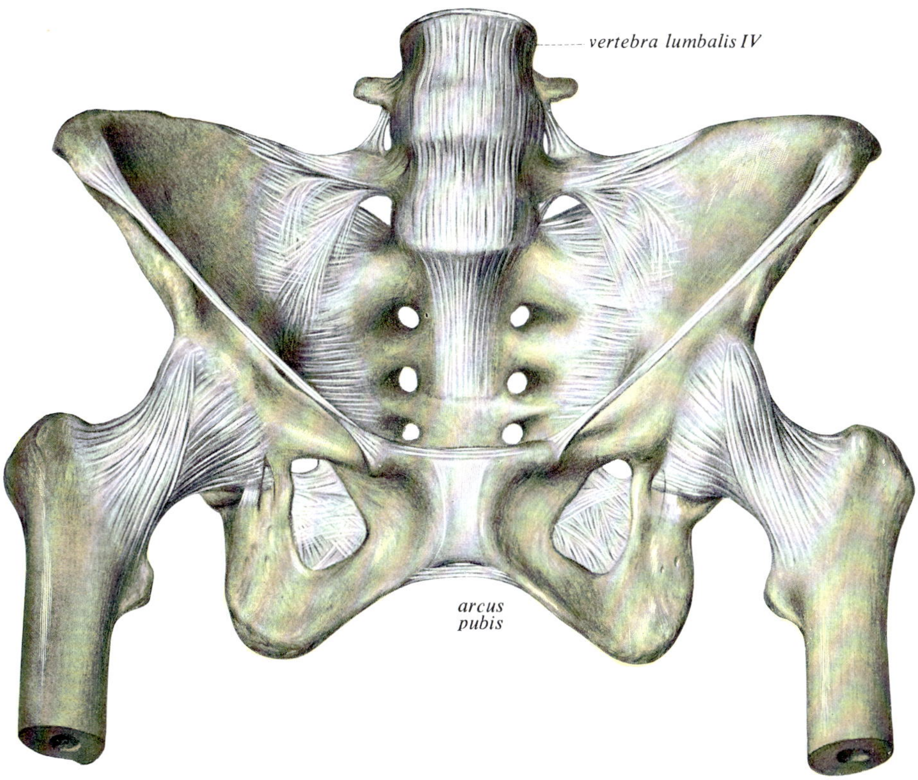

Fig. 225. Female pelvis with its ligaments *(ligamenta pelvis)*. Ventral view.

The Chief Differences between Male and Female Pelves: (Continued)

(7) The cavity of the true pelvis *(pelvis minor)* is wider and more shallow in the female than in the male.

(8) The outline of the *apertura superior* of the *pelvis minor* is more nearly circular in the female. This is, in part, related to the protrusion of the *promontorium* into the male pelvis minor to give it more of a heart shape.

(9) The inferior outlet of the *pelvis minor* is larger in the female.

(10) The sciatic notches are wider and more shallow in the female pelvis and the ischial spines do not protrude so far into the pelvis minor. The interspinous distance is, therefore, greater in the female.

(11) The *os coccygis* is more movable and able to accommodate for increased size of the birth canal near the termination of pregnancy (Fig. 147).

(12) The bones of the female pelvis are more delicate and lighter in weight than those of the male pelvis.

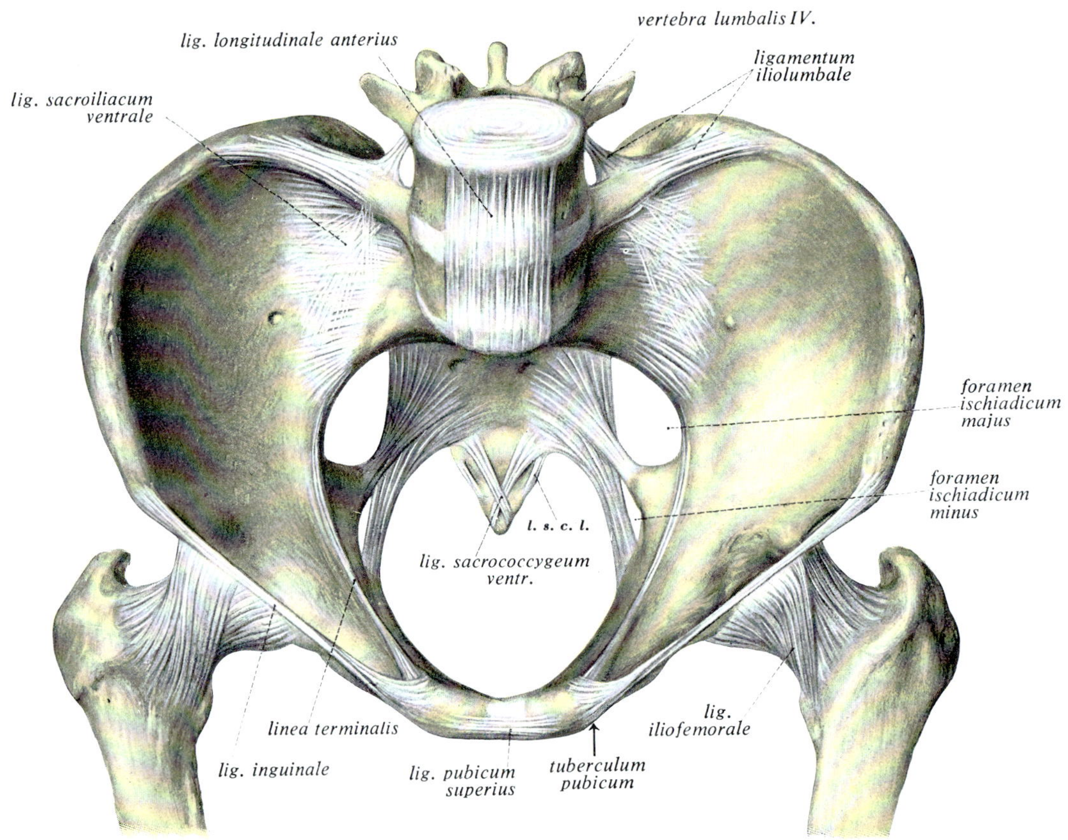

Fig. 226. Male pelvis with its ligaments *(ligamenta pelvis)*. Cranial view. l. s. c. l. = *ligamentum sacrococcygeum laterale*. Compare with Fig. 227.

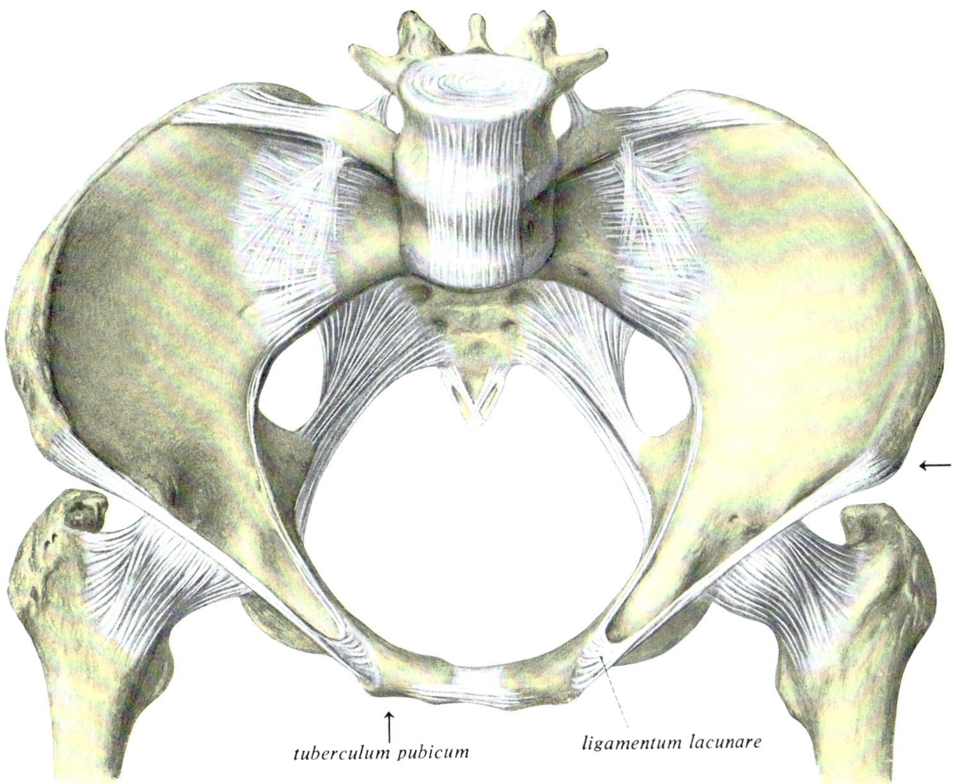

Fig. 227. Female pelvis with its ligaments *(ligamenta pelvis)*. Cranial view. Compare with Fig. 226.

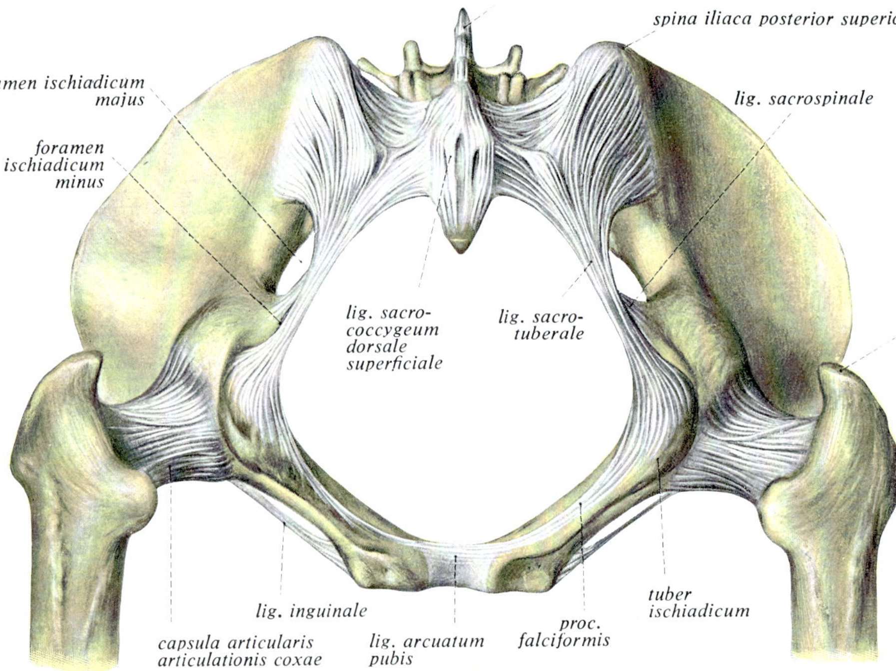

Fig. 228. Female pelvis with its ligaments *(ligamenta pelvis)*. Caudal view.

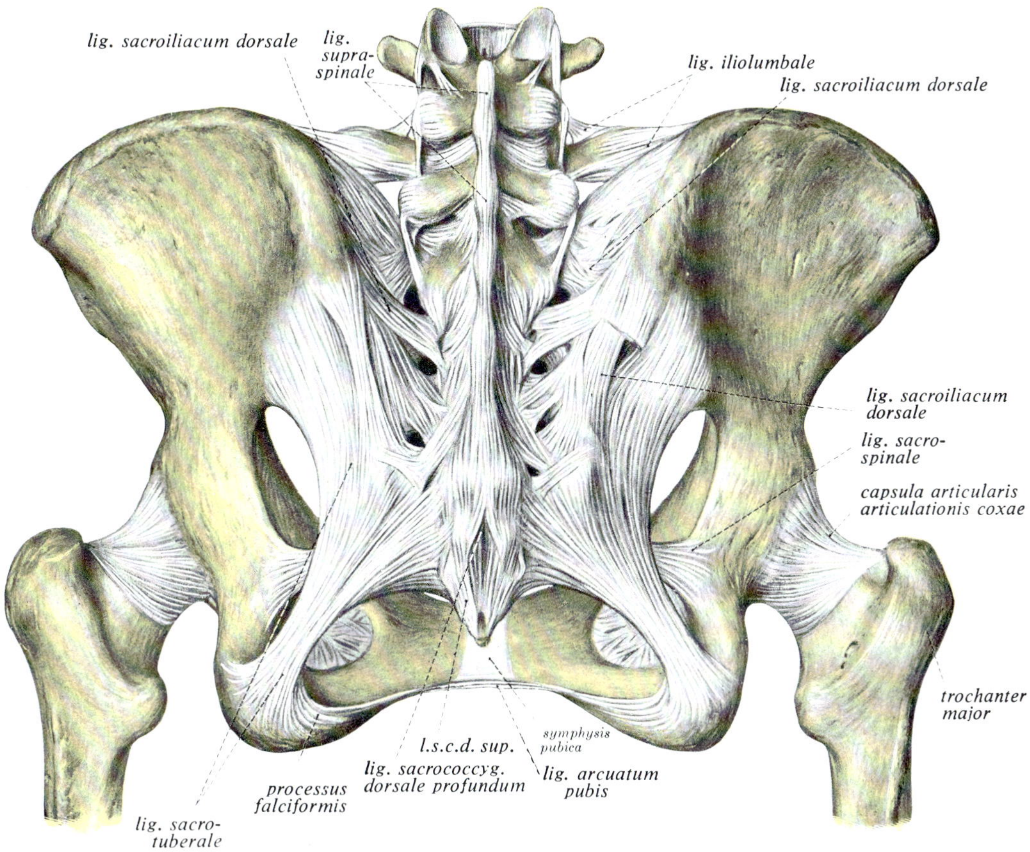

Fig. 229. Female pelvis with its ligaments *(ligamenta pelvis)*. Dorsal view. On the right, a superficial layer of the *ligamentum sacroiliacum dorsale* has been removed. l. s. c. d. sup. = *ligamentum sacrococcygicum dorsale superficiale.*

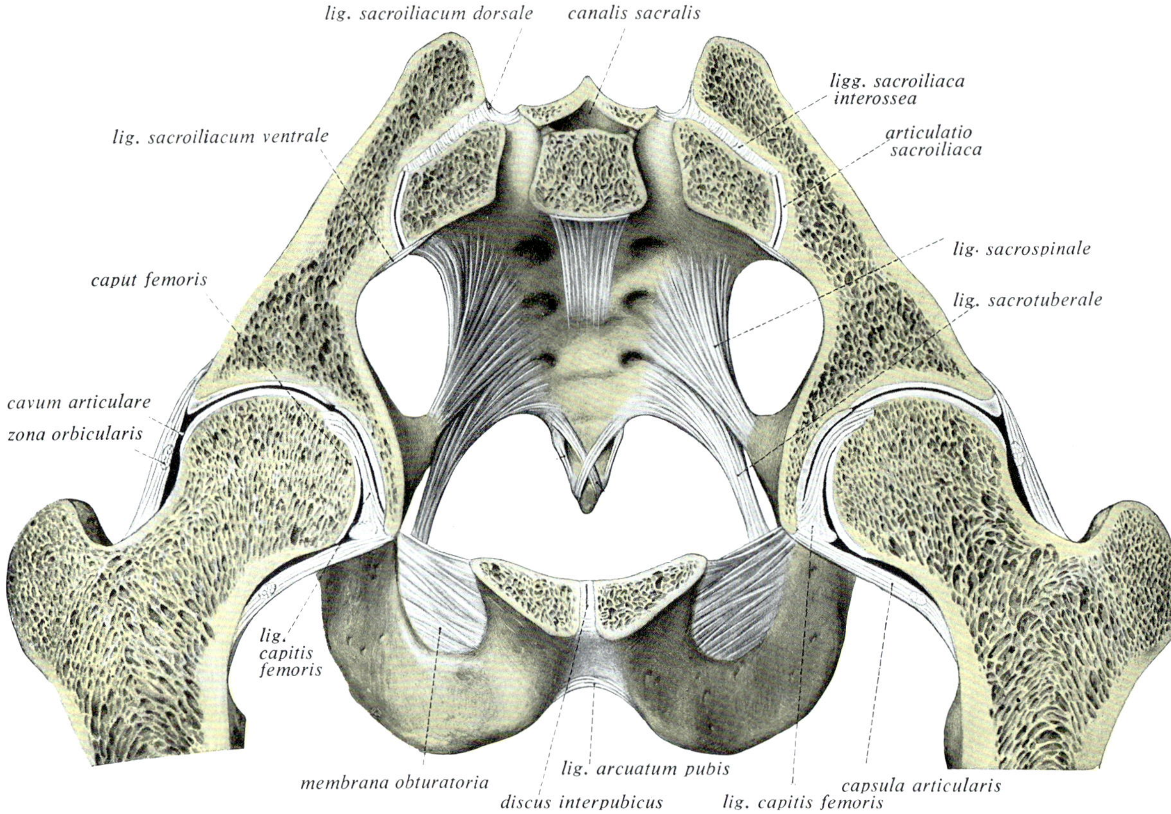

Fig. 230. Frontal section of the pelvis and both hip joints *(pelvis et articulationes coxae)*, somewhat perpendicular to the pelvic axis. The preparation shows, in addition to the hip joints, the *symphysis pubica* with its articular space, the *articulationes sacroiliacae*, the pelvic view of the *ligamenta sacrospinale et sacrotuberale*.

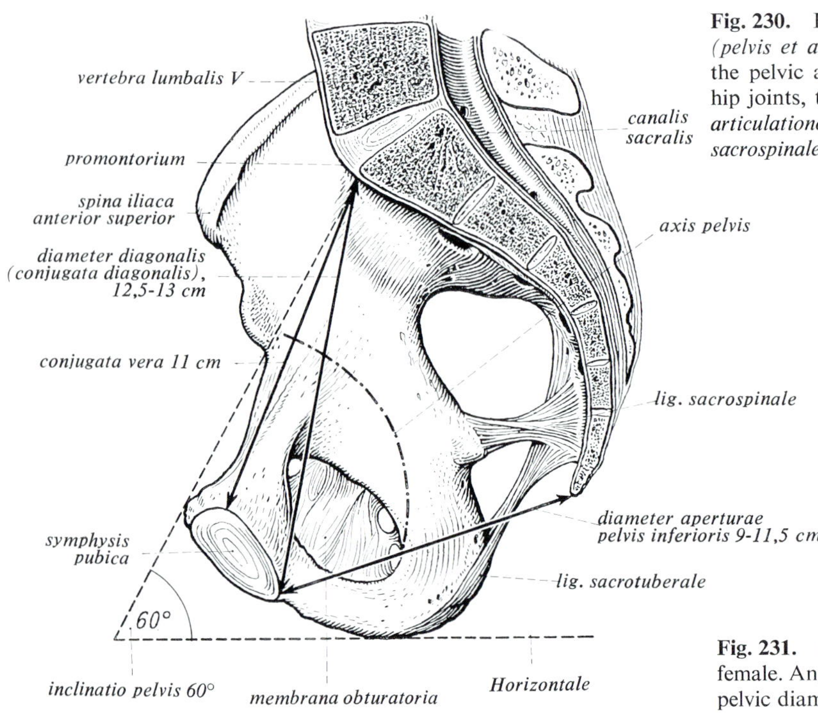

Fig. 231. Median sagittal section of the *pelvis* of an adult female. Angle of the pelvic inclination with the pelvic axis and pelvic diameter indicated.

Figs. 232 and 233. Right hip joint *(articulatio coxae)*.
Fig. 232. Ventral view. Fig. 233. Dorsal view.

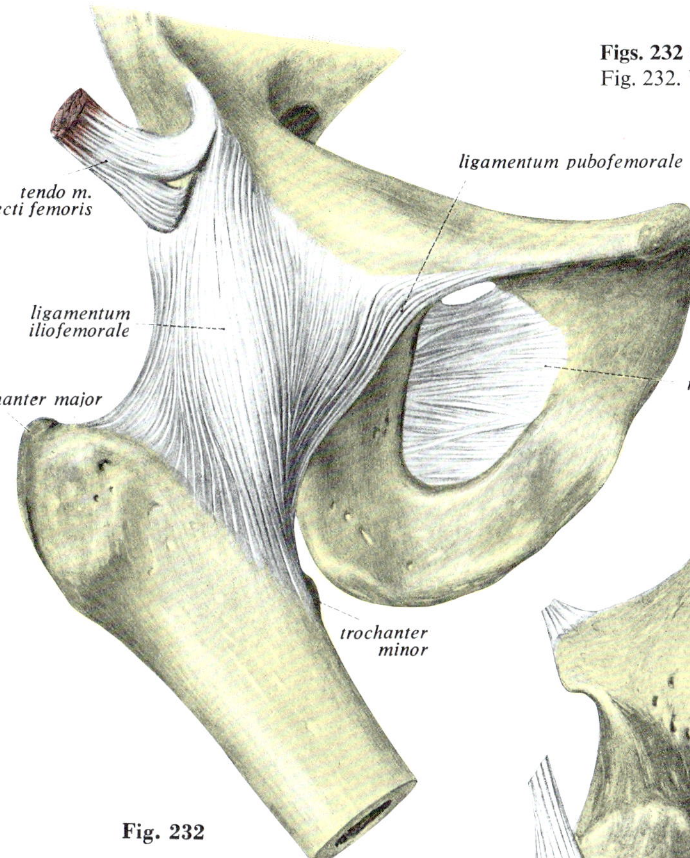

Fig. 232

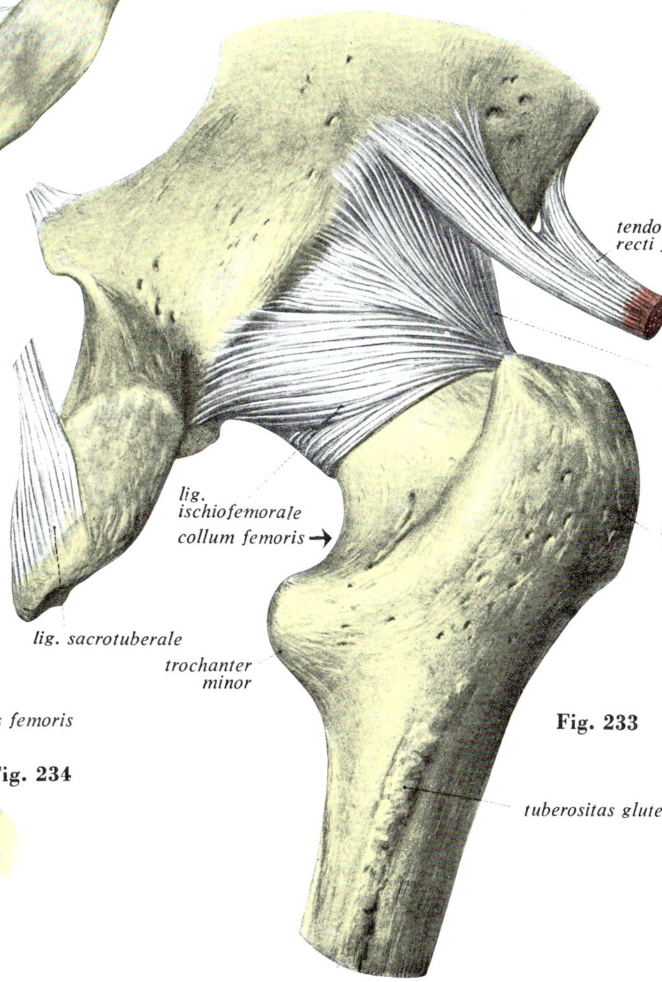

Fig. 233

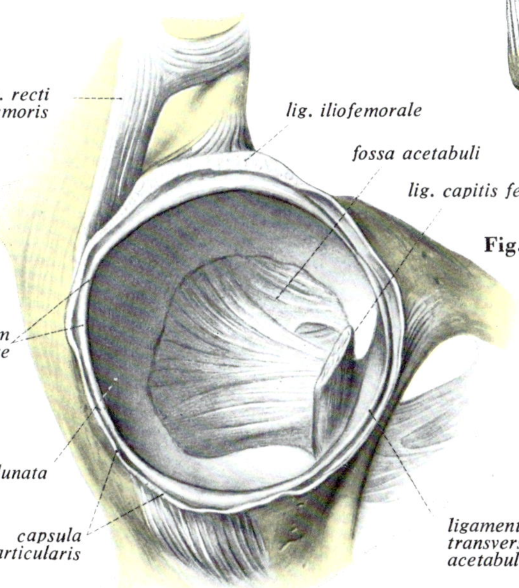

Fig. 234

Fig. 234. Socket of the right hip joint *(articulatio coxae)* after severing the joint capsule and the *ligamentum capitis femoris*. The head of the femur was removed from the *acetabulum*.

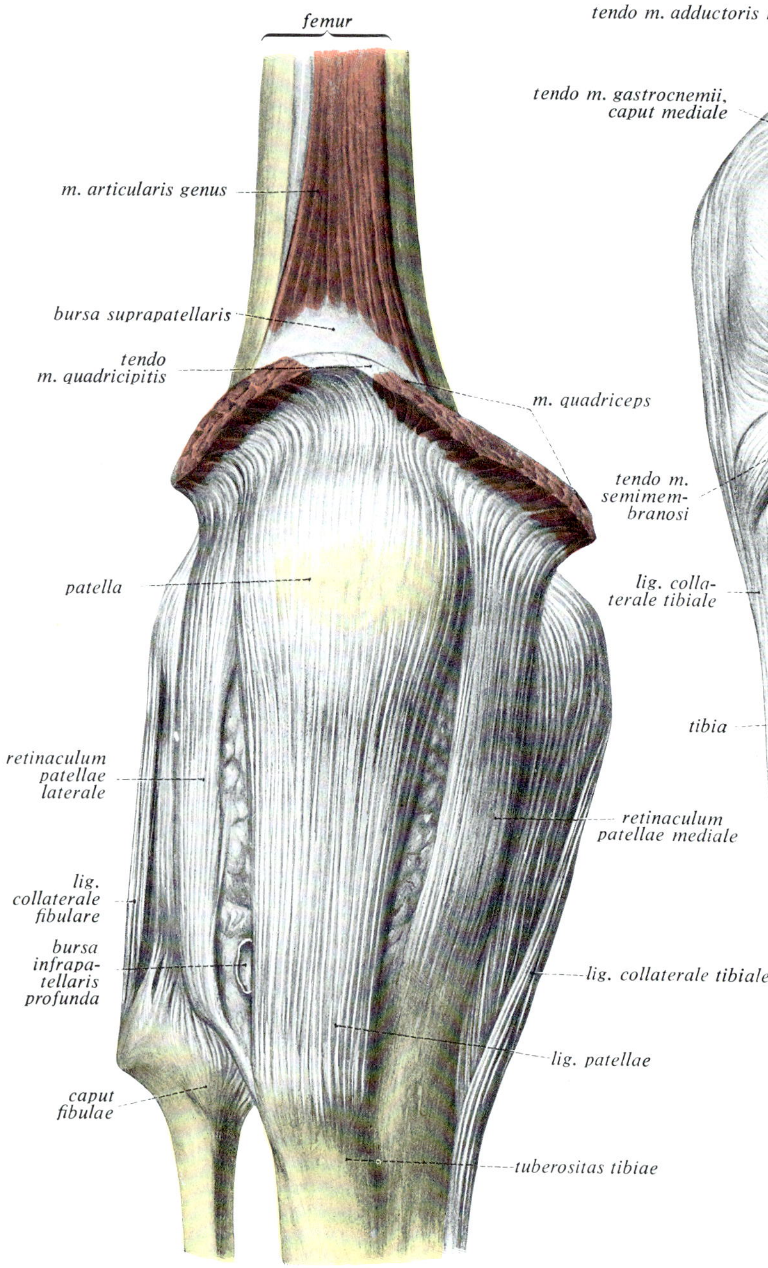

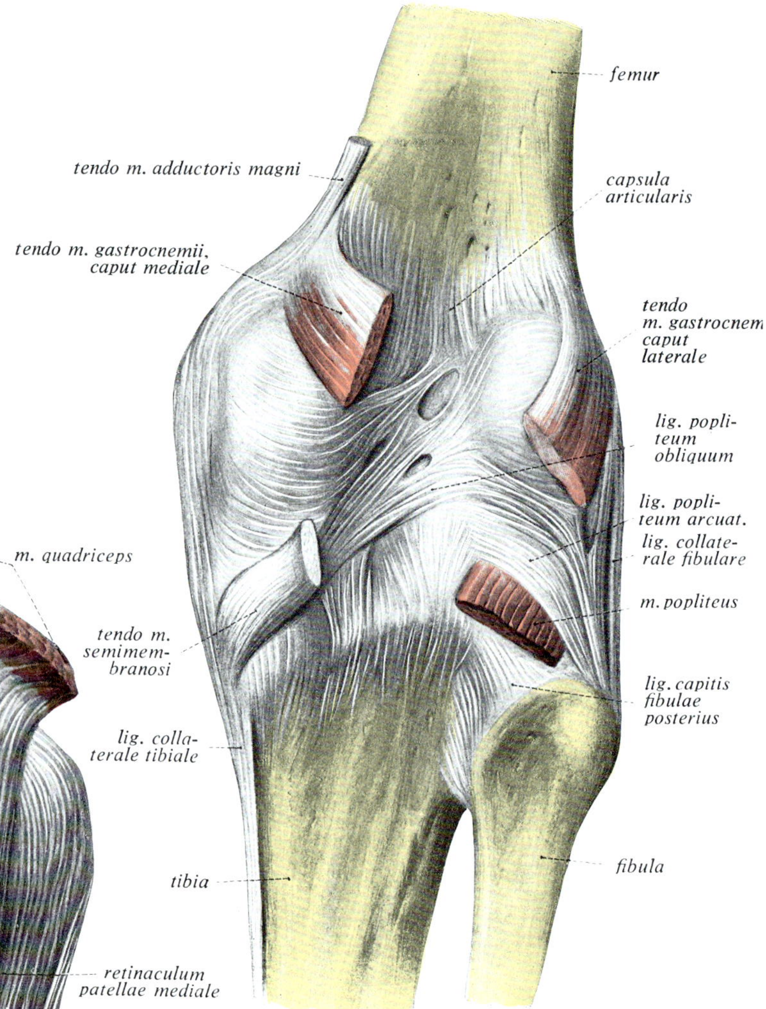

Fig. 235. Extended right knee joint *(articulatio genus)*. Anterior view.

Fig. 236. Extended right knee joint *(articulatio genus)*. Posterior view.

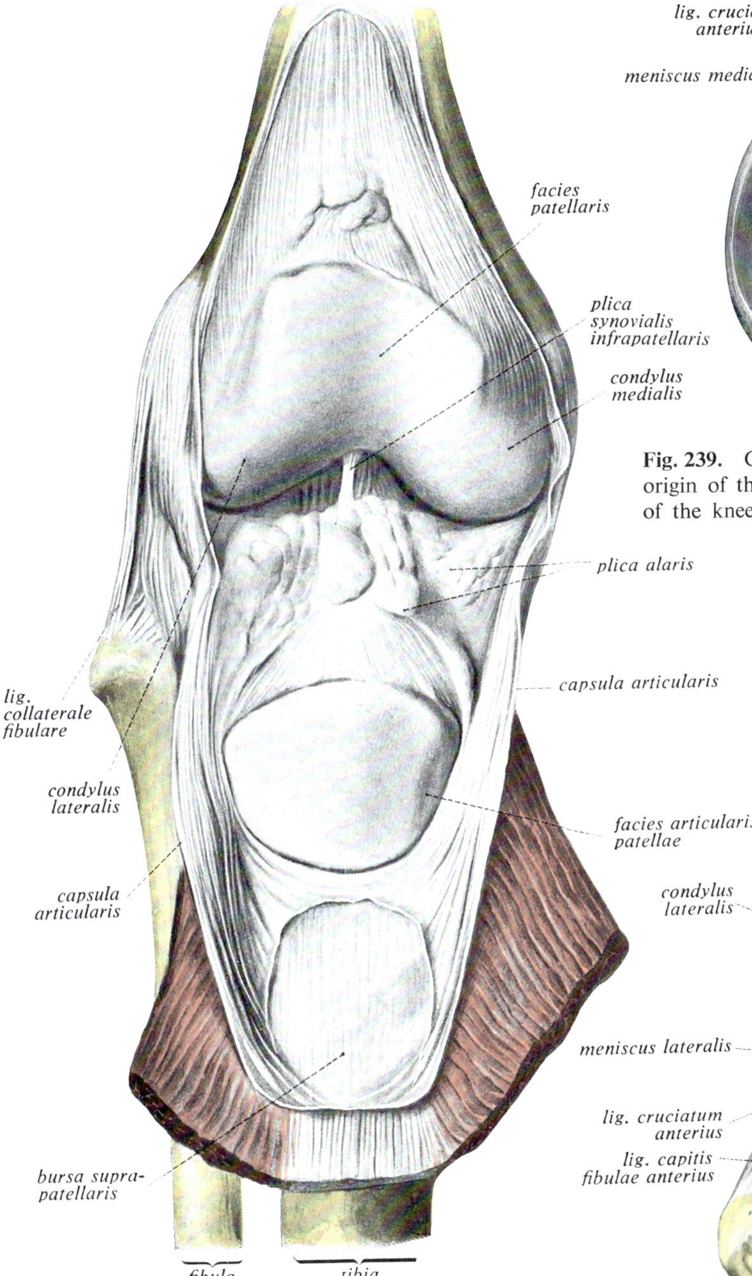

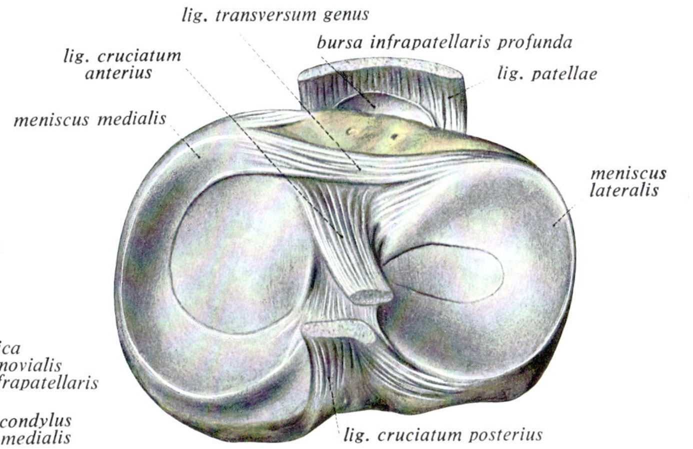

Fig. 239. Condyle of the tibia with both menisci and the origin of the cruciate ligaments *(ligamenta cruciata genus)* of the knee.

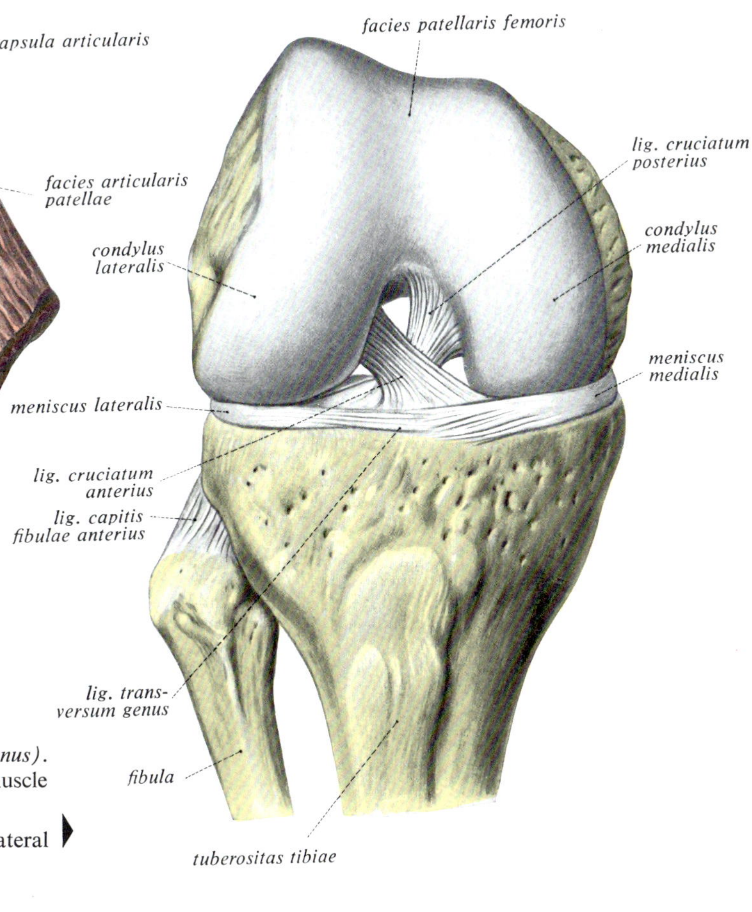

Fig. 237. Extended right knee joint *(articulatio genus)*. Opened by two lateral incisions and the Quadricep muscle with the patella pulled downward.

Fig. 238. Flexed right knee joint. Joint capsule and lateral ligaments removed. ▶

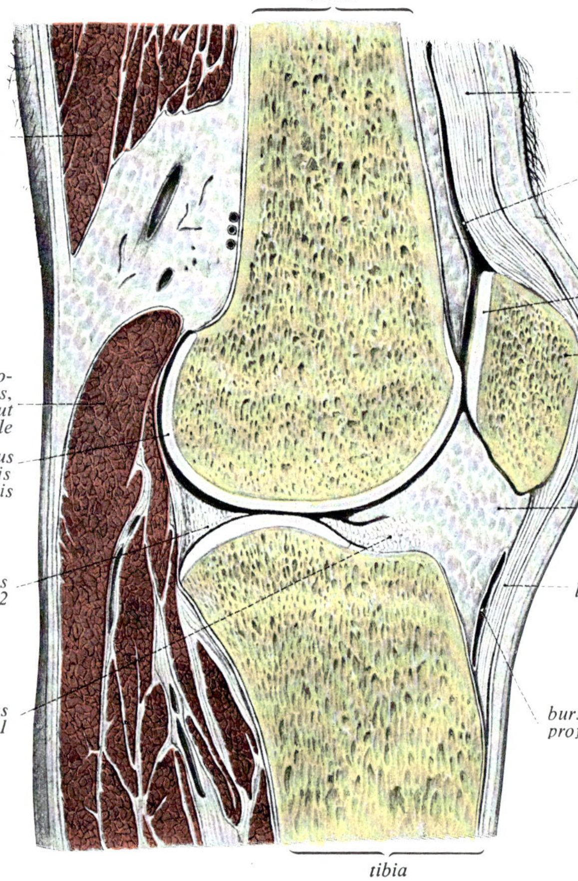

Fig. 240. Sagittal section of the right knee joint *(articulatio genus)* extension. The cut goes through the *condylus lateralis tibiae* and the *meniscus lateralis*. The latter was cut in two places: anterior and posterior. The congruity of the articular surfaces covered with cartilage are made possible by means of *menisci*, the *plicae alares* and the fat bodies of the joint. The articular cavity is enlarged through the communication with the labyrinthine bursa.

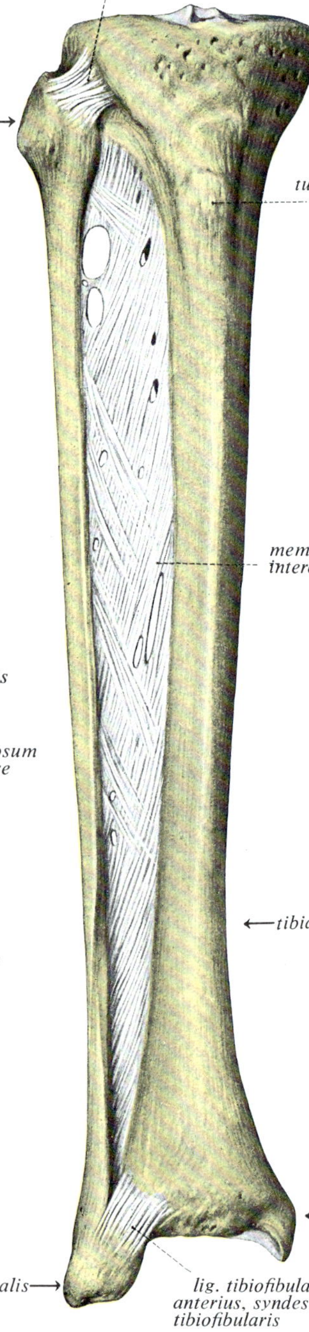

Fig. 241. The right tibiofibular articulation *(articulationes tibiofibulares)* with their ligaments. Anterior view.

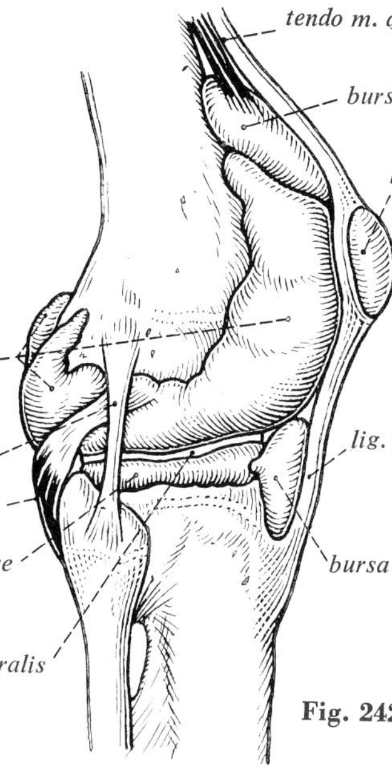

Fig. 242

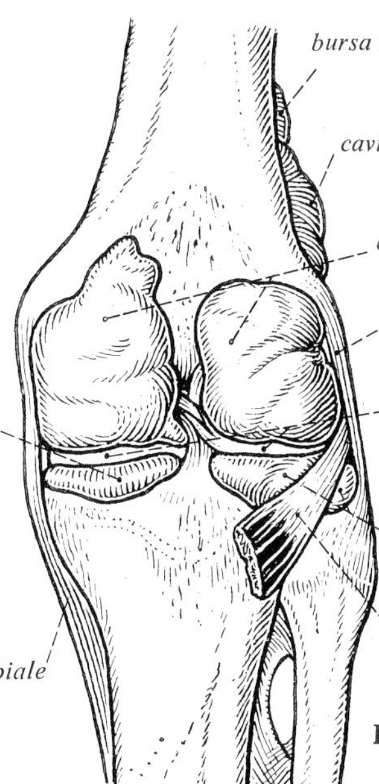

Fig. 243

Figs. 242 and 243. Joint effusion of the right knee joint *(articulatio genus)*. Fig. 242. Seen from lateral. Fig. 243. Seen from dorsal.

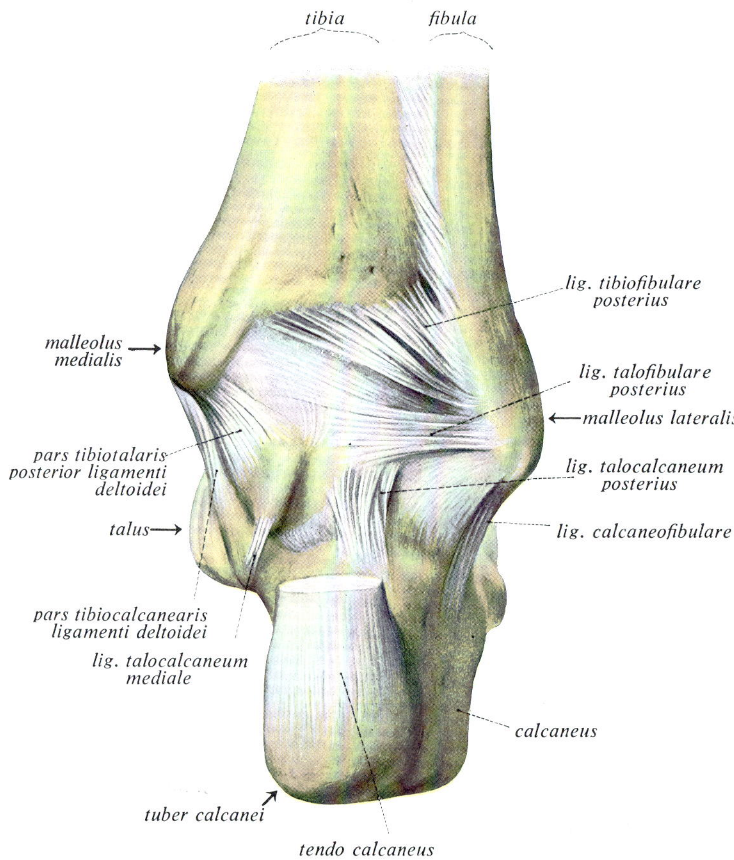

Fig. 244. The distal syndesmosis (articulatio) tibiofibularis and ankle joint *(articulatio talocruralis)*. Only a stump of the calcaneal tendon remains. Dorsal view.

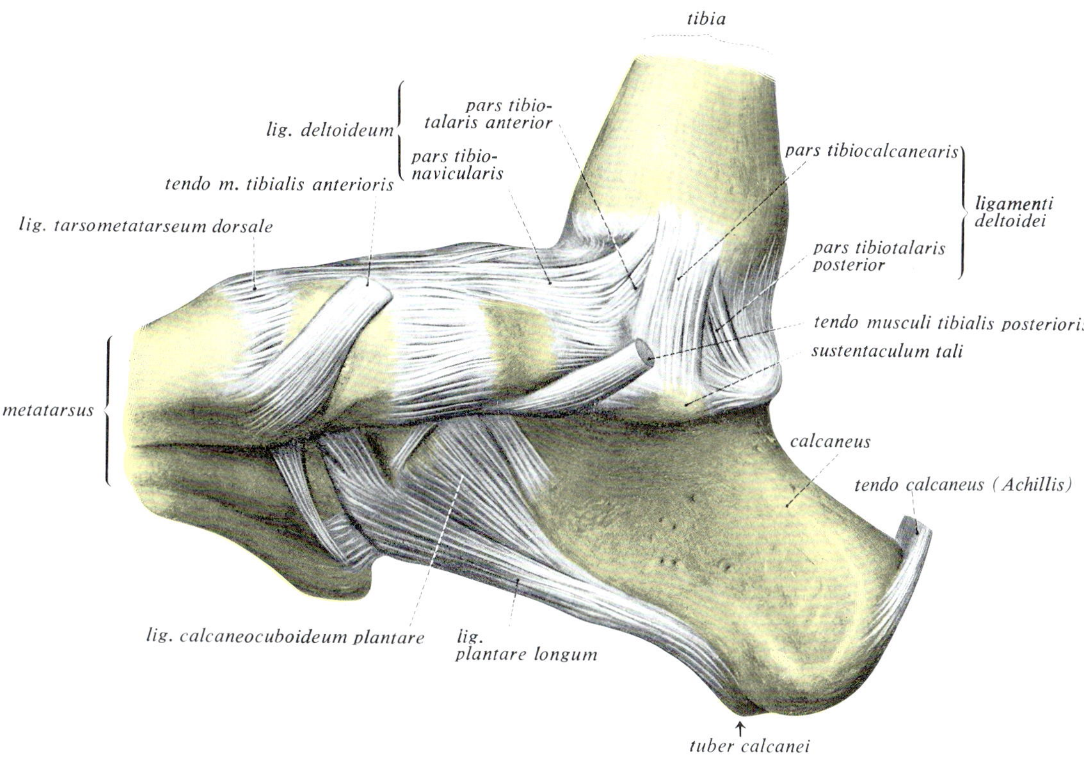

Fig. 245. Ligaments between the foot and the leg *(ligamenta tarsi)*. Medial view.

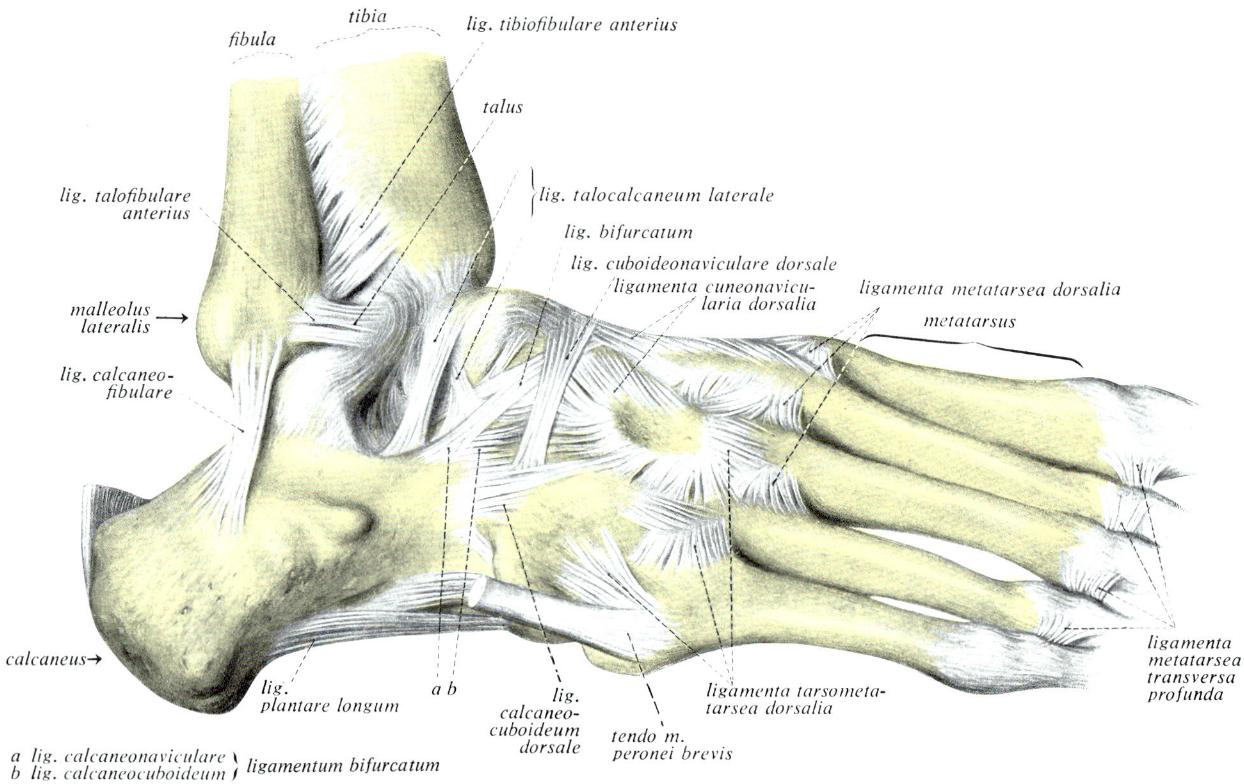

Fig. 246. Ligaments of the foot *(ligamenta pedis)*. Dorsolateral view.

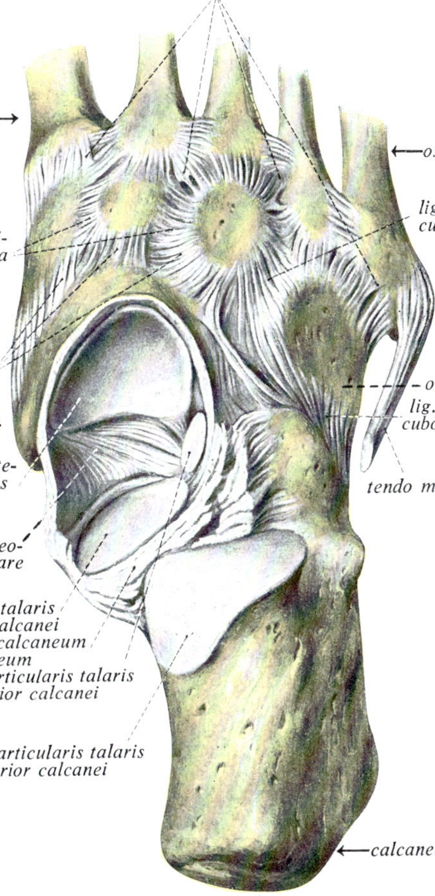

Fig. 247. *Articulatio talocalcaneonavicularis*, lower ankle joint. Viewed from above. The *talus* was disarticulated and removed to display its articulations, especially the navicular socket for its head.

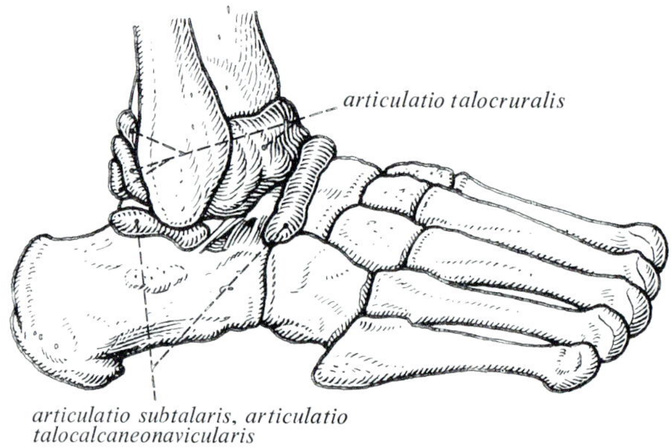

Fig. 248. Joint effusion of the upper and lower ankle joints on the right foot, *(articulatio talocruralis, articulatio subtalaris, articulatio talocalcaneonavicularis)*. Lateral view (after Benninghoff, Goerttler, Lehrbuch der Anatomie des Menschen. Vol. I).

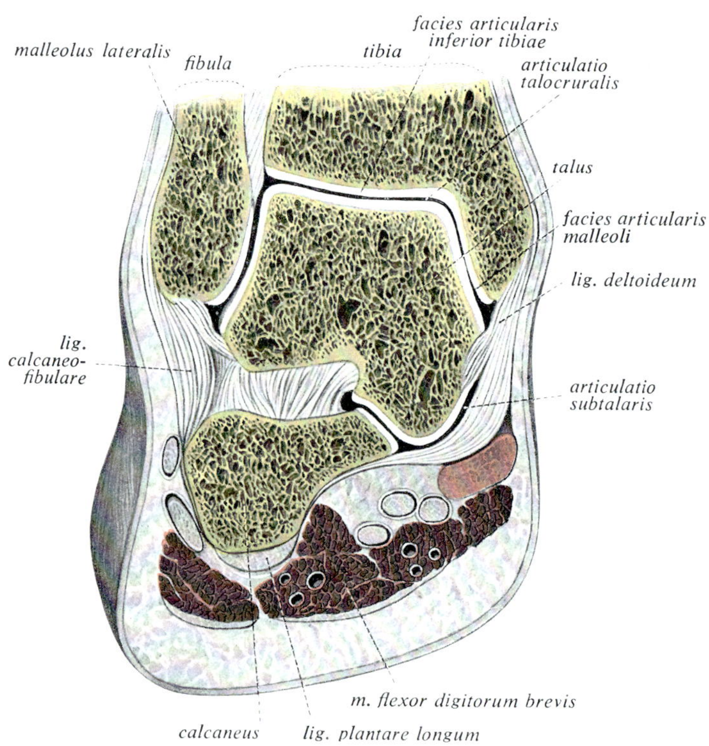

Fig. 249. Frontal frozen section through the upper ankle joint *(articulatio talocruralis)* and the dorsal compartment of the lower ankle joint *(articulatio subtalaris)*.

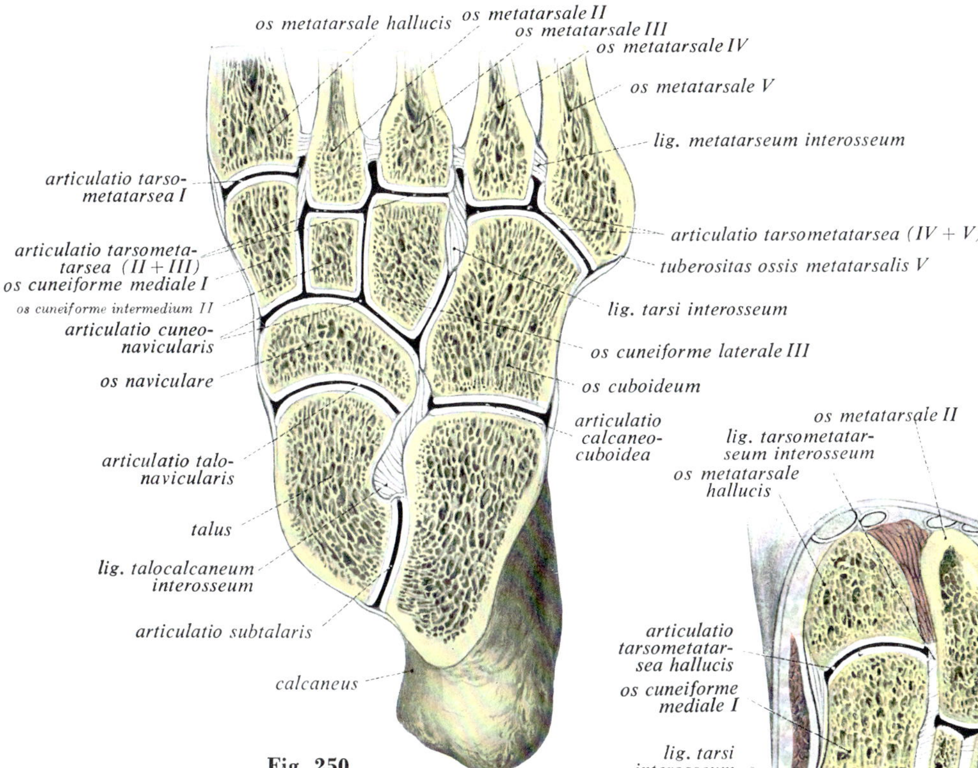

Fig. 250

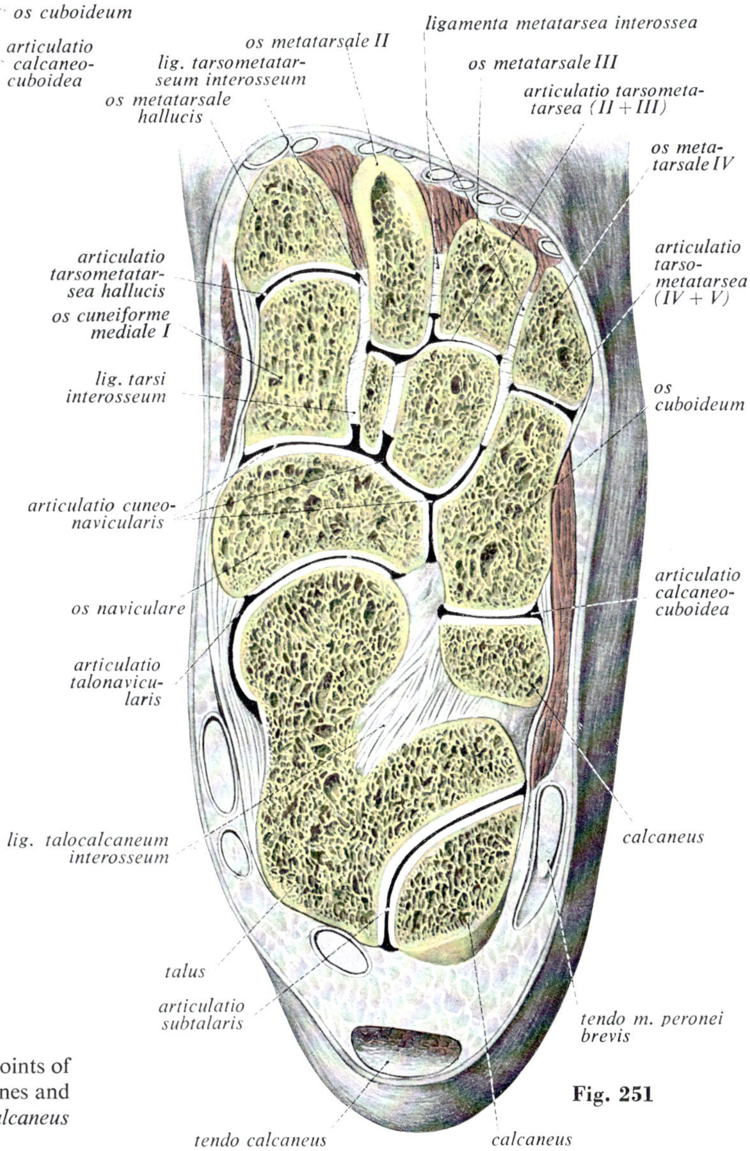

Fig. 251

Figs. 250 and 251. Horizontal sections through the joints of the ankle and foot *(articulationes tarsi)*. Fig. 250. Bones and joints. Fig. 251. The cut is at a higher level, so the *calcaneus* is cut in two places.

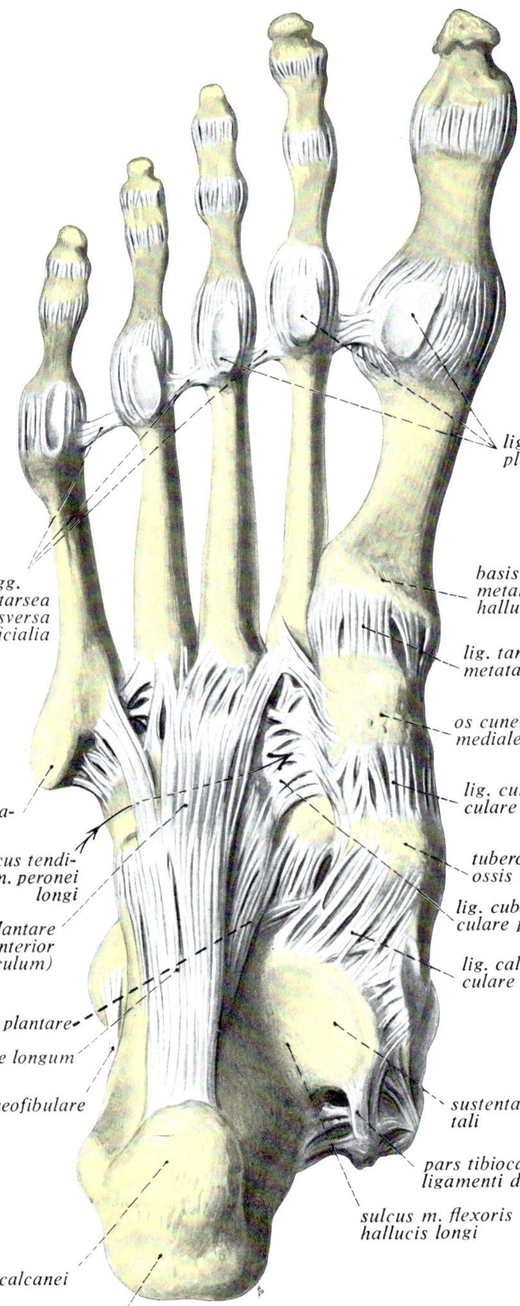

Fig. 252. Ligaments of the plantar surface of the foot *(planta pedis)*. Superficial layers.

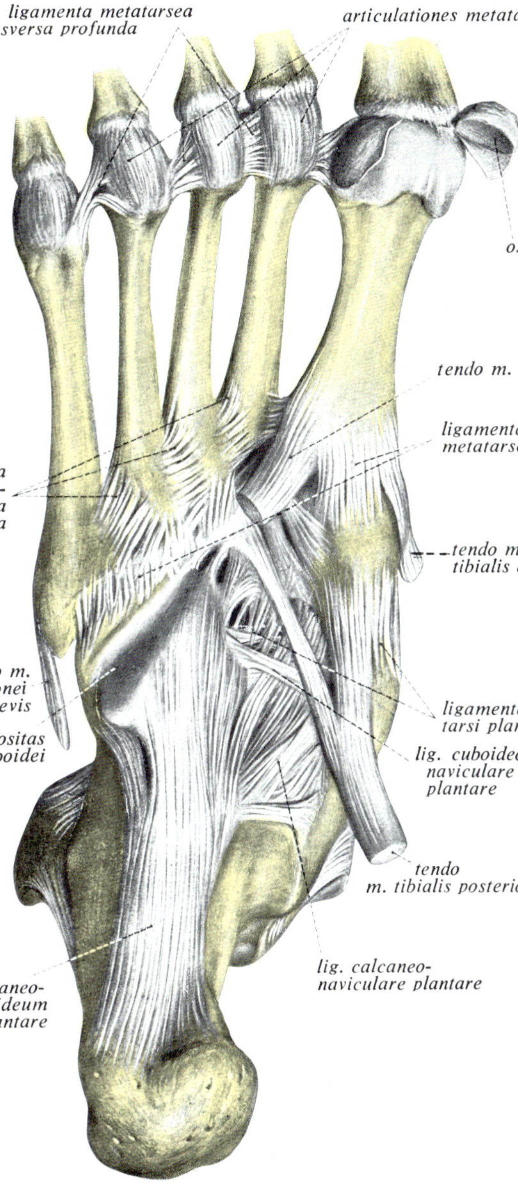

Fig. 253. Ligaments of the plantar surface of the foot *(planta pedis)*. Deep layers. The metatarsal joint of the great toe was opened, exposing a sesamoid bone.

Muscles

Neck, Trunk and Pelvis

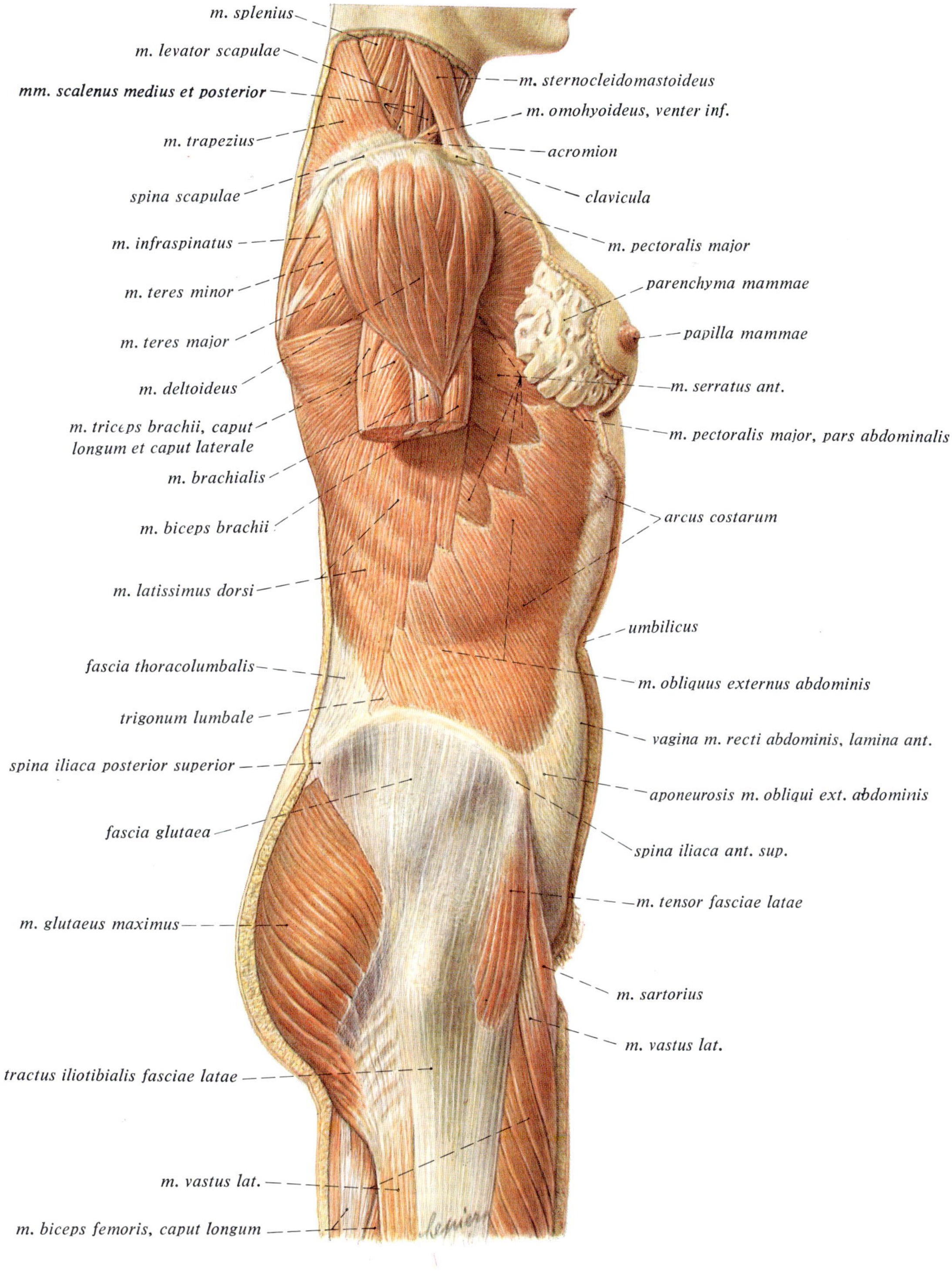

Fig. 254. Musculature of the neck, trunk, and thigh of an adult female. Mammary gland *(mamma)* dissected.

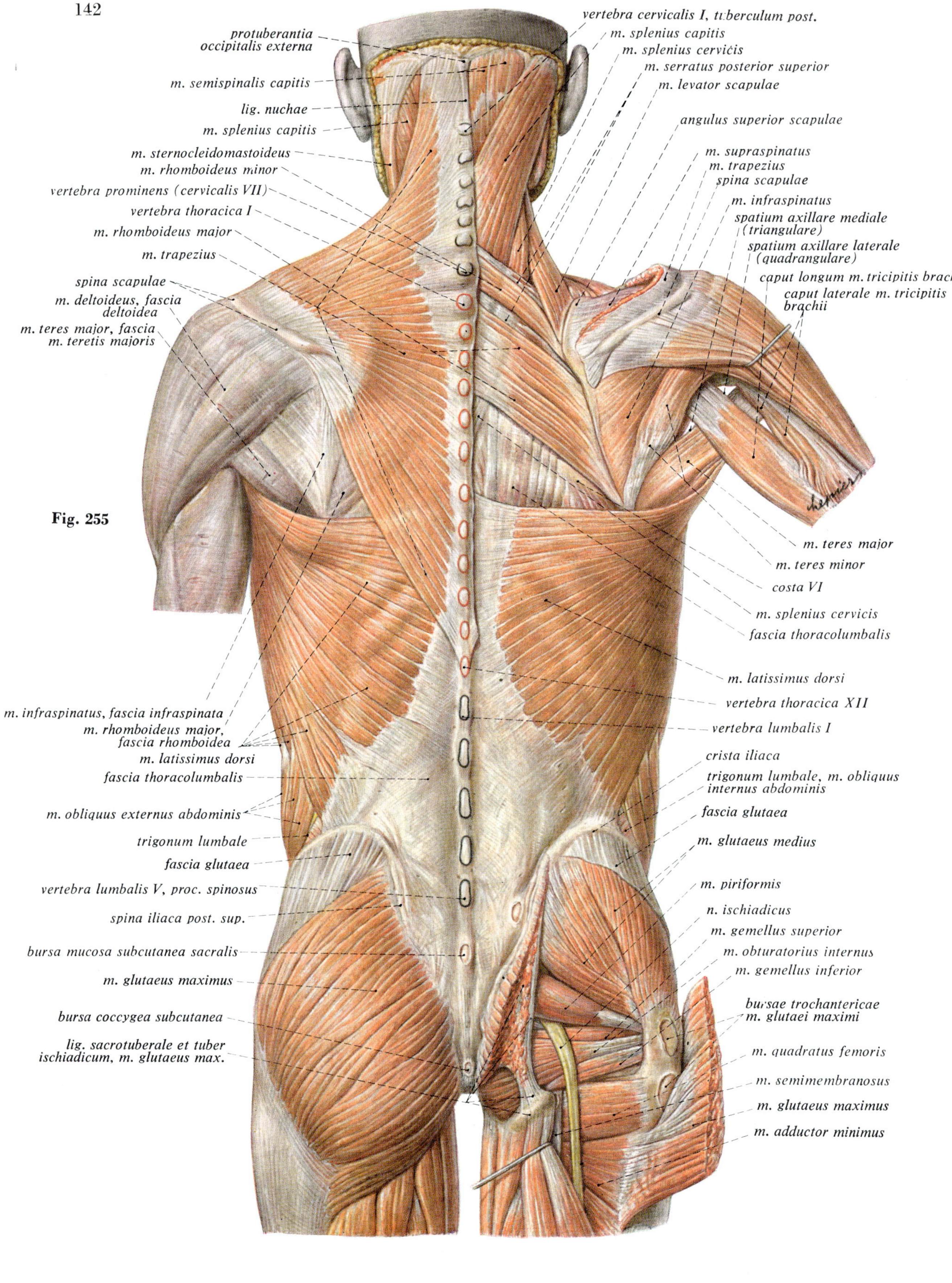

protuberantia occipitalis externa
m. semispinalis capitis
lig. nuchae
m. splenius capitis
m. sternocleidomastoideus
m. rhomboideus minor
vertebra prominens (cervicalis VII)
vertebra thoracica I
m. rhomboideus major
m. trapezius
spina scapulae
m. deltoideus, fascia deltoidea
m. teres major, fascia m. teretis majoris
m. infraspinatus, fascia infraspinata
m. rhomboideus major, fascia rhomboidea
m. latissimus dorsi
fascia thoracolumbalis
m. obliquus externus abdominis
trigonum lumbale
fascia glutaea
vertebra lumbalis V, proc. spinosus
spina iliaca post. sup.
bursa mucosa subcutanea sacralis
m. glutaeus maximus
bursa coccygea subcutanea
lig. sacrotuberale et tuber ischiadicum, m. glutaeus max.
vertebra cervicalis I, tuberculum post.
m. splenius capitis
m. splenius cervicis
m. serratus posterior superior
m. levator scapulae
angulus superior scapulae
m. supraspinatus
m. trapezius
spina scapulae
m. infraspinatus
spatium axillare mediale (triangulare)
spatium axillare laterale (quadrangulare)
caput longum m. tricipitis brachii
caput laterale m. tricipitis brachii
m. teres major
m. teres minor
costa VI
m. splenius cervicis
fascia thoracolumbalis
m. latissimus dorsi
vertebra thoracica XII
vertebra lumbalis I
crista iliaca
trigonum lumbale, m. obliquus internus abdominis
fascia glutaea
m. glutaeus medius
m. piriformis
n. ischiadicus
m. gemellus superior
m. obturatorius internus
m. gemellus inferior
bursae trochantericae m. glutaei maximi
m. quadratus femoris
m. semimembranosus
m. glutaeus maximus
m. adductor minimus

Fig. 255

Muscles of the Back – First Layer (Fig. 255)

Name	*Origin*	*Insertion*
1. m. trapezius A flat triangular muscle (see Fig. 254); tendinous tissue in region where the cervical and thoracic spinous processus meet	Medial third of linea nuchae superior; protuberantia occipitalis externa; cervical spinous processes via ligamentum nuchae; spines of thoracic vertebrae and their supraspinous ligaments	Lateral third of clavicle (Fig. 275); acromion scapulae; spina scapulae
Nerve: n. accessorius plus C 3, 4		
Action: Cranial fibers elevate the scapula, the caudal depress it; the middle fibers pull the scapula dorsally, suspend the shoulder girdle, help rotate the scapula. Normal tension helps maintain the square shoulder. When the n. accessorius is cut, the shoulder droops.		
2. m. latissimus dorsi A large triangular muscle	By way of the fascia thoracolumbalis (aponeurosis), from the 6 caudal thoracic, all lumbar spines, os sacrum, and labium externum cristae iliacae. Muscular slips from 3 or 4 caudal ribs and angulus inferior scapulae	By a flat tendon to floor of the sulcus intertubercularis humeri, ventral to insertion of m. teres major; bursa m. latissimi dorsi subtendinea
Nerve: n. thoracodorsalis of the plexus brachialis (C 6, 7, 8)		
Action: Extends and adducts the humerus and rotates it medially. Draws the arm and shoulder downward and backward		
3. m. rhomboideus major	Spines of the 2nd to 5th thoracic vertebrae	Margo medialis scapulae, caudal to the spina scapulae
4. m. rhomboideus minor	Spines of 7th cervical and 1st thoracic vertebra; ligamentum nuchae	Margo medialis scapulae, cranial to the spina scapulae
Nerve: For both: n. dorsalis scapulae from the plexus brachialis (C 4, 5)		
Action: Draws the scapula upward and medially. Holds scapula to trunk along with the m. serratus anterior		
5. m. levator scapulae Borders the m. scalenus posterior ventrally	The tubercula posteriora of the processus transversi of the upper 4 cervical vertebrae	Angulus superior scapulae (and the immediate adjacent region) to the base of the spina scapulae
Nerve: Plexus cervicalis and the n. dorsalis scapulae (C 3, 4)		
Action: Pulls the scapula upward and medially (along with the m. trapezius). If the scapula is fixed, it pulls the neck laterally		

◀ **Fig. 255.** Shoulder, neck, back, and gluteal muscles. *Left:* Superficial layers. *Right:* Deeper layers.

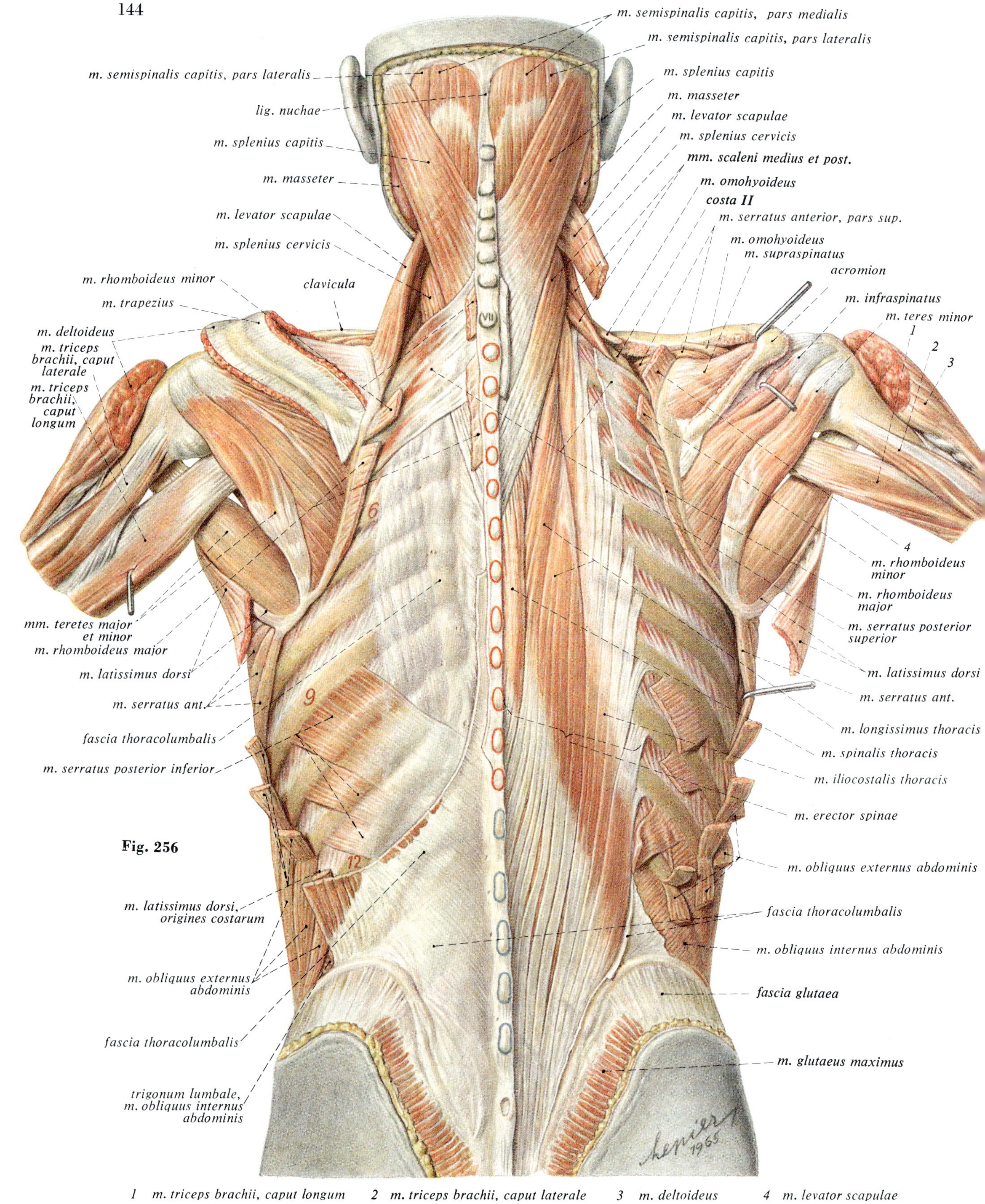

Fig. 256

1 m. triceps brachii, caput longum 2 m. triceps brachii, caput laterale 3 m. deltoideus 4 m. levator scapulae

Muscles of the Back – Respiratory Muscles (Fig. 256)

Name	*Origin*	*Insertion*
1. m. serratus posterior superior A thin, quadrilateral muscle	lig. nuchae, spinous processes of 7th cervical and the first 2 or 3 thoracic vertebrae	Ribs 2–5, lateral to their angles
2. m. serratus posterior inferior (more broad than above)	By way of fascia thoracolumbalis from last 2 thoracic and upper 2 lumbar spinous processes	Inferior borders of last 4 ribs, lateral to their angles

Nerve: For both: nn. intercostales (superior T 1–4; inferior T 9–12)

Action: m. serratus posterior superior elevates first 4 ribs, assists in inspiration; m. serratus posterior inferior pulls last 4 ribs caudally, helps in expiration

Deep Muscles of the Back – The True Back Muscles: Mm. splenius capitis and cervicis (Figs. 256, 257)

The two muscles are close together at their origin (from the spinous processes). Gradually, as they approach their individual insertions, they become separated into two specific muscles.

1. m. splenius capitis The mm. splenii get their innervations from the true back muscles	ligamentum nuchae, spinous processes of 3rd (4th) to 7th cervical and first 3 thoracic vertebrae	Lateral third of the linea nuchalis superior (and the processus mastoideus ossis temporalis)

Nerve: Rami dorsales of nerves C 2–4, lateral branches

Action: Muscles of both sides, acting together, extend the head and neck; one side acting alone, rotates the head to the same side

2. m. splenius cervicis	Spines of 3rd (or 4th) to 6th thoracic vertebrae	tubercula posteriora of the transverse processes of the first 3 cervical vertebrae

Nerve: Rami dorsales of nerves C 2–5, lateral branches (same as m. splenius capitis)

Action: Muscles of both sides acting together extend the neck and head. Muscles of one side rotates the upper cervical vertebrae and, by its action on the atlas, rotates the head to the same side

◀ **Fig. 256.** Shoulder, neck, and back musculature. Deeper layers of long back muscles.

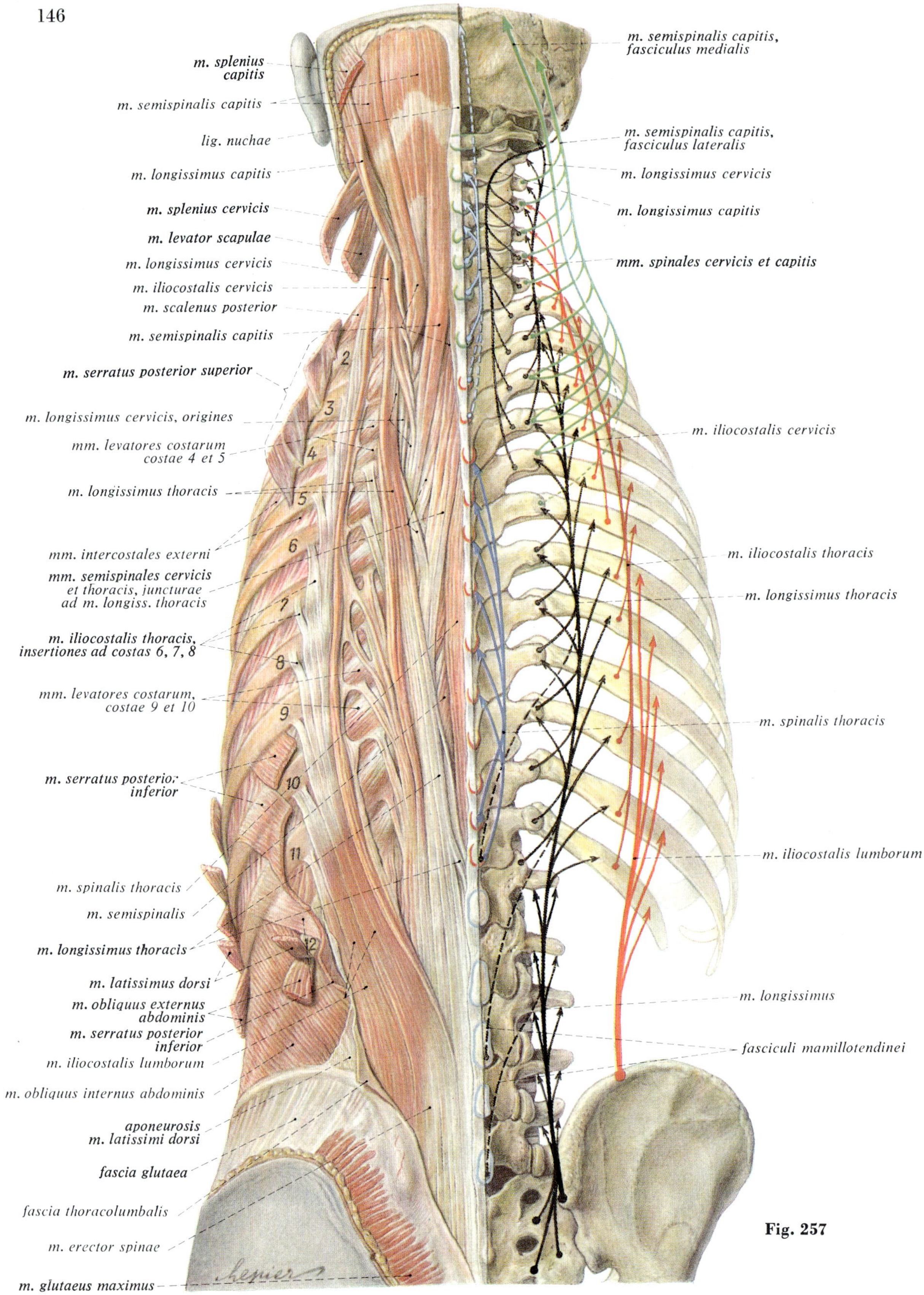
m. splenius capitis
m. semispinalis capitis
lig. nuchae
m. longissimus capitis
m. splenius cervicis
m. levator scapulae
m. longissimus cervicis
m. iliocostalis cervicis
m. scalenus posterior
m. semispinalis capitis
m. serratus posterior superior
m. longissimus cervicis, origines
mm. levatores costarum costae 4 et 5
m. longissimus thoracis
mm. intercostales externi
mm. semispinales cervicis et thoracis, juncturae ad m. longiss. thoracis
m. iliocostalis thoracis, insertiones ad costas 6, 7, 8
mm. levatores costarum, costae 9 et 10
m. serratus posterior inferior
m. spinalis thoracis
m. semispinalis
m. longissimus thoracis
m. latissimus dorsi
m. obliquus externus abdominis
m. serratus posterior inferior
m. iliocostalis lumborum
m. obliquus internus abdominis
aponeurosis m. latissimi dorsi
fascia glutaea
fascia thoracolumbalis
m. erector spinae
m. glutaeus maximus
m. semispinalis capitis, fasciculus medialis
m. semispinalis capitis, fasciculus lateralis
m. longissimus cervicis
m. longissimus capitis
mm. spinales cervicis et capitis
m. iliocostalis cervicis
m. iliocostalis thoracis
m. longissimus thoracis
m. spinalis thoracis
m. iliocostalis lumborum
m. longissimus
fasciculi mamillotendinei
2
3
4
5
6
7
8
9
10
11
12

Fig. 257

The Spinae Muscles (Sacrospinalis) (Fig. 257)

Name		*Origin*	*Insertion*
1. m. iliocostalis (lateral column): Os ilium to ribs to ribs (red lines)			
a–c continuous without sharp delineations	a) *Lumbar section:* m. iliocostalis lumborum	As the m. erector spinae joins with the m. longissimus from the labium externum cristae iliacae	The angles of ribs 5 to 12 Cranial: tendinous Caudal: fleshy
	b) *Dorsal section:* m. iliocostalis thoracis	Individual slips from the 12th to the 7th ribs	By thin tendons on angles of the upper 6 ribs and to the transverse process of the 7th cervical vertebra
	c) *Cervical section:* m. iliocostalis cervicis	Cranial and middle ribs (2nd to 6th)	Transverse processes of the 4th to the 7th cervical vertebrae
2. m. longissimus (intermediate column, the longest) Os sacrum to transverse process to transvers process (black lines)			
	a) *m. longissimus thoracis* blends with m. longissimus cervicis and then with the m. spinalis	As the m. erector spinae joins with the m. iliocostalis from the sacrum and transverse processes of lumbar vertebrae (tendinous) with some slips from transverse processes of thoracic vertebrae	*Cranial:* rounded tendons *Caudal:* fleshy *Medial:* processus accessorii of upper lumbar vertebrae; transverse processes of thoracic vertebrea *Lateral:* Slips to processus costarii of lumbar vertebrae and all ribs between the anguli et tubercula
	b) m. longissimus cervicis	Transverse processes of upper 4 or 5 thoracic vertebrae	Transverse processes of 2nd to 6th cervical vertebrae (tendinous)
	c) m. longissimus capitis	Transverse processes of the upper thoracic vertebrae and the transverse and articular processes of middle and lower cervical vertebrae	Dorsal margin of the processus mastoideus ossis temporalis
3. mm. spinalis (medial column): Spinous process to spinous process (blue lines)			
m. spinalis thoracis (continuation of m. sacrospinalis)		Spinous processes of the caudal thoracic vertebrae (blending with the m. longissimus)	Spinous processes of 3rd to 9th thoracic vertebrae
m. spinalis cervicis (inconstant)		Lower 2 cervical and first 2 thoracic spinous processes	Spinous processes of axis and 2nd and 3rd cervical vertebrae
m. spinalis capitis (Rarely a separate muscle, usually fused with the m. semispinalis capitis)		Spinous processes of the lower cervical and upper thoracic vertebrae	With m. semispinalis capitis between the linea superior and inferior nuchae on the occipital bone

Nerve: Rami dorsales of all spinal nerves (cervical, thoracic, and lumbar)

Action: Muscles of both sides, acting together, extend the vertebral column and assist in maintaining erect posture. Muscles of one side, acting alone, bend vertebral column to the side

Fig. 257. Neck and long back muscles. Left: Deeper layers. Right: Diagram of origins, course, and insertion of the back muscles. Outline of spinous processes of: lumbar vertebrae, bright blue; the thoracic vertebrae, red; the cervical vertebrae, green. The longissimus muscle column, black.

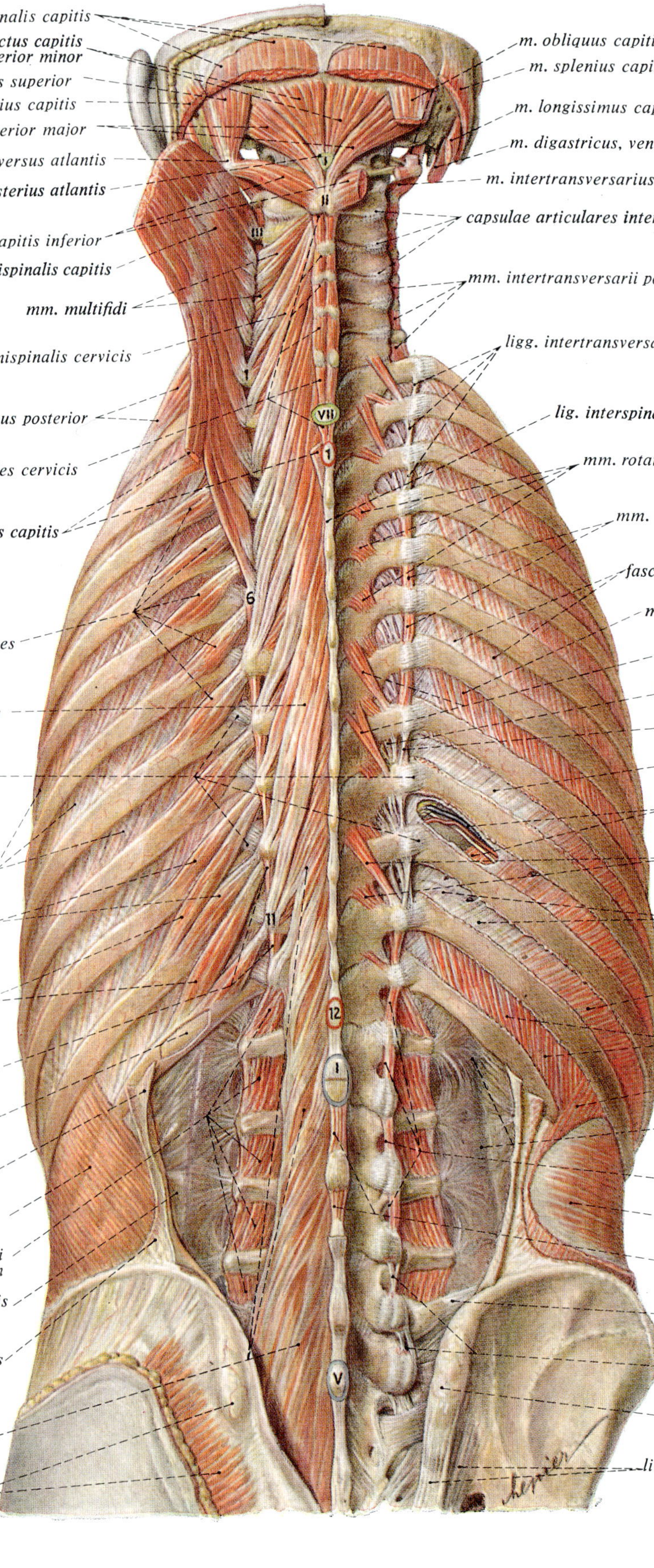
m. semispinalis capitis
m. rectus capitis posterior minor
m. obliquus capitis superior
m. splenius capitis
m. rectus capitis posterior major
processus transversus atlantis
tuberculum posterius atlantis
m. obliquus capitis inferior
m. semispinalis capitis
mm. multifidi
m. semispinalis cervicis
m. scalenus posterior
mm. interspinales cervicis
m. spinalis capitis
mm. levatores costarum breves
m. semispinalis thoracis
ligg. costotransversaria lateralia
fascia mm. intercostalium ext.
mm. levatores costarum breves
mm. levatores costarum longi
mm. intertransversarii thoracis
costa 12, periosteum depellatum
fascia thoracolumbalis
m. obliquus internus abdominis
mm. intertransversarii laterales lumborum
fascia transversalis
m. obliquus externus abdominis
mm. multifidi
spina iliaca post. sup. et m. glutaeus maximus
m. obliquus capitis superior
m. splenius capitis
m. longissimus capitis
m. digastricus, venter posterius
m. intertransversarius cervicis
capsulae articulares intervertebrales
mm. intertransversarii posteriores cervicis
ligg. intertransversaria
lig. interspinale
mm. rotatores thoracis breves
mm. intertransversarii
fascia mm. intercostalium ext.
mm. intercostales externi
mm. rotatores longi
lig. costotransversarium superius
lig. intertransversarium
membrana intercostalis interna
n. a. v. intercostales et m. intercostalis intimus
mm. rotatores longi et breves
membrana intercostalis interna
m. intercostalis internus
m. intercostalis externus
m. obliquus internus abd.
margo m. quadrati lumborum
mm. intertransversarii mediales lumborum
m. transversus abdominis
mm. interspinales lumborum
lig. iliolumbale
ligg. intertransversaria
spina iliaca post. sup.
lig. sacrotuberale
I
II
III
VII
1
6
11
12
V

Fig. 258

Deep Layer of Back Muscles, Transversospinal Muscles (Figs. 256–258, 260)

Name	*Origin*	*Insertion*
1. m. semispinalis thoracis **m. semispinalis cervicis** (without separate boundaries)	Pass obliquely upward and medially from the transverse process to the spinous processes, hence the name transversospinal. Absent in the lumbar vertebrae	
	Transverse processes of all thoracic vertebrae	Spinous processes 4 to 6 segments higher than their origin, including the spine of the axis
m. semispinalis capitis (transversooccipitalis, largest muscle in back of neck with 1 or 2 conspicuous tendinous intersections. Fig. 257)	Transverse processes of 3 cervical and 5 or 6 thoracic vertebrae	Between the linea nuchalis superior et inferior

Nerve: Rami dorsales of the cervical and thoracic nerves

Action: Extend vertebral column (especially the cervical vertebrae) and head, bending the head backwards. Unilateral innervation draws the muscle of the head toward the opposing side. Together, with the m. sternocleidomastoideus, supports the head

2. mm. multifidi (spans 2 or 3 vertebrae)	Dorsal surface of the sacrum; transverse processes of lumbar, thoracic, and lower cervical vertebrae	Spinous process of lumbar, thoracic, and cervical vertebrae up to the axis
3. mm. rotatores cervicis The mm. rotatores breves link adjacent vertebrae; the mm. rotatores longi skip one vertebra **mm. rotatores thoracis** **mm. rotatores lumborum**	Transverse process of the cervical vertebrae Transverse process of thoracic vertebrae Transverse process of the lumbar vertebrae	Roots of the spinous processes of the adjacent or the second vertebra above

Nerve: Rami dorsales of the spinal nerves: cervical, thoracic, and (lumbar) nerves

Action: Also of the transversospinal group. When acting bilaterally, they all extend the vertebral column. When acting individually and unilaterally, they bend the vertebral column to the side and rotate the vertebrae

Fig. 258. Deep neck and back musculature. Transversospinal group.

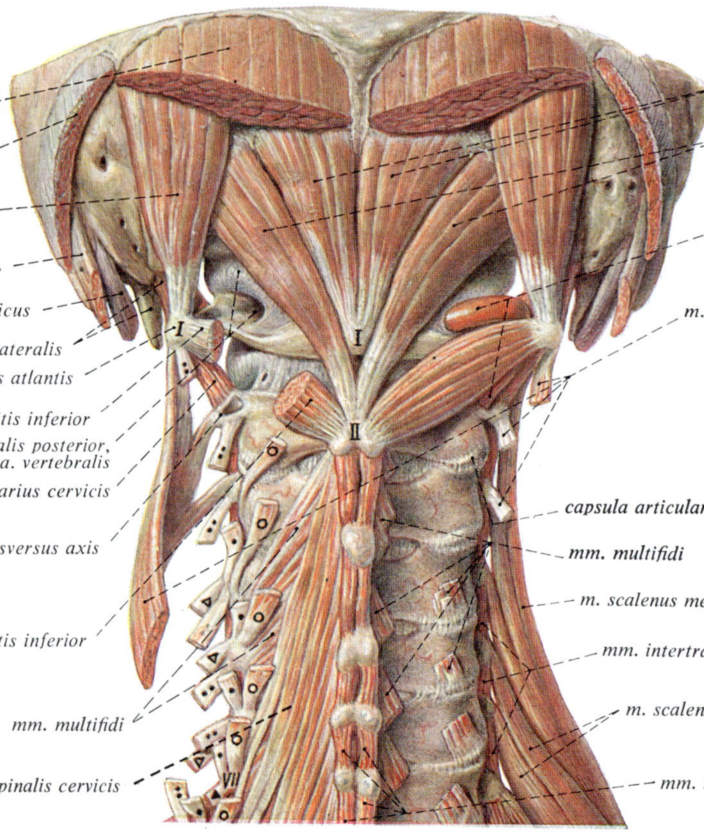

Fig. 259. Middle and deep layers of the neck musculature. The suboccipital triangle.

Note: The vertebral artery (Fig. 259) is deep in the suboccipital triangle, bounded by the *m. obliquus capitis superior* and *inferior* and the *m. rectus capitis posterior major*. After passing through the *foramen transversarium atlantis,* the vertebral artery runs directly medial in its groove in the *atlas*, and passes through the *membrana atlantooccipitalis posterior* and the *dura*, through the *foramen occipitale magnum* to supply part of the brain.

Short Suboccipital Muscles (Transversospinal muscles) (Figs. 258, 259)

Name	*Origin*	*Insertion*
1. m. rectus capitis posterior major	Spinous process of the axis (II)	linea nuchae inferior
2. m. rectus capitis posterior minor	tuberculum posterius atlantis	Medial part of the linea nuchae inferior of the os occipitale
3. m. rectus capitis lateralis (Fig. 281)	Processus transversus atlantis	Processus jugularis ossis occipitalis
4. m. obliquus capitis superior	Processus tranversus atlantis	Os occipitale, above the linea nuchalis inferior
5. m. obliquus capitis inferior	Spinous process of the axis (II)	Processus transversus atlantis

Nerve: n. suboccipitalis (ramus dorsalis of the first cervical nerve)

Action: Extend and rotate head. The mm. rectus capitis posterior major and obliquus capitis inferior turn the head to the same side; the m. rectus capitis lateralis bends the head laterally (unilateral innervation)

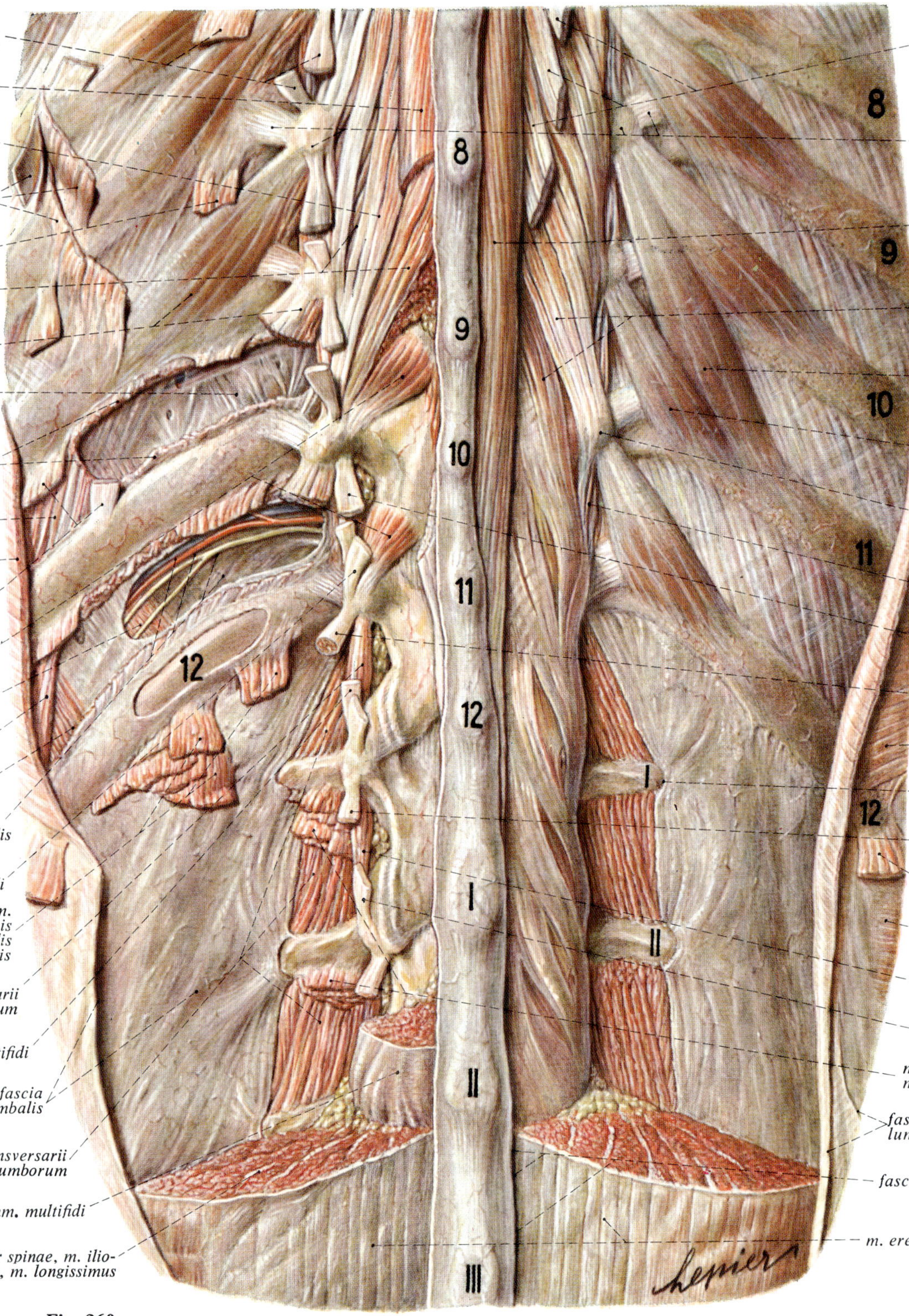
m. longissimus thoracis
m. spinalis
m. semispinalis thoracis
m. iliocostalis thoracis
m. longissimus thoracis
mm. multifidi
m. levator costae brevis
membrana intercostalis interna
mm. intercostales externi
mm. intercostales externi
m. serratus post. inferior
m. iliocostalis thoracis
mm. rotatores
mm. intercostales intimi
mm. intercostales externi
mm. intercostales interni
v. a. n. intercostalis
mm. multifidi
insertiones m. longissimi thoracis et m. iliocostalis thoracis
mm. intertransversarii lumborum
mm. multifidi
fascia thoracolumbalis
mm. intertransversarii lumborum
mm. multifidi
m. erector spinae, m. iliocostalis, m. longissimus
m. semispinali thoracis
lig. costotransversarium laterale, processus transversus vertebrae thoracicae 9
m. spinalis
mm. multific
m. levator costae longi
m. levator costae brev
proc. transversus vertebrae thoracicae
lig. intertra versarium
m. longissi thoracis
m. longissim thoracis
m. serratus post. inf.
processus tra versus verteb lumbalis I
m. longissimu
m. obliquus internus abdominis
m. transversu abdominis
mm. intertransversa lumboru
mm. multifidi
m. erector spinae m. longissimus
fascia thoraco-lumbalis
fascia thoracolumba
m. erector spinae
8
9
10
11
12
I
II
III
Lenier

Fig. 260

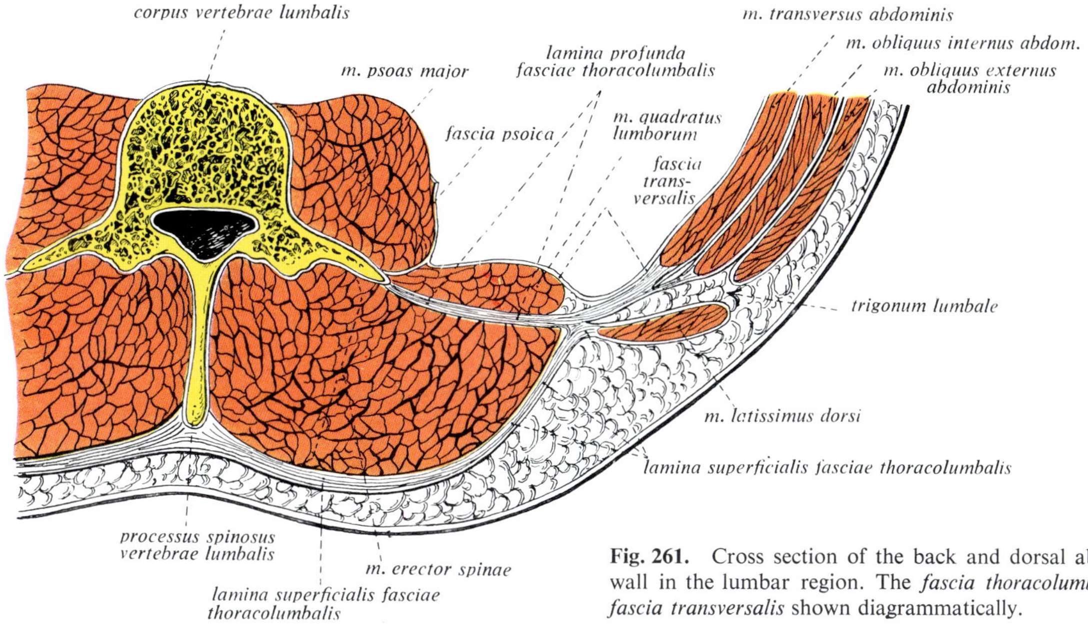

Fig. 261. Cross section of the back and dorsal abdominal wall in the lumbar region. The *fascia thoracolumbalis* and *fascia transversalis* shown diagrammatically.

Note: *Fascia thoracolumbalis (aponeurosis lumbodorsalis):* A tendonous sheath from the mm. *transversus abdominis, latissimus dors,* and *serratus posterior inferior.* It is fastened on the processus spinosus with the posterior layer *(lamina superficialis),* on the transverse processes of the lumbar vertebrae with the anterior layers *(lamina profunda)*, and is stretched between the 12th rib and *crista iliaca.*

Lumbar triangle *(trigonum lumbale)* is a small triangular interval of the back bordered by the *m. obliquus externus abdominis* and by the *m. latissimus dorsi* and the *crista iliaca* (Figs. 255, 261). Occasionally it is the site of a hernia.

Fascia transversalis: The inner surface of the peritoneal musculature is separated from the peritoneum by the *fascia transversalis.* Among other things, it strengthens the dorsal wall of the canalis inguinalis. The principal outpouching of the *fascia transversalis* is the *fascia spermatica interna (tunica vaginalis communis)* which invests the inner part of the spermatic cord and testis.

Vasa intercostalia, n. intercostalis (ramus ventralis): In the middle part of Fig. 260, the intercostal vessels and the intercostal nerve are displayed through a window in the intercostal muscles. They run lateral to the *sulcus costae:* the *vena intercostalis posterior* is above; the *arteria intercostalis posterior,* in the middle; and the *nervus intercostalis,* below.

Fig. 260. Deep back muscles: Rotatores, Multifidi, and Levator costae. The spinous processes of the vertebral column were designated in the thoracic region with Arabic numerals 8–12; in the lumbar region with Roman numerals I–III. The first two transverse processes of the lumbar vertebrae are also labeled I and II. The ribs 8–12 on the right are shown with Arabic numerals.

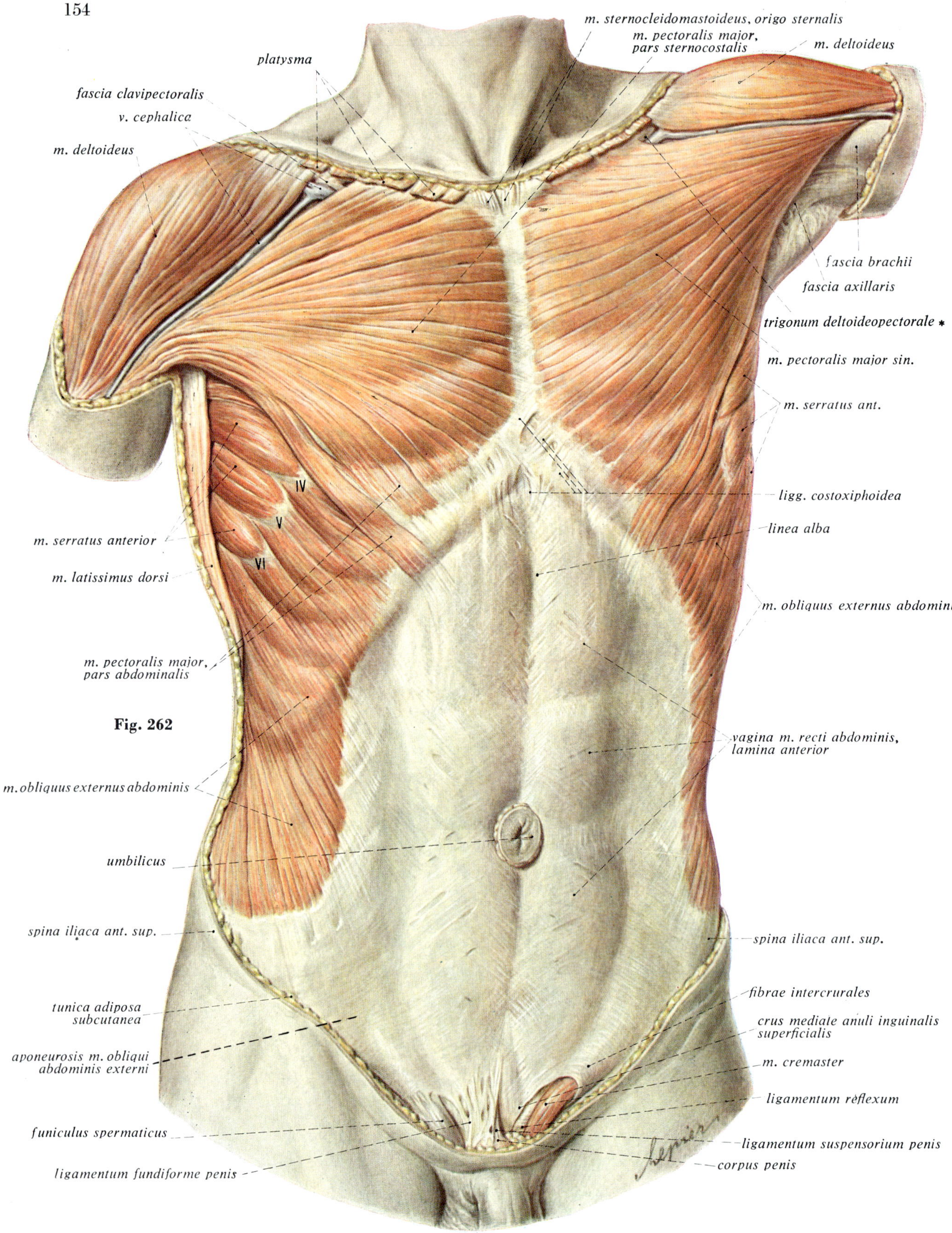

m. sternocleidomastoideus, origo sternalis
m. pectoralis major, pars sternocostalis
m. deltoideus
platysma
fascia clavipectoralis
v. cephalica
m. deltoideus
fascia brachii
fascia axillaris
trigonum deltoideopectorale *
m. pectoralis major sin.
m. serratus ant.
IV
V
VI
ligg. costoxiphoidea
linea alba
m. serratus anterior
m. latissimus dorsi
m. obliquus externus abdomini
m. pectoralis major, pars abdominalis
vagina m. recti abdominis, lamina anterior
m. obliquus externus abdominis
umbilicus
spina iliaca ant. sup.
spina iliaca ant. sup.
fibrae intercrurales
tunica adiposa subcutanea
crus mediale anuli inguinalis superficialis
aponeurosis m. obliqui abdominis externi
m. cremaster
ligamentum reflexum
funiculus spermaticus
ligamentum suspensorium penis
corpus penis
ligamentum fundiforme penis

Fig. 262

Thoracic and Abdominal Muscles (Figs. 262, 269)

Name	*Origin*	*Insertion*
1. m. pectoralis major Strong, predominantly fleshy; tendinous only at insertion	*Pars clavicularis:* Sternal half of clavicle *Pars sternocostalis:* Ventral surface of sternum and costal cartilages 2 to 6 *Pars abdominalis:* A slip from the aponeurosis of the m. obliquus externus abdominis	All fibers converge toward a flat tendon (5 cm broad) which is inserted into the crista tuberculi majoris humeri

Nerve: Rami pectorales lat. et med. from the plexus brachialis (C 5 – T 1)

Action: Flexes, adducts, and rotates the arm medially. Powerful adduction (lowering the raised arm). In many cases, works with other muscles (mm. latissimus dorsi and trapezius)

2. m. pectoralis minor (Weak and moderately flat)	Ribs 2 to 5 near the cartilage-bone junction	Processus coracoideus scapulae (medial border)

Nerve: Rami pectorales mediales (C 8 – T 1)

Action: Depresses the shoulder, raises ribs in forced inspiration; seldom functions alone, but with the mm. serratus anterior and trapezius, etc.

3. m. subclavius	Short, thick tendon on 1st rib at junction of cartilage and bone	Acromial end of clavicle

Nerve: n. subclavius from the plexus brachialis

Action: Adequate for such a small muscle; assists in drawing the shoulder forward and downward

4. m. serratus anterior	With fleshy digitations from first 9 ribs, consisting of 3 parts. The middle is the weakest; the caudal, the strongest	
(Pars superior)	Ribs 1 and 2, somewhat converging	angulus superior scapulae
(Pars media)	Ribs 2–4, diverging	margo medialis scapulae
(Pars inferior)	Ribs 5–9, strongly converging	angulus inferior scapulae

Nerve: N. thoracicus longus from the plexus brachialis (C 5, 6, 7)

Action: Holds scapula closely to the body, draws scapula forward as in a pushing action. Assists in flexion and abduction of the arm

◀ **Fig. 262.** Pectoral and abdominal musculature. Ventral view of superficial layer. Ribs: IV–VI.

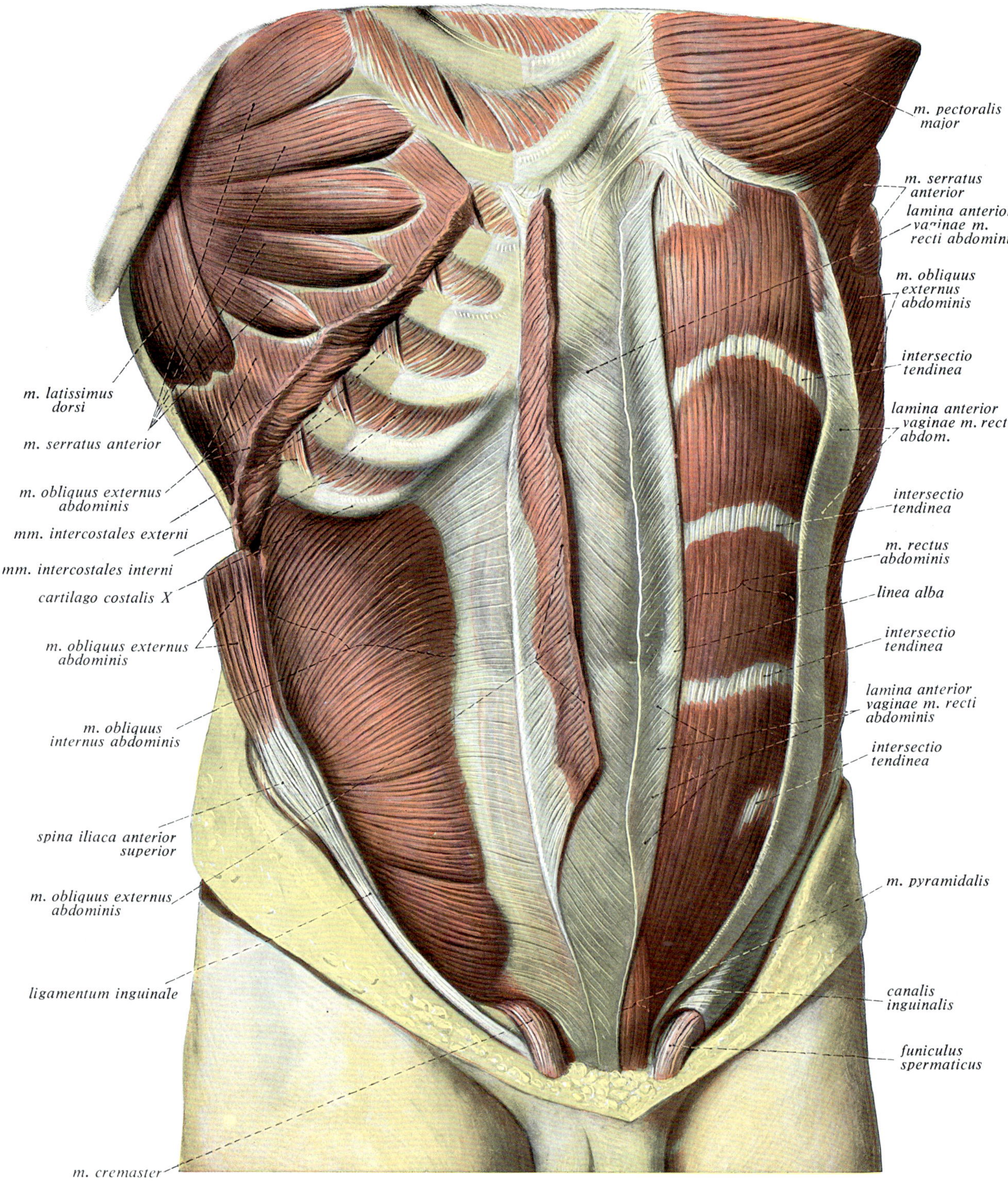

Fig. 263. Abdominal musculature, second layer (from ventral and right). *Left:* The outer layer of rectus sheath has been opened along its midline, to display the *mm. rectus abdominis* and *pyramidalis*. *Right:* The *m. obliquus abdominalis externus* has been transected and 3 flaps reflected to display the *m. obliquus abdominalis internus*.

Muscles of the Abdomen, Superficial Layers (Figs. 262, 263)

Name	*Origin*	*Insertion*
1. m. obliquus externus abdominis Course of the fibers from lateral-cranial toward the medial-caudal	Fleshy digitations from lower 8 ribs. The dorsal border is free	On labium externum cristae iliacae, on the inguinal ligament and outer layer of the rectus sheath

Nerve: Intercostal nerves, branches of lumbar plexus (n. iliohypogastricus and n. ilioinguinalis)

Action: Maintains abdominal pressure to keep viscera in position; forces viscera up to elevate diaphragm during expiration; increases abdominal pressure to initiate and aid the rectum in evacuation of its contents; both sides flex vertebral column; one side bends it laterally and rotates it

Name	*Origin*	*Insertion*
2. m. obliquus internus abdominis Course of fibers at right angles to the External oblique	Linea intermedia cristae iliacae; fascia thoracolumbalis; lateral two-thirds of the ligamentum inguinale	Fleshy digitations to lower 3 ribs (9–12), the linea alba, aponeurosis helps in formation of rectus sheath (see Fig. 263)

Nerve: Same as above

Action: Same as for External, but rotates toward the same side, supports the External of the opposing side, bends the body laterally

Name	*Origin*	*Insertion*
3. m. cremaster	Caudal fibers of the m. obliquus internus abdominalis (often from m. transversus abdominis)	Goes with the spermatic cord to the testis

Nerve: Ramus genitalis n. genitofemoralis

Action: Supports and elevates the testis

Name	*Origin*	*Insertion*
4. m. transversus abdominis	1. *Costal:* Deep surfaces of costal cartilages of lower 6 ribs 2. *Vertebral:* The fascia thoracolumbalis from the processus transversi of the lumbar vertebrae 3. *Pelvic:* Labium internum cristae iliacae; lateral third of ligamentum inguinale	Aponeurosis helps form rectus sheath; attaches to processus xiphoideus and linea alba; helps form falx inguinalis which attaches to superior border of the pubis and the linea pectinea

Nerve: Nn. intercostales, branches of plexus lumbalis (n. iliohypogastricus, n. ilioinguinalis, n. genitofemoralis)

Action: Contraction and expansion of abdominal wall, and maintains abdominal pressure to keep viscera in position

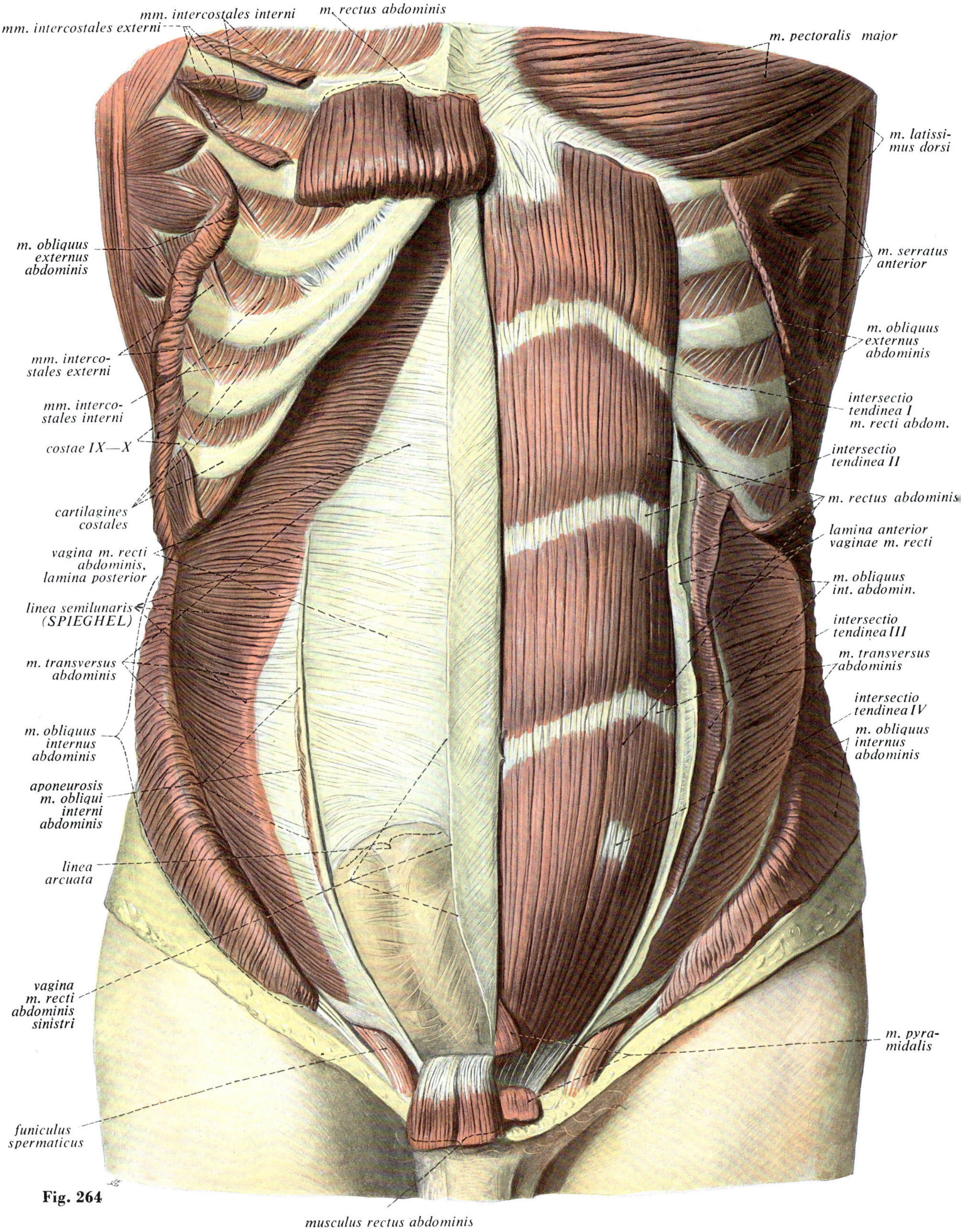
mm. intercostales interni
m. rectus abdominis
mm. intercostales externi
m. pectoralis major
m. latissimus dorsi
m. obliquus externus abdominis
m. serratus anterior
m. obliquus externus abdominis
mm. intercostales externi
intersectio tendinea I m. recti abdom.
mm. intercostales interni
costae IX—X
intersectio tendinea II
m. rectus abdominis
cartilagines costales
lamina anterior vaginae m. recti
vagina m. recti abdominis, lamina posterior
m. obliquus int. abdomin.
linea semilunaris (SPIEGHEL)
intersectio tendinea III
m. transversus abdominis
m. transversus abdominis
intersectio tendinea IV
m. obliquus internus abdominis
m. obliquus internus abdominis
aponeurosis m. obliqui interni abdominis
linea arcuata
vagina m. recti abdominis sinistri
m. pyramidalis
funiculus spermaticus
musculus rectus abdominis

Fig. 264

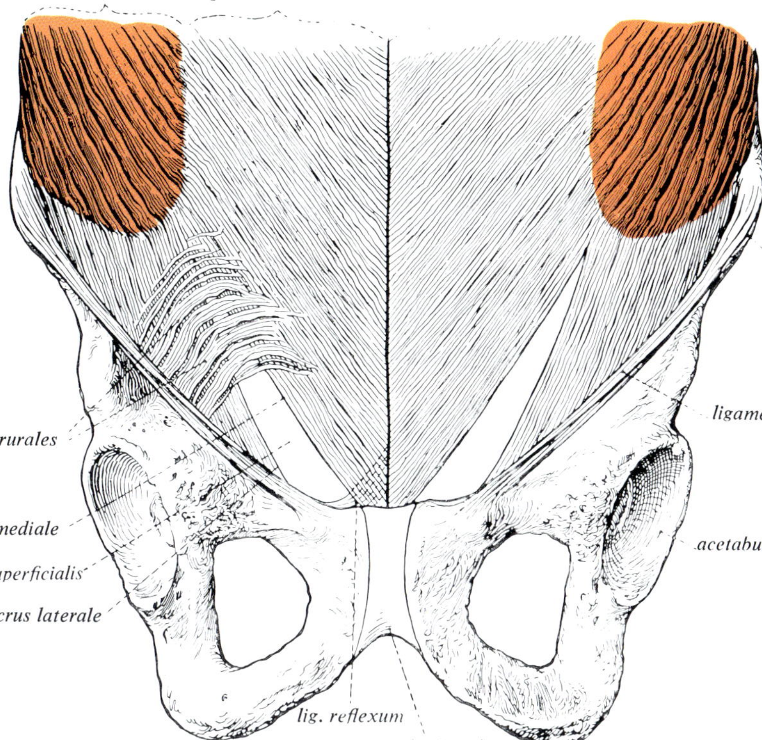

Fig. 265. A diagrammatic view of the aponeurosis of the *m. obliquus externus abdominis*, including the *fibrae intercrurales* that form the *anulus inguinalis superficialis*.

Straight Muscles of the Abdomen (Figs. 263–264)

Name	*Origin*	*Insertion*
1. m. rectus abdominis Contains 3 or 4 tendinous intersections	5th to 7th cartilage, processus xiphoideus	Cranial border of the os pubis between the tuberculum pubicum and the symphysis

Nerves: Middle and caudal nn. intercostales (T 7 – T 12) (rarely upper lumbar nerves)

Action: Flexes the vertebral column; pulls the sternum toward the pubis (antagonist of long back muscles); tenses anterior abdominal wall; and assists in compressing the abdominal contents

2. m. pyramidalis (inconstant)	Ventral surface of pubis and ligamentum pubicum anterior	Linea alba cranial to symphysis

Nerve: Branch of 12th thoracic nerve

Action: Tenses the linea alba. The size of the triangular muscle varies

Fig. 264. Deep layers of the muscles of the abdomen. *Left:* The m. rectus abdominis exposed, m. pyramidalis is cut to show the rectus tendon; in addition, the *m. obliquus internus abdominis* is cut. *Right:* The mm. rectus abdominis and obliquus internus were resected to display all the *m. transversus abdominis* and the dorsal layer of the rectus sheath with the *linea arcuata* and *linea semilunaris*.

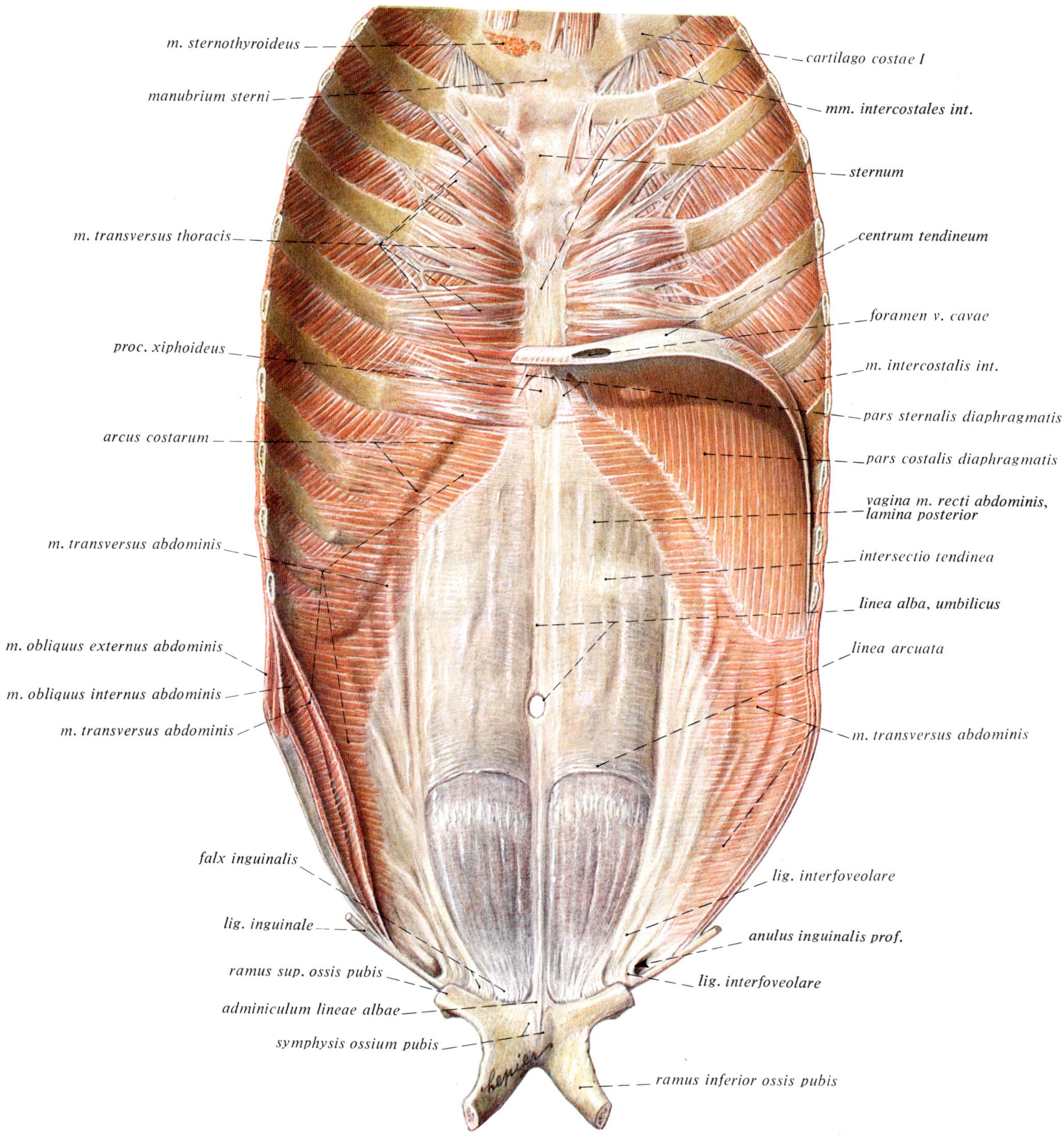

Fig. 266. Inner view of the ventral thoracic and abdominal musculature.

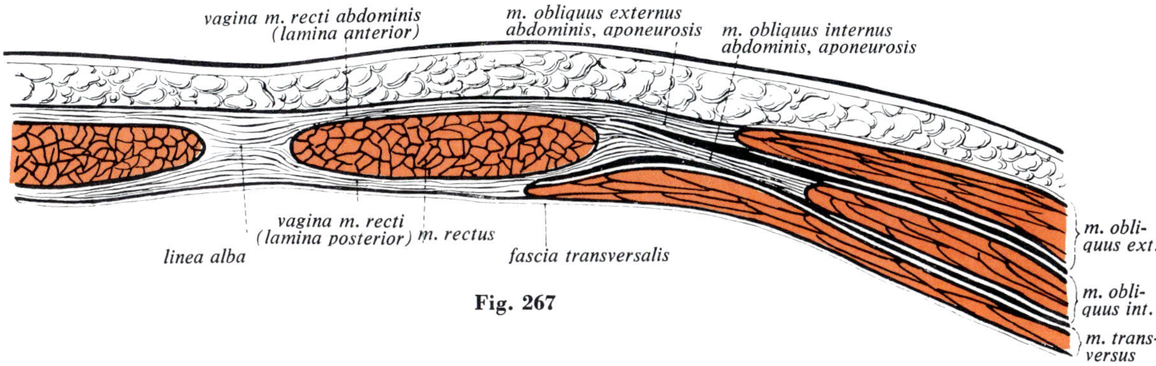

Fig. 267

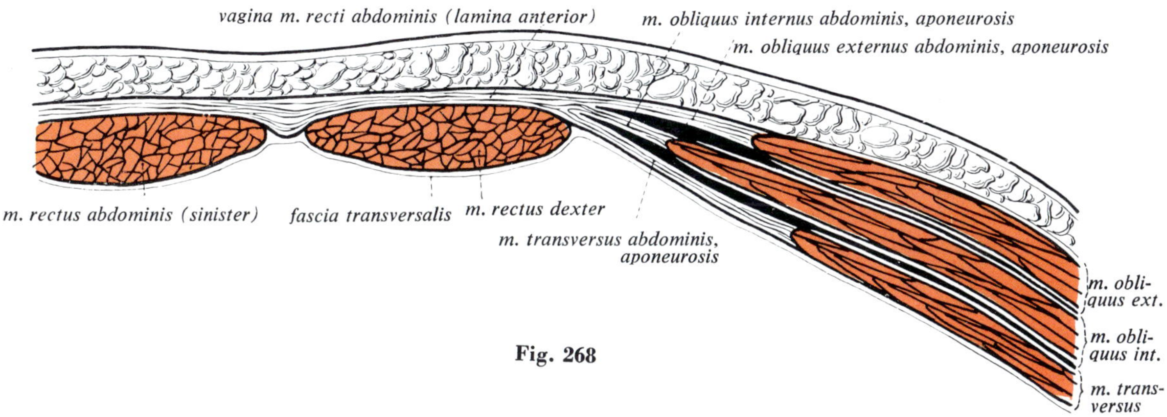

Fig. 268

Figs. 267 and 268. Diagrams of cross sections of the ventral abdominal wall. Formation and relationship of the rectus sheath and the aponeurotic tendons of the flat abdominal muscles. Fig. 267. Cranial to the *umbilicus*. Fig. 268. In the middle between the *umbilicus* and the *symphysis pubis*.

Note: The rectus sheath above the *linea arcuata* is made up of the aponeurosis of 3 wide abdominal muscles: the *m. obliquus ext.* and half of the *m. obliquus int.* form the ventral layer; the other half of the *m. obliquus internus* and the *m. transversus abdominis* form the dorsal layer. Below the *linea arcuata,* all 3 aponeuroses pass ventral to the *m. rectus*; the dorsal wall of the sheath is formed here by only the *fascia transversalis.*

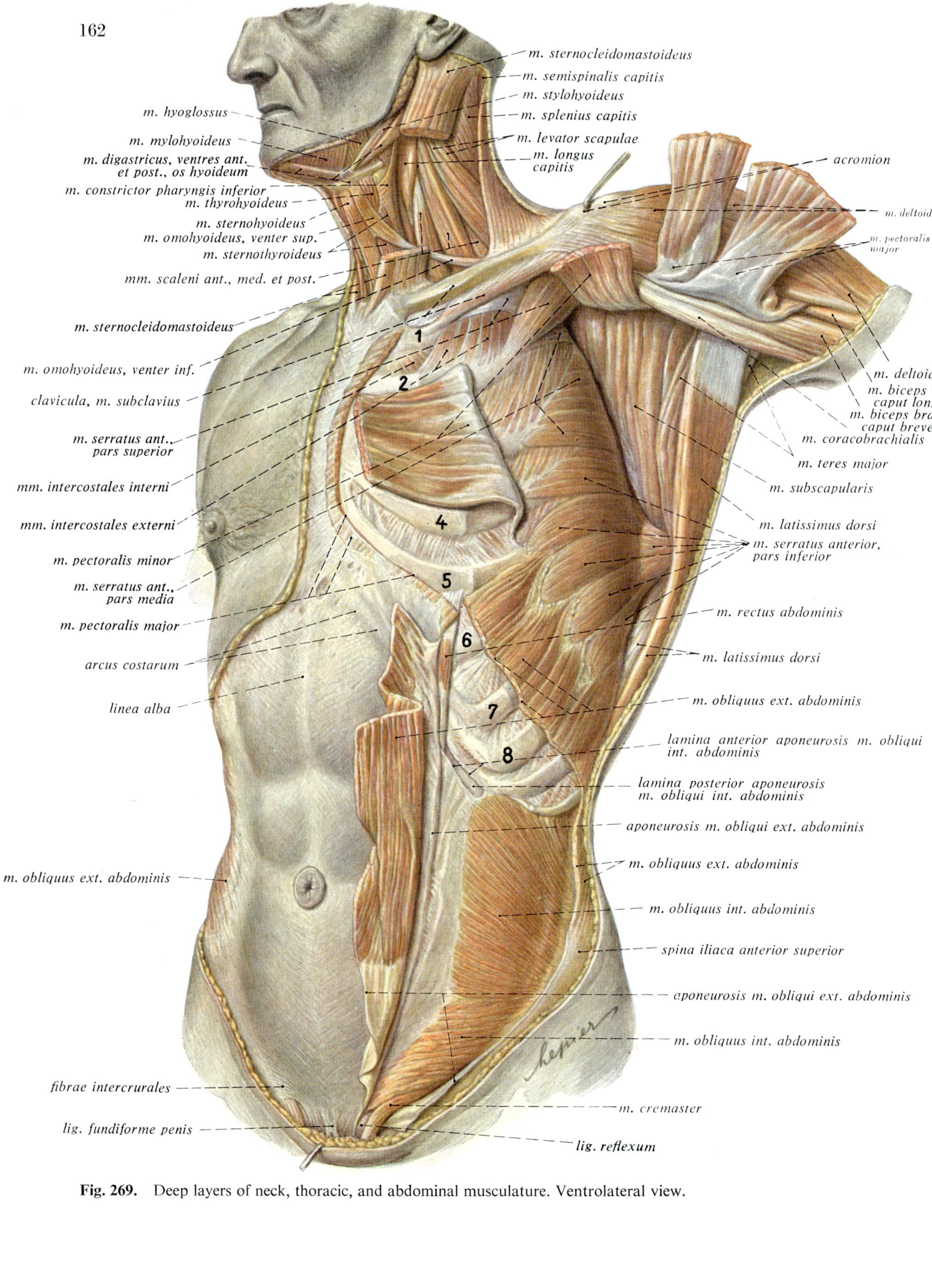

Fig. 269. Deep layers of neck, thoracic, and abdominal musculature. Ventrolateral view.

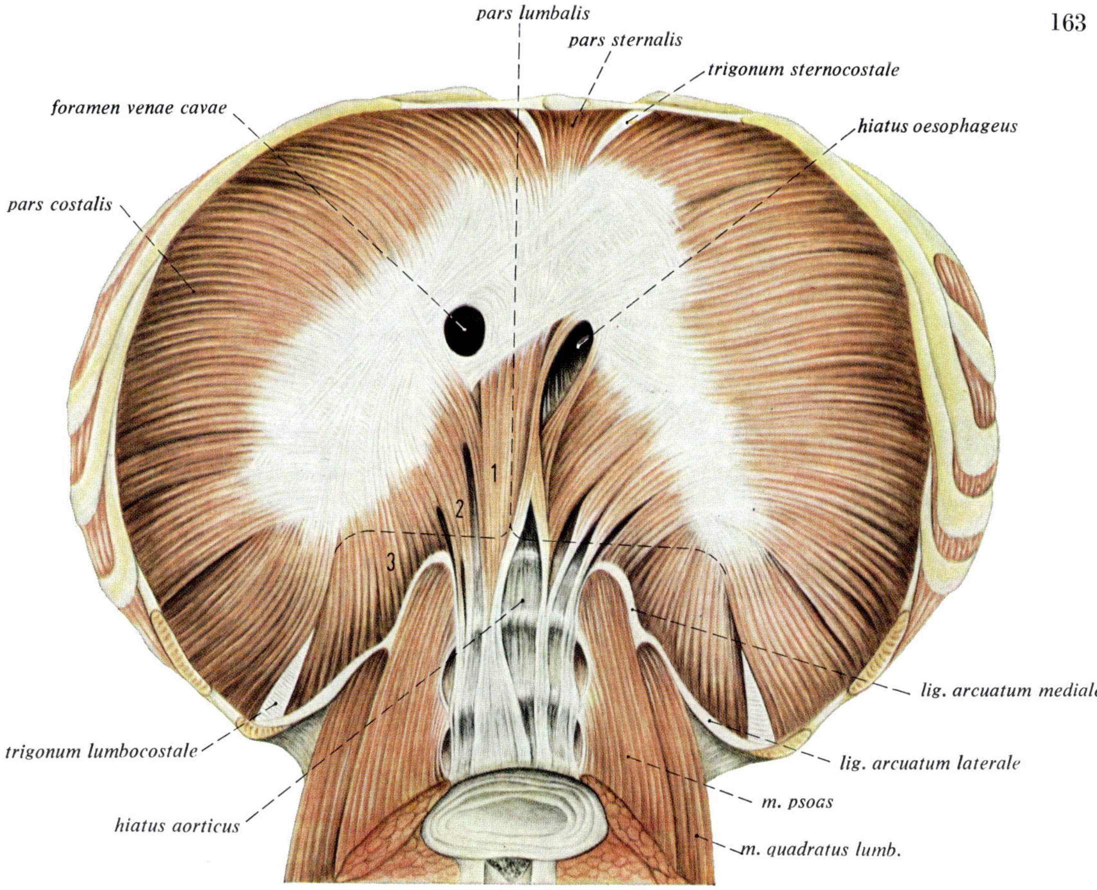

Fig. 270. Diaphragma from abdominal view: 1. *crus mediale.* 2. *crus intermedium.* 3. *crus laterale*

Diaphragma (Figs. 266, 270)

Name	*Origin*		*Insertion*
pars sternalis	Inner surface of processus xiphoideus		
pars costalis	Inner surface of 6 caudal ribs (cartilages)		
pars lumbalis	*crus mediale + crus inter-medium* (tendinous)	Ventral surface of lumbar vertebrae 2–4 (tendon), between the component of both sides: hiatus aorticus	In the central tendon: foramen v. cavae In the lumbar portion: the hiatus oesophagicus
	crus laterale	Transverse process of lumbar vertebra 1 (2); medial and lateral lumbar costal arches	

Nerve: n. phrenicus from the plexus cervicalis C 4 (3–5)

Action: Respiratory muscle (diaphragmatic breathing) produces inspiration, sustains abdominal muscular pressure

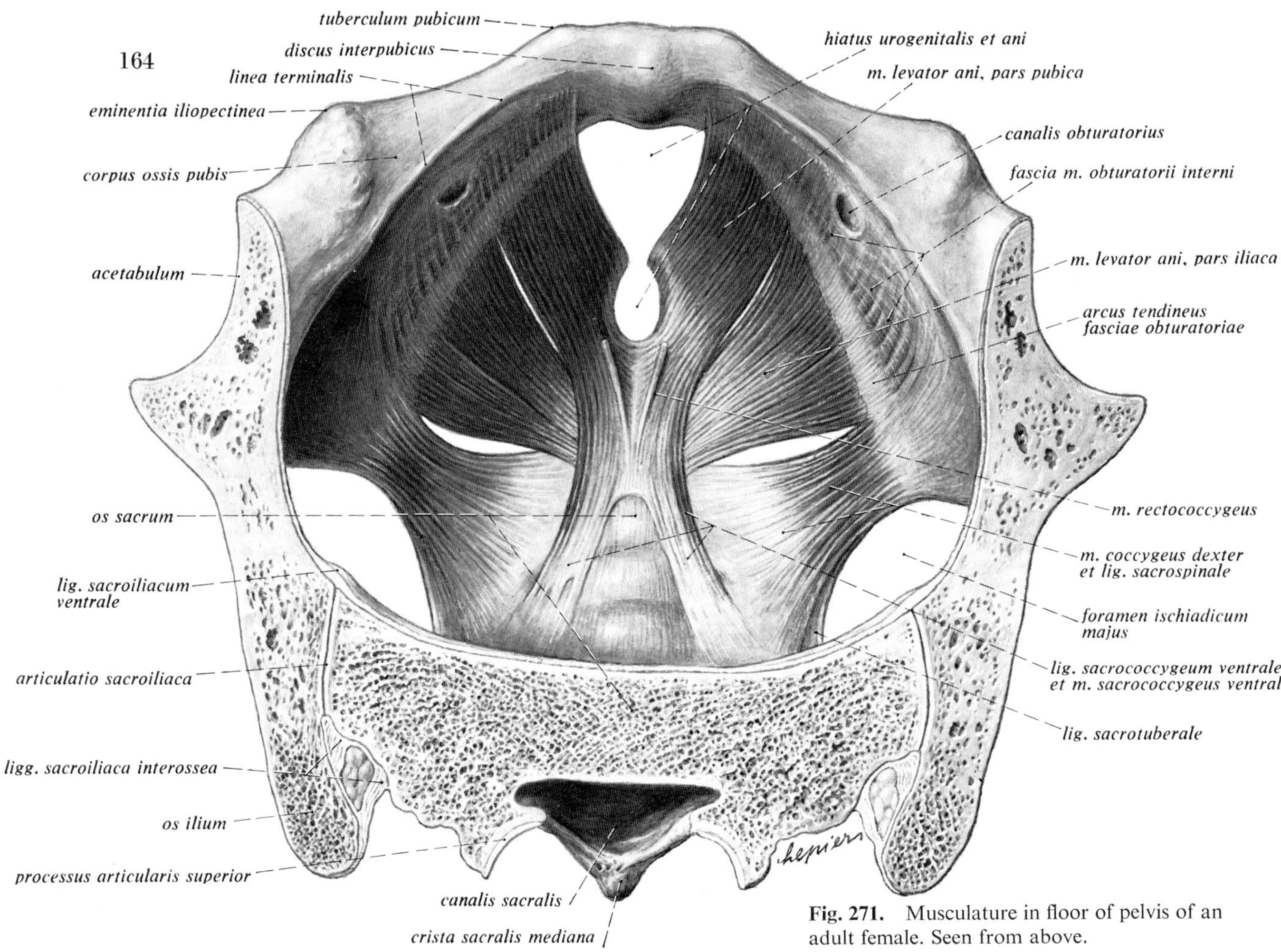

Fig. 271. Musculature in floor of pelvis of an adult female. Seen from above.

Name	*Origin*	*Insertion*
m. quadratus lumborum 4-sided muscle in dorsal wall of abdomen (Fig. 273)	Labium internum cristae iliacae, ligamentum iliolumbale	12th rib, (medial border); transverse processes of upper 4 lumbar vertebrae
Nerve: Branches of 12th thoracic and upper 3 lumbar nerves (T 12; L 1–4)		
Action: Depresses and fixes last rib (expiration); abducts or bends trunk to same side, when acting unilaterally		

Muscles of the Pelvic Floor (Figs. 271, 272)

I. diaphragma pelvis		
1. m. levator ani, funnel-shaped, made up of several muscle parts: mm. pubococcygicus, puborectalis, iliococcygicus, levator prostatae	arcus tendineus m. levatoris ani (spans the m. obturator internus from the symphysis to the spina ischiadica)	os sacrum, os coccygicum, m. sphincter ani externus
Nerve: Plexus pudendalis, nn. sacrales (S 3–5)		
Action: Supports and slightly raises the pelvic floor		
2. m. coccygeus	spina ischiadica	os sacrum and os coccygis

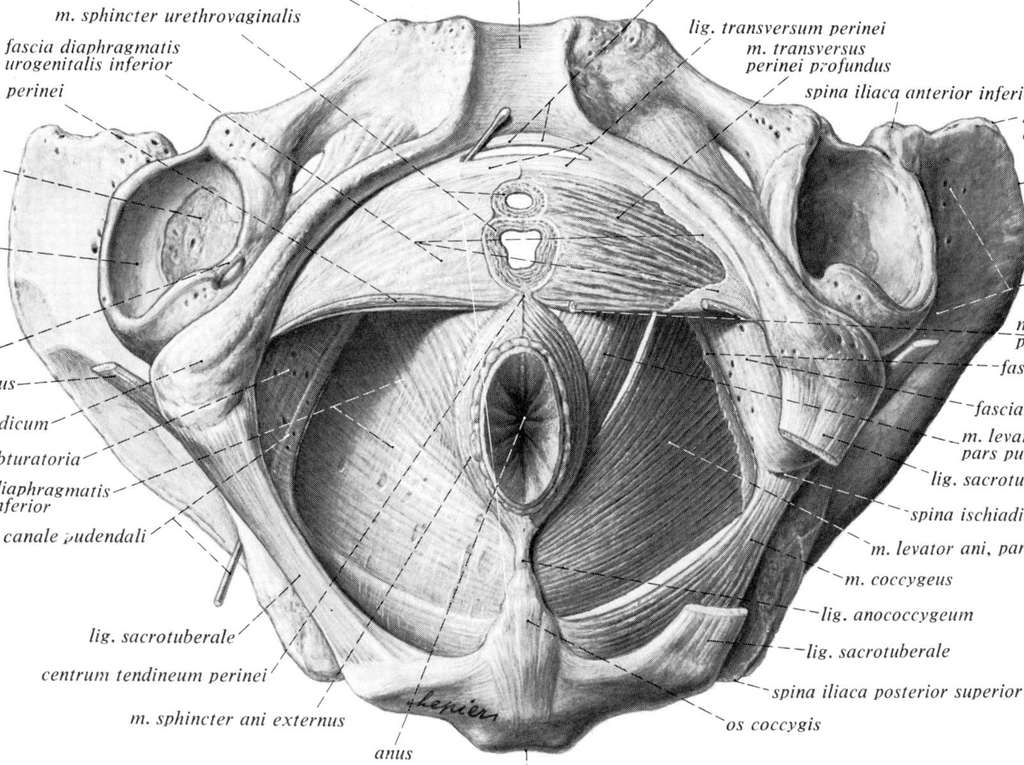

Fig. 272. Musculature in floor of pelvis of an adult female. Perineal view. Sound in pudendal canal (ALCOCK).

Muscles of the Pelvic Floor (continued)

II. m. sphincter ani externus
(pars subcutanea, pars superficialis, pars profunda)

III. diaphragma urogenitale

1. **m. transversus perinei profundus:** Stretches between the *rami ischiadici*, completed by the *ligamentum transversum perinei* and *ligamentum arcuatum pubis*. The male urethra or the urethra and vagina pass through this.
2. **m. transversus perinei superficialis (variable)**
   Nerve: both muscles perineal branches of *n. pudendus* (S 2–4)

centrum tendineum perinei: A knotty-like tendinous tissue for all muscles of the pelvic floor. It is interlaced anteriorly with the *m. sphincter ani externus*, with the dorsal border of the *m. transversus perinei profundus*, involving in addition, the *mm. levator ani* and *bulbospongiosus*.

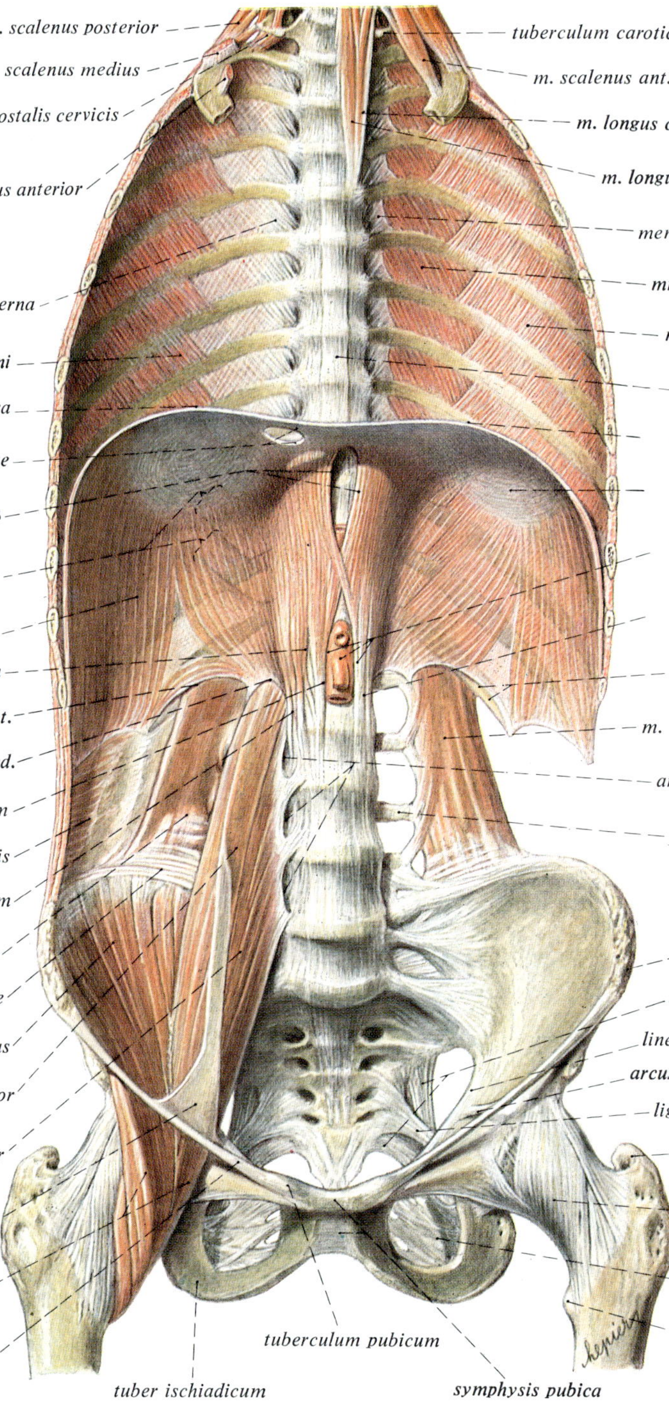

Fig. 273. The thoracic cavity *(cavum thoracis)*, the *diaphragma*, the dorsal psoas musculature, and the *pelvis*. Ventral view.

Muscles

Head and Neck

Fig. 274. *Platysma.* The skin and subcutaneous fatty tissue were removed from the lower jaw region of the right side of the neck and upper thorax.

Fig. 275. Head, neck, and upper thorax, showing triangles of the neck. The facial muscles for expression and part of the muscles of mastication, cervical muscles, the *mm. deltoideus*, *pectoralis major*, *trigonum caroticum* and *plexus brachialis*. The lower part of the parotid gland is pulled back with a hook.

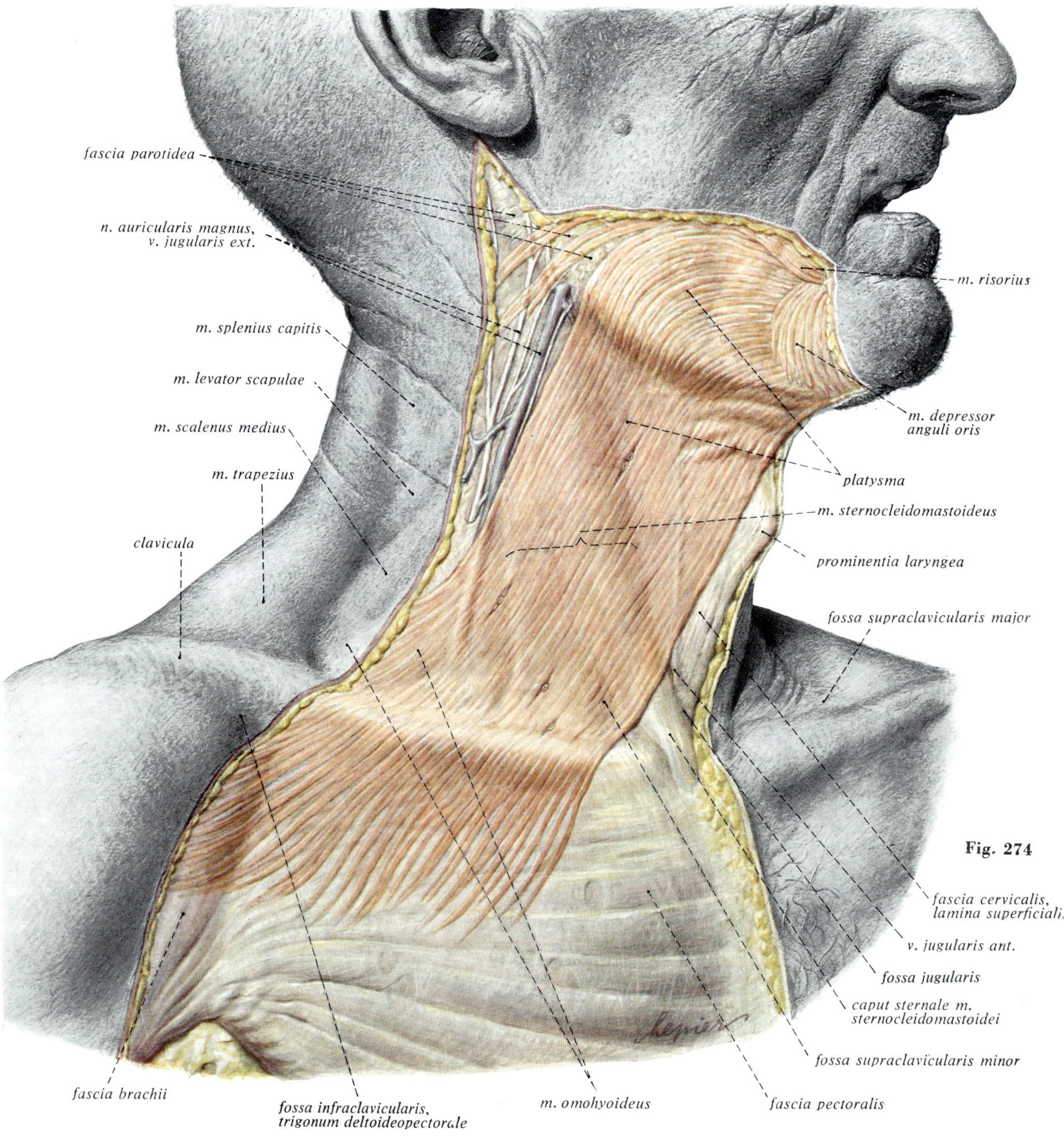

Fig. 274

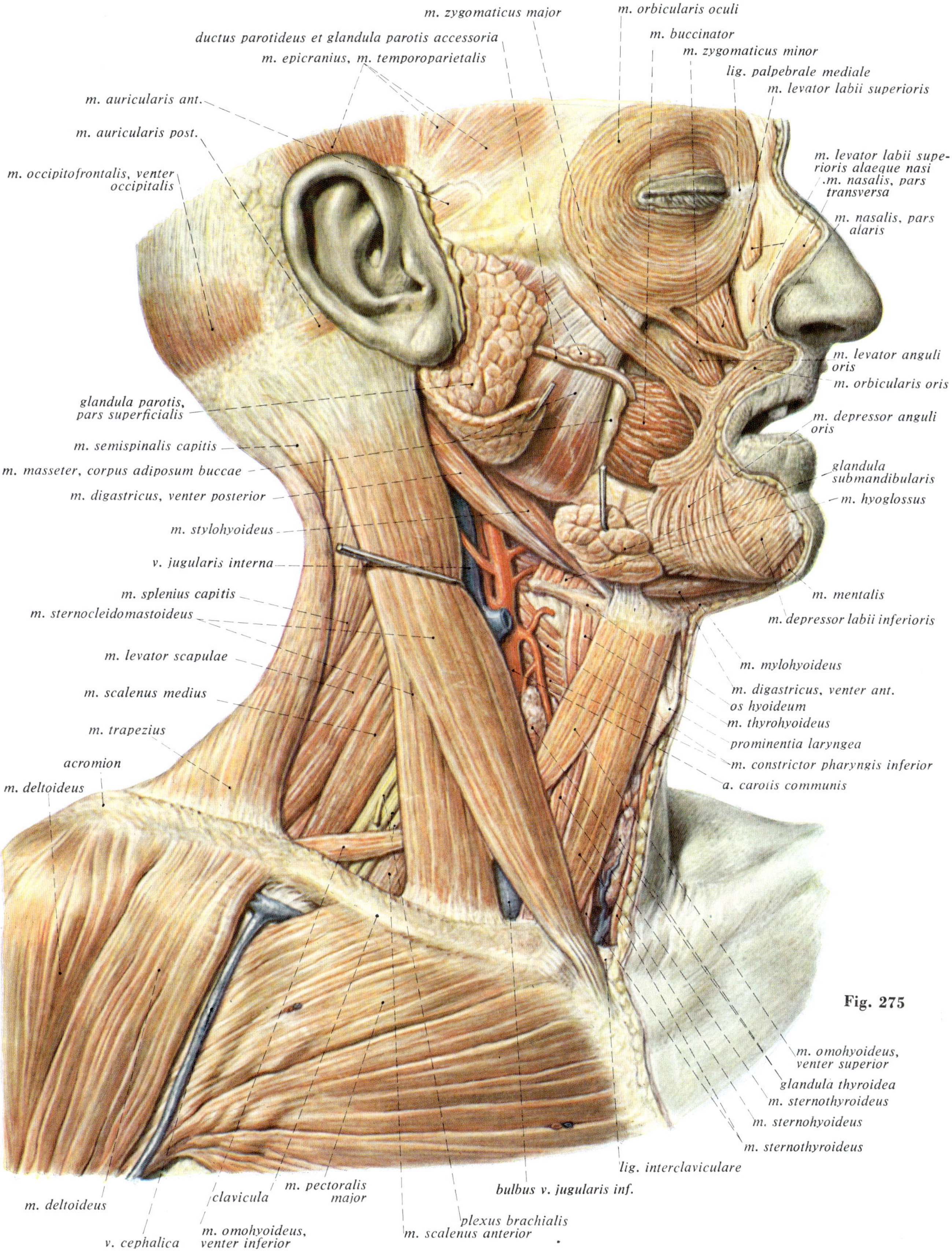
m. zygomaticus major
m. orbicularis oculi
ductus parotideus et glandula parotis accessoria
m. buccinator
m. zygomaticus minor
m. epicranius, m. temporoparietalis
lig. palpebrale mediale
m. levator labii superioris
m. auricularis ant.
m. auricularis post.
m. levator labii superioris alaeque nasi
m. nasalis, pars transversa
m. occipitofrontalis, venter occipitalis
m. nasalis, pars alaris
m. levator anguli oris
m. orbicularis oris
glandula parotis, pars superficialis
m. depressor anguli oris
m. semispinalis capitis
glandula submandibularis
m. masseter, corpus adiposum buccae
m. hyoglossus
m. digastricus, venter posterior
m. stylohyoideus
v. jugularis interna
m. mentalis
m. splenius capitis
m. sternocleidomastoideus
m. depressor labii inferioris
m. levator scapulae
m. mylohyoideus
m. digastricus, venter ant.
m. scalenus medius
os hyoideum
m. thyrohyoideus
m. trapezius
prominentia laryngea
acromion
m. constrictor pharyngis inferior
m. deltoideus
a. carotis communis
m. omohyoideus, venter superior
glandula thyroidea
m. sternothyroideus
m. sternohyoideus
m. sternothyroideus
lig. interclaviculare
m. pectoralis major
bulbus v. jugularis inf.
m. deltoideus
clavicula
plexus brachialis
m. omohyoideus, venter inferior
m. scalenus anterior
v. cephalica

Fig. 275

The Suprahyoid Muscles* (Figs. 276, 277, 279, 289)

Name	*Origin*	*Insertion*
1. m. digastricus Divided into 2 bellies by a tendon. These are fastened through a short tendon to the margin of the hyoid bone	Incisura mastoidea ossis temporalis (venter posterior)	Fossa digastrica mandibulae (venter anterior)
Nerve: Venter anterior: n. mylohyoideus. Venter posterior: n. facialis		
Action: Opens jaws (depresses lower jaw); elevates (fixes) the hyoid bone		
2. m. stylohyoideus Passes on either side of tendon of the m. digastricus	Processus styloideus ossis temporalis	Lateral margin of the body of the hyoid bone near the cornu majus
Nerve: n. facialis		
Action: Fixes hyoid bone; it pulls the hyoid bone backward and upward during deglutition		
3. m. mylohyoideus The muscles of both sides in midline are united by a raphe	Linea mylohyoidea mandibulae. The muscles form a fleshy plate across the mandibular arch	Raphe mylohyoidea and cranial margin of body of hyoid bone
Nerve: n. mylohyoideus from mandibular division of trigeminal nerve		
Action: Elevates oral floor and tongue during deglutition; depresses mandible, or elevates hyoid bone		
4. m. geniohyoideus It borders directly on the tongue muscles, especially the m. genioglossus	Spina mentalis mandibulae, short tendon	Ventral margin of body of hyoid bone
	Muscles on both sides lie close together, a thin connective tissue-like septum separates them in the midline	
Nerve: n. hypoglossus		
Action: Supports the action of m. mylohyoideus (elevates the tongue); elevates and fixes hyoid bone; depresses mandible		

* In contrast to the Infrahyoid muscles, the Suprahyoid muscles belong to the muscles of the head, since they connect only bones of the head. The *m. digastricus* is not a true Hyoid muscle, since it is only indirectly connected with the hyoid bone.

Name		*Origin*	*Insertion*
1. m. sternocleidomastoideus (Fig. 275)			
	Sternal head:	Ventral surface of the manubrium sterni	Lateral surface of processus mastoideus and linea nuchae superior
	Clavicular head:	Cranial surface of medial third of clavicle	

Nerve: n. accessorius; fibers from second cervical nerve

Action: Various: Both sides together, holds head, moves chin upward and pulls back of head down. One side alone, turns chin upward and to opposite side. The understanding of this muscle clarifies the anatomy of the neck

Infrahyoid Muscles (Figs. 275, 279, 280)

1. m. sternohyoideus (thin, narrow muscle)	Inner surface of manubrium sterni and sternoclavicular joint	Corpus ossis hyoidei
2. m. sternothyroideus (shorter, wider muscle)	1st costal cartilage; dorsal surface of manubrium sterni, caudal to m. sternohyoideus	Outer surface of thyroid cartilage (opposite the origin of m. thyrohyoideus)
3. m. thyrohyoideus (small quadrilateral muscle)	Outer surface of the thyroid cartilage	Inferior border of cornu majus of hyoid bone
4. m. omohyoideus (two fleshy bellies united in middle by a single tendon)	Margo superior scapulae between angulus superior and incisura scapulae (venter inferior)	Caudal border of lateral section of body of hyoid bone (venter superior)

Nerve: Ansa cervicalis

Action: Fixes hyoid bone firmly; with Suprahyoid muscles, assist in movements of tongue, hyoid bone, and larynx in swallowing and phonation. With the m. thyrohyoideus (and hyoid bone fixed) elevates larynx in act of swallowing and production of high notes. The m. sternothyroideus does the opposite in drawing down the larynx to produce low notes. Muscles assist in respiration (pull sternum cranially in inspiration)

Musculi auriculares (Fig. 275)

m. auricularis anterior	Fascia temporalis, lamina superficialis	Base of cartilaginous external ear
m. auricularis posterior	Tendon of insertion of m. sternocleidomastoideus	

Nerve: n. facialis

Action: Moves the external ear (pinna)

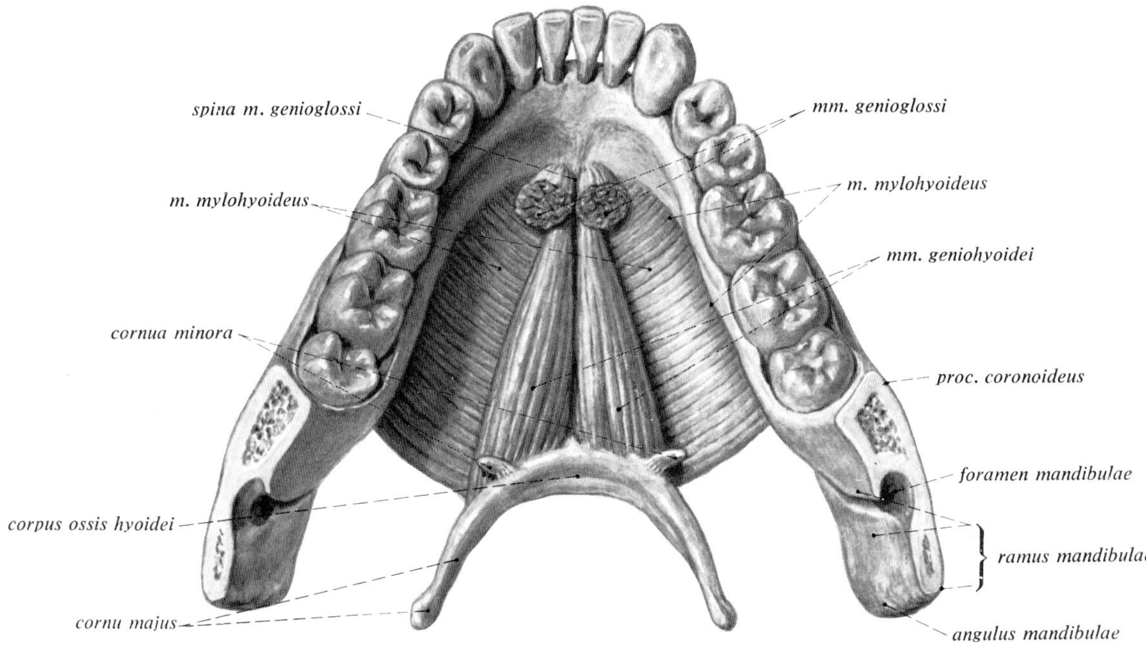

Fig. 276. *Mm. mylohyoideus* and *geniohyoideus*, seen from occlusal surface *(diophragma oris)* (1/1). Hyoid bone with *cornu majus et minus, mm. mylohyoideus* and *geniohyoideus*. Genioglossus muscle stumps of origin were preserved.

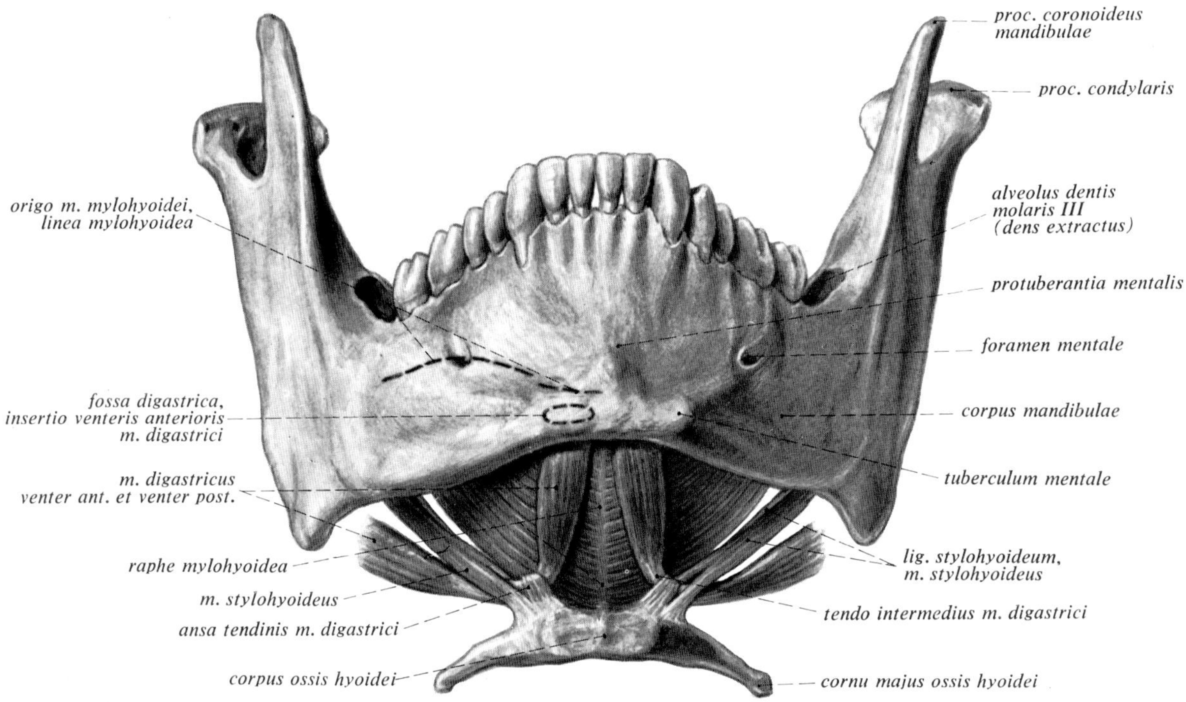

Fig. 277. *Mandibula, os hyoideum, mm. ossis hyoidei* seen from in front and below. The origin of the *m. mylohyoideus* and the *fossa digastrica* on the inner surface of the mandible are indicated by interrupted lines.

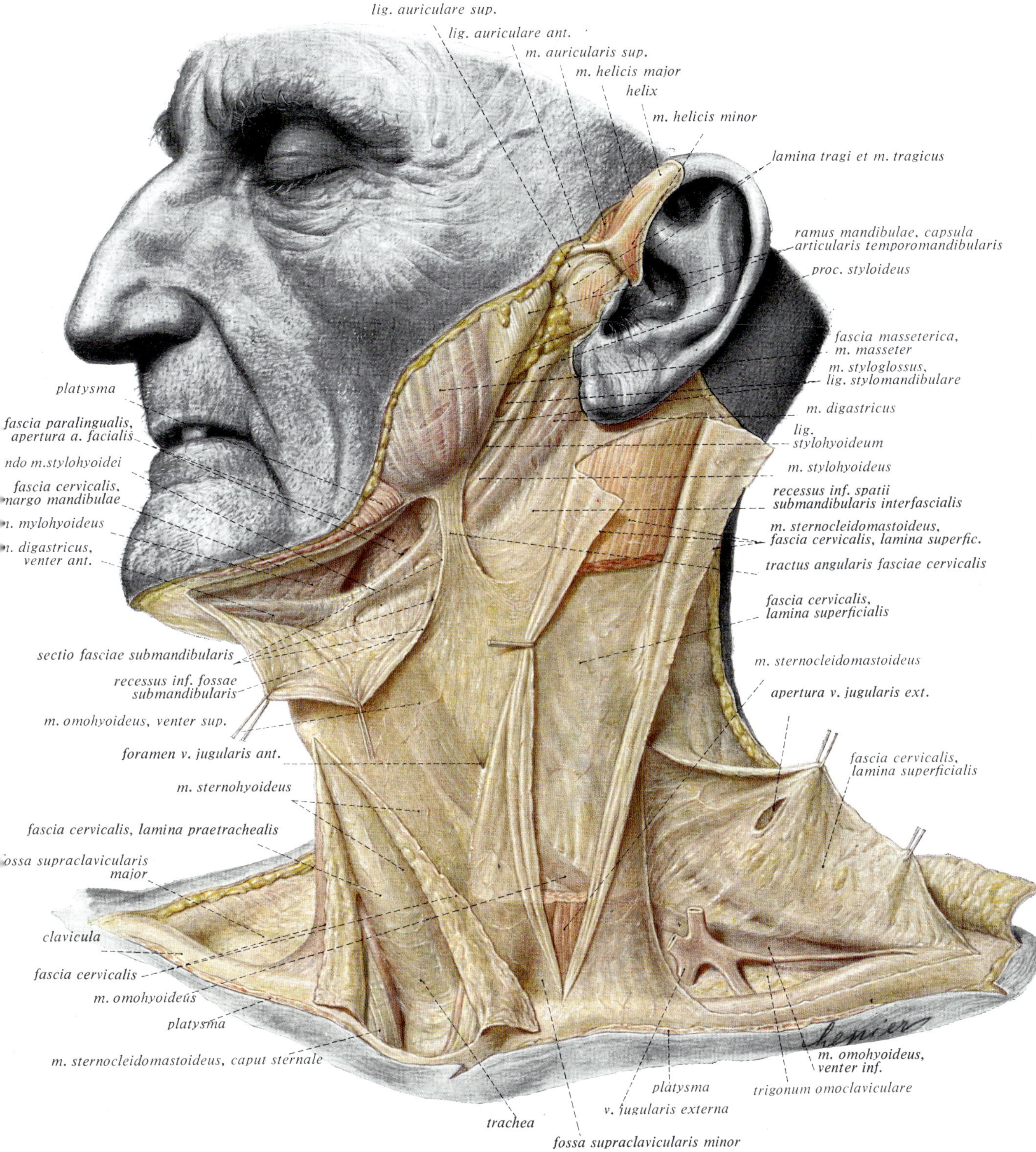

Fig. 278. The cervical fascia and the exposed areas after the removal of a greater portion of the musculature of the neck and submandibular region, including the vessels and nerves. Ventrolateral view.

Fig. 279. Neckmusculature.
Ventral view.
Left: Superficial layer.
Right: Deeper layer with cervical vessels and nerves of the neck and *trigonum deltoideopectorale.*

* *fascia cervicalis, lamina praetrachealis*

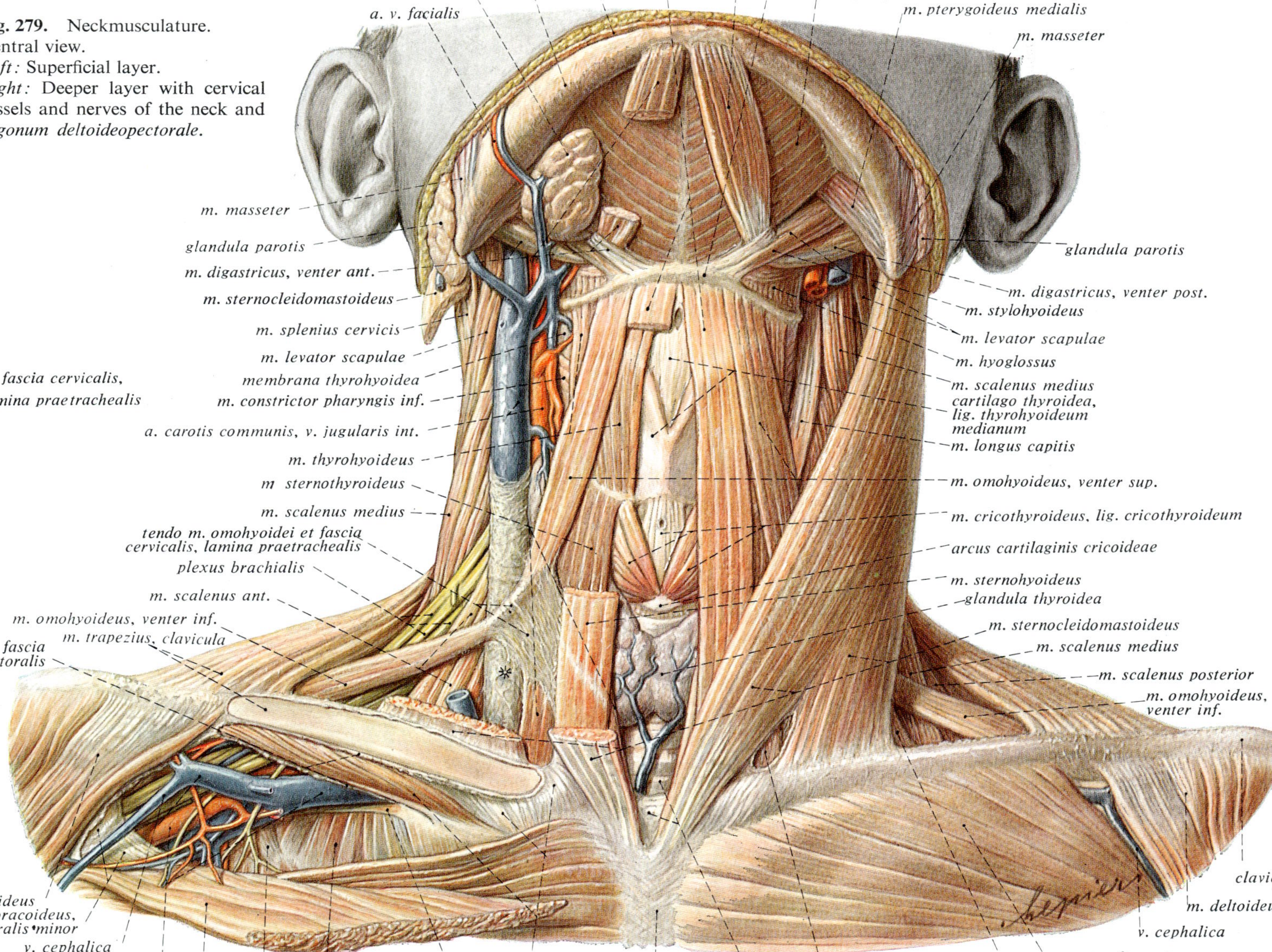

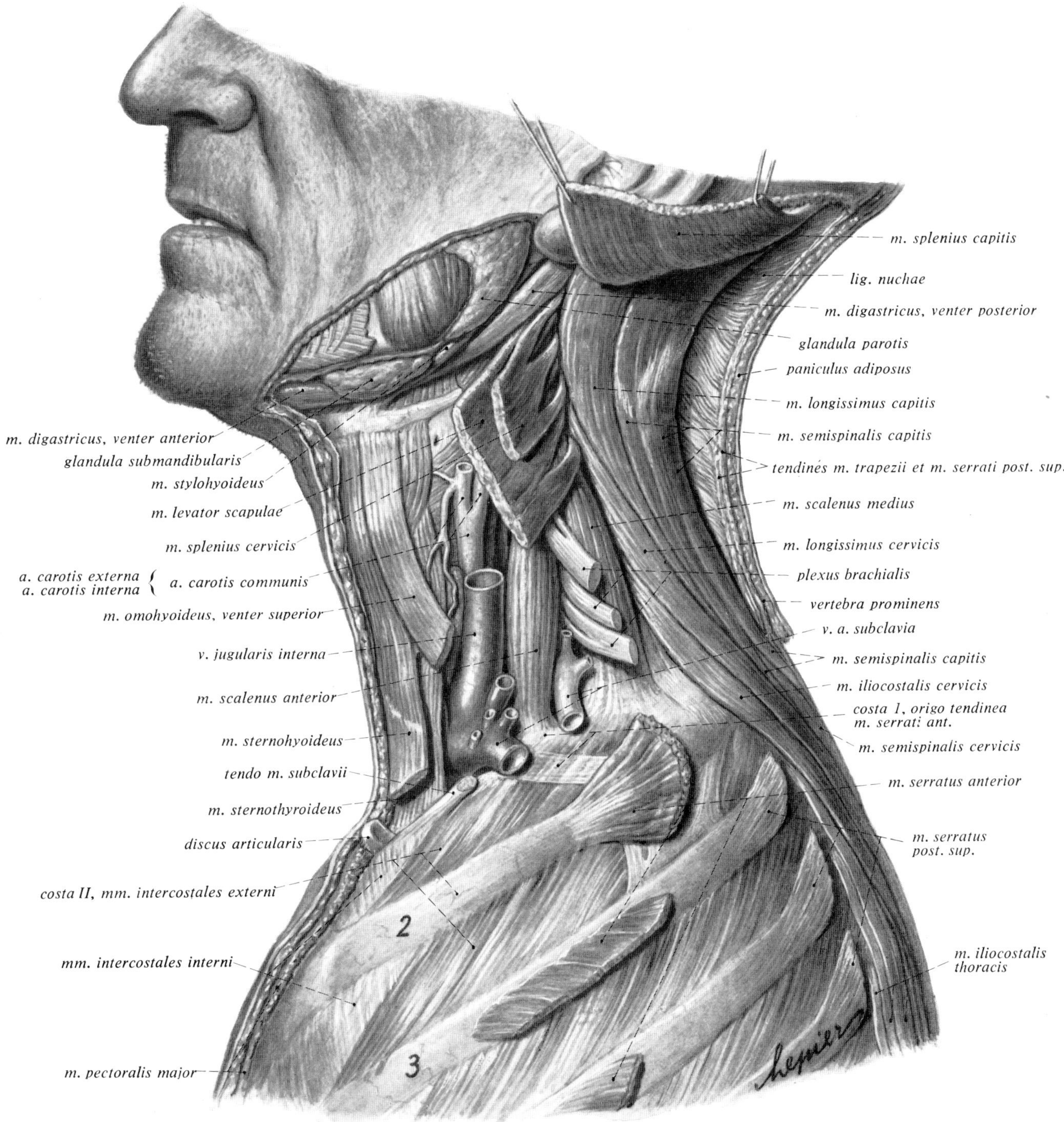

Fig. 280. Neck, upper thorax, deeper layers. *Mm. levator scapulae* and *splenius cervicis* were cut in front. Observe the *a. subclavia* and *plexus brachialis* in the scalene hiatus.

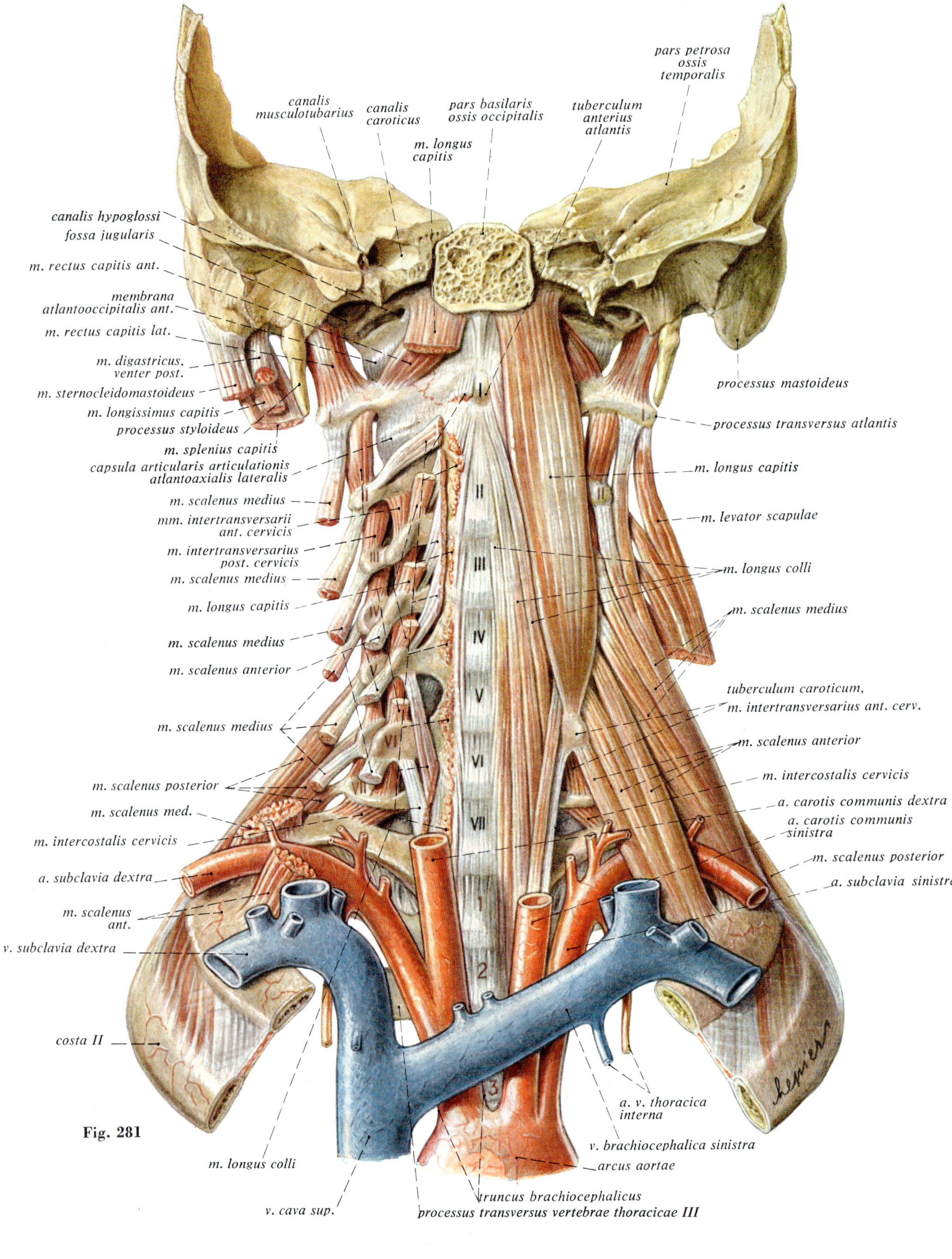
canalis musculotubarius
canalis caroticus
pars basilaris ossis occipitalis
tuberculum anterius atlantis
pars petrosa ossis temporalis
m. longus capitis
canalis hypoglossi
fossa jugularis
m. rectus capitis ant.
membrana atlantooccipitalis ant.
m. rectus capitis lat.
m. digastricus, venter post.
m. sternocleidomastoideus
m. longissimus capitis
processus styloideus
m. splenius capitis
capsula articularis articulationis atlantoaxialis lateralis
m. scalenus medius
mm. intertransversarii ant. cervicis
m. intertransversarius post. cervicis
m. scalenus medius
m. longus capitis
m. scalenus medius
m. scalenus anterior
m. scalenus medius
m. scalenus posterior
m. scalenus med.
m. intercostalis cervicis
a. subclavia dextra
m. scalenus ant.
v. subclavia dextra
costa II
m. longus colli
v. cava sup.
processus mastoideus
processus transversus atlantis
m. longus capitis
m. levator scapulae
m. longus colli
m. scalenus medius
tuberculum caroticum, m. intertransversarius ant. cerv.
m. scalenus anterior
m. intercostalis cervicis
a. carotis communis dextra
a. carotis communis sinistra
m. scalenus posterior
a. subclavia sinistra
a. v. thoracica interna
v. brachiocephalica sinistra
arcus aortae
truncus brachiocephalicus
processus transversus vertebrae thoracicae III

Fig. 281

Lateral Vertebral Group (Prevertebral) of Deep Cervical Muscles (Figs. 269, 281)

Name	*Origin*	*Insertion*
1. m. scalenus anterior	Tubercula anteriora of transverse processes of 3rd to 6th cervical vertebrae	Scalene tubercle on 1st rib
2. m. scalenus medius	Tubercula anteriora of transverse processes of last six cervical vertebrae	Cranial surface of 1st rib, dorsal to subclavian groove
3. m. scalenus posterior	Tubercula posteriora of transverse processes of last three cervical vertebrae	Outer surface of 2nd rib

Nerve: Plexus cervicalis (and plexus brachialis)

Action: mm. scaleni, acting together, elevate 1st and 2nd ribs or flex the vertebral column (muscles of inspiration); acting one side at a time, they bend neck to side

Anterior Vertebral Group (Prevertebral) of Deep Cervical Muscles (Fig. 281)

1. m. longus colli		
Vertical portion	Body of first 3 thoracic and last 3 cervical vertebrae	Bodies of cervical vertebrae C_2–C_4
Superior oblique	Tubercula anteriora of transverse process of cervical vertebrae C_3–C^5	Tuberculum anterius atlantis and body of next cervical vertebra
Inferior oblique	Anterior surface of bodies of first 2 or 3 thoracic vertebrae	Tubercula anteriora of the transverse processes of 5th and 6th cervical vertebrae
2. m. longus capitis	Tubercula anteriora of transverse processes of 3rd–6th cervical vertebrae	Inferior border of pars basilaris of occipital bone
3. m. rectus capitis anterior	Lateral mass of atlas and root of its transverse process	as bone

Nerve: Cervical plexus

Action: Bends the cervical vertebrae column, or the head forward, by unilateral innervation, inclines and rotates the head toward the same side

Fig. 281. Deep cervical muscles after removal of the cervical viscera. Ventral view. Cervical vertebrae: I–VII; upper thoracic vertebrae: 1–3. The base of the skull cut off almost frontally near the level of the basilar portion. First and second ribs were cut near the bone-cartilage junction. The *vena cava superior* and *arcus aorticus* are shown with their large trunks; the *truncus brachiocephalicus*, the *a. carotis communis*, the left *a. subclavia* with its passage through the scalene hiatus.

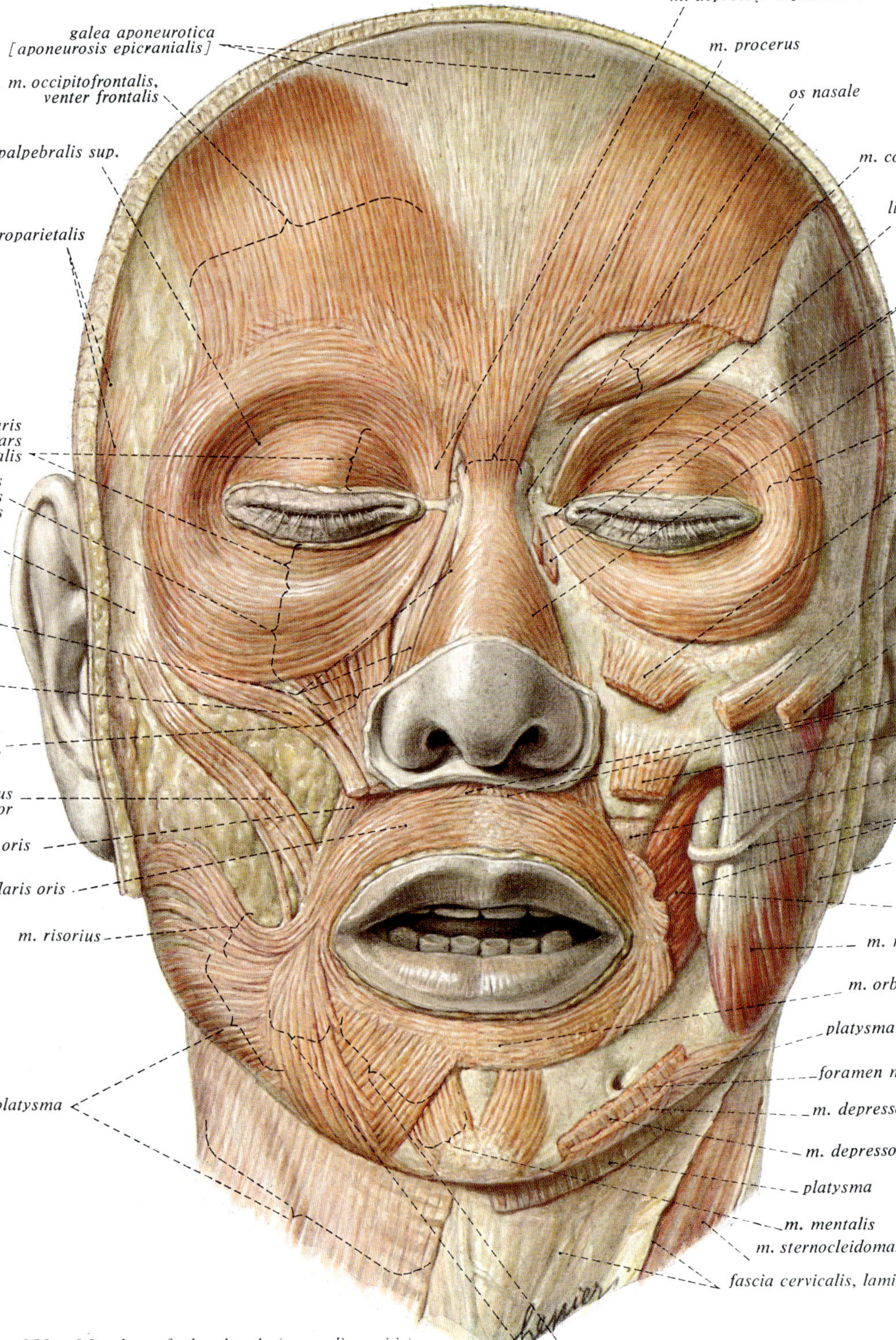

Fig. 282. Muscles of the head *(musculi capitis)*. *Right:* Superficial (expression) layer. *Left:* Deeper layers (muscles of expression and chewing) of the facial muscles.

Muscles of the Eyelids (Fig. 282)

Name	*Origin*	*Insertion*
1. m. orbicularis oculi		
pars orbitalis	processus frontalis maxillae; medial angle of eye; ligamentum palpebrae mediale	Surrounds orbital opening as a sphincter, some fibers go to eyebrow
pars palpebralis	ligamentum palpebrae mediale	raphe palpebralis lateralis
pars lacrimalis	crista lacrimalis posterior	Tarsus of each eyelid
2. m. depressor supercilii	processus nasalis ossis frontalis	Skin of eyebrow
Nerve: n. facialis, rami temporales et zygomatici		
Action: Closes lids, compresses lacrimal sac, moves eyebrows		
3. m. corrugator supercilii	processus nasalis ossis frontalis	Skin of eyebrow
4. m. procerus	Bridge of nose and lateral nasal cartilage	Skin of forehead between eyebrows
Nerve: n. facialis, rami temporales		
Action: Acts upon skin of forehead (glabella) and eyebrows		

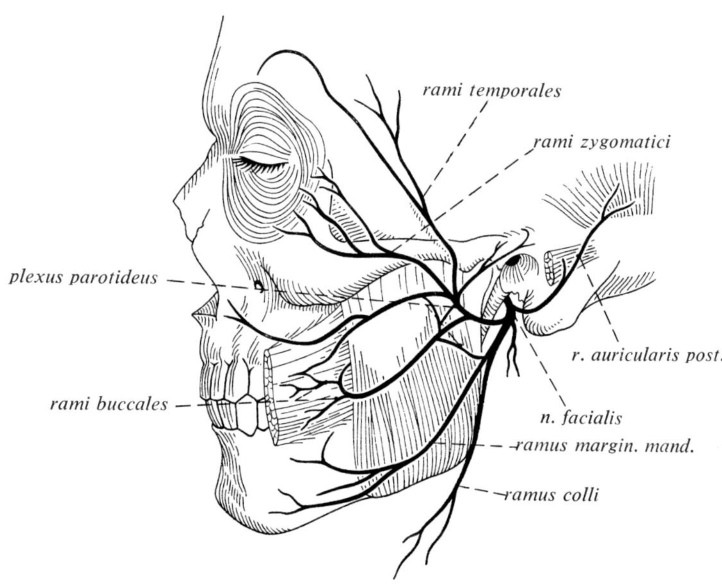

Fig. 283. *Rami temporales, zygomatici, buccales, marginalis mandibulae* and *ramus colli* from the *n. facialis* for the facial musculature. (Feneis, 1967).

Musculi Epicranii (Figs. 282, 284)

Name	*Origin*	*Insertion*
m. occipitofrontalis, venter frontalis:	margo supraorbitalis, skin of forehead and eyebrows	galea aponeurotica
m. occipitofrontalis, venter occipitalis:	linea nuchalis suprema	galea aponeurotica
m. temporoparietalis	fascia temporalis, lamina superficialis near ear	On skin and fascia temporalis above and in front of ear

Nerve: n. facialis

Action: Moves scalp, wrinkles forehead

Muscles of the Nose (Figs. 282, 284)

1. m. nasalis

pars transversa:	Area over canine teeth (the maxilla)	Aponeurosis over bridge of nose
pars alaris:	Area over the lateral incisors (alar cartilage)	Skin at tip of nose
2. m. depressor septi	fossa incisiva maxillae	Alar cartilage and septum of nose

Nerve: n. facialis

Action: Slightly moves nose, namely, ala of the nose (dilates and contracts nostrils)

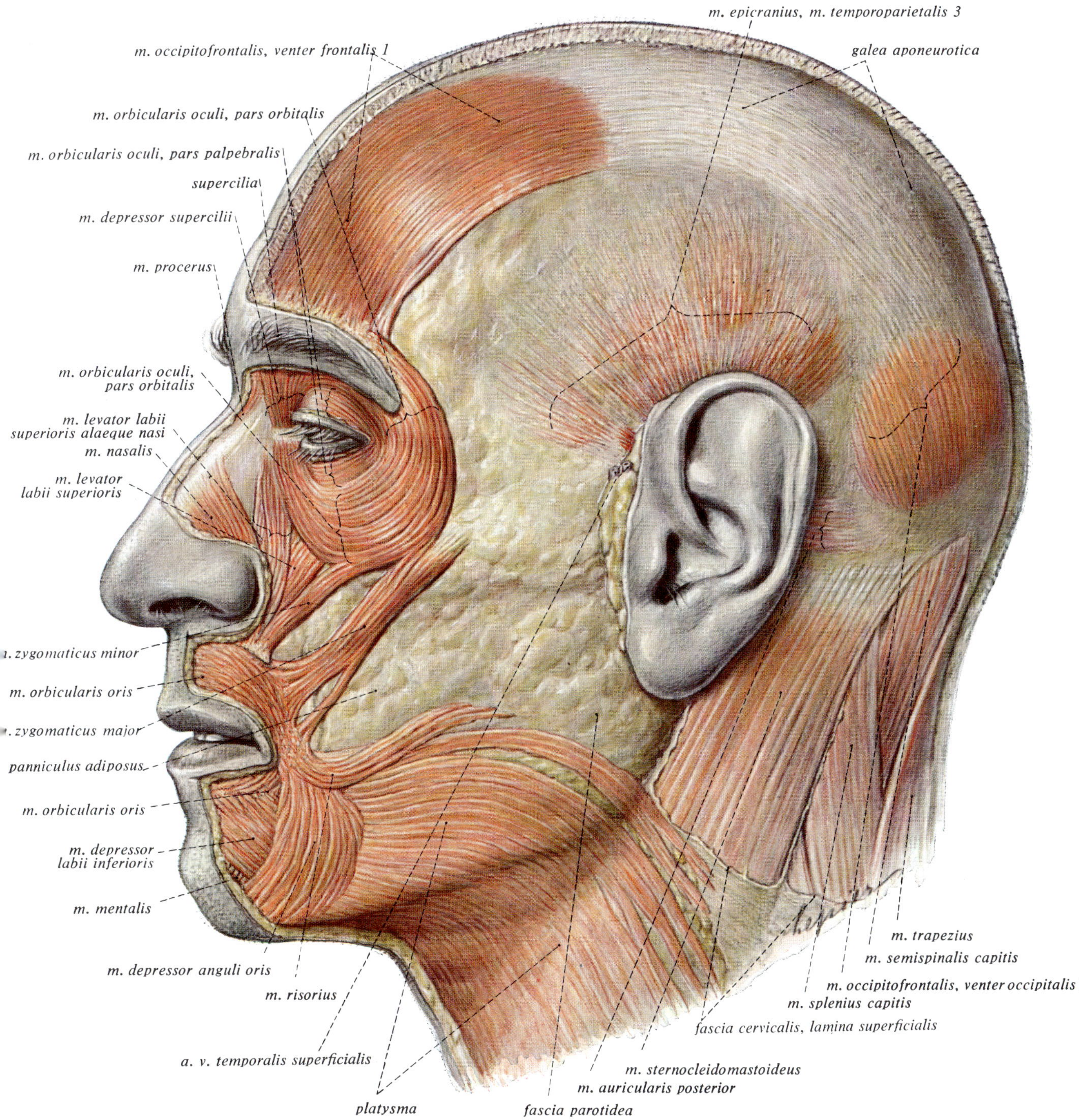

Fig. 284. Lateral aspect of the head with mimetic musculature and superficial layers of the cervical musculature. The three parts of the *m. epicranius* are designated 1, 2, 3.

Muscles of the Oral Region (Figs. 282–286)

Name	*Origin*	*Insertion*
1. m. levator labii superioris alaeque nasi	processus frontalis maxillae	Ala of nose and upper lip
2. m. levator labii superioris	margo infraorbitalis	Ala of nose and upper lip
3. m. zygomaticus minor	Malar surface of zygomatic bone	Near angle of mouth
4. m. zygomaticus major	Lateral surface of zygomatic bone	Angle of mouth
5. m. risorius (a part of the Platysma)	fascia masseterica	Angle of mouth
6. m. depressor anguli oris	linea obliqua mandibulae	Angle of mouth; lower lip
7. m. levator anguli oris	fossa canina maxillae	Musculature of upper lip; angle of mouth
8. m. depressor labii inferioris	Mandible between symphysis and foramen mentale	Lower lip
9. m. orbicularis oris	The following specifications: pars marginalis: fibers blended with adjacent muscles pars labialis: fibers restricted to lips	Protrudes and shapes lips
10. m. buccinator	Outer surface of mandible; processus alveolaris maxillae; fascia buccopharyngea	Angle of mouth and lips; its interlacing fibers contribute to m. orbicularis oris
11. m. mentalis	Incisive fossa of mandible	Skin of chin

Nerve: n. facialis (Fig. 283)

Action: Moves lips, ala of nose, cheeks, skin of chin. m. risorius: draws angle of mouth laterally (smiling)

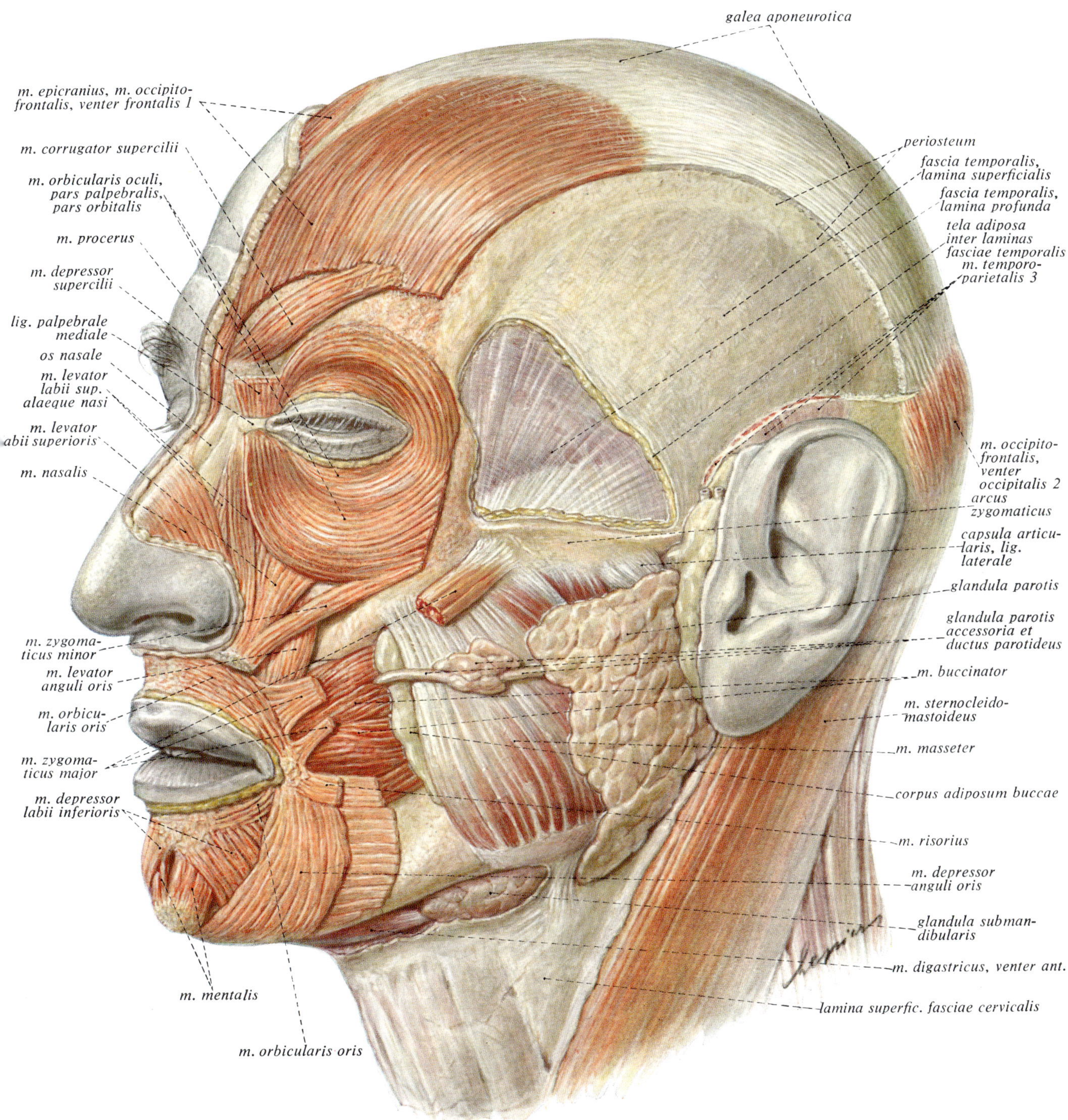

Fig. 285. The head and upper cervical region from the left side. Mimetic musculature, part of the Masseter muscles, salivary glands, the *m. sternocleidomastoideus* and some of the upper cervical muscles. The three parts of the *m. epicranius* designated 1, 2, 3.

Muscles of Mastication (Figs. 286, 287, 289)

The muscles of mastication are invested by fasciae. They are the only cranial muscles resembling the true skeltal muscles with distinct separate muscles with well defined fascia. These 4 muscles (Masseter, Temporal and both Pterygoid muscles) move the mandible in the temporomandibular articulation.

Name	*Origin*	*Insertion*
1. m. masseter pars superficialis	processus zygomaticus maxillae; lower margin of arcus zygomatici	angulus and ramus mandibulae; base of processus coronoideus mandibulae
pars profunda	From posterior part of lower margin and medial surface of arcus zygomatici	
Nerve: n. massetericus from mandibular division of n. trigeminus		
Action: Closes jaws, elevates mandible		
2. m. temporalis	fossa temporalis and fascia temporalis (lamina profunda)	Anterior border and medial surface of processus coronoideus mandibulae
Nerve: nn. temporales profundi from mandibular division of n. trigeminus		
Action: Elevates mandible (closes jaws); posterior fibers retract mandible		
3. m. pterygoideus lateralis	Main lower head: Lateral surface of lamina lateralis processus pterygoidei. Accessory upper head: facies temporalis alae majoris ossis sphenoidalis	Fovea pterygoidea processus condylaris mandibulae; discus articularis of temporomandibular joint
4. m. pterygoideus medialis	Fossa pterygoidea; processus pyramidalis ossis palatini; lamina lateralis processus pterygoidei	Medial surface of angulus mandibulae; opposite of m. masseter (on tuberositas pterygoidea)
Nerve: n. pterygoideus lateralis et medialis, respectively, from mandibular division of n. trigeminus		
Action: Opens jaws, protrudes mandible, moves mandible from side to side, grinding motion (lateral); closes jaws (medial)		

Fig. 286. Lateral view of head and upper neck muscles with mimetic and masticator muscles. The external ear and part of the *arcus zygomaticus* were removed. A wide piece of the upper half of the *m. sternocleidomastoideus* was removed to display the large vessels. The *m. masseter* was partly removed to display its tendinous insertions between the muscle bundles. A few mimetic muscles were cut off near their origins.

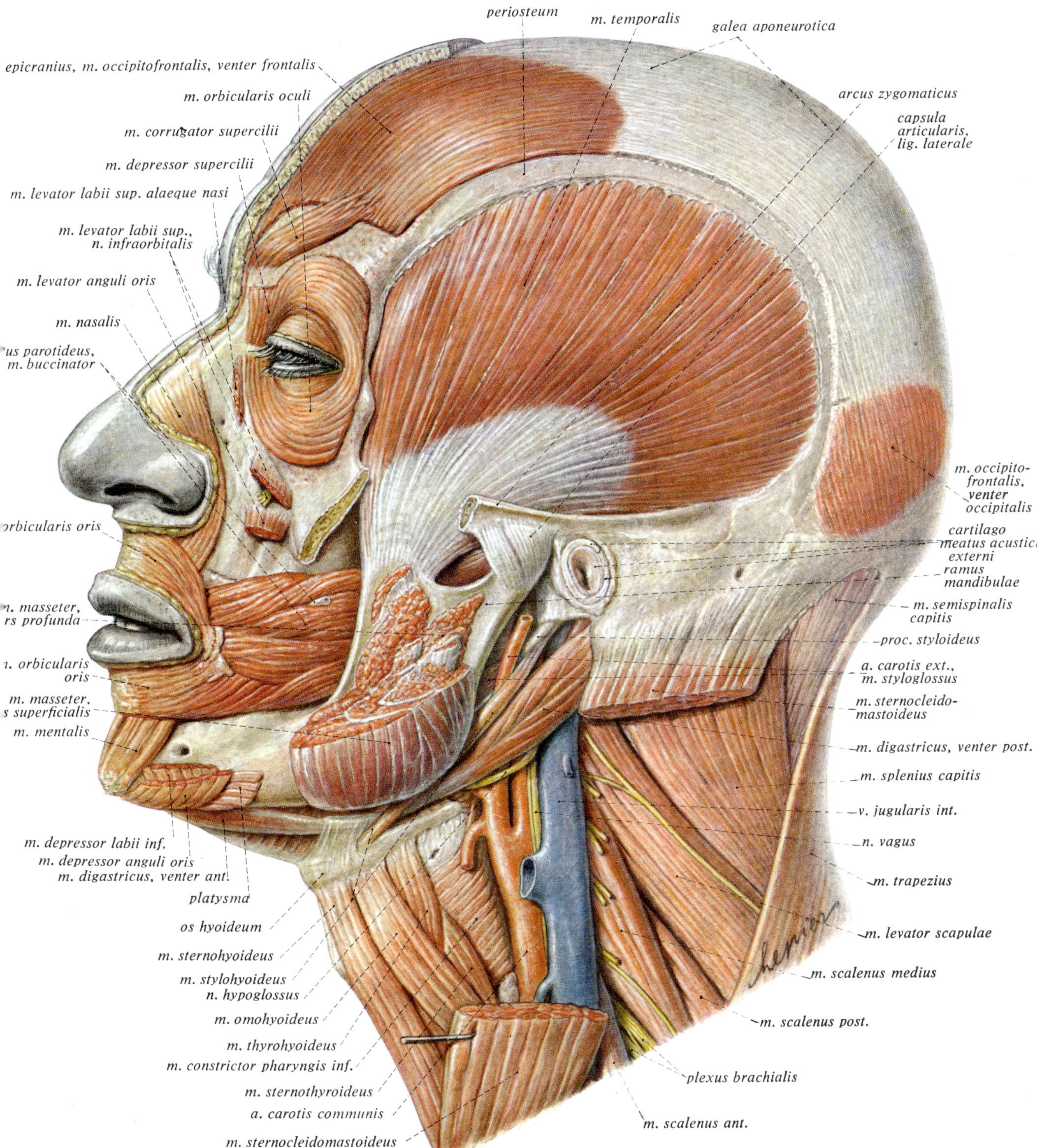
periosteum
m. temporalis
galea aponeurotica
epicranius, m. occipitofrontalis, venter frontalis
m. orbicularis oculi
m. corrugator supercilii
m. depressor supercilii
m. levator labii sup. alaeque nasi
m. levator labii sup.,
n. infraorbitalis
m. levator anguli oris
m. nasalis
us parotideus,
m. buccinator
orbicularis oris
n. masseter,
rs profunda
ı. orbicularis
oris
m. masseter,
s superficialis
m. mentalis
m. depressor labii inf.
m. depressor anguli oris
m. digastricus, venter ant.
platysma
os hyoideum
m. sternohyoideus
m. stylohyoideus
n. hypoglossus
m. omohyoideus
m. thyrohyoideus
m. constrictor pharyngis inf.
m. sternothyroideus
a. carotis communis
m. sternocleidomastoideus
arcus zygomaticus
capsula
articularis,
lig. laterale
m. occipito-
frontalis,
venter
occipitalis
cartilago
meatus acustici
externi
ramus
mandibulae
m. semispinalis
capitis
proc. styloideus
a. carotis ext.,
m. styloglossus
m. sternocleido-
mastoideus
m. digastricus, venter post.
m. splenius capitis
v. jugularis int.
n. vagus
m. trapezius
m. levator scapulae
m. scalenus medius
m. scalenus post.
plexus brachialis
m. scalenus ant.

Fig. 286.

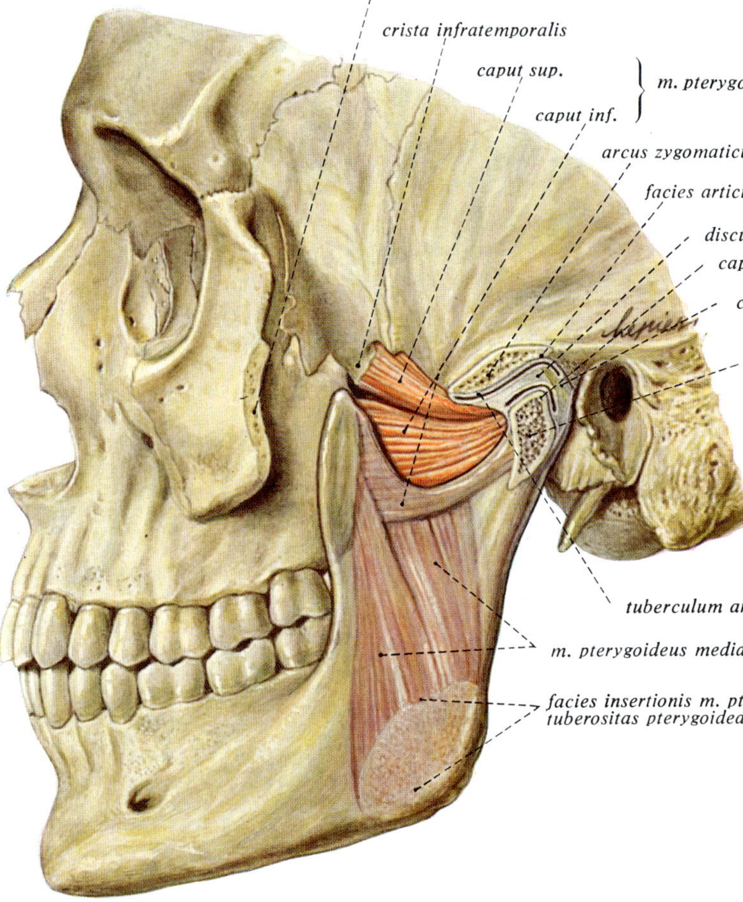

Fig. 287. Mandibular articulation *(articulatio temporomandibularis)*. The temporomandibular joint was opened. The cut was made near the *tuberculum articulare* in a sagittal direction so that the *collum mandibulae* and the capsular ligament may be seen with the *discus articularis*. The *ramus mandibulae* is displayed as being transparent in order to show the origin and course of the *mm. pterygoidei lat. et med.*

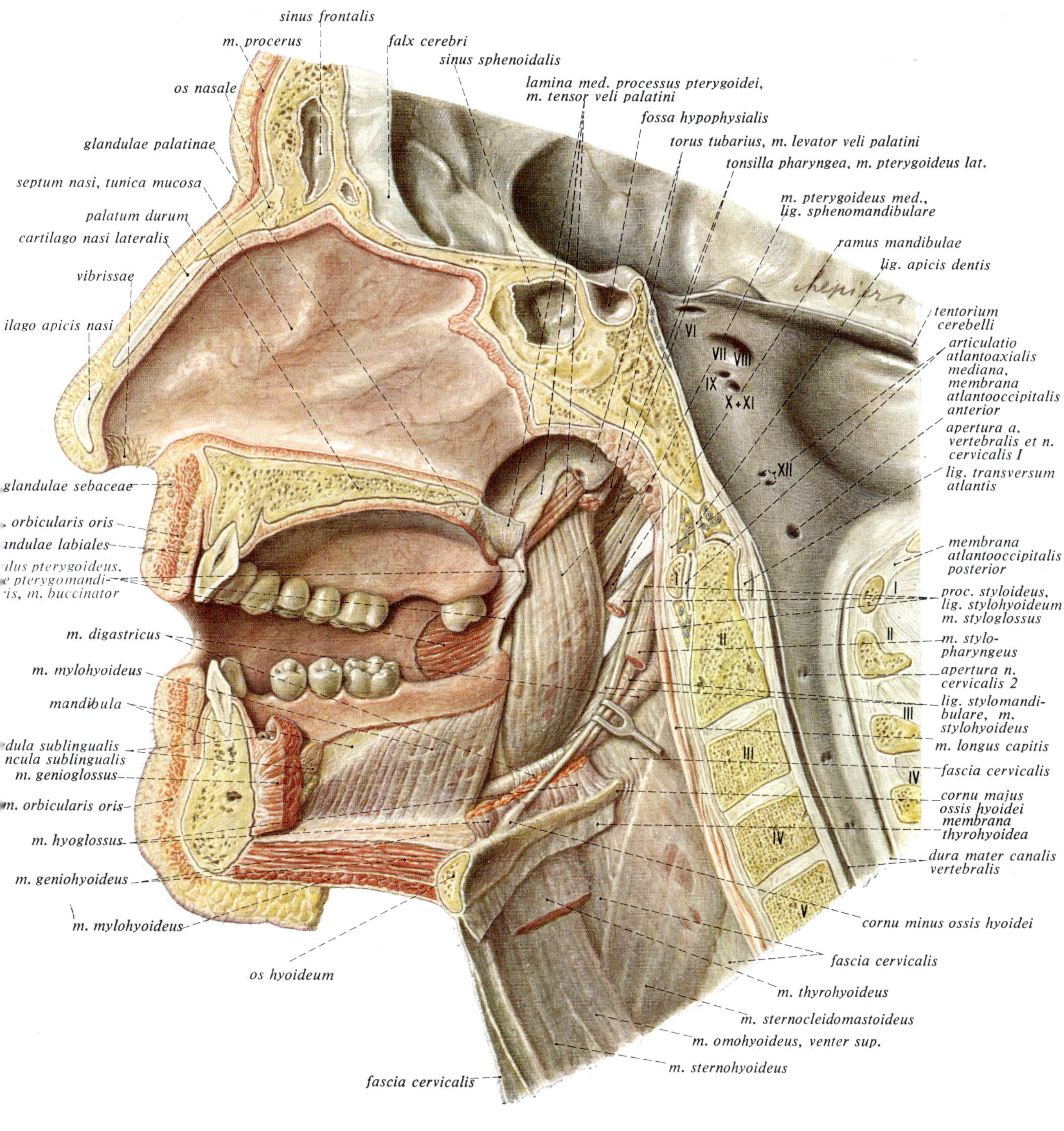

Fig. 288. Paramedian sagittal section through the face and neck. The nasal and oral cavities, as well as some muscles of the floor of the mouth and upper cervical region are displayed. Cervical vertebrae, I–V. The points of exits of the cranial nerves through the dura mater, VI–XII.

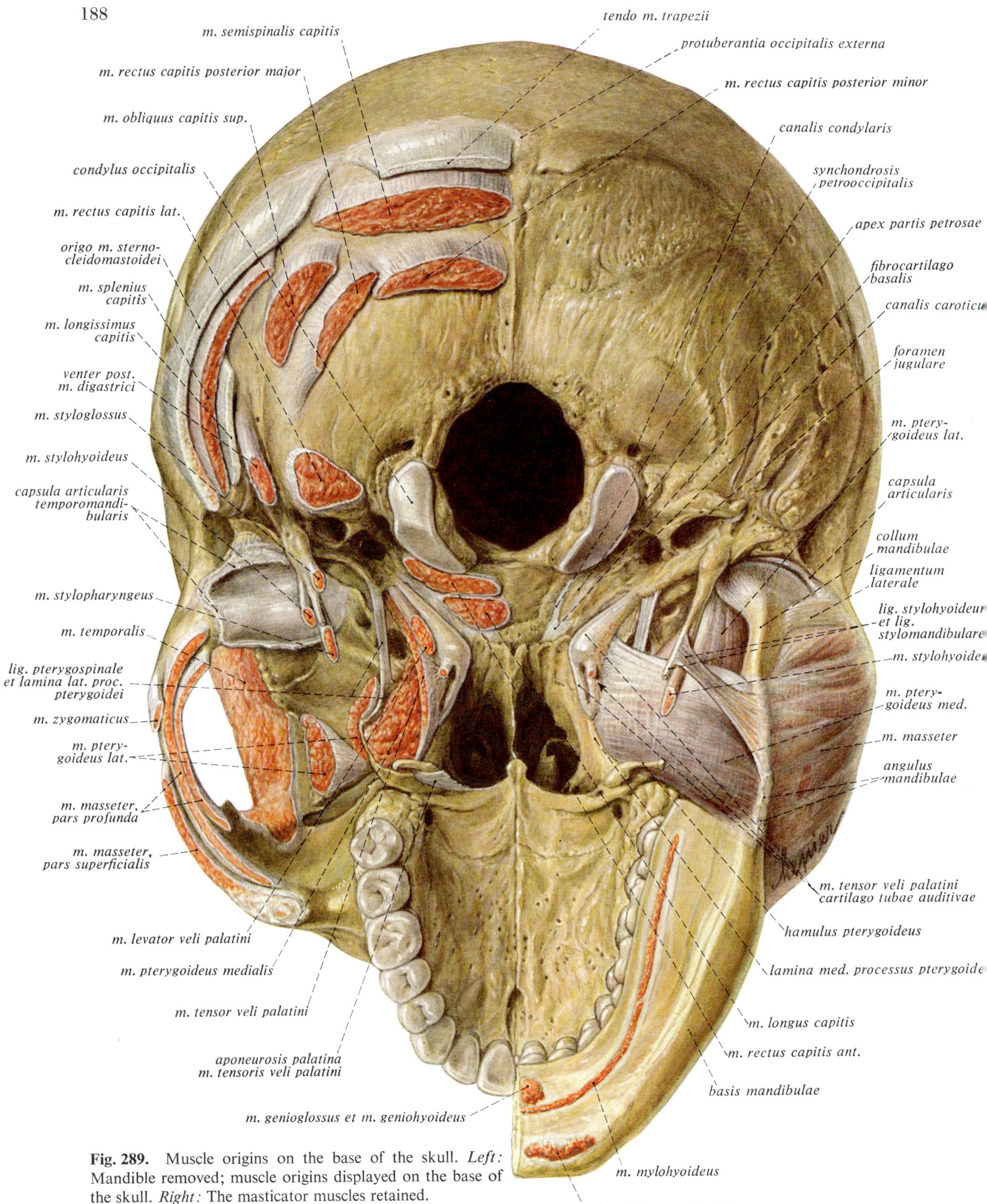

Fig. 289. Muscle origins on the base of the skull. *Left:* Mandible removed; muscle origins displayed on the base of the skull. *Right:* The masticator muscles retained.

Muscles

The Upper Limb

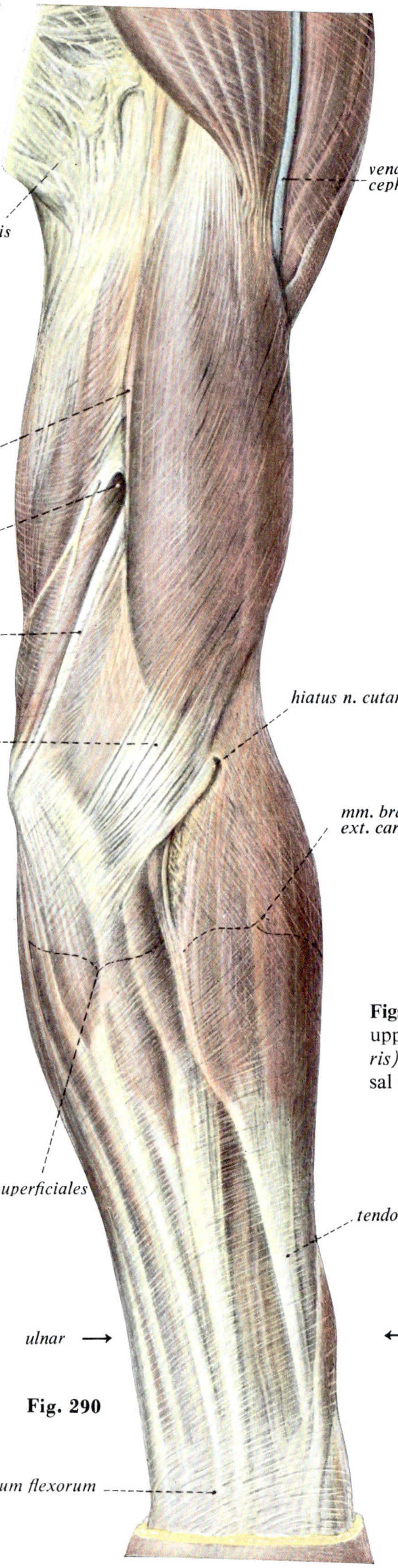

Fig. 290

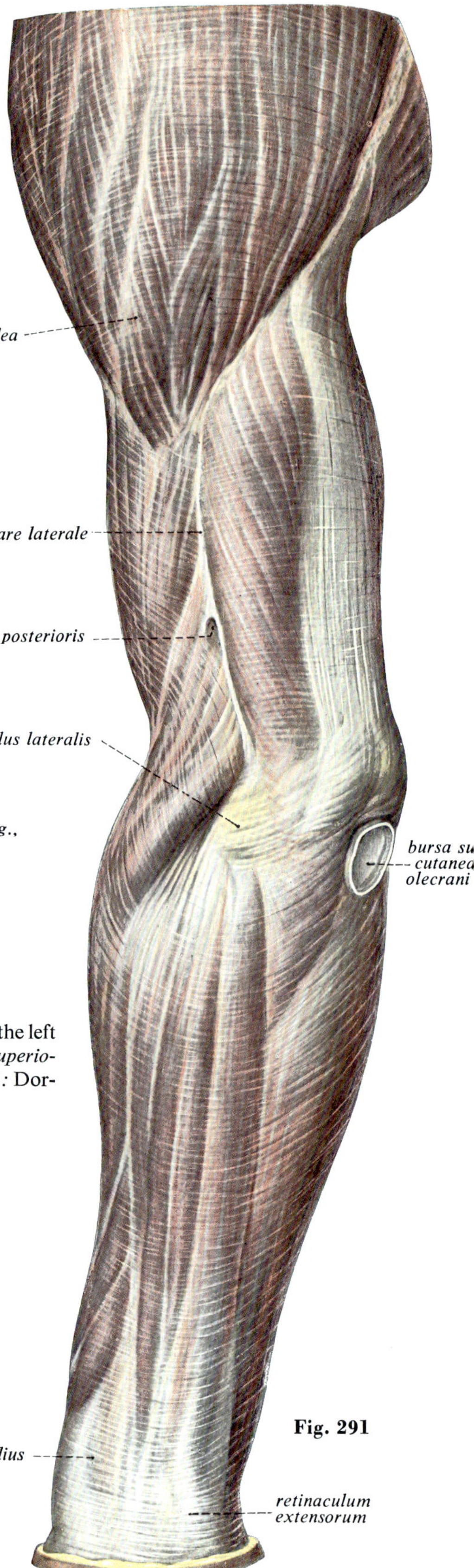

Fig. 291

Figs. 290 and 291. Fascia of the left upper limbs *(fascia membri superioris)*. *Left:* Palmar view. *Right:* Dorsal view.

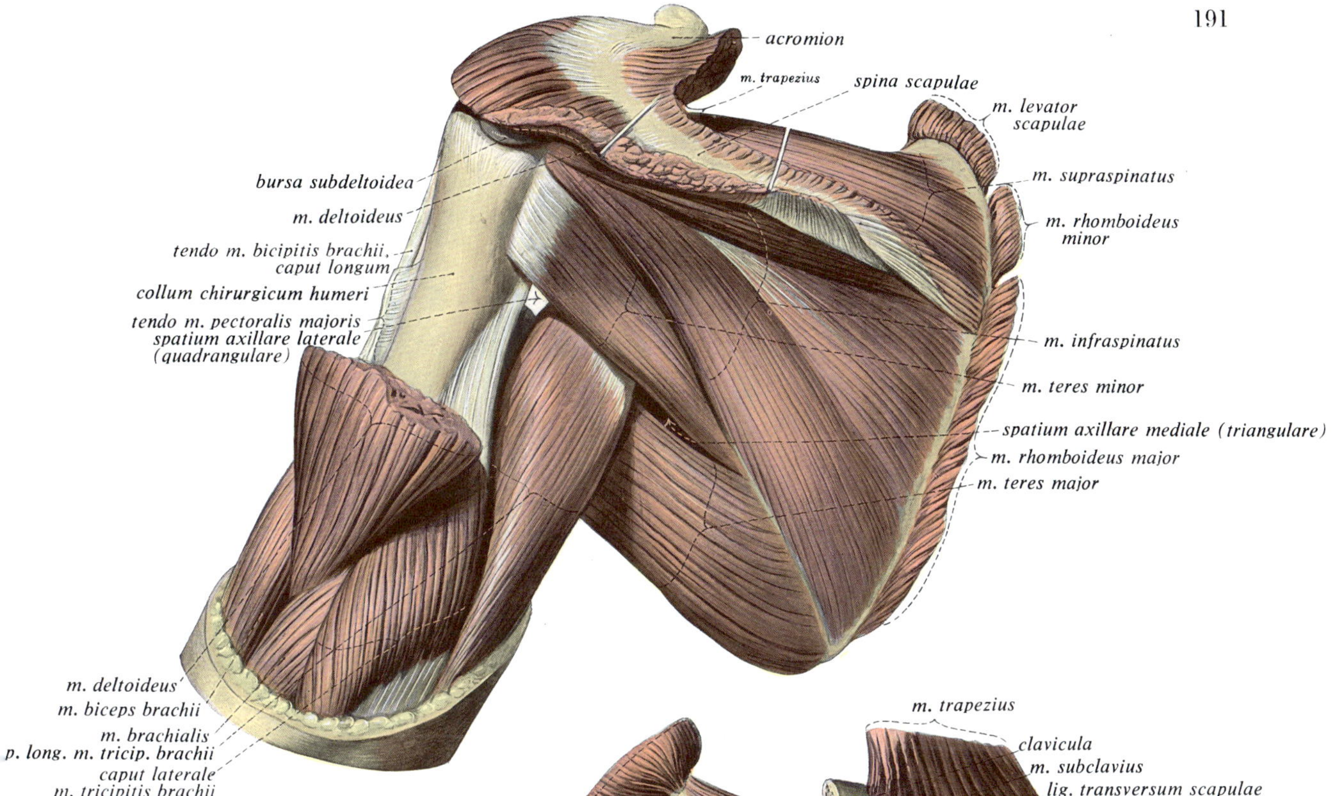

Fig. 292. Muscles of the dorsal surface of the *scapula*. Note the lateral and medial axillary spaces. See Figs. 293, 296, 297.

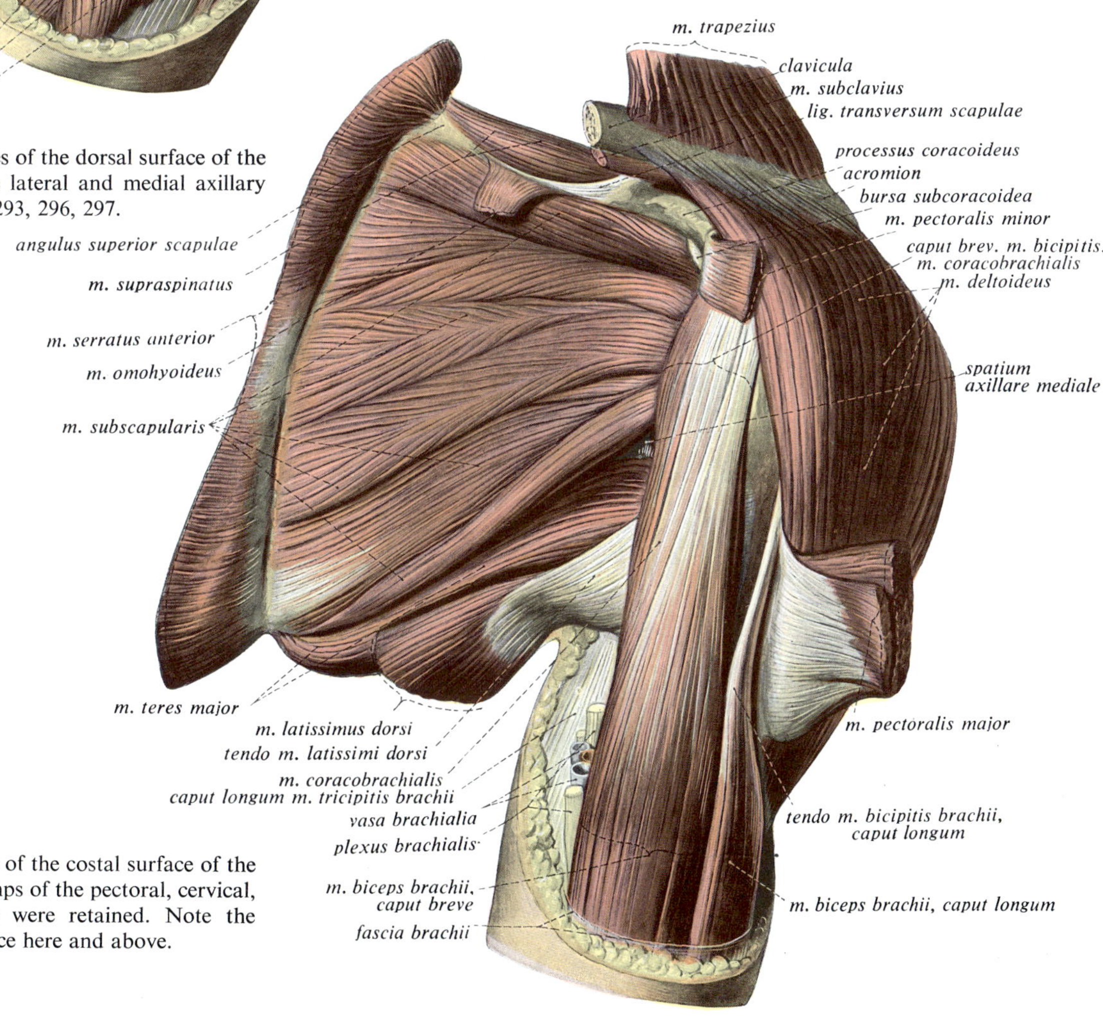

Fig. 293. Muscles of the costal surface of the *scapula*. Short stumps of the pectoral, cervical, and back muscles were retained. Note the medial axillary space here and above.

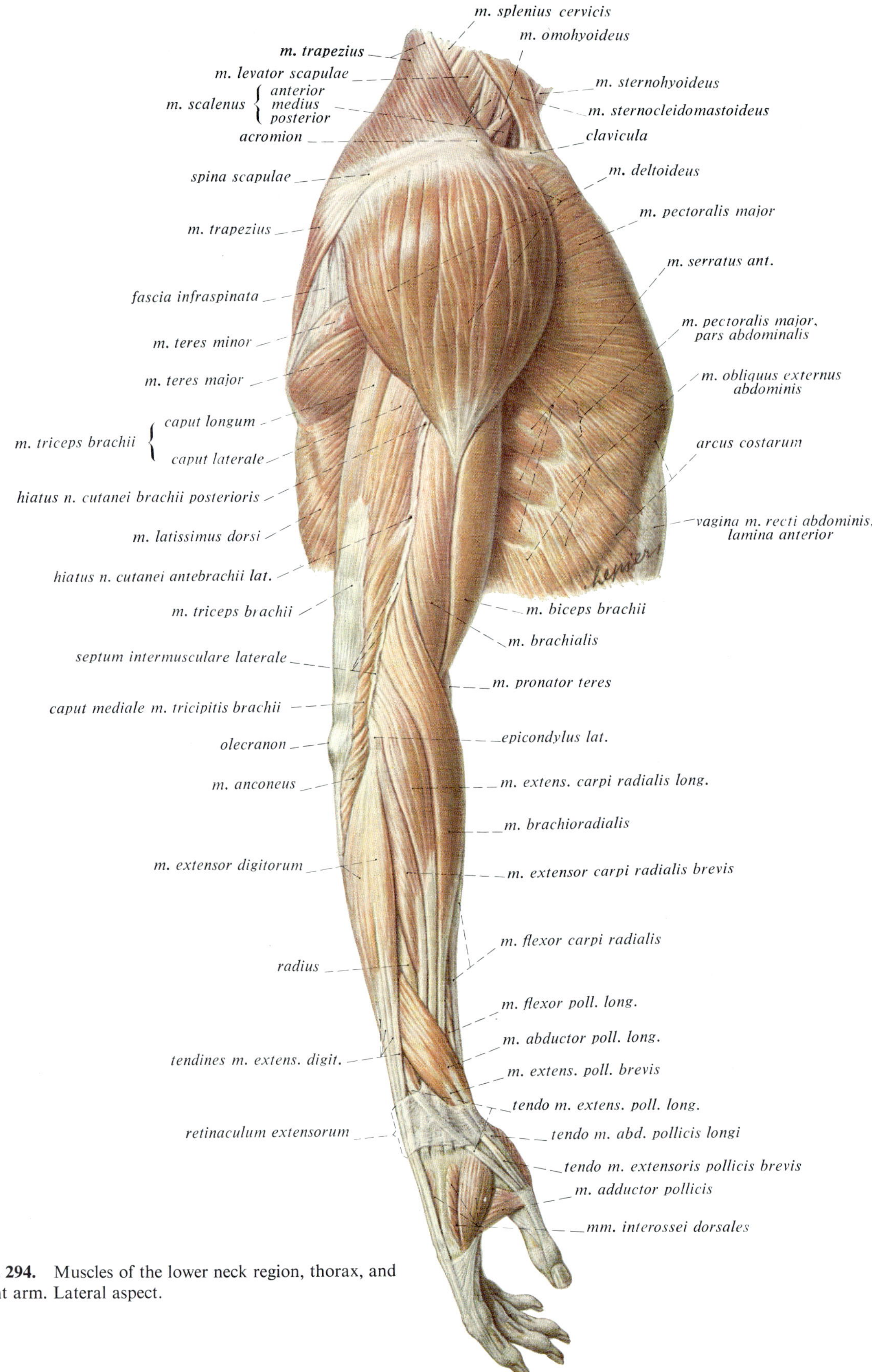

Fig. 294. Muscles of the lower neck region, thorax, and right arm. Lateral aspect.

Shoulder Muscles (Figs. 293, 295, 296, 302, 303)

Name	*Origin*	*Insertion*
1. m. supraspinatus	Fossa supraspinata scapulae	Highest facet of tuberculum majus humeri (tendinous)
2. m. infraspinatus	Caudal margin of the spina scapulae, fossa et fascia infraspinata	Middle facet of tuberculum majus humeri (tendinous)
Nerve: n. suprascapularis from plexus brachialis (C 4, 5, 6)		
Action: m. supraspinatus abducts humerus; starts abduction and assists the m. deltoideus; m. infraspinatus rotates humerus laterally; assists in holding head of humerus		
3. m. teres minor	Caudal section of fossa infraspinata and lateral margin (2/3) of scapula, fascia infraspinata	Lower facet of tuberculum majus humeri (tendinous)
Nerve: n. axillaris from plexus brachialis (C 4, 5)		
Action: Lateral rotator and adductor of humerus		
4. m. teres major	Lateral border of scapula near angulus inferior (medial third)	Tendon on crest of tuberculum minus humeri, dorsal to that of the m. latissimus dorsi (the 2 tendons separated by bursa)
Nerve: n. subscapularis (C 5, 6, 7) of the plexus brachialis		
Action: Adductor, medial rotator and extensor of arm		
5. m. subscapularis (under the insertion: the bursa subscapularis)	Facies costalis scapulae; fossa subscapularis	Short, broad tendon into the tuberculum minus and its adjacent crest; blends with capsule of shoulder joint
Nerve: n. subscapularis (C 5, 6, 7) from plexus brachialis		
Action: Adductor and medial rotator of arm; assists in flexion and extension		
6. m. deltoideus	Acromial third of clavicle, the acromion and spina scapulae	tuberositas deltoidea humeri (subdeltoid bursa between muscle and tuberculum majus humeri)
Nerve: n. axillaris (C 5, 6)		
Action: Ventral (clavicular) fibers assist in flexion and medial rotation of humerus. Dorsal (scapular) fibers assist in extension and lateral rotation of humerus. Middle or central part is a powerful abductor of humerus, lifting it to the horizontal		

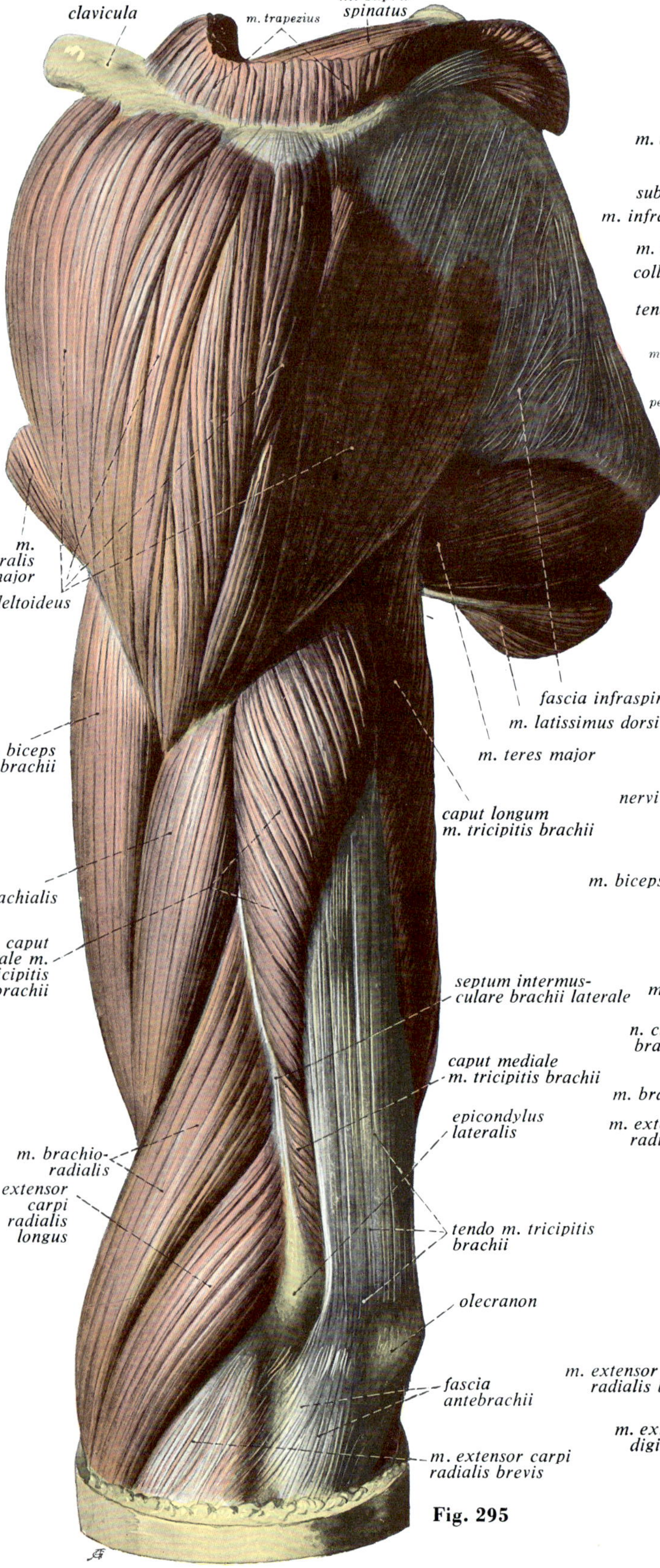
clavicula
m. trapezius
m. supra-
spinatus
m.
pectoralis
major
m. deltoideus
m. biceps
brachii
m. brachialis
caput
laterale m.
tricipitis
brachii
m. brachio-
radialis
m. extensor
carpi
radialis
longus
fascia infraspinata
m. latissimus dorsi
m. teres major
caput longum
m. tricipitis brachii
septum intermus-
culare brachii laterale
caput mediale
m. tricipitis brachii
epicondylus
lateralis
tendo m. tricipitis
brachii
olecranon
fascia
antebrachii
m. extensor carpi
radialis brevis

Fig. 295

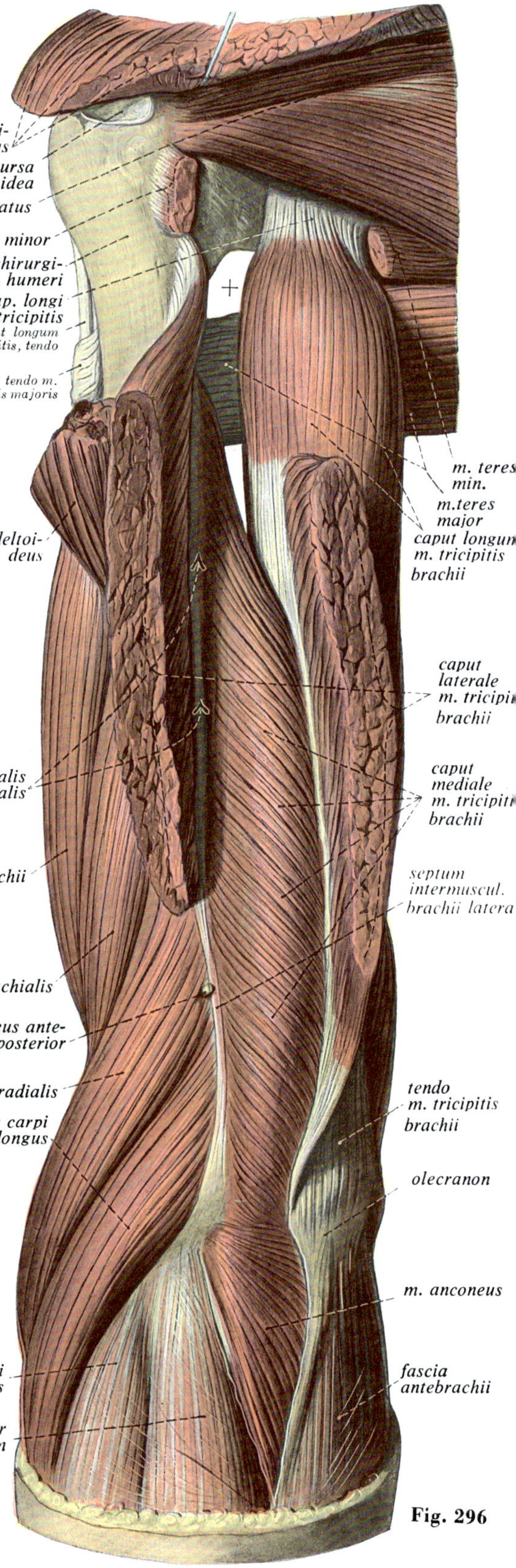
m. deltoi-
deus
bursa
subdeltoidea
m. infraspinatus
m. teres minor
collum chirurgi-
cum humeri
tendo cap. longi
m. tricipitis
caput longum
m. bicipitis, tendo
tendo m.
pectoralis majoris
m. deltoi-
deus
canalis
nervi radialis
m. biceps brachii
m. brachialis
n. cutaneus ante-
brachii posterior
m. brachioradialis
m. extensor carpi
radialis longus
m. extensor carpi
radialis brevis
m. extensor
digitorum
m. teres
min.
m.teres
major
caput longum
m. tricipitis
brachii
caput
laterale
m. tricipi
brachii
caput
mediale
m. tricipit
brachii
septum
intermuscul.
brachii latera
tendo
m. tricipitis
brachii
olecranon
m. anconeus
fascia
antebrachii

Fig. 296

Extensor Muscle of the Upper Arm (Figs. 294–296, 302, 308, 313)

Name	*Origin*	*Insertion*
m. triceps brachii *caput longum:* (Operates 2 joints)	tuberculum infraglenoidale scapulae	Verticle muscle fibers running distalward to the olecranon
caput laterale: (Operates 1 joint)	Lateral and dorsal side of humerus, lateral $^{2}/_{3}$ of septum intermusculare laterale	Joins the common tendon of insertion to the olecranon
caput mediale: (Operates 1 joint)	Dorsal side of humerus, lateral and distal to radial groove; septum intermusculare mediale et laterale	Posterior aspect of olecranon and into deep fascia on both sides of the forearm
m. anconeus (Situated in the forearm)	epicondylus lateralis humeri. Developmentally, it appears to be a part of the m. triceps brachii	Posterior surface of ulna, slightly distal to olecranon

Nerve: n. radialis (C 7, 8)

Action: Extends forearm; adducts and extends arm, braces extended elbow joint (when pushing an object)

Quadrangular and triangular spaces:

1. *Quadrangular Space:* Bounded by tendon of caput longum m. triceps brachii, medially; m. teres major, inferiorly; the humerus, laterally; m. teres minor and capsule of shoulder joint, superiorly (Fig. 292).
   Transmits: n. axillaris, a., v. circumflexa humeri posterior.
2. *Triangular space:* Bounded by m. teres minor, superiorly; m. teres major, inferiorly; caput longum m. triceps brachii, laterally (Fig. 292).
   Transmits: a. circumflexa scapulae.

Fig. 295. The *m. deltoideus* and muscles of the left upper arm. Dorsolateral view.

Fig. 296. Muscles of the left upper arm, deeper layer. Dorsolateral view. The m. deltoideus has been removed except for attachments. The *fascia antebrachii* was removed where it covered the *m. anconeus;* the *m. teres minor* and caput laterale m. triceps brachii were cut and reflected.
+ the lateral axillary space, quadrangular; beneath is the medial axillary space, triangular.

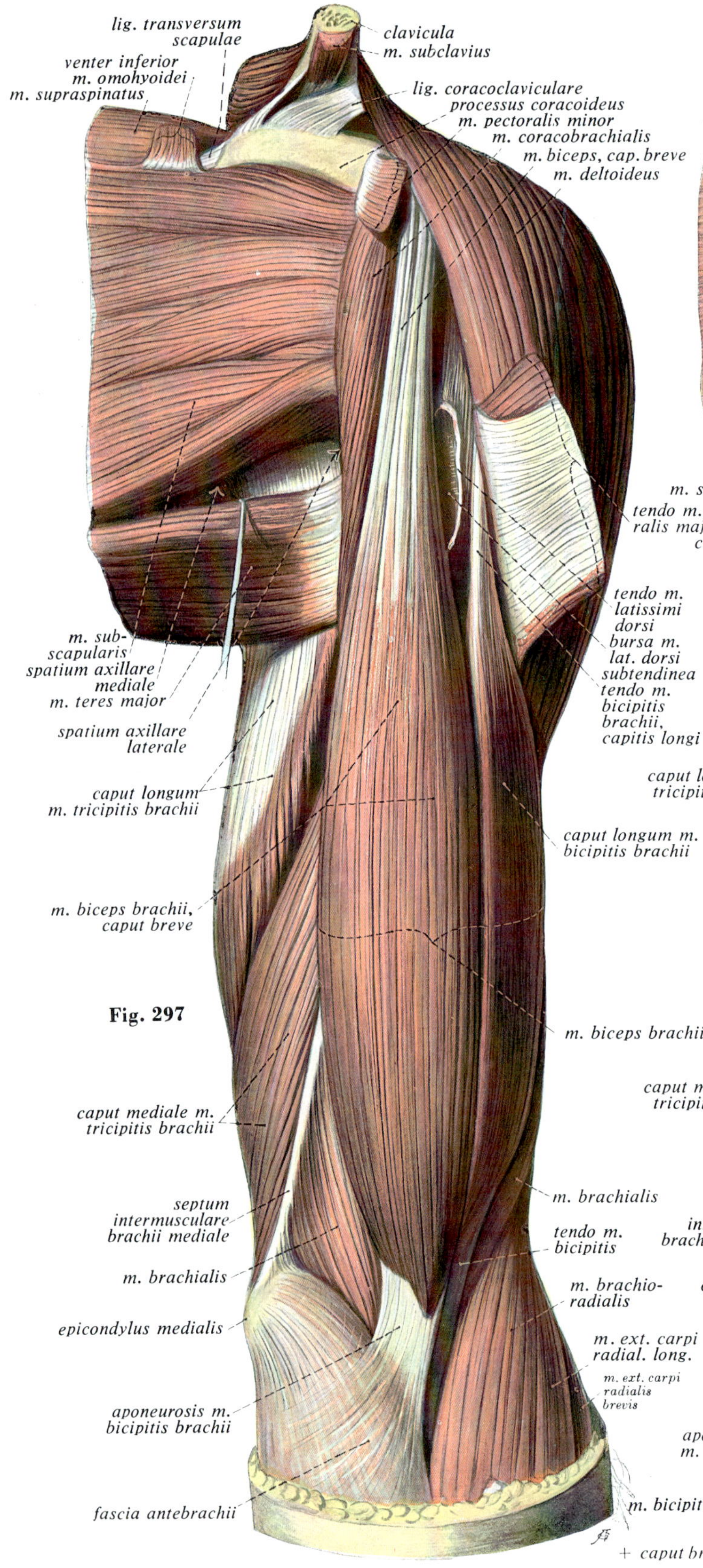

Fig. 297

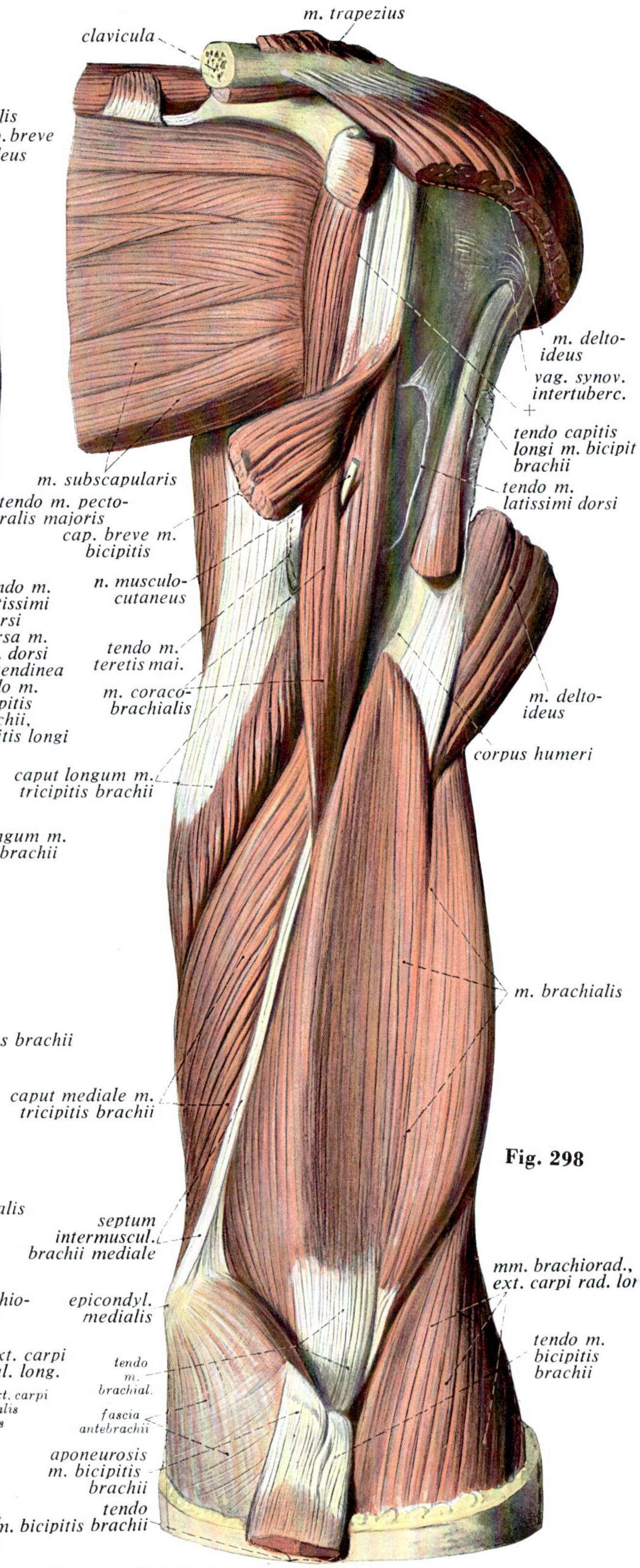

Fig. 298

+ caput breve m. bicipitis et m. coracobrachialis, origo communis

Flexor Surface of the Muscles of the Arm (Figs. 294, 297, 298, 300, 303, 312)

Name		*Origin*	*Insertion*
1. m. biceps brachii (Operates 2 joints)	*caput longum:*	Tendon through shoulder joint to tuberculum supraglenoidale scapulae (long tendon)	Posterior half of tuberositas radialis. Bicipital aponeurosis to fascia antebrachii
	caput breve:	Short tendon from tip of processus coracoideus scapulae	

Action: Flexes and supinates the forearm. Tenses fascia antebrachii. Caput longum aids in flexion of the shoulder joint and holds head of humerus in place

Name	*Origin*	*Insertion*
2. m. coracobrachialis (sometimes pierced by n. musculocutaneus)	Tip of the processus coracoideus (fused with caput breve m. tricipitis)	Ventral and medial side of humerus near middle of shaft

Action: Flexes and adducts the arm

Name	*Origin*	*Insertion*
3. m. brachialis (Operates 1 joint)	Distal half of anterior aspect of humerus and the septa intermuscularia mediale et laterale	tuberositas ulnae (short tendon) and rough impression on anterior surface of processus coronoideus ulnae

Action: Primary flexor of forearm

Nerve: n. musculocutaneus for all three muscles

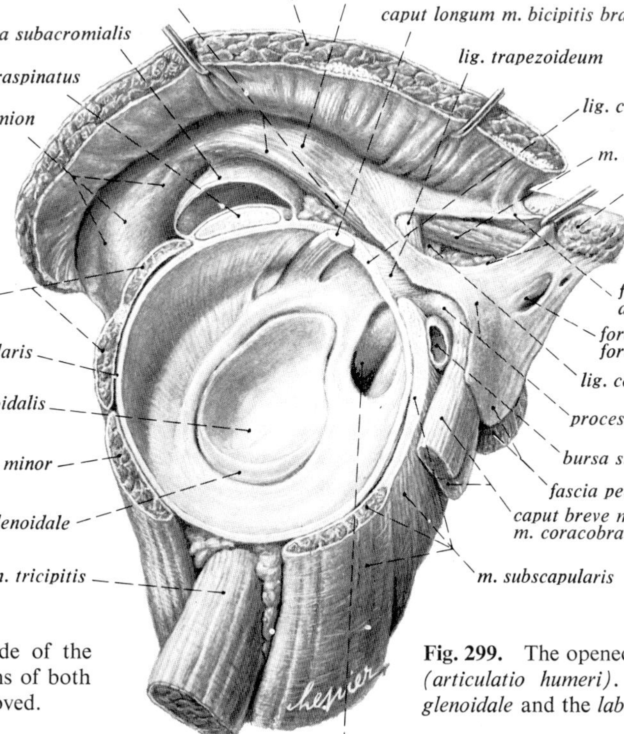

Fig. 297. Muscles of the flexor side of the left arm. Superficial layer.

Fig. 298. Muscles of the flexor side of the arm. Deep layer. The middle sections of both *mm. deltoideus* and *biceps* were removed.

Fig. 299. The opened right shoulder joint *(articulatio humeri)*. Notice the *cavitas glenoidale* and the *labrum glenoidale.*

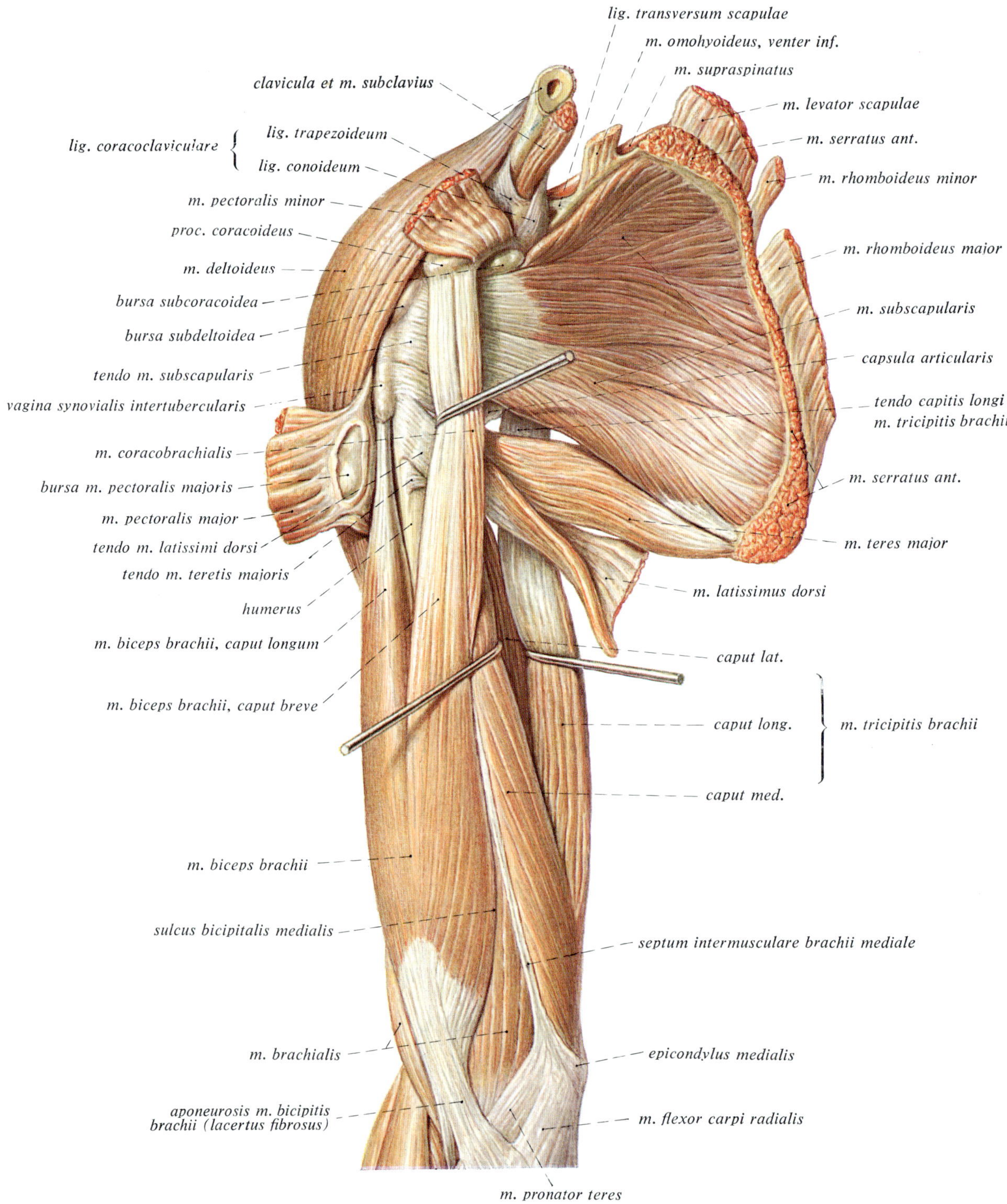

Fig. 300. The muscles of the costal surface of the *scapula* and muscles of the flexor side of the upper arm. Superficial layer.

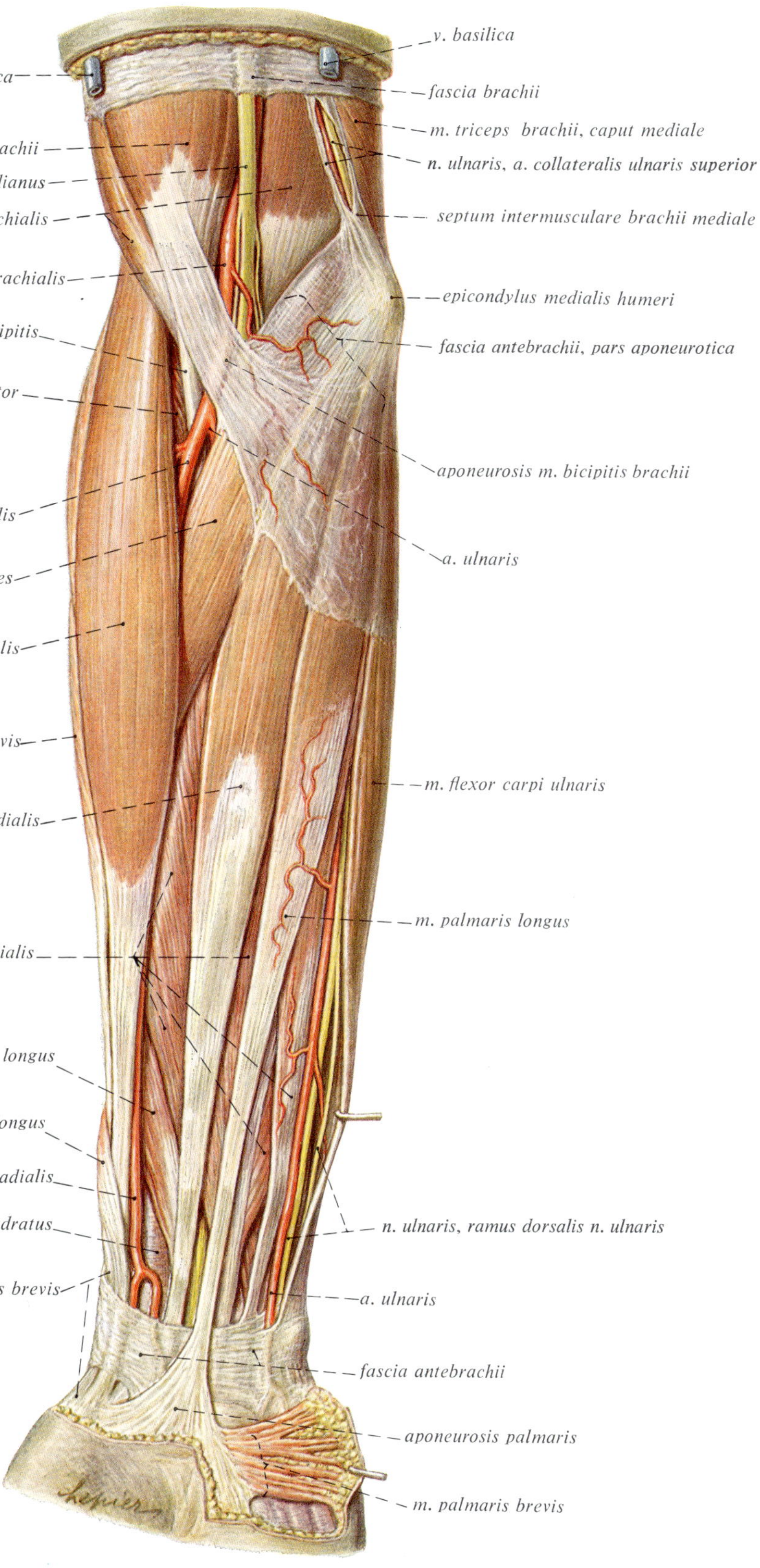

Fig. 301. Muscles (superficial layers) of the flexor side of the forearm and the *m. brachioradialis*. Palmar view.

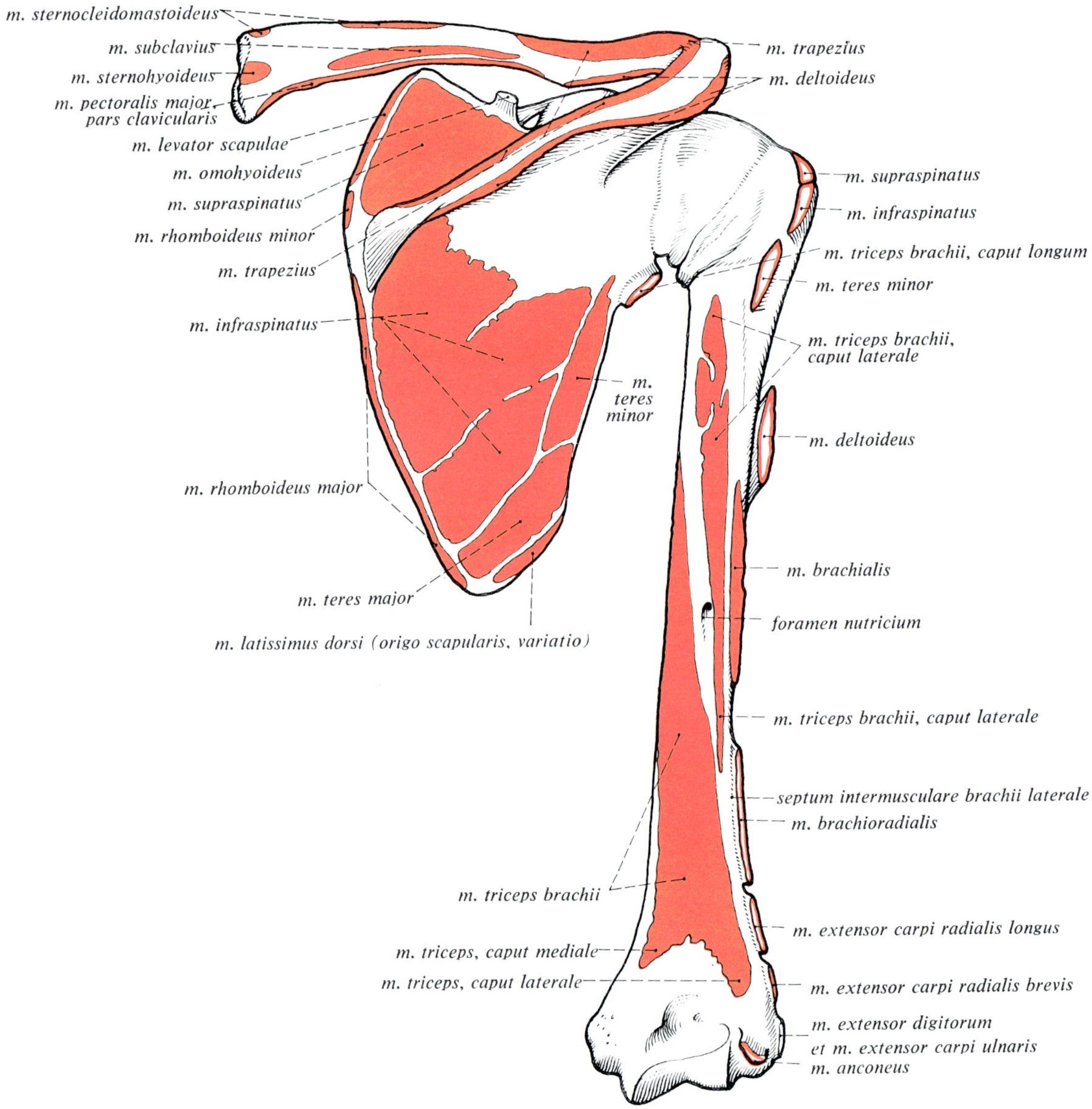

Fig. 302. Diagram of muscle origins and insertions of *clavicula, scapula,* and *humerus*. Dorsal view of right upper arm.

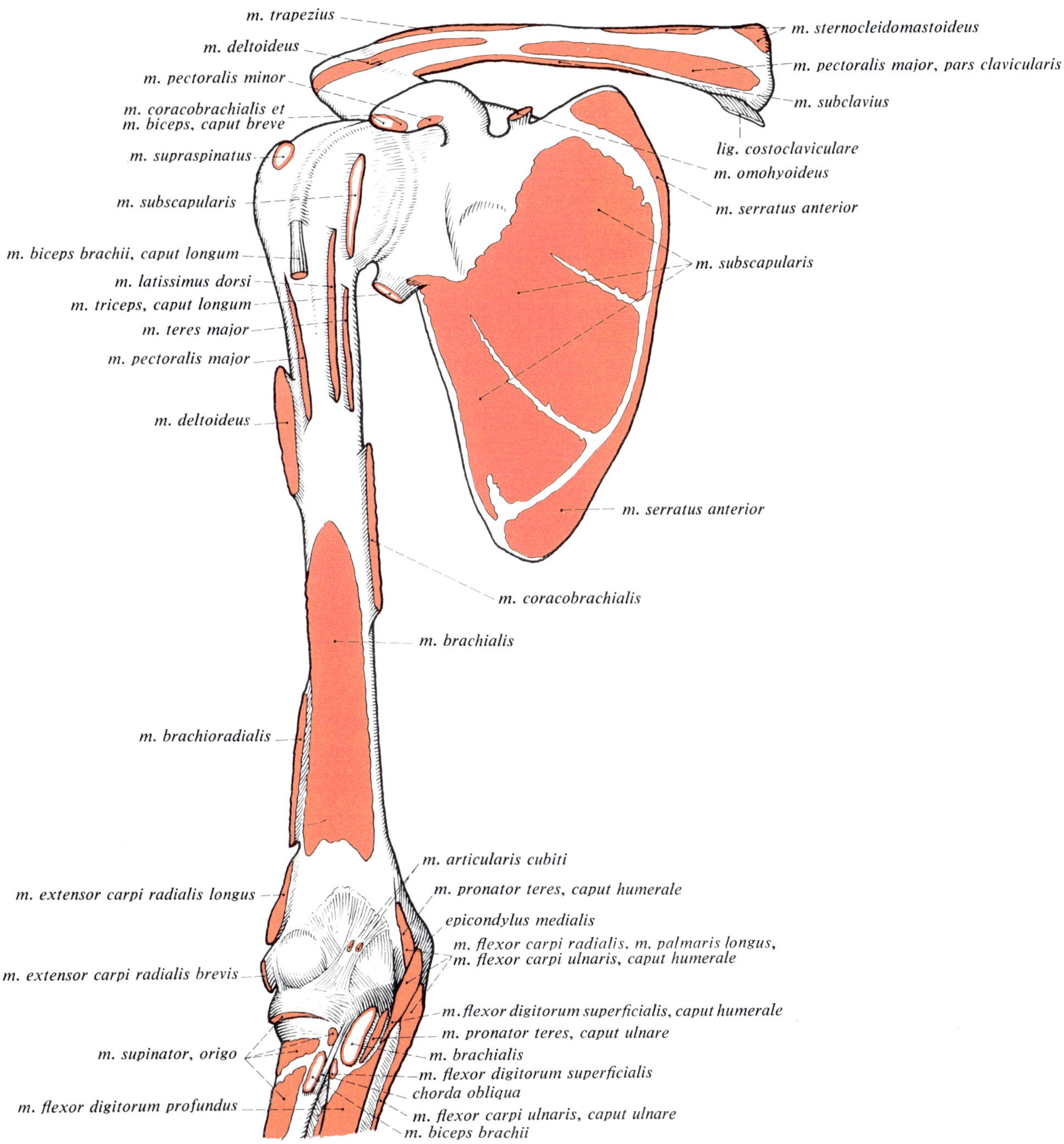

Fig. 303. Diagram of muscle origins and insertions on the *clavicula, scapula, humerus,* and cranial end of the *ulna* and *radius.* Ventral view of the right upper arm.

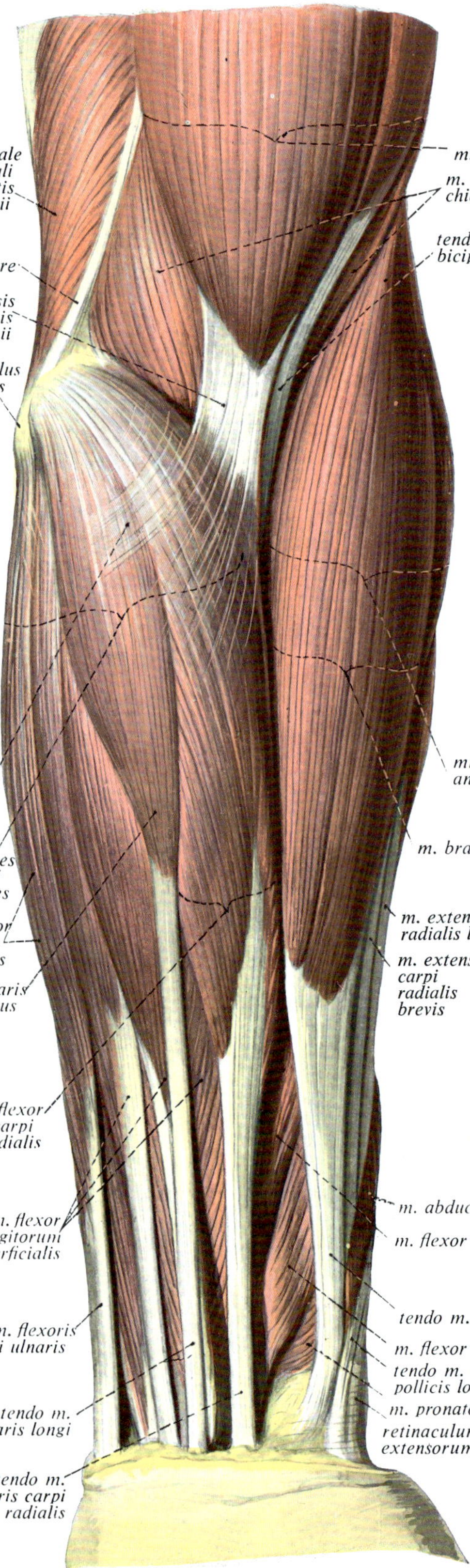

caput mediale musculi tricipitis brachii
m. biceps brachii
m. brachialis
tendo m. bicipitis
septum intermusculare brachii mediale
aponeurosis m. bicipitis brachii
epicondylus medialis
fascia antebrachii
mm. radiales antebrachii
m. brachioradialis
mm. flexores antebrachii superficiales
m. flexor carpi ulnaris
m. extens. carpi radialis longus
m. extensor carpi radialis brevis
m. palmaris longus
m. flexor carpi radialis
m. abductor pollicis longus
m. flexor digitorum superficialis
m. flexor digitorum superficialis
tendo m. brachioradialis
tendo m. flexoris carpi ulnaris
m. flexor pollicis longus
tendo m. abductoris pollicis longi
tendo m. palmaris longi
m. pronator quadratus
retinaculum extensorum
tendo m. flexoris carpi radialis

Fig. 304

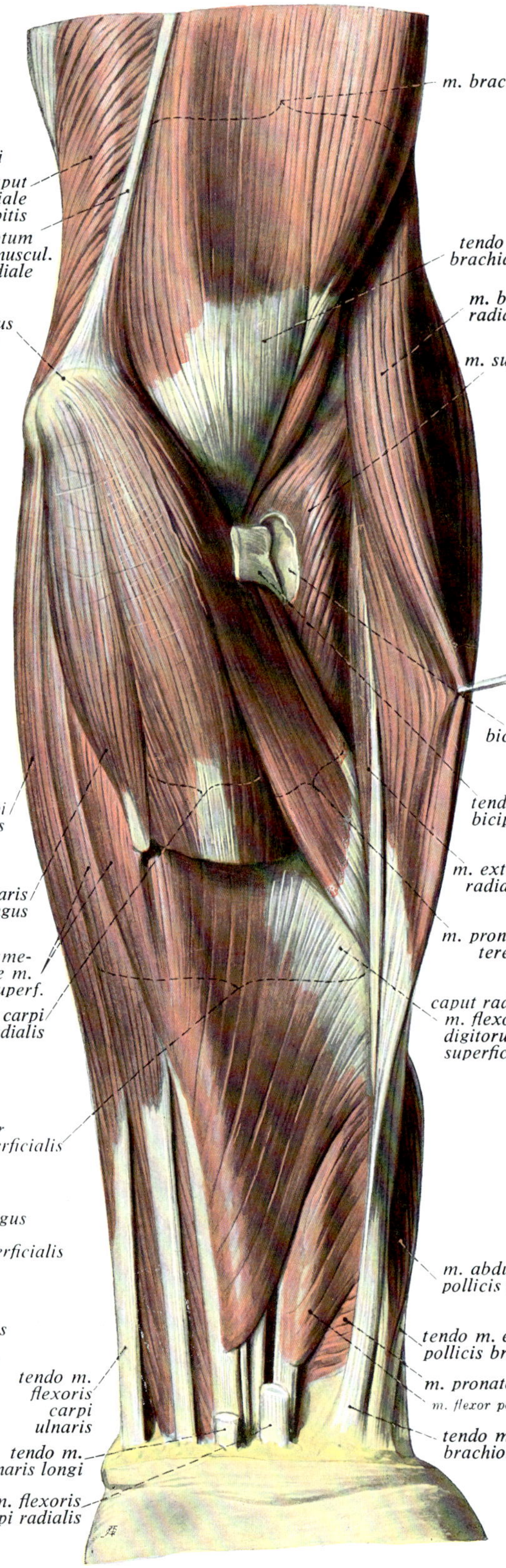

m. brachialis
caput mediale m. tricipitis
septum intermuscul. brachii mediale
tendo m. brachialis
m. brachioradialis
epicondylus medialis
m. supinator
bursa bicipitorad.
mm. flexor carpi ulnaris
tendo m. bicipitis
m. palmaris longus
m. extensor carpi radialis longus
m. pronator teres
caput humeroulnare m. flex. dig. superf.
m. flexor carpi radialis
caput radiale m. flexoris digitorum superficialis
m. flexor digitorum superficialis
m. abductor pollicis longus
tendo m. extensoris pollicis brevis
tendo m. flexoris carpi ulnaris
m. pronator quadr.
m. flexor pollic. long.
tendo m. palmaris longi
tendo m. brachioradialis
tendo m. flexoris carpi radialis

Fig. 305

Flexor Muscles of Forearm, Superficial Group (Figs. 301, 304, 305, 312, 315, 318)

Name	*Origin*	*Insertion*
1. m. pronator teres		
caput humerale (strong)	epicondylus medialis humeri, fascia antebrachii	On the lateral and dorsal surface of radius (middle 1/3)
caput ulnare (weak)	processus coronoideus ulnae	
Nerve: n. medianus (passes through between the two heads; C 5–T 1)		
Action: Pronates and flexes the forearm		
2. m. flexor carpi radialis	epicondylus medialis humeri, fascia antebrachii	Base of 2nd metacarpal bone, palmar surface
Nerve: n. medianus (C 5–T 1)		
Action: Flexes wrist and elbow; abducts wrist, pronates forearm		
3. m. palmaris longus (inconstant)	epicondylus medialis humeri, fascia antebrachii	aponeurosis palmaris
Nerve: n. medianus (C 5–T 1)		
Action: Tenses aponeurosis palmaris; weak flexor of elbow and wrist		
4. m. flexor digitorum superficialis		
caput humeroulnare:	epicondylus medialis humeri and processus coronoideus ulnae	4 long tendons to the middle phalanges of fingers 2 to 5
caput radiale:	Upper half, anterior border of radius	
Nerve: n. medianus (C 5–T 1)		
Action: Flexes middle phalanges of 4 medial fingers; assists in flexion of forearm; medial abduction of hand		
5. m. flexor carpi ulnaris		
caput humerale:	epicondylus medialis humeri	os pisiforme and, by ligaments, to 5th metacarpal bone and os hamatum
caput ulnare:	olecranon and, via the fascia antebrachii, posterior border of ulna	
Nerve: n. ulnaris (C 7, 8; T 1)		
Action: Flexes and adducts wrist joint; flexor of elbow		

Fig. 304. Flexor muscles of the left forearm, superficial layer. Palmar view.

Fig. 305. The same, after severing the *mm. palmaris longus* and *flexor carpi radialis.*

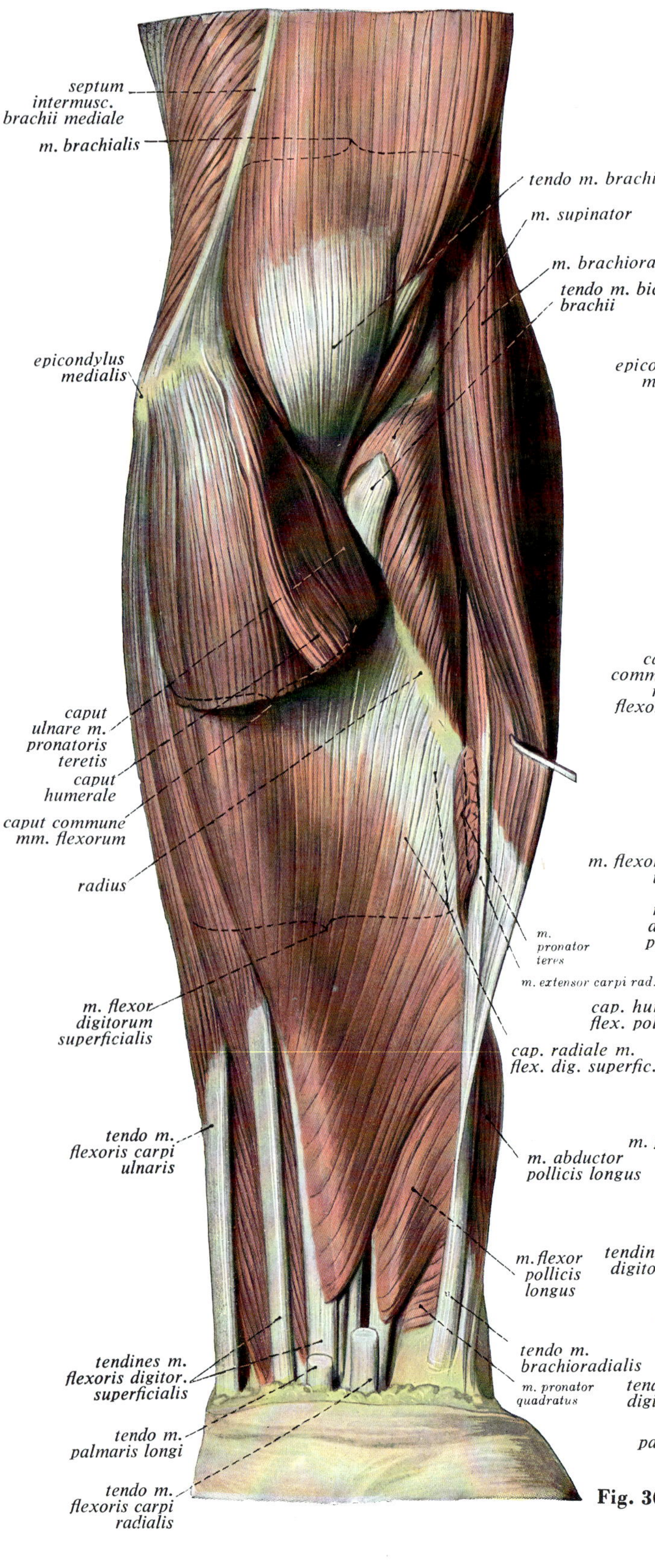
septum
intermusc.
brachii mediale
m. brachialis
tendo m. brachialis
m. supinator
m. brachioradialis
tendo m. bicipitis
brachii
epicondylus
medialis
caput
ulnare m.
pronatoris
teretis
caput
humerale
caput commune
mm. flexorum
radius
m.
pronator
teres
m. extensor carpi rad. long.
m. flexor
digitorum
superficialis
cap. radiale m.
flex. dig. superfic.
tendo m.
flexoris carpi
ulnaris
m. abductor
pollicis longus
m. flexor
pollicis
longus
tendines m.
flexoris digitor.
superficialis
tendo m.
brachioradialis
m. pronator
quadratus
tendo m.
palmaris longi
tendo m.
flexoris carpi
radialis

Fig. 306

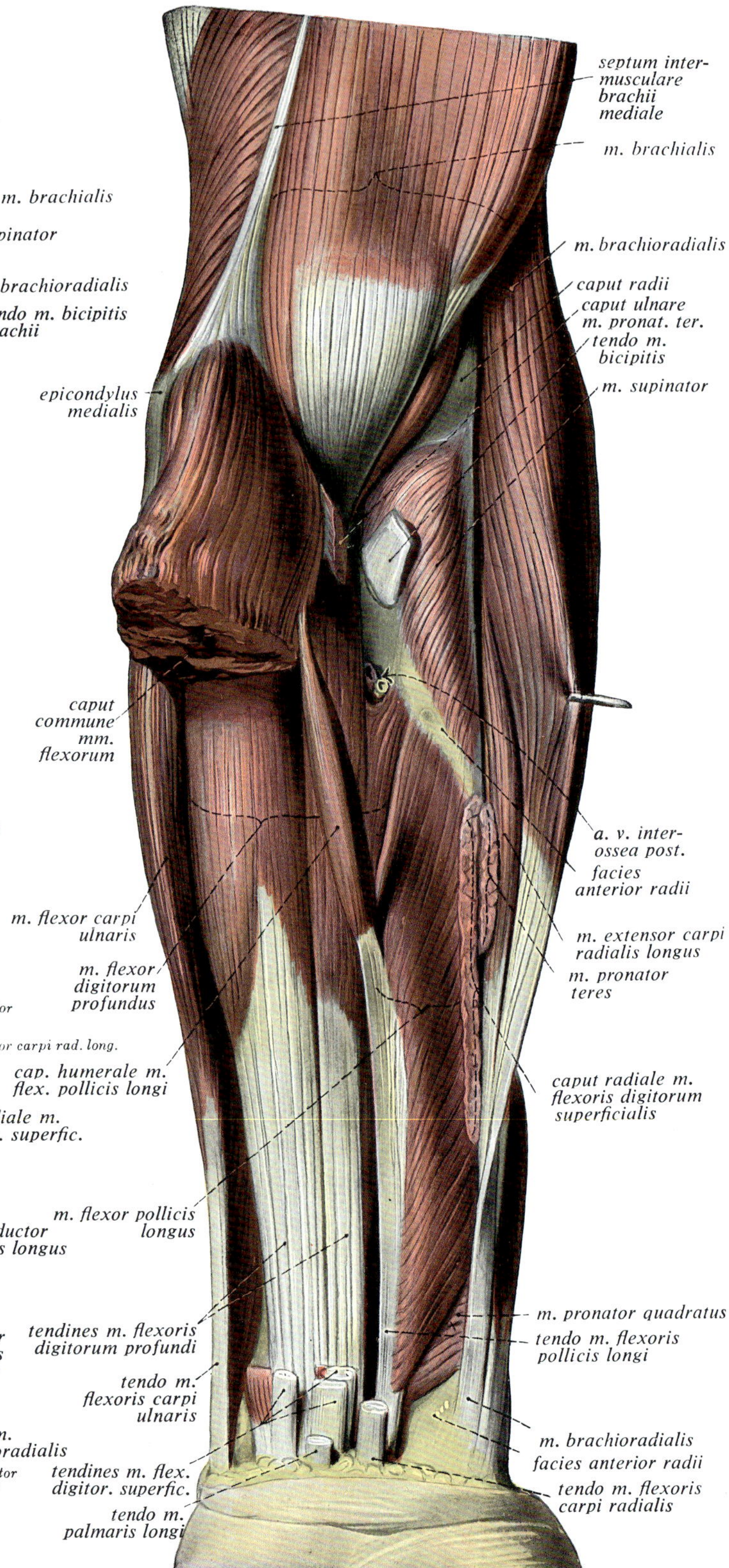
septum inter-
musculare
brachii
mediale
m. brachialis
m. brachioradialis
caput radii
caput ulnare
m. pronat. ter.
tendo m.
bicipitis
m. supinator
epicondylus
medialis
caput
commune
mm.
flexorum
a. v. inter-
ossea post.
facies
anterior radii
m. flexor carpi
ulnaris
m. extensor carpi
radialis longus
m. flexor
digitorum
profundus
m. pronator
teres
cap. humerale m.
flex. pollicis longi
caput radiale m.
flexoris digitorum
superficialis
m. flexor pollicis
longus
tendines m. flexoris
digitorum profundi
m. pronator quadratus
tendo m. flexoris
pollicis longi
tendo m.
flexoris carpi
ulnaris
m. brachioradialis
facies anterior radii
tendines m. flex.
digitor. superfic.
tendo m. flexoris
carpi radialis
tendo m.
palmaris longi

Fig. 307

Flexor Muscles of the Forearm, Deep Group (Figs. 306, 307, 312)

Name	*Origin*	*Insertion*
1. m. flexor digitorum profundus	Anterior and medial surfaces of ulna; membrana interossea	Distal phalanges of fingers 2 to 5
Nerve: n. ulnaris for ulnar side, n. medianus for radial side (C 7, 8; T 1)		
Action: Flexes joints of fingers 2 to 5 (especially the terminal phalanges but also the other phalanges) and wrist joint		
2. m. flexor pollicis longus *caput radiale* (the main part)	Anterior surface of radius; adjacent part of membrana interossea	Terminal phalanx of thumb
caput humerale	processus coronoideus ulnae or epicondylus medialis humeri	
Nerve: Anterior interosseous branch of n. medianus (C 8; T 1)		
Action: Flexes terminal phalanx of thumb; aids in flexion of proximal phalanx and adduction of metacarpal		
3. m. pronator quadratus	Anterior surface of ulna, distal ¼	Anterior surface of distal fourth of radius
Nerve: Anterior interosseous branch of n. medianus (C 8; T 1)		
Action: Pronates the hand		

Fig. 306. Flexor muscles of the left forearm, middle layer. *mm. pronator teres, flexor carpi radialis* and the *palmaris longus* were divided to display the *m. flexor digitorum superficialis;* the *m. brachioradialis* was pulled back laterally.

Fig. 307. Deep layers of the flexor muscles of the left forearm. All superficial flexor muscles were cut and partially resected with the exception of the *m. flexor carpi ulnaris.*

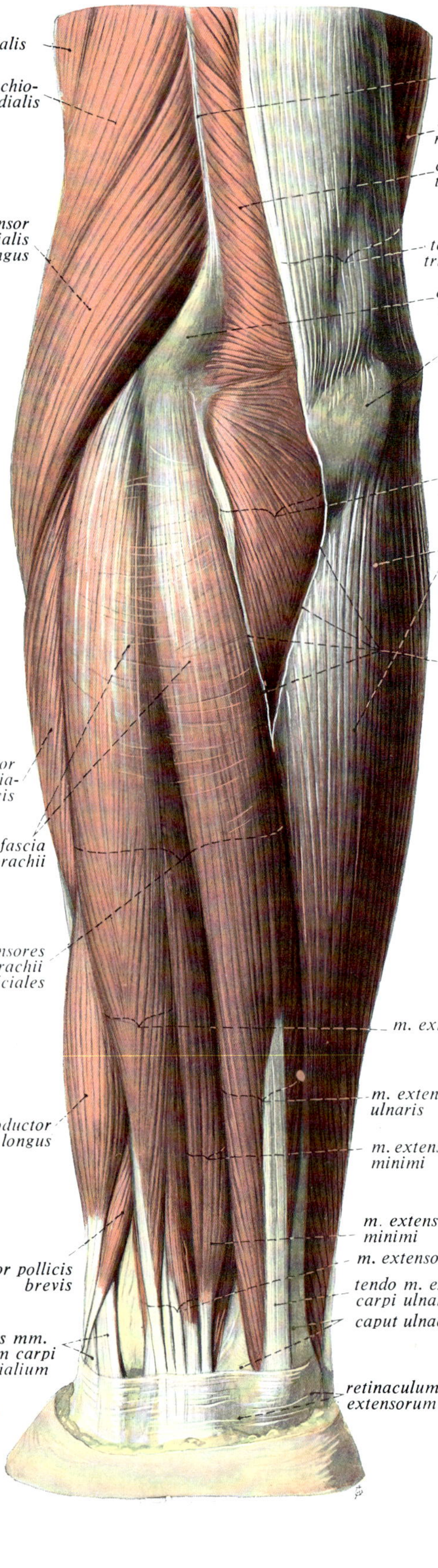
m. brachialis
m. brachio-radialis
m. extensor carpi radialis longus
septum intermusculare brachii laterale
caput mediale m. tricipitis brachii
caput mediale m. tricipitis brachii
tendo m. tricipitis brachii
epicondylus lateralis
olecranon
m. anconeus
m. flexor carpi ulnaris
fascia ante-brachii
m. extensor carpi radia-lis brevis
fascia antebrachii
mm. extensores antebrachii superficiales
m. extensor digitorum
m. extensor carpi ulnaris
m. abductor pollicis longus
m. extensor digiti minimi
m. extensor digiti minimi
m. extensor digitor.
m. extensor pollicis brevis
tendo m. extensoris carpi ulnaris
caput ulnae
tendines mm. extensorum carpi radialium
retinaculum extensorum

Fig. 308

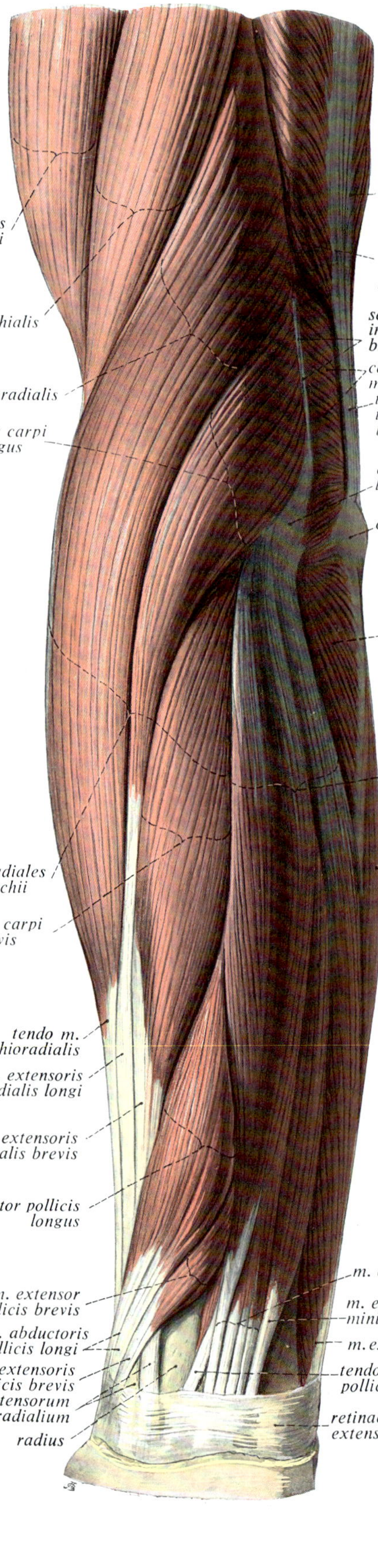
m. biceps brachii
m. brachialis
m. brachioradialis
m. extensor carpi radialis longus
m. triceps brachii
caput laterale m. tricipitis brachii
septum intermusculare brachii laterale
caput mediale m. tricipitis
tendo m. tricipitis brachii
epicondylus lateralis
olecranon
m. anconeus
mm. exten-sores super-ficiales antebrachii
m. flexor carpi ulnaris
mm. radiales antebrachii
m. extensor carpi radialis brevis
tendo m. brachioradialis
tendo m. extensoris carpi radialis longi
tendo m. extensoris carpi radialis brevis
m. abductor pollicis longus
m. extensor pollicis brevis
m. extensor digit.
m. extensor digiti minimi
tendo m. abductoris pollicis longi
m. ext. carpi ulnaris
tendo m. extensoris pollicis brevis
tendo m. extensoris pollicis longi
tendines mm. extensorum carpi radialium
retinaculum extensorum
radius

Fig. 309

Extensor Muscles of the Forearm (Figs. 302–304, 308, 309, 312, 313)

Name	*Origin*	*Insertion*
1. m. brachioradialis	Lateral supracondylar ridge of humerus; septum intermusculare laterale	Proximal end of processus styloideus radii
Nerve: n. radialis (C 5, 6)		
Action: Flexes forearm; pronates forearm if supinated; supinates, if forearm is pronated		
2. m. extensor carpi radialis longus	Distal $^1/_3$ of lateral supracondylar ridge of humerus and septum intermusculare laterale	Base of 2nd metacarpal bone
3. m. extensor carpi radialis brevis	epicondylus lateralis humeri	Base of 3rd metacarpal bone
Nerve: n. radialis (C 6, 7)		
Action: Extends and abducts the hand		

Superficial Layers of Extensor Muscles (Figs. 308, 309, 316)

1. m. extensor digitorum	epicondylus lateralis humeri; fascia antebrachii	By 4 tendons to middle and distal phalanges of the fingers
2. m. extensor digiti minimi		Joins extensor tendon to little finger
Nerve: deep n. radialis (C 6, 7, 8)		
Action: Extends the little finger (proximal phalanges, in particular); indirectly the entire hand, also medial abduction		
3. m. extensor carpi ulnaris Separated from above by an intermuscular septum	epicondylus lateralis humeri; fascia antebrachii	Base of 5th metacarpal, dorsal surface
Nerve: deep n. radialis (C 6, 7, 8)		
Action: Extends (slightly) and adducts hand		

Fig. 308. Superficial group of extensor muscles of the left forearm and the distal part of the arm. Dorsal view.

Fig. 309. Superficial muscles of the left forearm and the distal part of the arm. As seen from the lateral (radial) side.

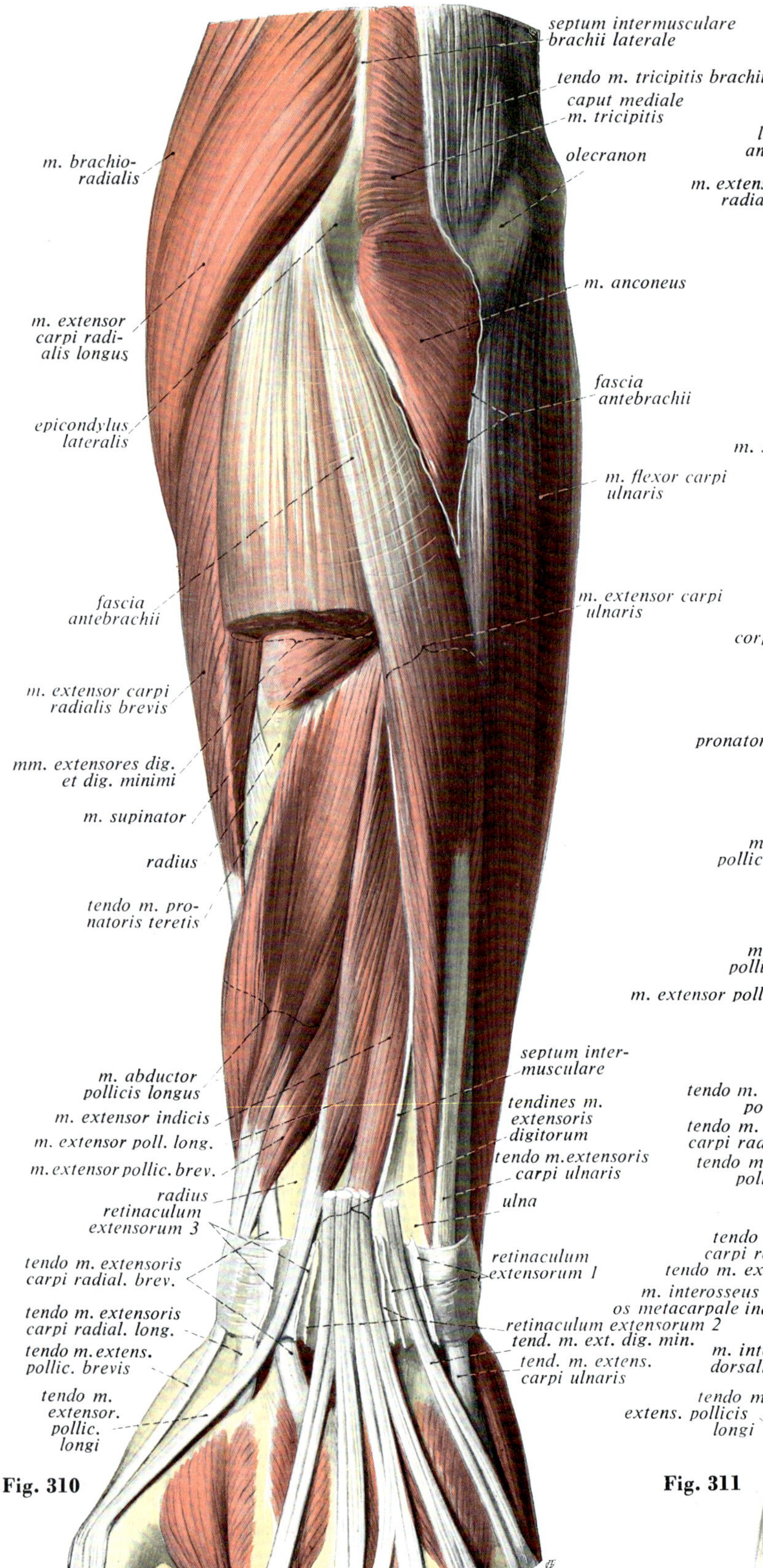

septum intermusculare brachii laterale
tendo m. tricipitis brachii
caput mediale m. tricipitis
olecranon
m. anconeus
fascia antebrachii
m. flexor carpi ulnaris
m. extensor carpi ulnaris
septum inter- musculare
tendines m. extensoris digitorum
tendo m.extensoris carpi ulnaris
ulna
retinaculum extensorum 1
retinaculum extensorum 2
tend. m. ext. dig. min.
tend. m. extens. carpi ulnaris
m. brachio- radialis
m. extensor carpi radi- alis longus
epicondylus lateralis
fascia antebrachii
m. extensor carpi radialis brevis
mm. extensores dig. et dig. minimi
m. supinator
radius
tendo m. pro- natoris teretis
m. abductor pollicis longus
m. extensor indicis
m. extensor poll. long.
m. extensor pollic. brev.
radius
retinaculum extensorum 3
tendo m. extensoris carpi radial. brev.
tendo m. extensoris carpi radial. long.
tendo m. extens. pollic. brevis
tendo m. extensor. pollic. longi

Fig. 310

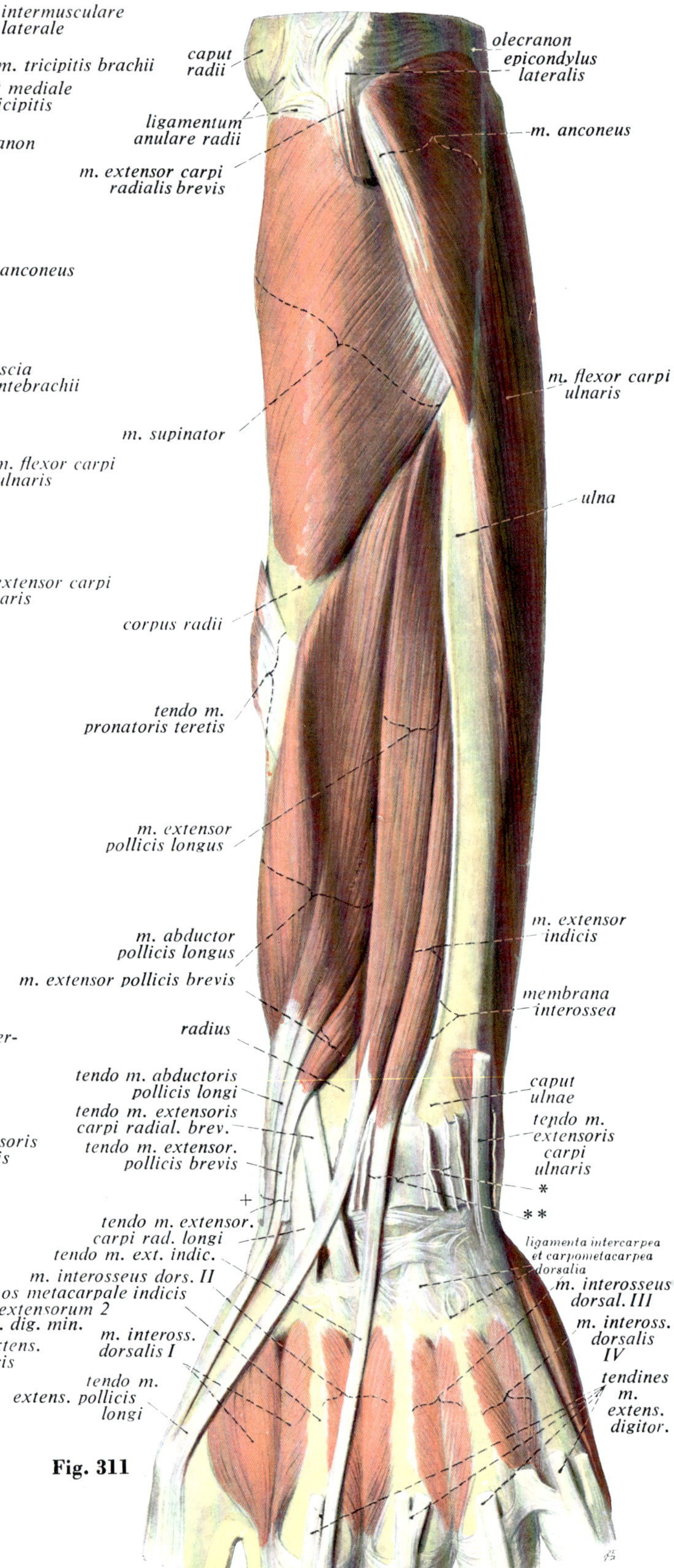

caput radii
ligamentum anulare radii
m. extensor carpi radialis brevis
olecranon
epicondylus lateralis
m. anconeus
m. flexor carpi ulnaris
m. supinator
ulna
corpus radii
tendo m. pronatoris teretis
m. extensor pollicis longus
m. abductor pollicis longus
m. extensor pollicis brevis
m. extensor indicis
membrana interossea
radius
tendo m. abductoris pollicis longi
tendo m. extensoris carpi radial. brev.
tendo m. extensor. pollicis brevis
caput ulnae
tendo m. extensoris carpi ulnaris
*
+
**
tendo m. extensor. carpi rad. longi
tendo m. ext. indic.
ligamenta intercarpea et carpometacarpea dorsalia
m. interosseus dors. II
os metacarpale indicis
m. interosseus dorsal. III
m. inteross. dorsalis I
m. inteross. dorsalis IV
tendo m. extens. pollicis longi
tendines m. extens. digitor.

Fig. 311

Extensor Muscles of the Forearm (continued) **and Supinator Muscle (Figs. 310, 311, 313, 316)**

Name	*Origin*	*Insertion*
1. m. abductor pollicis longus	Posterior surface of ulna and radius; membrana interossea	Base of 1st metacarpal of thumb, radial side
2. m. extensor pollicis brevis	Posterior surface of radius; membrana interossea	Base of proximal phalanx of thumb
Nerve: Deep n. radialis (C 6, 7, 8)		
Action: Abducts thumb; extends 1st phalanx of thumb, and abducts hand		
1. m. extensor pollicis longus	Posterior surface of ulna; membrana interossea	Distal phalanx of thumb
2. m. extensor indicis		Dorsal extensor expansion to 1st phalanx of index finger
Nerve: Deep n. radialis (C 6, 7, 8)		
Action: Extends thumb and index finger, somewhat adducts index finger		
m. supinator (Figs. 306, 311–313) Two layers (superficial and deep) between which the deep branch of n. radialis lies	epicondulus lateralis humeri; ligamentum collaterale radii; ligamentum anulare radii; supinator crest of ulna	Lateral surface and posterior border of radius, proximal and distal to tuberositas radii
Nerve: Deep n. radialis (C 6)		
Action: Supinates hand and forearm		

Fig. 310. Extensor muscles of the left forearm. Dorsal view. The *mm. extensor digitorum* and *digiti minimi* were severed; the tendon compartments of the *retinaculum extensorum* were partly opened: 1. the *m. extensor digiti minimi;* 2. *m. extensor digitorum* and *extensor indicis;* 3. the *m. extensor pollicis longus.*

Fig. 311. Deep layer of extensor muscles of the left forearm. Dorsolateral view. The superficial layer of the extensors and the muscles of the radial group were removed with the exception of the tendon stumps. The tendon compartments of the *retinaculum extensorum* were completely opened: * the *m. extensor digiti minimi;* ** *mm. extensor digitorum* and *extensor indicis;* + *mm. abductor pollicis longus* and *extensor pollicis brevis.*

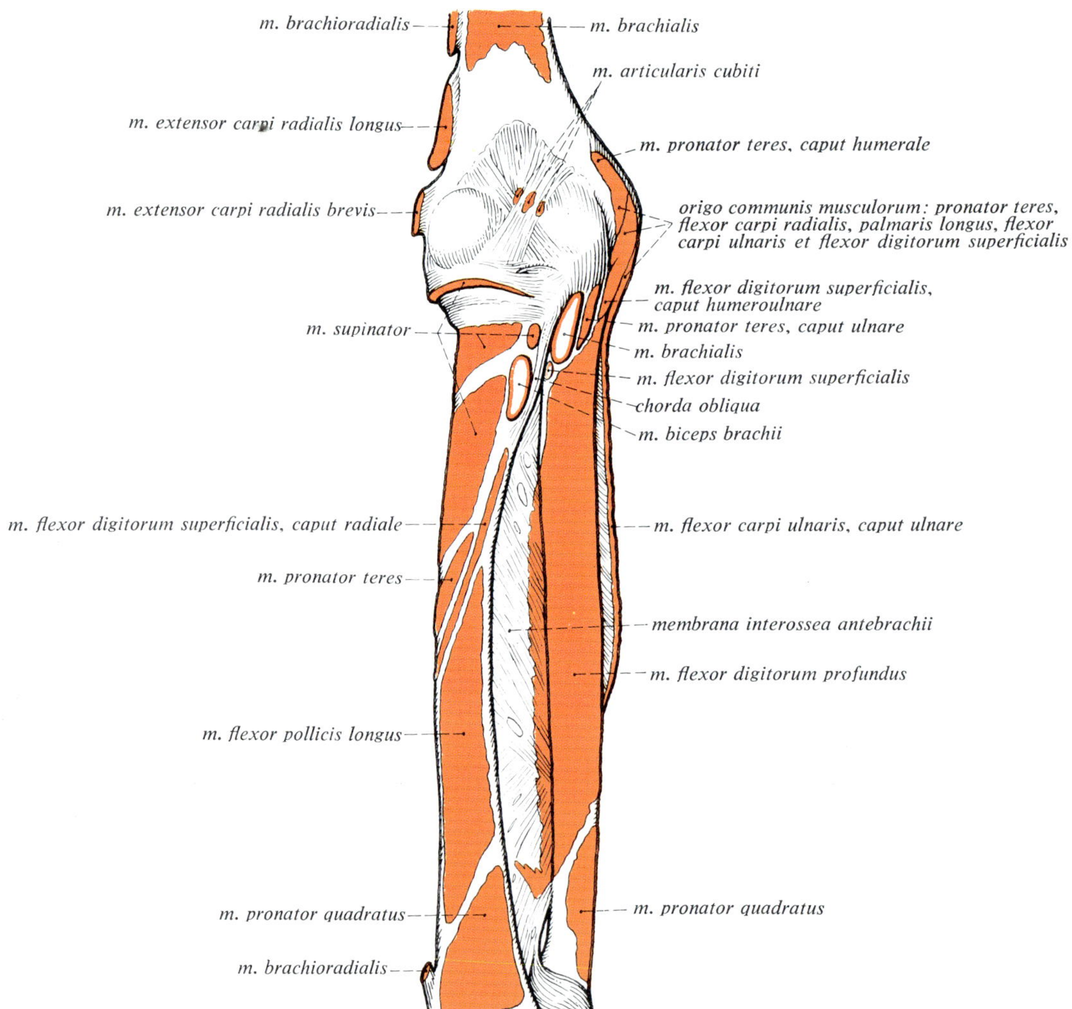

Fig. 312. Diagram of muscle attachments to the *radius, ulna*, and distal end of the *humerus*. Anterior or palmar view of right forearm. (2/3).

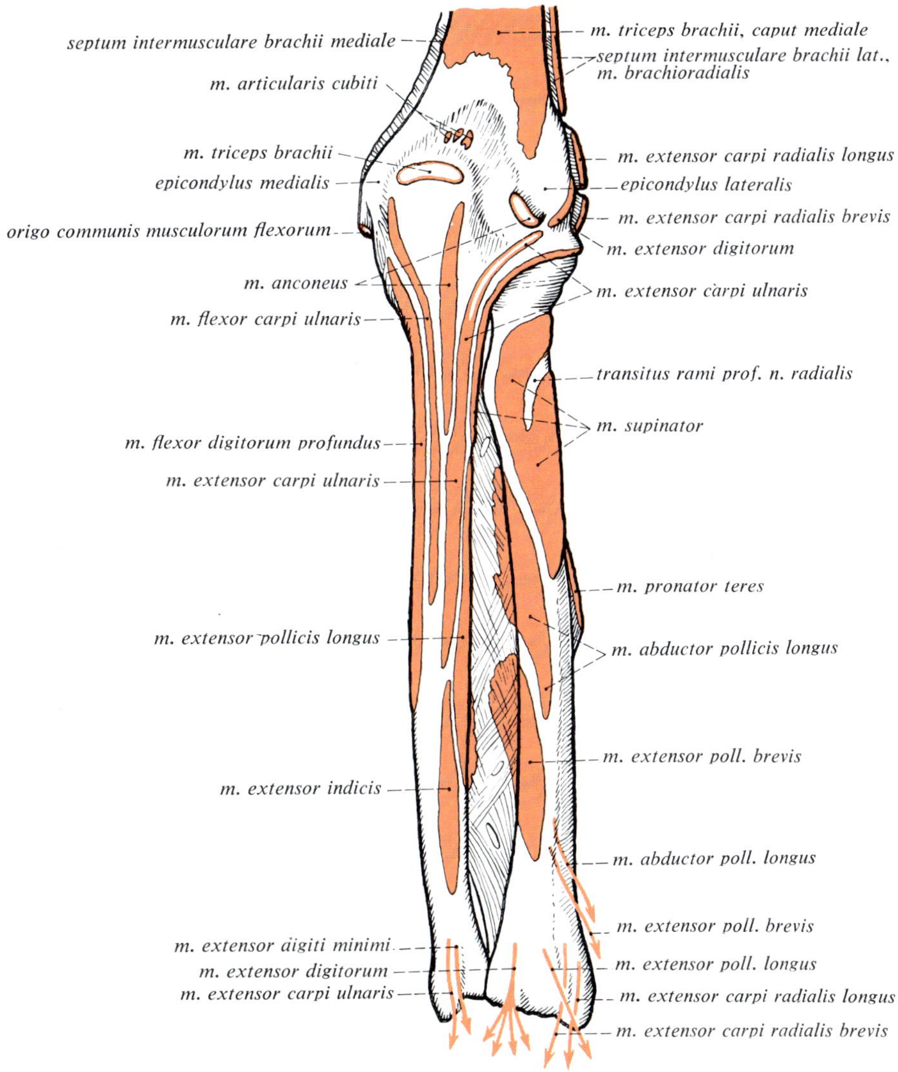

Fig. 313. Muscle attachments mapped out on the *radius, ulna,* and distal end of the *humerus.* Posterior or dorsal view of the right forearm. Arrows at distal end of the *ulna* and *radius* indicate the tendon compartments.

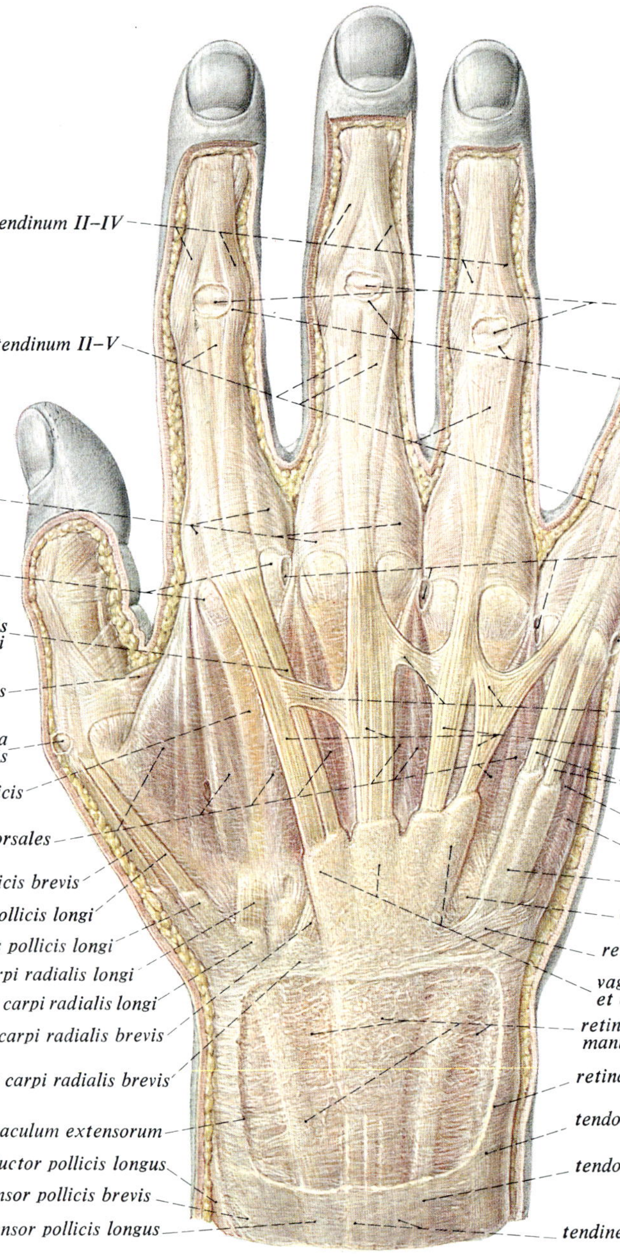

Fig. 314. Tendons and tendon sheaths of the dorsal aspect of the right hand. The *retinaculum extensorum* partly removed.

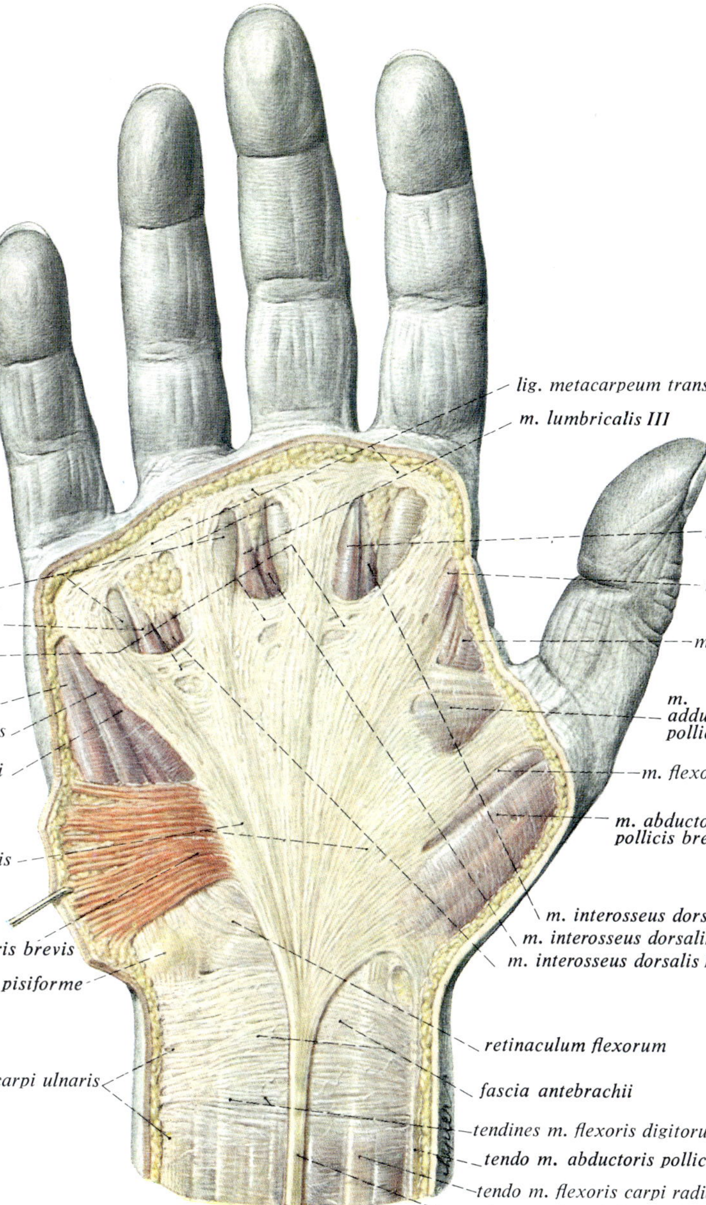

Fig. 315. Muscles and fascia of the right palm. The *mm. interossei,* the *aponeurosis palmaris* and *m. palmaris brevis* after removal of the skin and subcutaneous fatty tissues of the palm of the hand.

Name	*Origin*	*Insertion*
m. palmaris brevis Cutaneous muscle, numerous separated fasciculi	aponeurosis palmaris, medial margin	Skin over medial border of palm

Nerve: n. ulnaris, r. superficialis (C 8)

Action: Tenses skin of medial side of palm

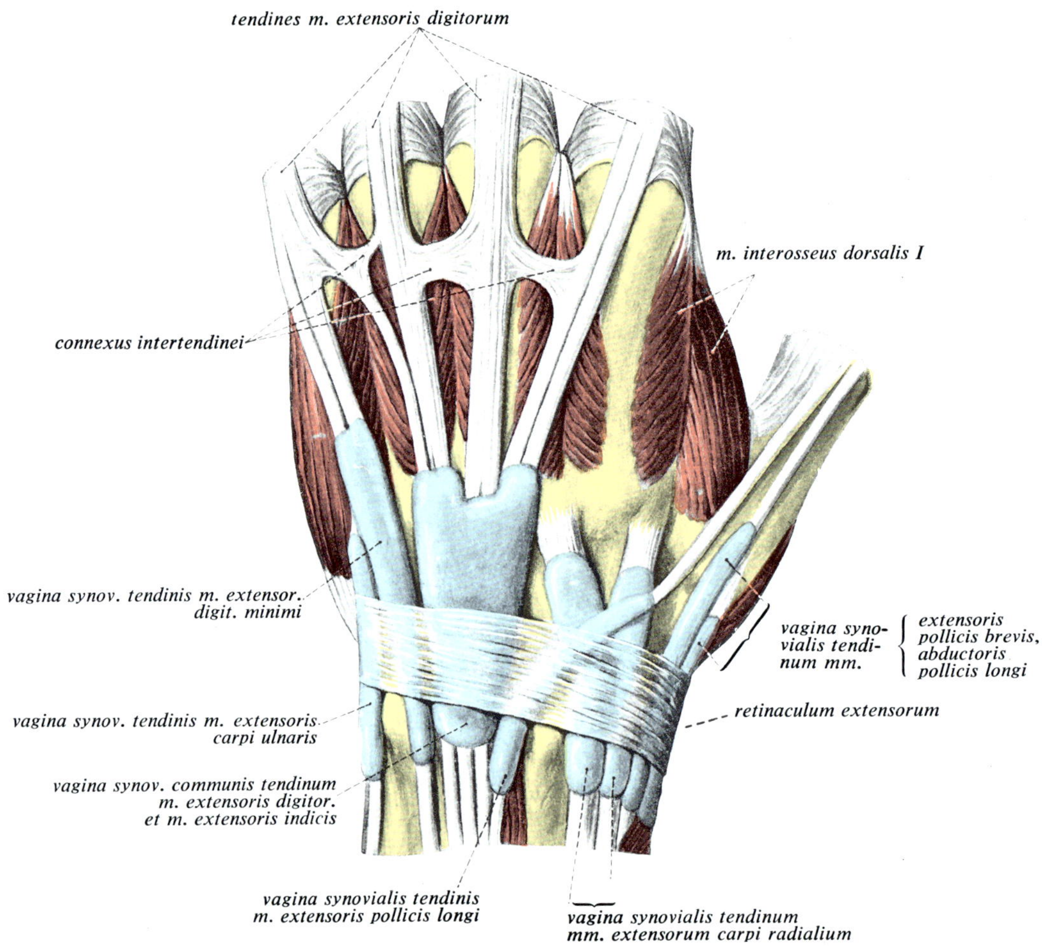

Fig. 316. Semidiagram of the tendons and tendon sheaths of the extensor tendons of the dorsal aspect of the hand and wrist.

The tendon sheaths *(vaginae synoviales)* for the tendons of the *mm. extensor pollicis brevis* and *abductor pollicis longus* as well as those of the *mm. extensor carpi longus and brevis* are mostly or partly held in common. Six tendon compartments hold tendons in position on the dorsum of the hand: (1) the most lateral or radial, the tendons of the *mm. abductor pollicis longus* and the *extensor pollicis brevis*; (2) the tendons of the *mm. extensor carpi radialis longus* and *brevis*; (3) the tendon of the *m. extensor pollicis longus;* (4) the tendons of the *mm. extensor digitorum* and *extensor indicis;* (5) the tendon of the *m. extensor digiti minimi;* and (6) the most medial or ulnar, the tendon of the *m. extensor carpi ulnaris.*

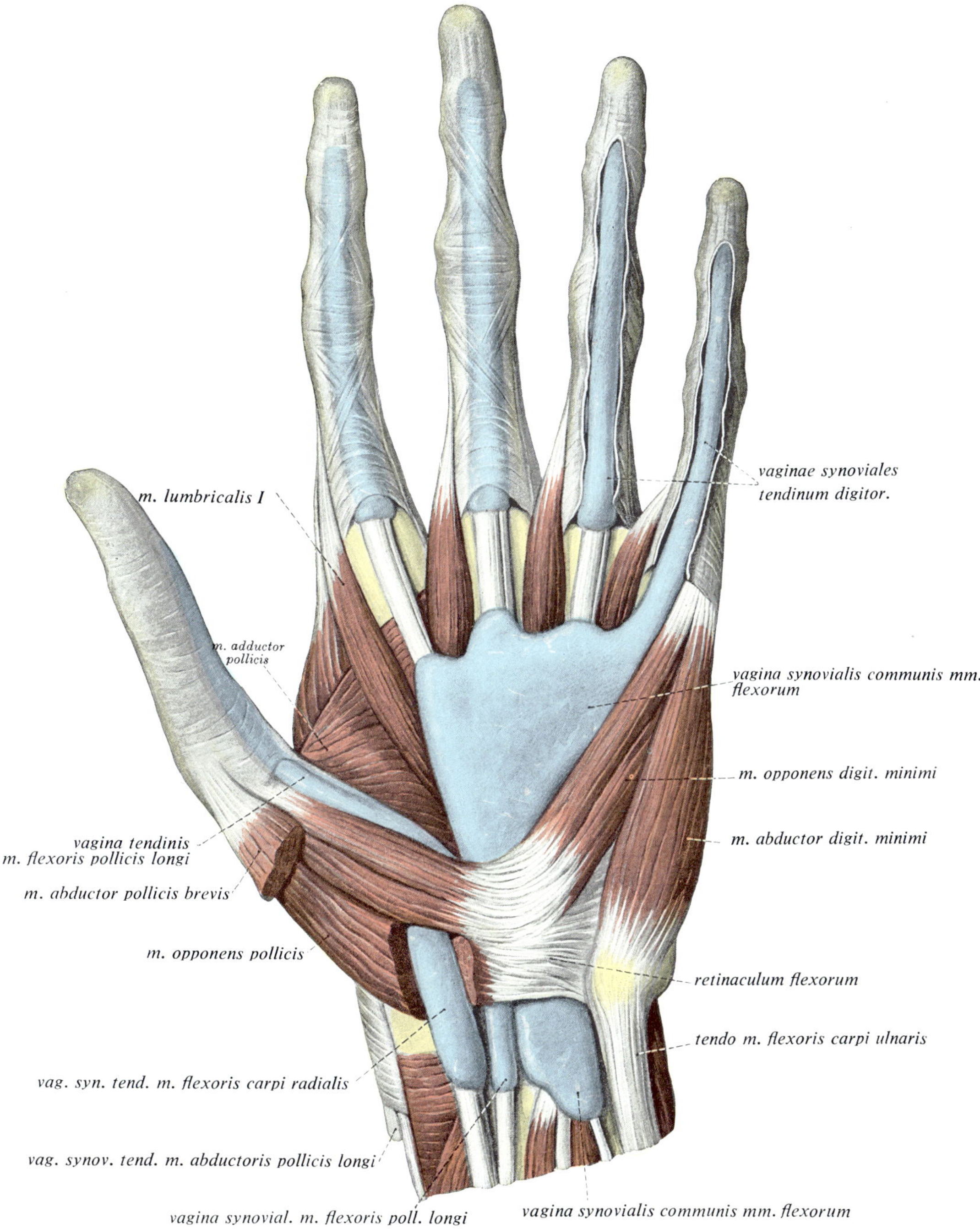

Fig. 317. Semidiagram of the synovial sheaths *(vaginae synoviales)* of the tendons of the palmar aspect of the left hand and wrist. The synovial tendon sheath of the *m. flexor carpi radialis* has been exposed by removing a short segment of the muscles of the thenar eminence. The ligamentous fibrous sheath of the 4th and 5th fingers were split. The tendon sheaths were displayed by injecting them with a blue latex. In the living, they are filled with a clear, colorless fluid.

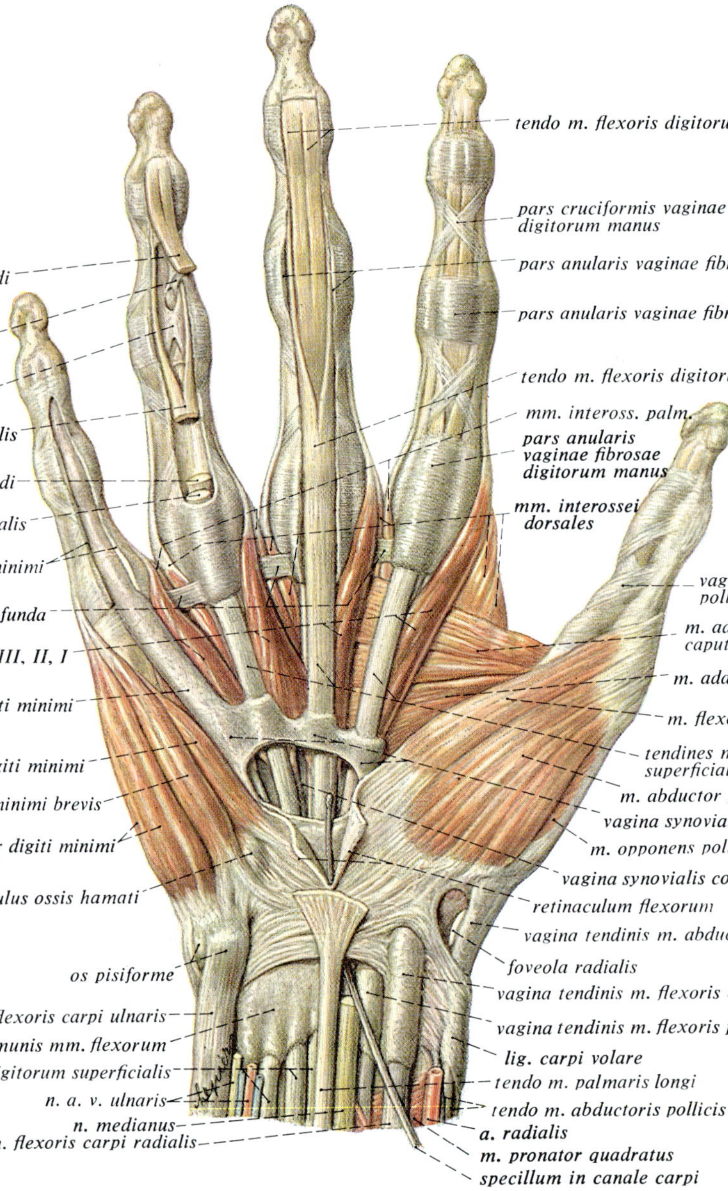

Fig. 318. Muscles of the palm after removal of the larger part of the *aponeurosis palmaris*. The tendon sheath of the middle finger was split along its entire length. The *retinaculum flexorum* was partially opened.

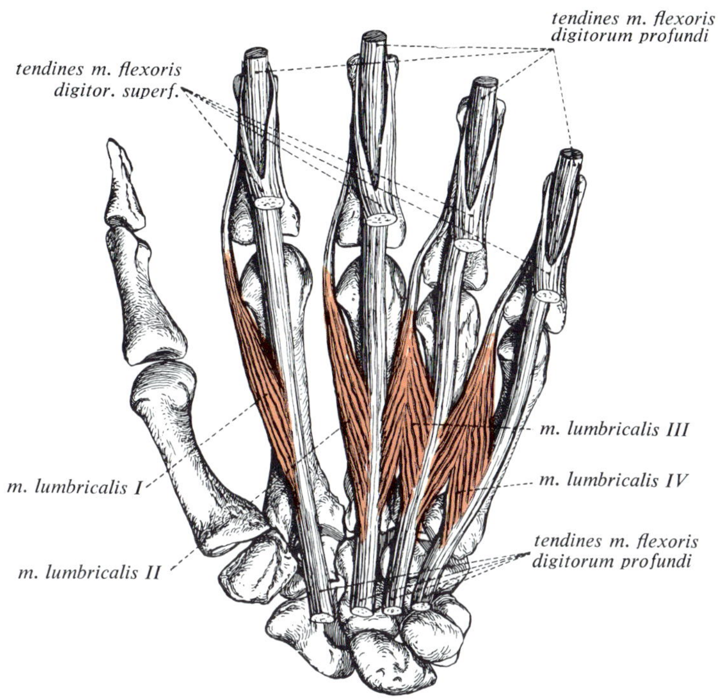

Fig. 319. Diagram of the *mm. lumbricales.* Palmar view of the left hand.

Mm. lumbricales (Figs. 319, 320)

Origin:	Tendons of m. flexor digitorum profundus
Insertion:	Dorsal aponeurosis of the proximal phalanx of fingers II to V
Nerve:	Two lateral lumbricals: n. medianus Two medial lumbricals: n. ulnaris
Action:	Flexes the metacarpophalangeal joints; extends the two distal phalanges

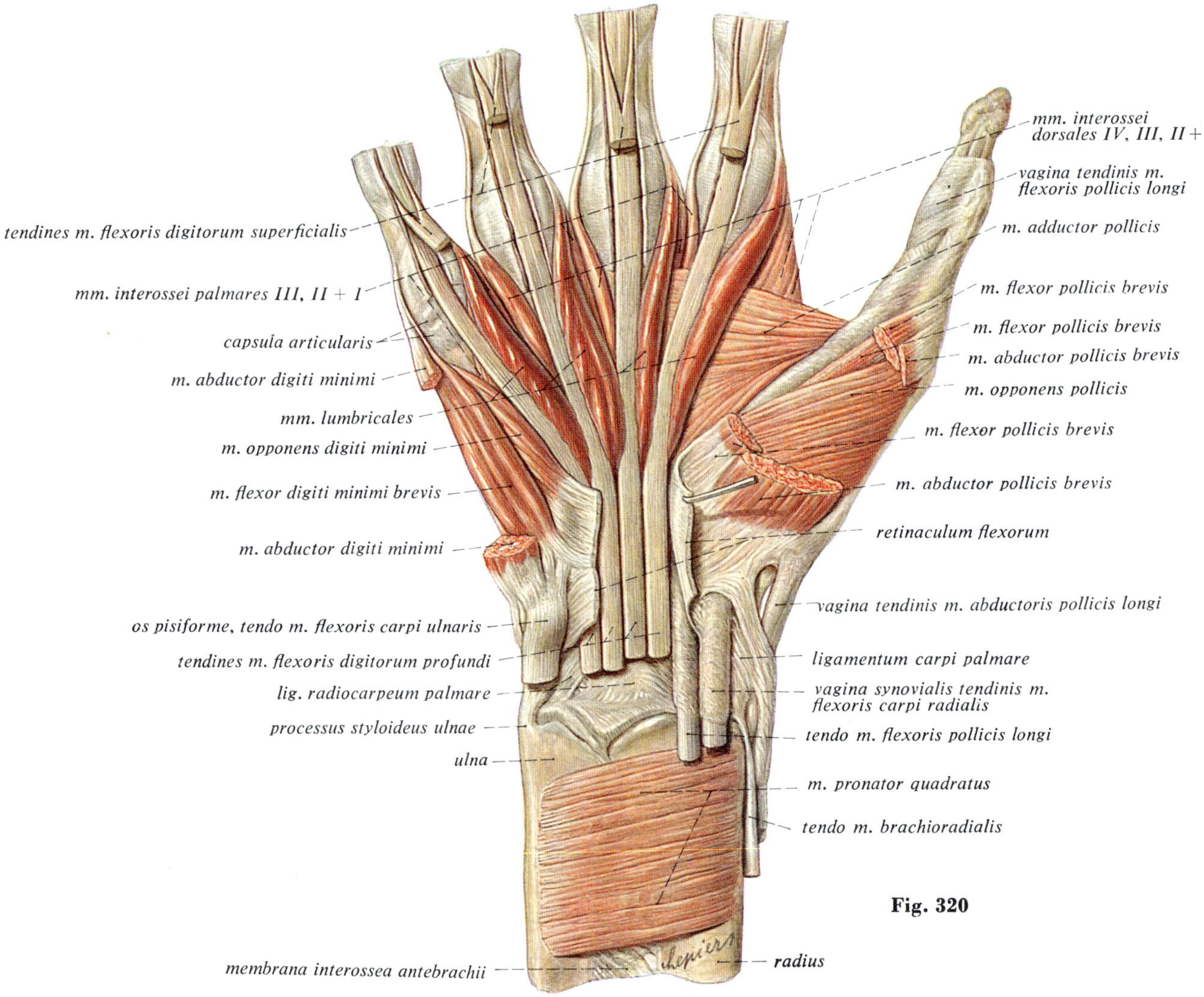
mm. interossei dorsales IV, III, II + I
vagina tendinis m. flexoris pollicis longi
m. adductor pollicis
m. flexor pollicis brevis
m. flexor pollicis brevis
m. abductor pollicis brevis
m. opponens pollicis
m. flexor pollicis brevis
m. abductor pollicis brevis
retinaculum flexorum
vagina tendinis m. abductoris pollicis longi
ligamentum carpi palmare
vagina synovialis tendinis m. flexoris carpi radialis
tendo m. flexoris pollicis longi
m. pronator quadratus
tendo m. brachioradialis
radius
tendines m. flexoris digitorum superficialis
mm. interossei palmares III, II + I
capsula articularis
m. abductor digiti minimi
mm. lumbricales
m. opponens digiti minimi
m. flexor digiti minimi brevis
m. abductor digiti minimi
os pisiforme, tendo m. flexoris carpi ulnaris
tendines m. flexoris digitorum profundi
lig. radiocarpeum palmare
processus styloideus ulnae
ulna
membrana interossea antebrachii

Fig. 320

Muscles of the Hypothenar Eminence (Figs. 318, 320, 321, 325, 326)

Name	*Origin*	*Insertion*
1. m. abductor digiti minimi	os pisiforme and tendon of m. flexor carpi ulnaris	Proximal phalanx of little finger, ulnar side
2. m. flexor digiti minimi brevis (variable)	retinaculum flexorum, hamulus ossis hamati	Ulnar side of proximal phalanx of little finger
3. m. opponens digiti minimi	retinaculum flexorum, hamulus ossis hamati	Ulnar margin of 5th metacarpal

Nerve: ramus profundus n. ulnaris (C 8; T 1)

Action: As their names indicate: Abducts and reflexes little finger; m. opponens digiti minimi also rotates 5th metacarpal and brings it out of plane of palm to meet the thumb and cup the hand

Fig. 320. Deeper layers of the musculature of the palm and the *m. pronator quadratus.* The *retinaculum flexorum* was severed. The flexor tendons of fingers 2–5 were severed to display the *mm. lumbricales.* The muscles of the *thenar* and *hypothenar* eminences were partly removed.

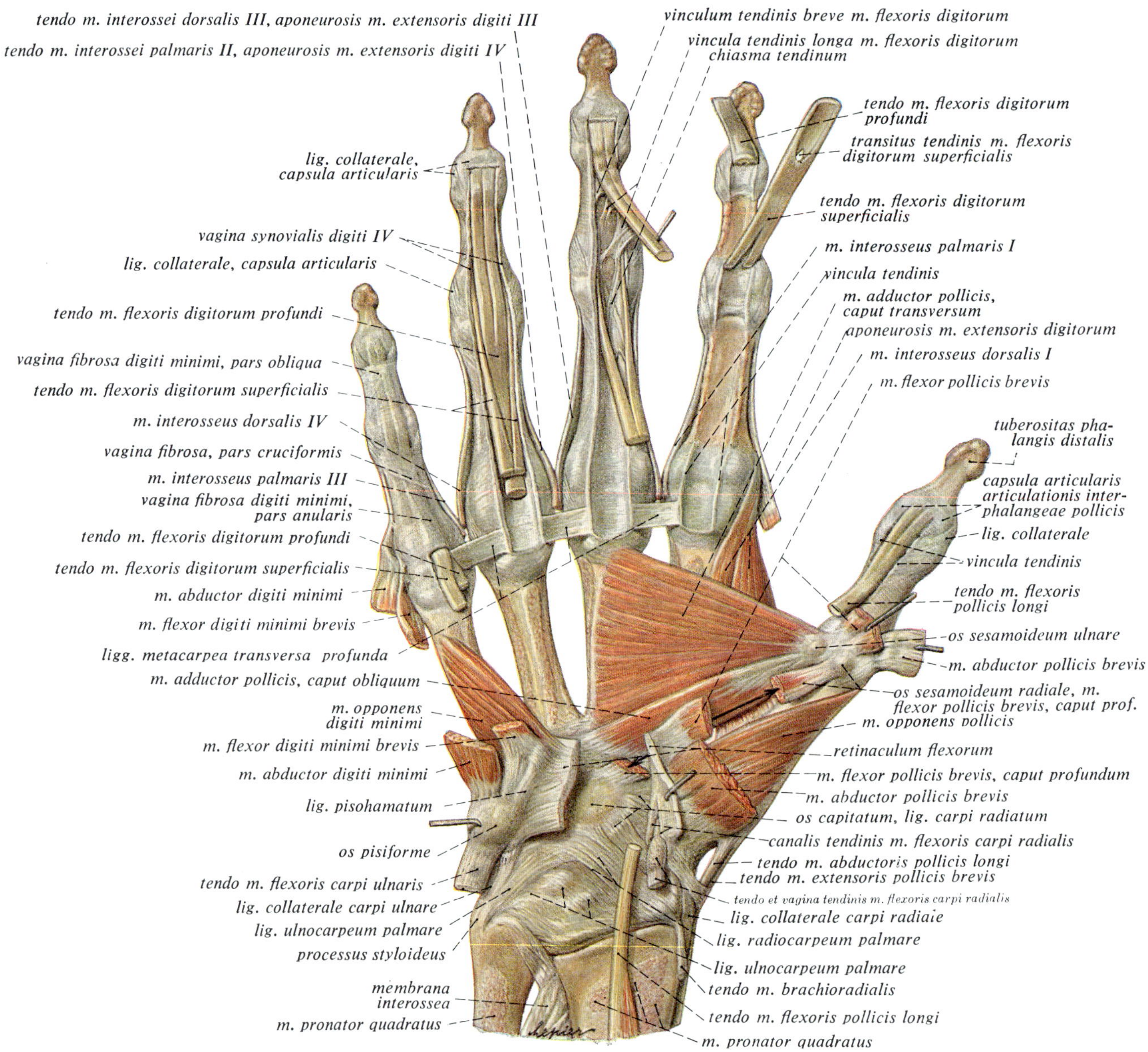

Fig. 321. Deepest layer of the musculature of the palm. The *canalis carpi* was opened by cutting the *retinaculum flexorum*. The origin and insertion of the *m. pronator quadratus* was severed at the distal end of the *radius* and *ulna*. The tendon of the *m. flexor pollicis longus* was kept in place. The flexor tendons of the fingers (after opening the tendon sheaths) were dissected to their insertion.

Muscles of the Thenar Eminence (Figs. 318, 320, 321, 325, 326)

The superficial layer of the thenar eminence is formed by the *mm. abductor pollicis brevis, opponens pollicis,* and the superficial or lateral portion of the *m. flexor pollicis brevis.* The deep layers of the thenar eminence muscles are composed of the deep or medial portion of the *mm. flexor pollicis brevis* and the *adductor pollicis.*

Name	*Origin*	*Insertion*
1. m. abductor pollicis brevis	retinaculum flexorum; tuberositas ossis scaphoidei; ridge of os trapezium	Radial side, proximal phalanx of thumb
Nerve: n. medianus (C 6–T 1)		
Action: Abducts thumb		
2. m. opponens pollicis	retinaculum flexorum; os trapezium	Entire length of radial border of 1st metacarpal of thumb
Nerve: n. medialis (C 6–T 1)		
Action: Opposes thumb to other fingers, abducts, flexes, rotates first metacarpal		
3. m. flexor pollicis brevis *Superficial portion*	retinaculum flexorum	Radial side of proximal phalanx of thumb; lateral sesamoid bone
Deeper portion	os trapezium	
Nerve: Lateral portion: n. medianus (C 6, 7). Deep or medial portion: n. ulnaris, deep branch (C 8, T 1)		
Action: Flexes proximal phalanx of thumb		
4. m. adductor pollicis a) *caput obliquum*	a) os capitatum; bases of 2nd and 3rd metacarpals	Medial (ulnar) side of proximal phalanx of thumb, sesamoid bone
b) *caput transversum*	b) Anterior surface of 3rd metacarpal	
Nerve: ramus profundus n. ulnaris (C 8; T 1)		
Action: Adducts the thumb; aids in opposition		

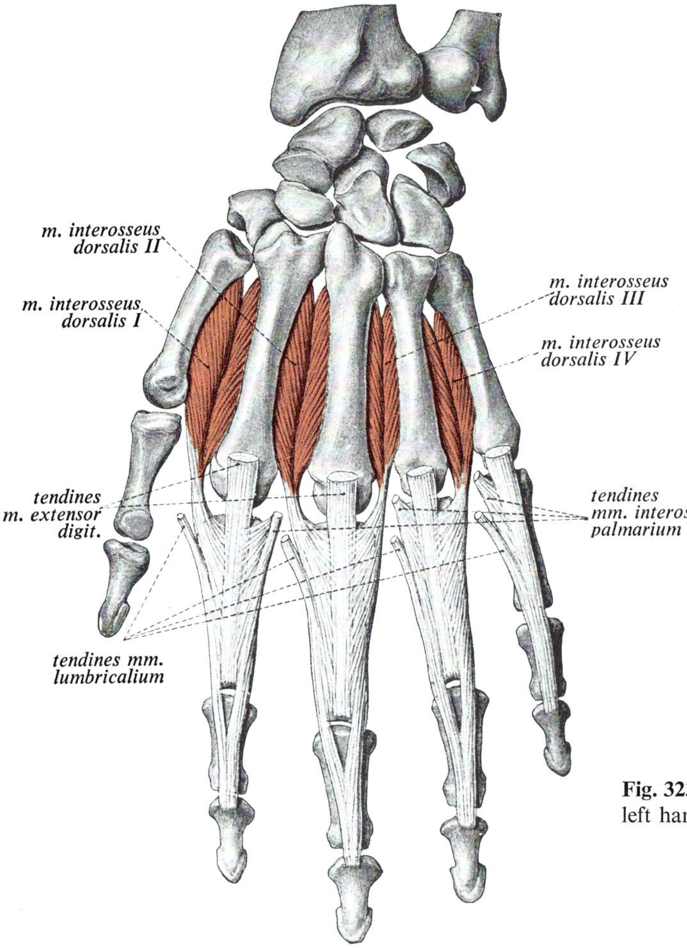

Fig. 322. Diagram of the *mm. interossei dorsales* and expanded extensor tendons of the fingers of the left hand.

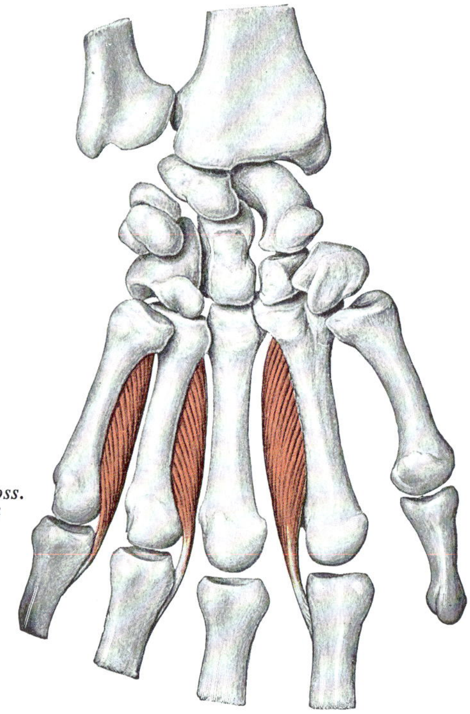

Fig. 323. Diagram of the *mm. interossei palmares* of the left hand.

Mm. interossei dorsales et palmares (Figs. 316, 322–326)

Nerve:	*n. ulnaris*
Action:	The mm. interossei dorsales abduct; the mm. interossei palmares adduct the fingers

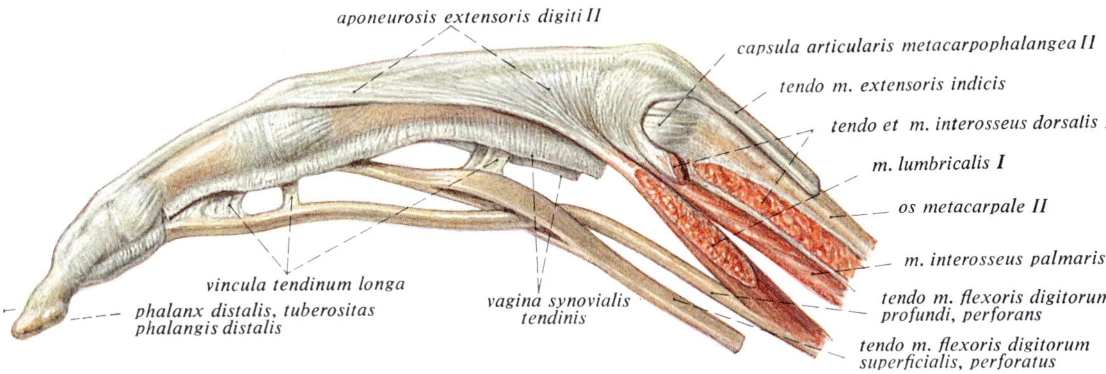

Fig. 324. Index finger of the right hand with the dorsal aponeurosis as well as the tendons of its flexor and extensor muscles.

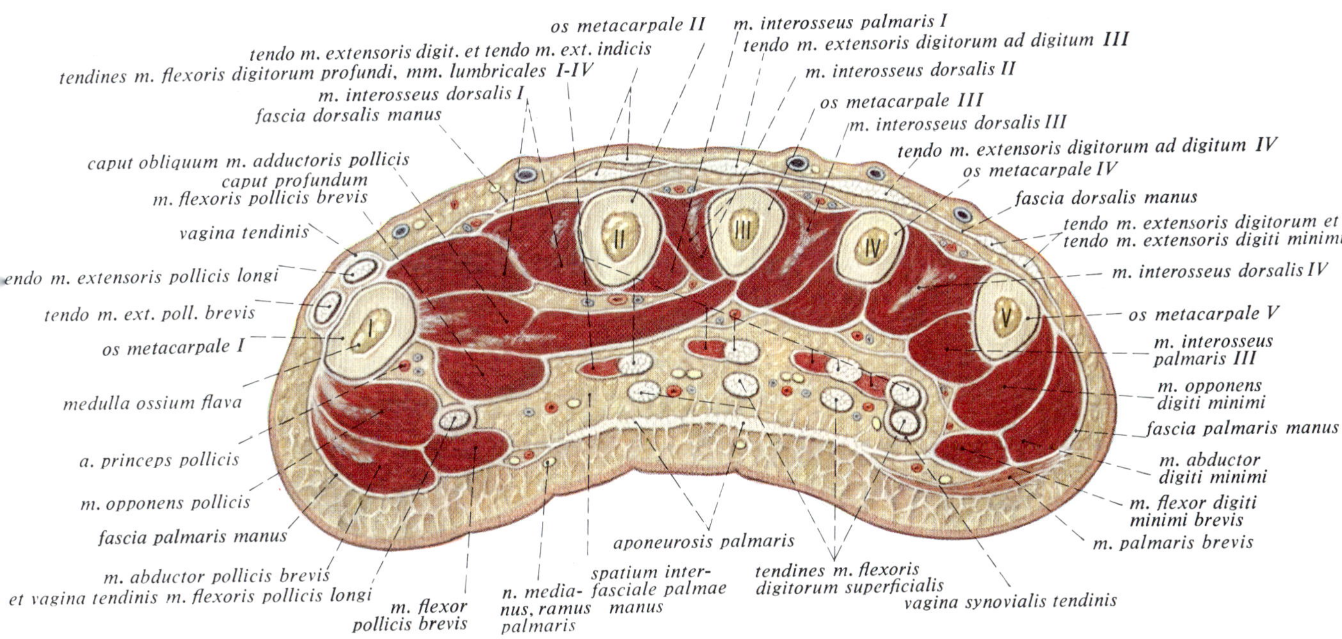

Fig. 325. Cross section of the right hand in the region of the *ossa metacarpalia* (I–V).

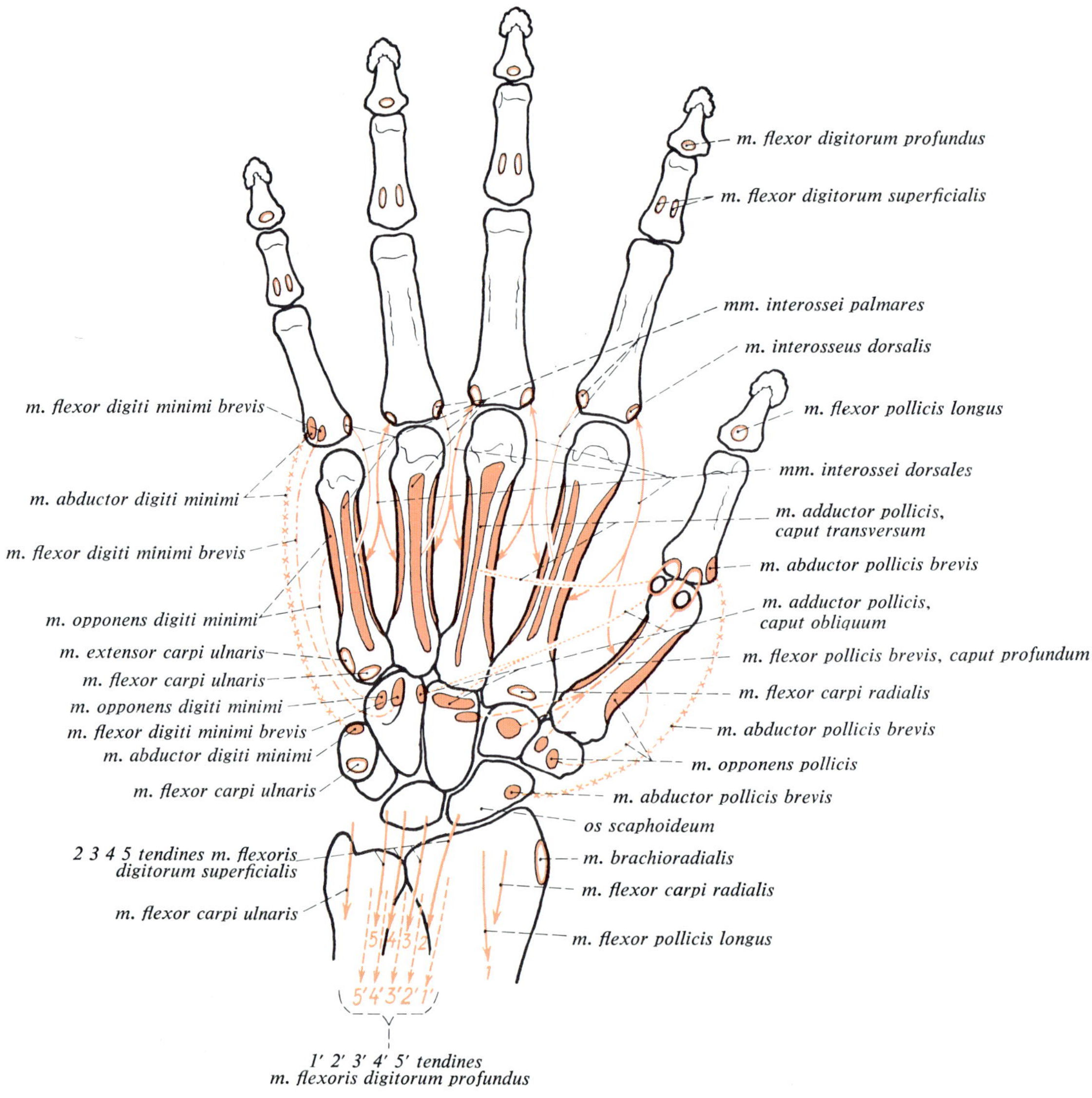

Fig. 326. Muscle origins and insertions mapped out on the palmar aspect of the right hand and wrist. The tendon sheath of the *articulatio radiocarpea* (1–7, two are not numbered) shown by the proximal placed arrows.

The tendons of the *m. flexor digitorum superficialis* (2–5): solid red arrows. The tendons of the *m. flexor digitorum profundus* (1'–5'): broken red arrows.

Muscles

The Lower Limb

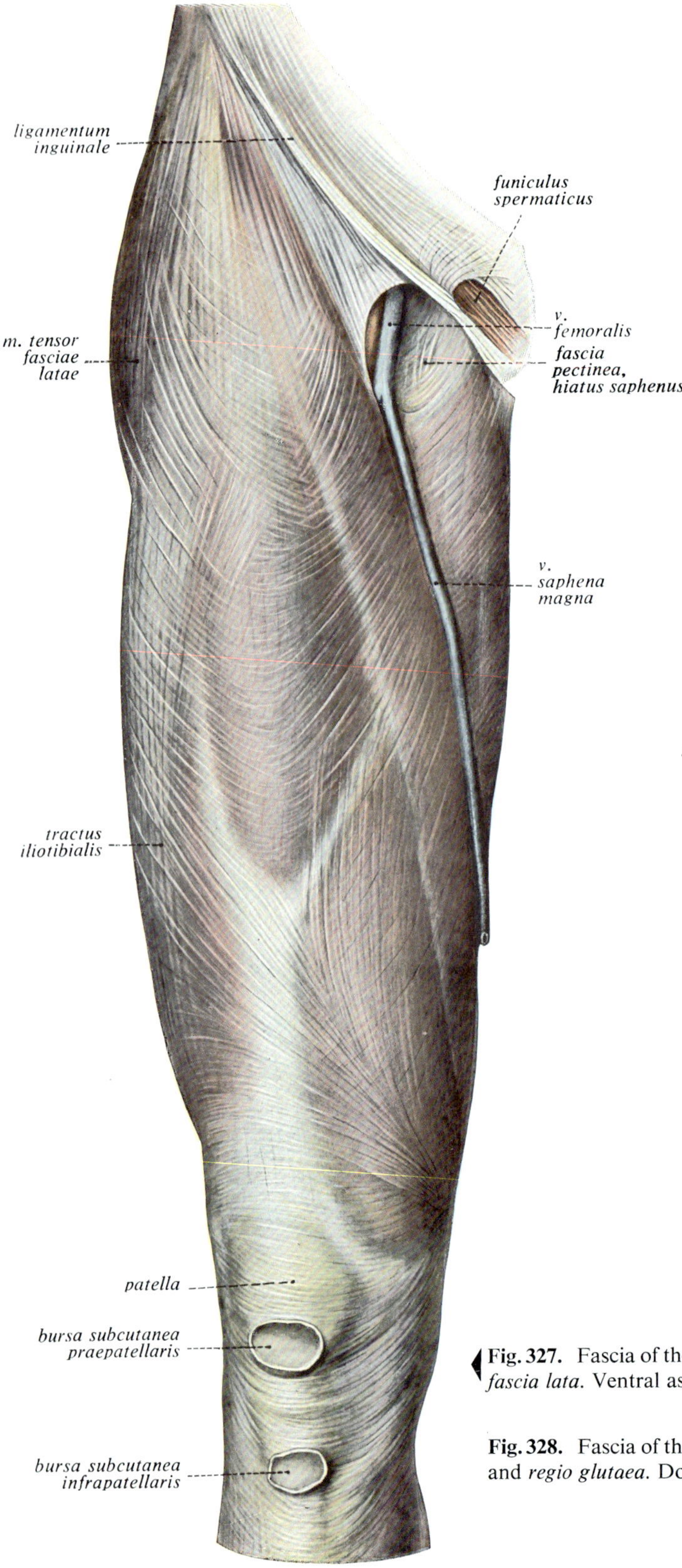

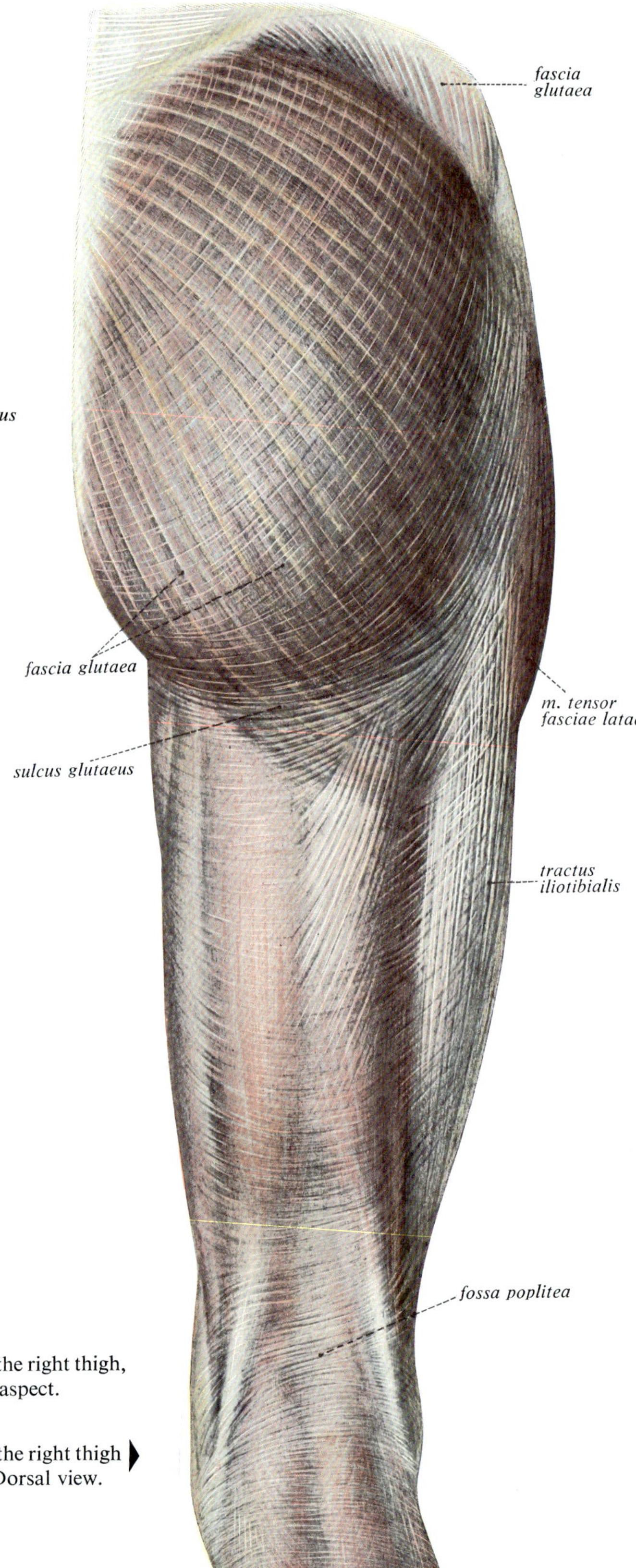

Fig. 327. Fascia of the right thigh, *fascia lata*. Ventral aspect.

Fig. 328. Fascia of the right thigh and *regio glutaea*. Dorsal view.

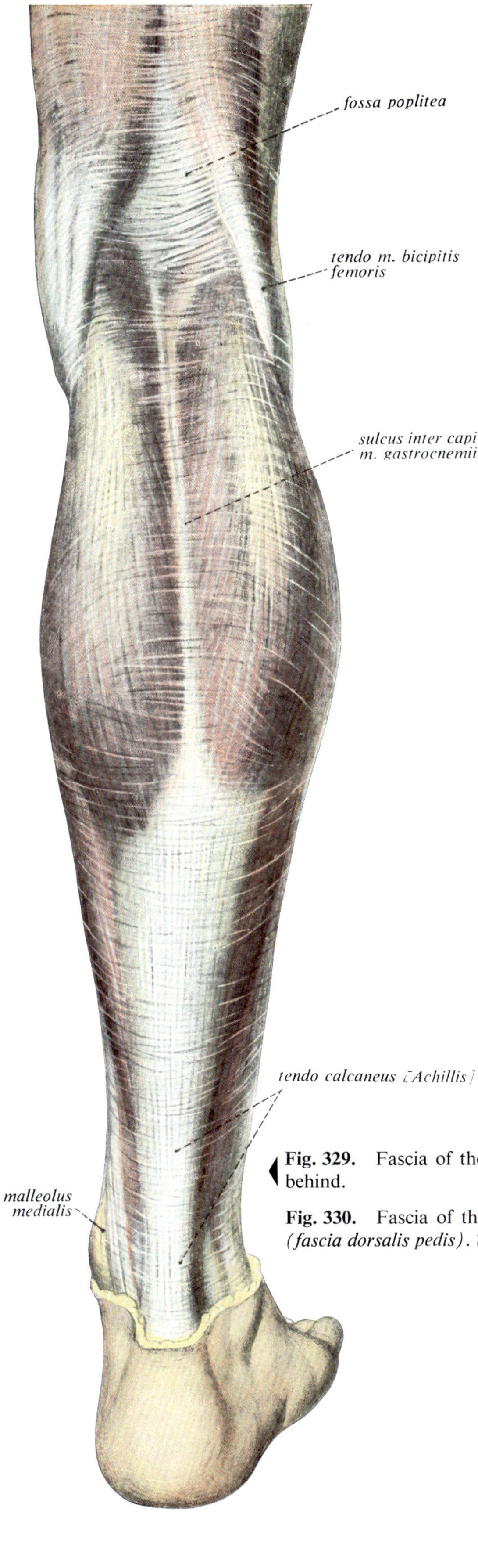

Fig. 329. Fascia of the leg, *fascia cruris*. Seen from behind.

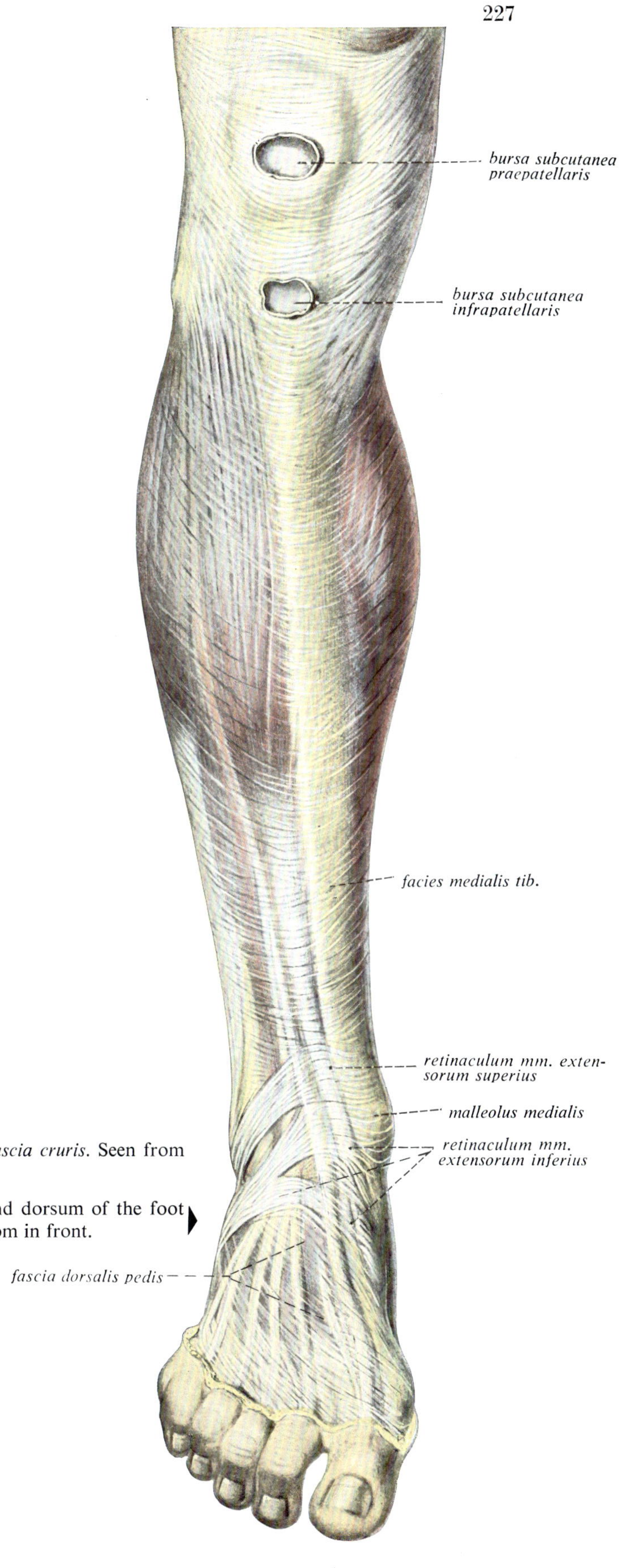

Fig. 330. Fascia of the leg and dorsum of the foot *(fascia dorsalis pedis)*. Seen from in front.

* Fracture of ramus superior ossis pubis.

Fig. 331. Musculature of the true pelvis and the medial side of the thigh. The pelvis and vertebral column are cut in the midline: The viscera, fascia, and peritoneum have been removed.

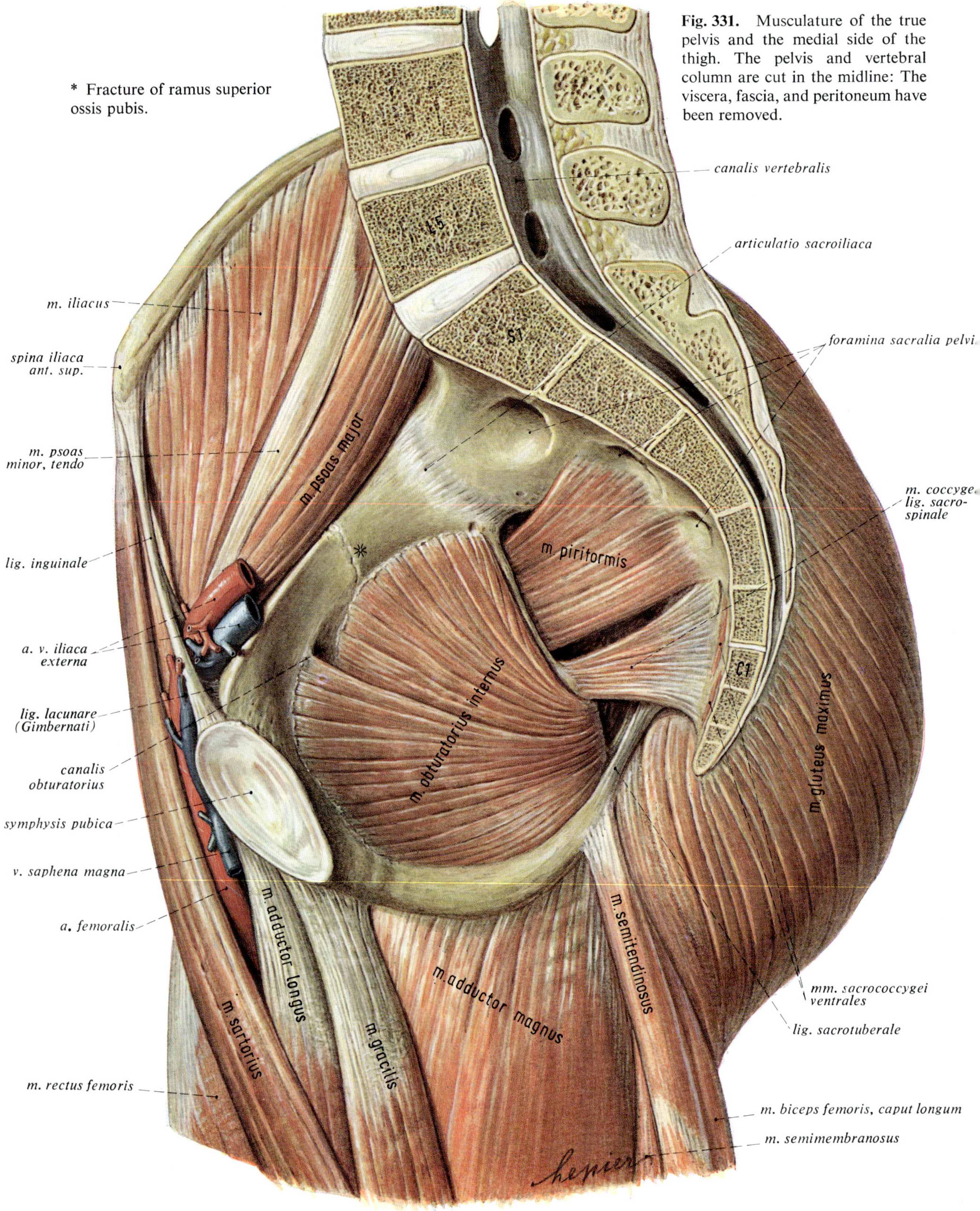

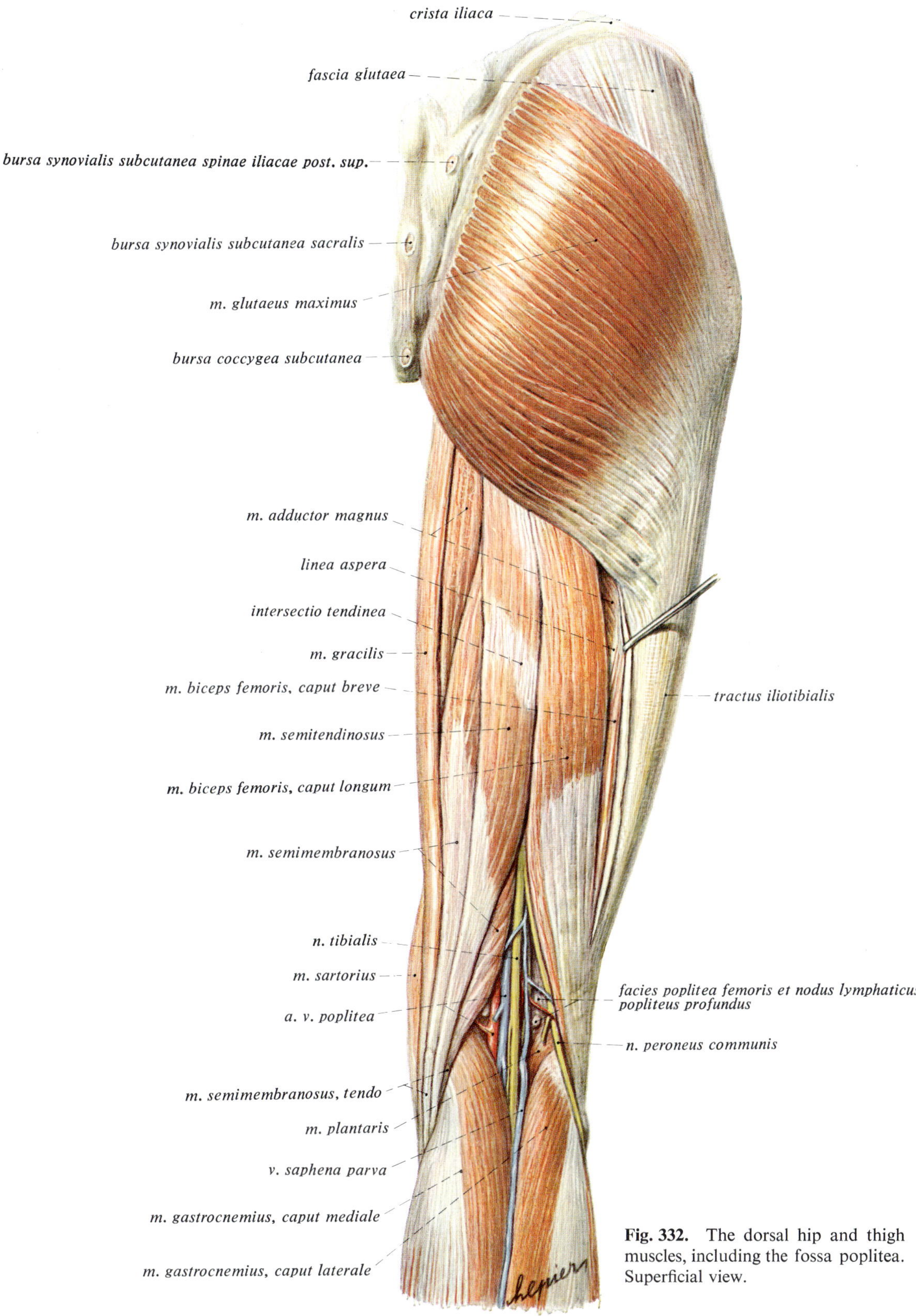

Fig. 332. The dorsal hip and thigh muscles, including the fossa poplitea. Superficial view.

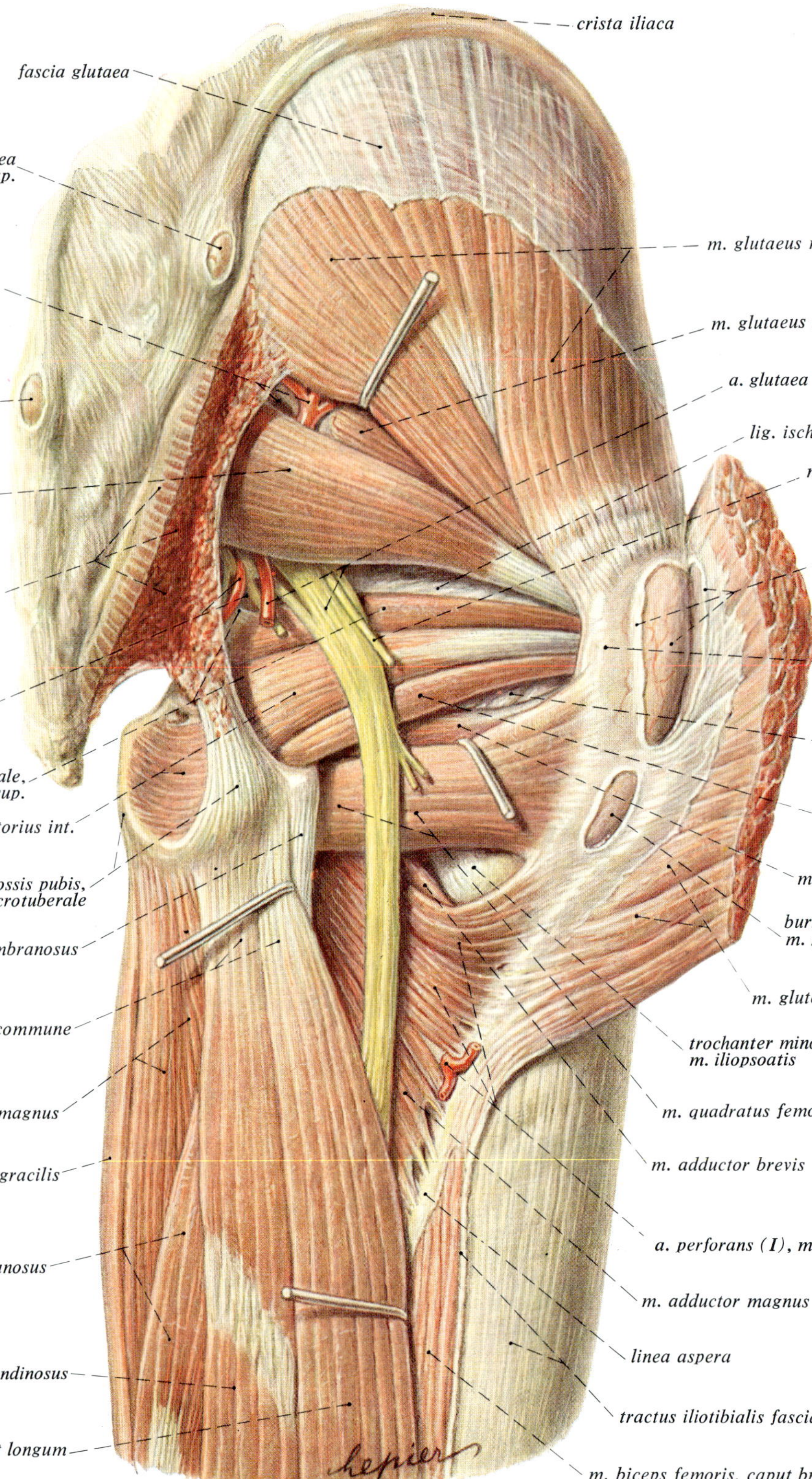

Fig. 333. Middle and deep layers of the regio glutaea and a superficial layer of the flexors on the thigh. The *m. gluteus maximus* is severed and reflected.

Dorsal Hip Muscles of Gluteal Region (Figs. 331, 338–340)

Name	*Origin*	*Insertion*
1. m. gluteus maximus (powerful, with coarse fasciculi)	linea glutaea posterior os ilii; posterior aspects of os sacrum; side of os coccygis; ligamentum sacrotuberale	tuberositas glutaea femoris and tractus iliotibialis of fascia lata
Nerve: n. glutaeus inferior (L 5; S 1, 2)		
Action: Extensor and powerful lateral rotator of thigh; inferior fibers assist in adduction of thigh; balances trunk on femur; fibers to tractus iliotibialis braces knee joint		
2. m. gluteus medius	External aspects of ilium; linea glutaea anterior et posterior; aponeurosis glutaea	Oblique ridge on lateral surface of trochanter major femoris
Nerve: n. glutaeus superior (L 4, 5; S 1)		
Action: Abducts femur, posterior fibers extend and rotate laterally, anterior fibers flex and rotate medially		
3. m. gluteus minimus	Outer aspect of ilium between linea glutaea ant. et post.	Tip (tendinous) of trochanter major femoris and capsule of hip joint
Nerve: n. glutaeus superior (L 4, 5; S 1)		
Action: Rotates thigh medially, abducts femur and, to some extent, flexes it		
4. m. piriformis	Pelvic surface of sacrum, lateral to sacral foramina 2, 3, and 4	A long tendon to upper border of trochanter major femoris
Nerve: n. ischiadicus or direct branches from the plexus sacralis (S 1, 2)		
Action: Rotates femur laterally; assists in abduction		
5. m. obturator internus	Margin of foramen obturatorium; membrana obturatoria	Medial surface of trochanter major femoris, proximal to fossa trochanterica
6. m. gemellus superior	spina ischiadica	With tendon of m. obturatorius to trochanter major
7. m. gemellus inferior	tuberositas ischiadica	
Nerve: Direct branches from the plexus sacralis		
Action: Rotates femur laterally, m. obturator internus extends and abducts when femur is flexed		
8. m. quadratus femoris	Lateral of tuber ischiadicum	crista intertrochanterica
Nerve: n. ischiadicus, branch from plexus sacralis (L 4, 5; S 1)		
Action: Rotates femur laterally; assists in adduction		
9. m. tensor fasciae latae	spina iliaca anterior superior	tractus iliotibialis fasciae latae
Nerve: n. glutaeus superior (L 4, 5; S 1)		
Action: Tenses the fascia lata; adduct the femur and, to some extend, flexes it; extends the leg		

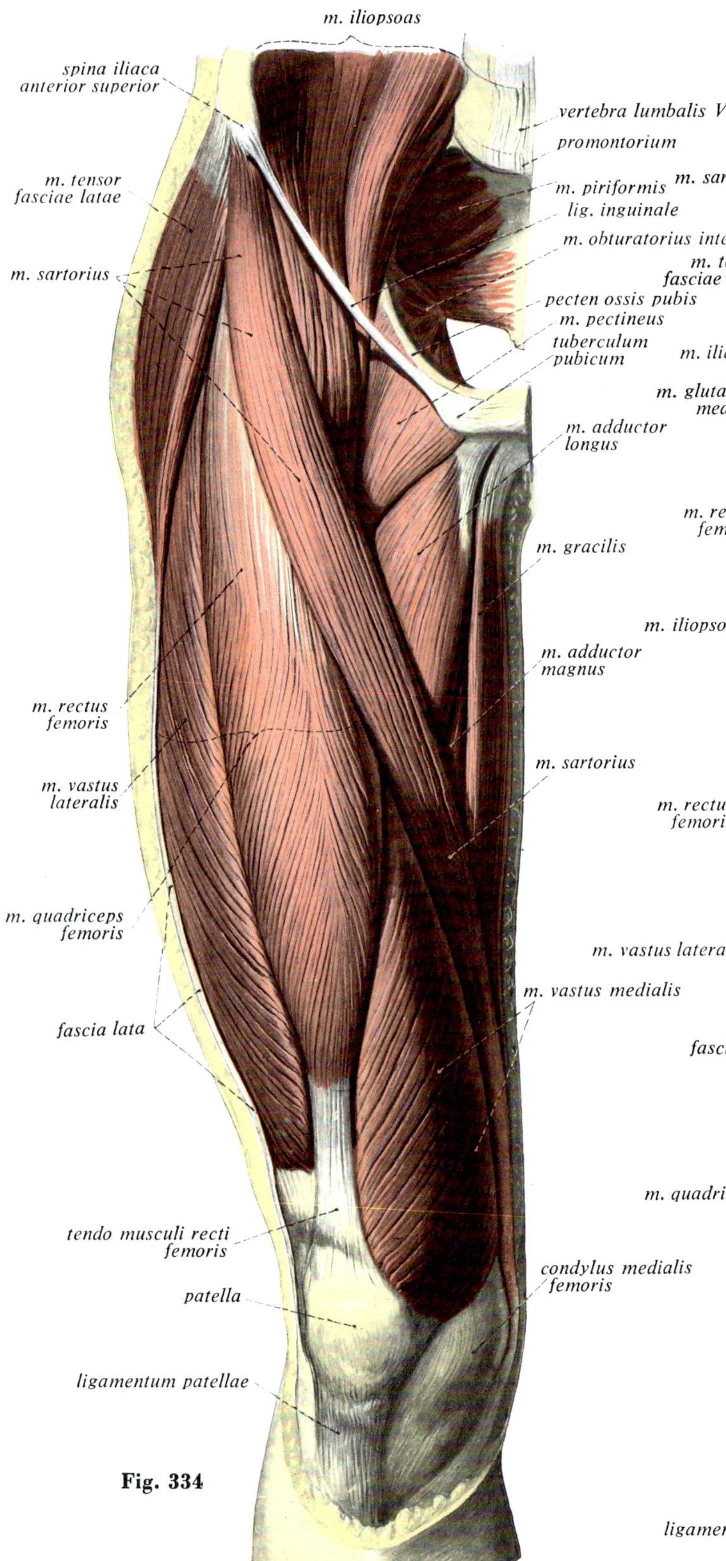
m. iliopsoas
spina iliaca anterior superior
vertebra lumbalis V
promontorium
m. tensor fasciae latae
m. piriformis
lig. inguinale
m. obturatorius internus
m. sartorius
pecten ossis pubis
m. pectineus
tuberculum pubicum
m. adductor longus
m. gracilis
m. adductor magnus
m. rectus femoris
m. vastus lateralis
m. sartorius
m. quadriceps femoris
m. vastus medialis
fascia lata
tendo musculi recti femoris
condylus medialis femoris
patella
ligamentum patellae

Fig. 334

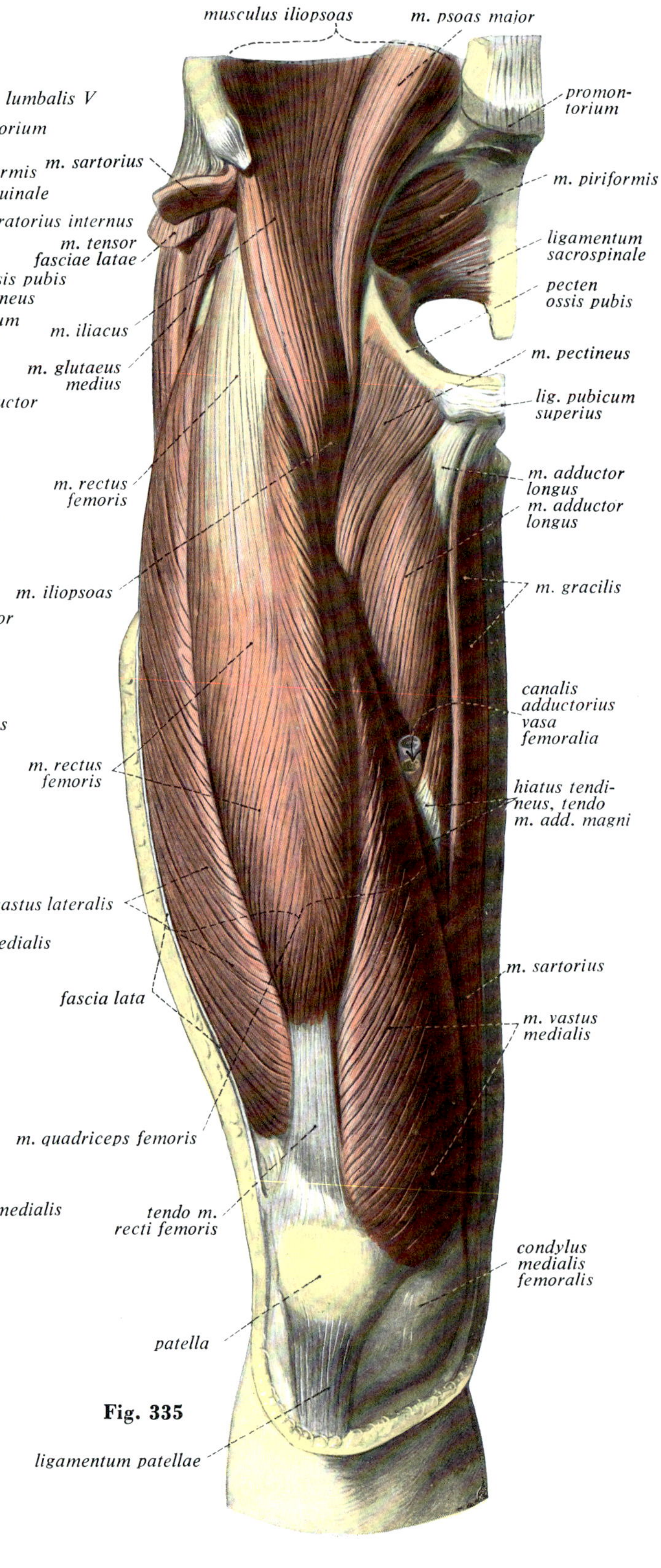
musculus iliopsoas
m. psoas major
promontorium
m. sartorius
m. piriformis
m. tensor fasciae latae
ligamentum sacrospinale
pecten ossis pubis
m. iliacus
m. pectineus
m. glutaeus medius
lig. pubicum superius
m. rectus femoris
m. adductor longus
m. adductor longus
m. iliopsoas
m. gracilis
canalis adductorius
vasa femoralia
m. rectus femoris
hiatus tendineus, tendo m. add. magni
m. vastus lateralis
m. sartorius
fascia lata
m. vastus medialis
m. quadriceps femoris
tendo m. recti femoris
condylus medialis femoralis
patella
ligamentum patellae

Fig. 335

Anterior Femoral Muscles (Figs. 334–336)

Name	*Origin*	*Insertion*
m. sartorius		Medial margin of tuberositas tibiae
Nerve: n. femoralis (L 2, 3)		
Action: Flexes, laterally rotates, abducts thigh; flexes leg; rotates leg medially in knee joint when leg is flexed		
m. quadriceps femoris (Extensor muscles)		
m. rectus femoris (operates 2 joints) Straight (anterior) head	Tendon from spina iliaca ant. inf.	The common tendon of the m. quadriceps femoris (which is the most powerful muscle in the entire human body) attaches to the cranial, medial, and lateral margins of the patella and, through intermediation of the ligamentum patellare, is inserted on the tuberositas tibiae
Reflected (posterior) head	Cranial margin of acetabulum	
m. vastus medialis	labium mediale linea aspera; linea intertrochanterica (distal end thicker than proximal)	
m. vastus lateralis	labium laterale linea aspera as far proximally as trochanter major	
m. vastus intermedius	Anterior and lateral surfaces of the shaft of the femur; septum intermusculare laterale	
m. articularis genus	From anterior surface of femur	Synovial membrane of knee joint
Nerve: n. femoralis (L 2, 3, 4)		
Action: Extends leg. m. rectus femoris aids in flexion of hip joint; m. articularis genus draws articular capsule proximally		

The Lacuna of the Inguinal Region:

The *ligamentum inguinale* stretches from the *spina iliaca anterior superior* to the *symphysis pubis.* The two lacuna are between the inguinal ligament and the pelvic bones and are separated by the *arcus iliopectineus* as follows:

1. *Lacuna musculorum:* lateral for the passage of the *m. iliopsoas* and *n. femoralis.*
2. *Lacuna vasorum:* medial, for the passage of the femoral vessels and lymph vessels of the *trigonum femorale.*

Boundaries: Ventrally, *ligamentum inguinale;* dorsally, periosteum of the bone; medially, the *ligamentum lacunare.*

Topographical arrangement: Lymph vessels are entirely medial; then the *v. femoralis* and, laterally, the *a. femoralis.*

Femoral hernia: The inner aperture, through which a hernia passes, is a weak space between the *v. femoralis* and the *ligamentum lacunare.* It is filled with lymph vessels and connective tissue. The outer aperture through which a hernia passes in the hiatus saphenous *(fossa ovalis)* of the *fascia lata* for the entrance of the *v. saphena magna* and the superficial lymph vessels.

◀ **Fig. 334.** The muscles of the ventral side of the right thigh. Superficial layer. The *ligamentum inguinale* is retained to show its attachments.

Fig. 335. Muscles of the ventral side of the right thigh. The *m. sartorius* and the *ligamentum inguinale* have been removed.

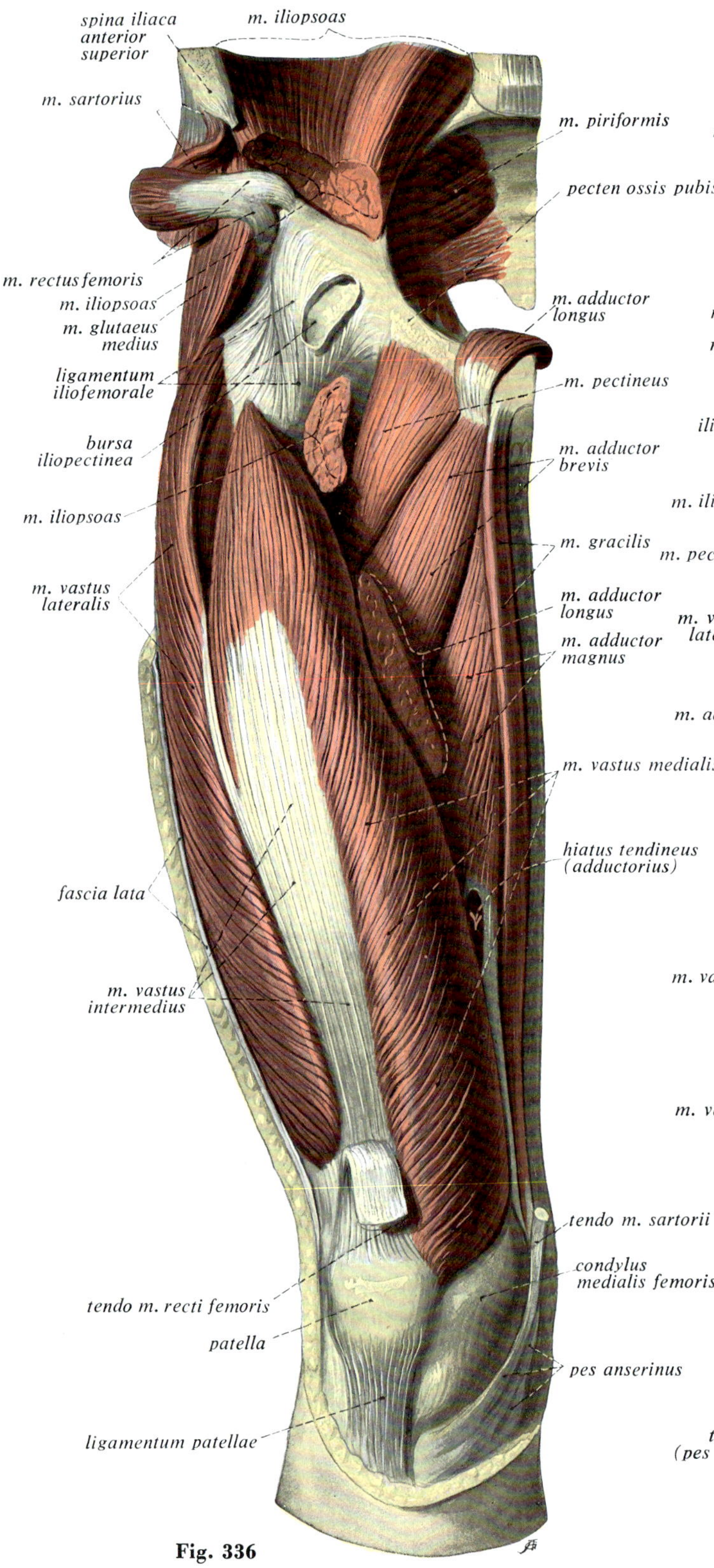

spina iliaca anterior superior
m. iliopsoas
m. sartorius
m. piriformis
pecten ossis pubis
m. rectus femoris
m. iliopsoas
m. glutaeus medius
m. adductor longus
ligamentum iliofemorale
m. pectineus
bursa iliopectinea
m. adductor brevis
m. iliopsoas
m. gracilis
m. vastus lateralis
m. adductor longus
m. adductor magnus
m. vastus medialis
hiatus tendineus (adductorius)
fascia lata
m. vastus intermedius
tendo m. sartorii
condylus medialis femoris
tendo m. recti femoris
patella
pes anserinus
ligamentum patellae

Fig. 336

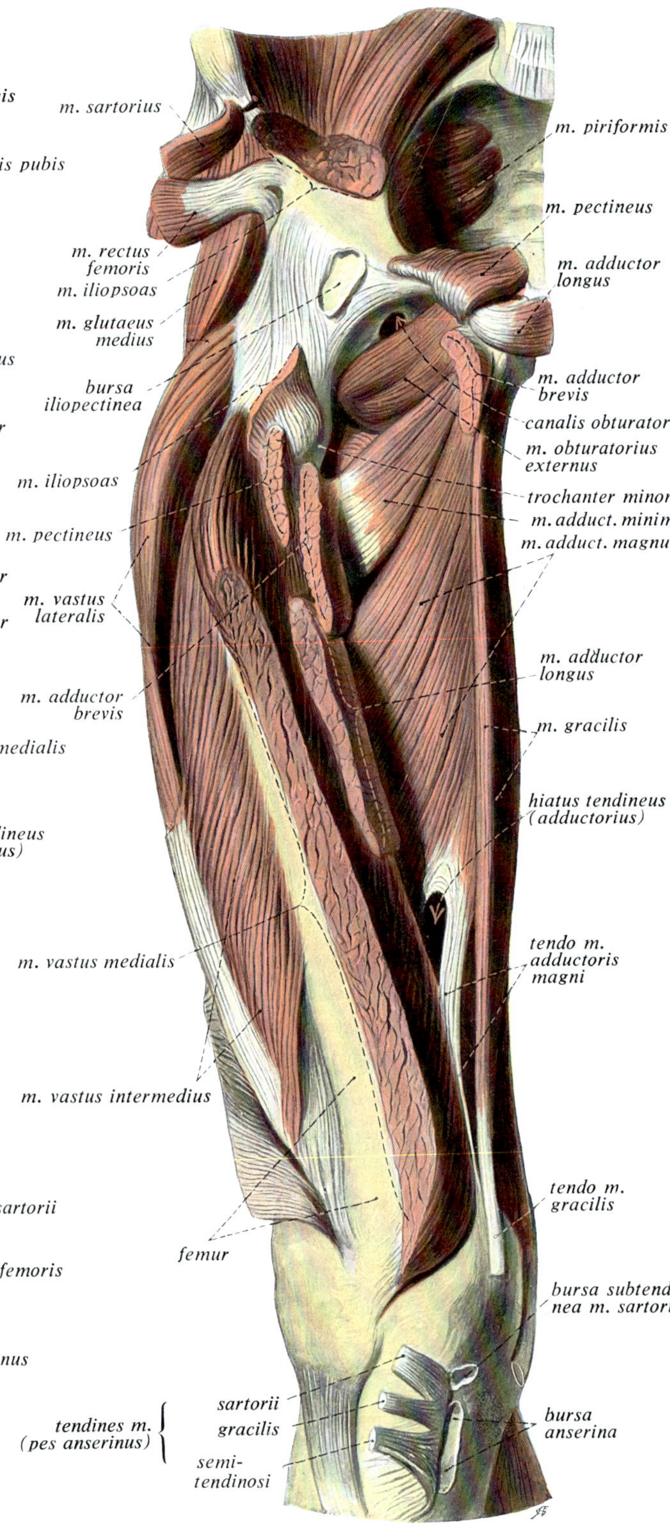

m. sartorius
m. piriformis
m. pectineus
m. rectus femoris
m. iliopsoas
m. adductor longus
m. glutaeus medius
bursa iliopectinea
m. adductor brevis
canalis obturator.
m. obturatorius externus
m. iliopsoas
trochanter minor
m. adduct. minim.
m. pectineus
m. adduct. magnus
m. vastus lateralis
m. adductor longus
m. adductor brevis
m. gracilis
hiatus tendineus (adductorius)
m. vastus medialis
tendo m. adductoris magni
m. vastus intermedius
tendo m. gracilis
femur
bursa subtendinea m. sartorii
tendines m. (pes anserinus)
sartorii
gracilis
semitendinosi
bursa anserina

Fig. 337

Medial Femoral Muscles (Adductor) (Figs. 338, 339, 344, 345, 352)

Name	*Origin*	*Insertion*
1. m. pectineus	Pecten ossis pubis	linea pectinea femoris
Nerve: n. femoralis (L 2, 3) and the accessory n. obturatorius		
Action: Adducts the thigh; also aids in flexion and lateral rotation in the hip joint		
2. m. adductor longus	Tendon from the border of ramus superior et inferior ossis pubis near symphysis	Middle third of labium mediale lineae asperae
Nerve: n. obturatorius (L 3; 4)		
Action: Adducts, aids flexion, and rotates thigh laterally		
3. m. gracilis (forms middle tendon of pes anserinus)	Flat tendon from ramus inferior ossis pubis near symphysis	Long tendon on medial borders of the shaft of the tibia near the tuberositas tibiae (pes anserinus)
Nerve: n. obturatorius (L 3; 4)		
Action: Adducts thigh, aids in flexion of the knee; rotates the leg medially		
4. m. adductor brevis	ramus inferior ossis pubis	Proximal third of labium mediale lineae asperae; and pectineal line
Nerve: n. obturatorius (L 3, 4)		
Action: Adducts thigh, aids in flexion and in lateral rotation of the thigh		
5. m. adductor magnus* (This and also the m. adductor brevis, lie in deeper layers than 1 to 3 above)	Lower part of ramus inferior ossis pubis; ramus ossis ischii; tuber ischiadicum	Fleshy: proximal $^2/_3$ of linea aspera, labium mediale tuberositas glutaea Tendinous: epicondylus medialis femoris *(hiatus tendineus)*
Nerve: n. obturatorius (L 3, 4) and n. ischiadicus (L 4, 5; S 1)		
Action: Powerful adductor of thigh; aids in flexion and assists in lateral rotation in hip joint. Lower portion of muscle extends the thigh and rotates it medially		
6. m. obturator externus	Medial margin of foramen obturatorium; outer surface of membrana obturatoria	fossa trochanterica femoris
Nerve: n. obturatorius (L 3, 4)		
Action: Rotates femur laterally; also aids in flexing the hip joint		

* The proximal, almost transverse part of the *m. adductor magnus* was formerly called (BNA) the *m. adductor minimus*. It works somewhat irregularly from the main muscle and aids in the lateral rotation of the hip joint.

Fig. 336. Middle layer of muscles of the ventral surface of the thigh. The *mm. sartorius, iliopsoas, rectus femoris* and *adductor longus* were partially resected.

Fig. 337. Deep layers of muscles of the ventral surface of the thigh. Preparation same as in 336, in addition, the *mm. pectineus, adductor brevis, vastus medialis,* and *gracilis* were cut.

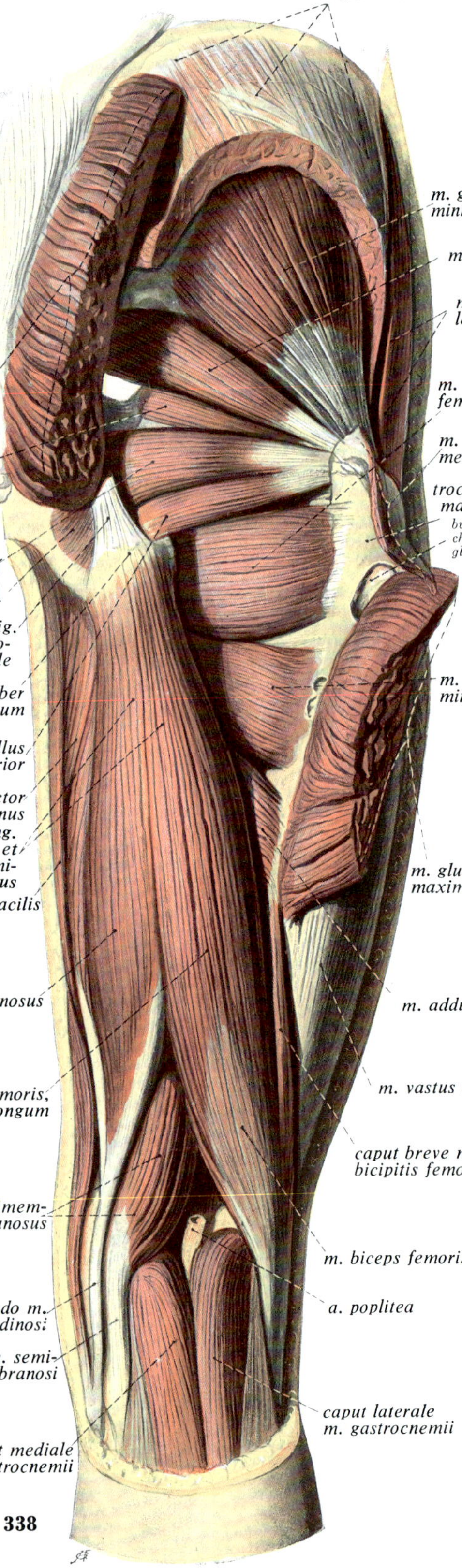
m. glutaeus medius
m. glutaeus minimus
m. piriformis
m. tensor fasciae latae
m. quadratus femoris
m. glutaeus medius
trochanter major
bursa trochanterica m. glut. max.
m. adductor minimus
m. glutaeus maximus
m. adductor magnus
m. vastus lateralis
caput breve m. bicipitis femoris
m. biceps femoris
a. poplitea
caput laterale m. gastrocnemii
m. glutaeus maximus
m. gemellus superior
m. obturat. internus
lig. sacrotuberale
tuber ischiadicum
m. gemellus inferior
m. adductor magnus
caput long. m. bicipit. et m. semitendinosus
m. gracilis
m. semitendinosus
m. biceps femoris, caput longum
m. semimembranosus
tendo m. semitendinosi
tendo m. semimembranosi
caput mediale m. gastrocnemii

Fig. 338

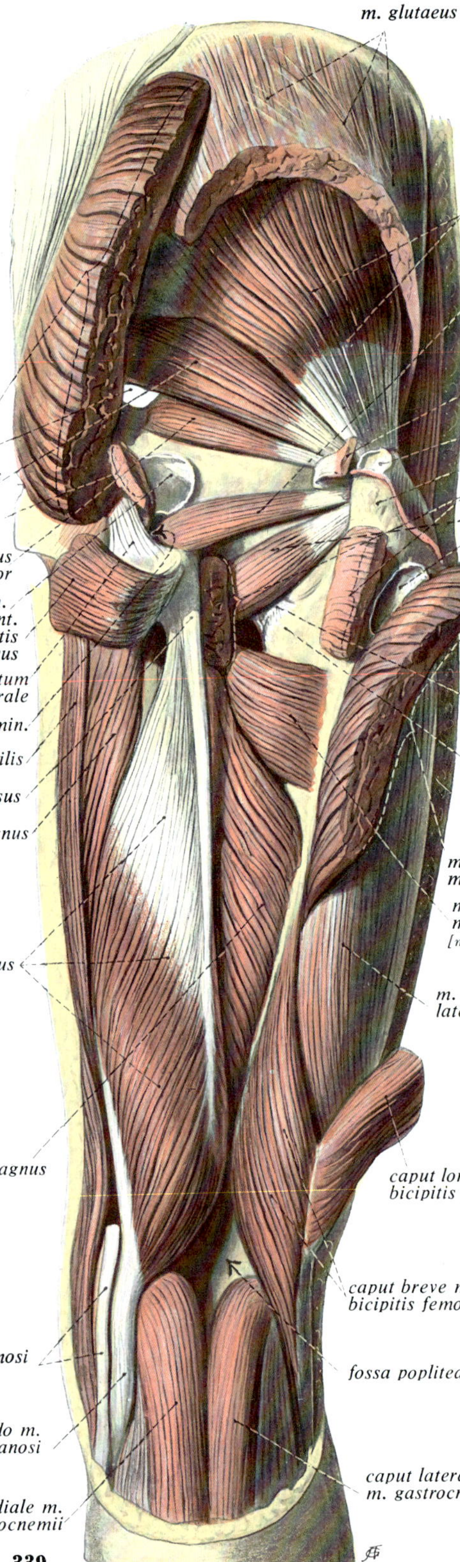
m. glutaeus medius
m. glutaeus minimus
m. gemellus inferior
tendo m. obturatorii interni
bursa synov.
troch. major
m. quadratus femoris
m. obtur. ext.
bursa trochanterica m. glutaei maximi
tendo m. iliopsoatis
trochanter minor
m. glutaeus max.
m. adductor. magn. [m. adductor minim.]
m. vastus lateralis
caput longum m. bicipitis femoris
caput breve m. bicipitis femoris
fossa poplitea
caput laterale m. gastrocnemii
m. glutaeus max.
foramen infrapirif.
m. piriformis
m. obturatorius internus
m. gemellus superior
bursa ischiadica m. obtur. int.
cap. long. m. bicipitis et m. semitendinosus
ligamentum sacrotuberale
for. ischiadic. min.
m. gracilis
m. semimembranosus
m. adductor magnus
m. semimembranosus
m. adductor magnus
tendo m. semitendinosi
tendo m. semimembranosi
caput mediale m. gastrocnemii

Fig. 339

The Posterior Femoral Muscles (Hamstring Muscles) (Flexors) (Figs. 338–345)

Name	*Origin*	*Insertion*
1. m. biceps femoris *caput longum* – operates 2 joints	tuber ischiadicum (short tendon fuses with m. semitendinosus)	caput fibulae by strong tendon, condylus lateralis tibiae (small slip)
caput breve – operates 1 joint	Distal half of labium laterale lineae asperae	

Nerve: *caput longum:* n. tibialis (S 1–3) *caput breve:* n. peroneus communis (L 5; S 1, 2)

Action: Both heads flex the leg, then rotate it laterally; long head also extends the thigh

2. m. semitendinosus (forms the 3rd tendon of the pes anserinus) (operates 2 joints)	Short tendon from tuber ischiadicum, fused with the caput longum m. bicipitis femoris	Long tendon: the terminal ramification (pes anserinus) of the tendon takes place on medial margin of the tuberositas tibiae

Nerve: n. tibialis (L 4, 5; S 1, 2)

Action: Extends thigh: flexes the leg (medial rotation)

3. m. semimembranosus (operates 2 joints)	tuber ischiadicum (by broad tendon; in the inner space with No. 1 and No. 2 above and the m. adductor magnus)	Thick, short tendon of condylus medialis tibiae (via lig. popliteum obliquum, to condylus lateralis femoris)

Nerve: n. tibialis (L 5; S 1, 2)

Action: Flexes the leg, medial rotation of the flexed leg; extends the thigh

I. foramen ischiadicum majus. Boundaries: *incisura ischiadica major, ligamentum sacrospinale* and *sacrotuberale*. The *m. piriformis* passes through this foramen.

1. Caudal to the *m. piriformis* (the *foramen infrapiriforme)* is the passage for the *n. ischiadicus, vasa glutaea inferiora,* the *n. cutaneus femoris posterior, vasa pudenda interna,* the *n. pudendus.*
2. Cranial to the *m. piriformis* (the *foramen suprapiriforme)* is the passage for the *vasa glutaea superiora* and the *n. glutaeus superius.*

II. foramen ischiadicum minus. Boundaries: *incisura ischiadica minor, ligamentum sacrospinale* and *sacrotuberale* transmit the *vasa pudenda interna* and the tendon of the *m. obturator internus* and its nerve into the *canalis pudendalis* (ALCOCK). The *canalis pudendalis* lies in the deep of the *fossa ischiorectalis* and is formed from the fascia of the *m. obturator internus* (Fig. 272).

Fig. 338. Deep layer of the dorsal muscles of the hip and superficial layers of the flexors on the thigh, the muscles of the *fossa poplitea.* The *mm. gluteus maximus* and *medius* were transected and reflected.

Fig. 339. Deep layer of posterior hip muscles and flexors of the thigh. Besides the *mm. gluteus maximus* and *medius,* the *quadratus femoris, obturator internus, biceps femoris* (long head), and the *semitendinosus* were cut. (The latter was cleaned away so that only the terminal tendons remain.)

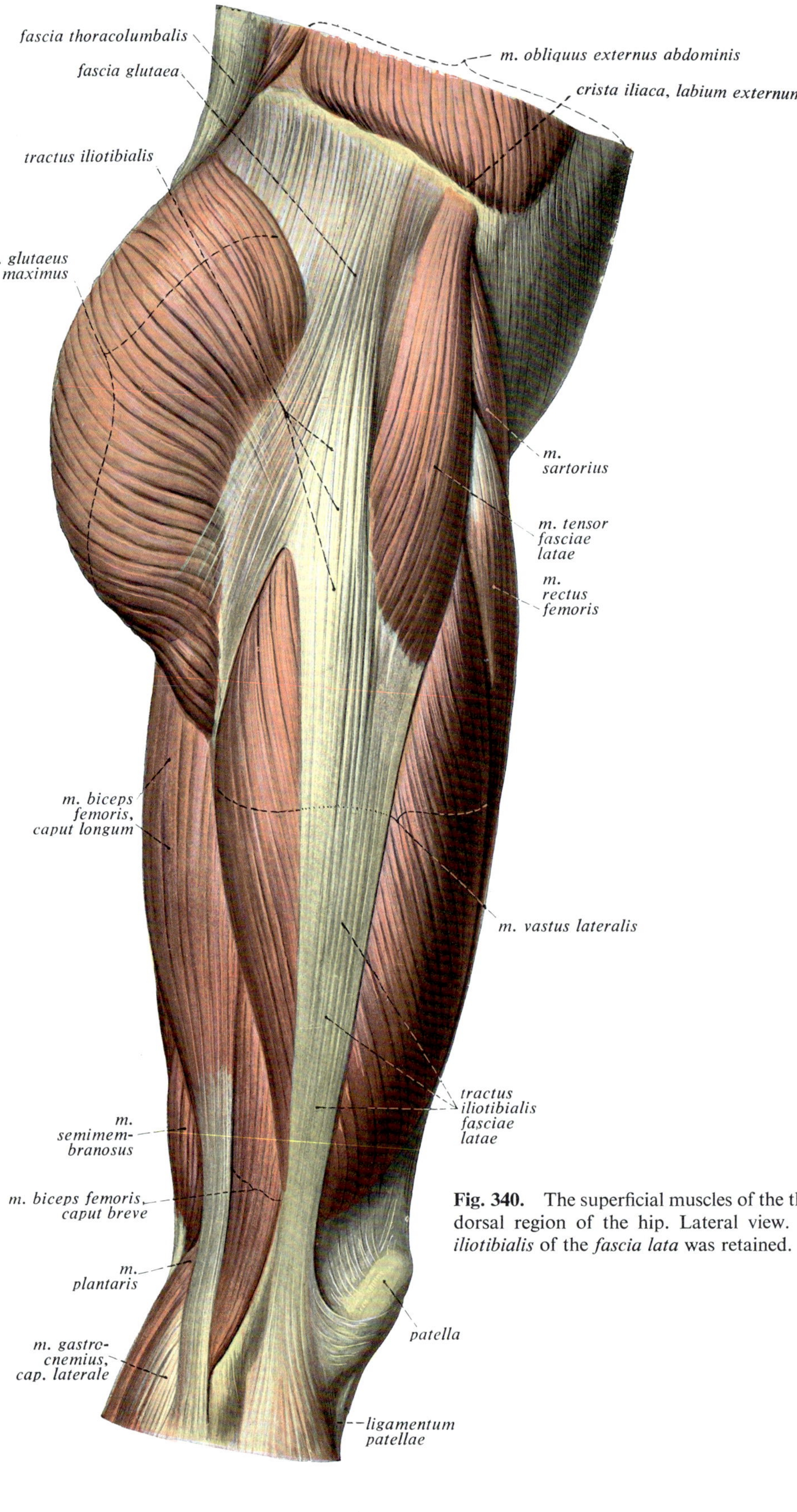

Fig. 340. The superficial muscles of the thigh and the dorsal region of the hip. Lateral view. The *tractus iliotibialis* of the *fascia lata* was retained.

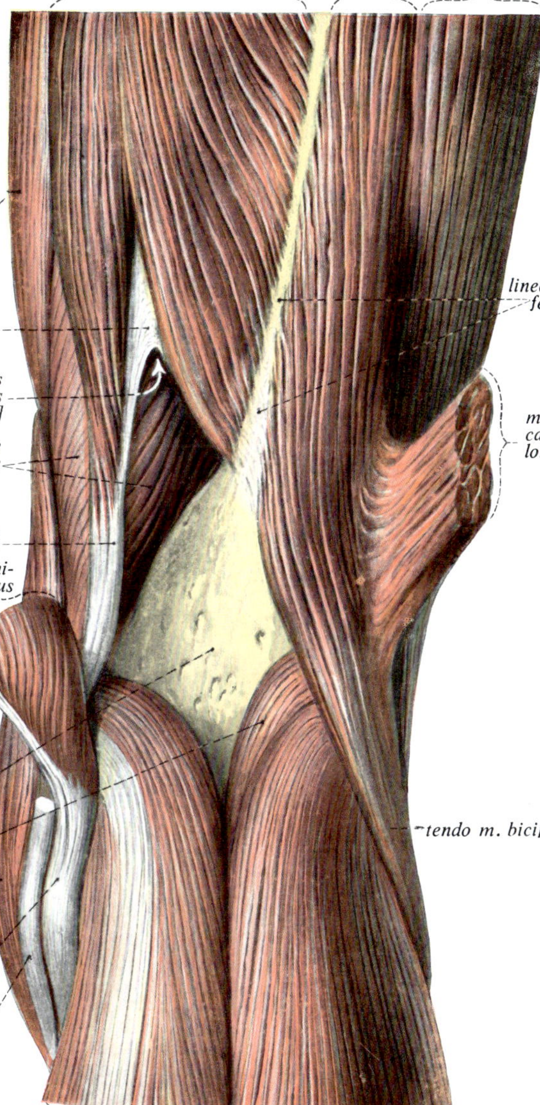

Fig. 341. The deep muscles of the *fossa poplitea*. Dorsal view. The *m. adductor magnus* and the *hiatus tendineus (adductorius)* have been exposed by cutting the *mm. semimembranosus, semitendinosus*, and the *caput longum m. bicipitis*.

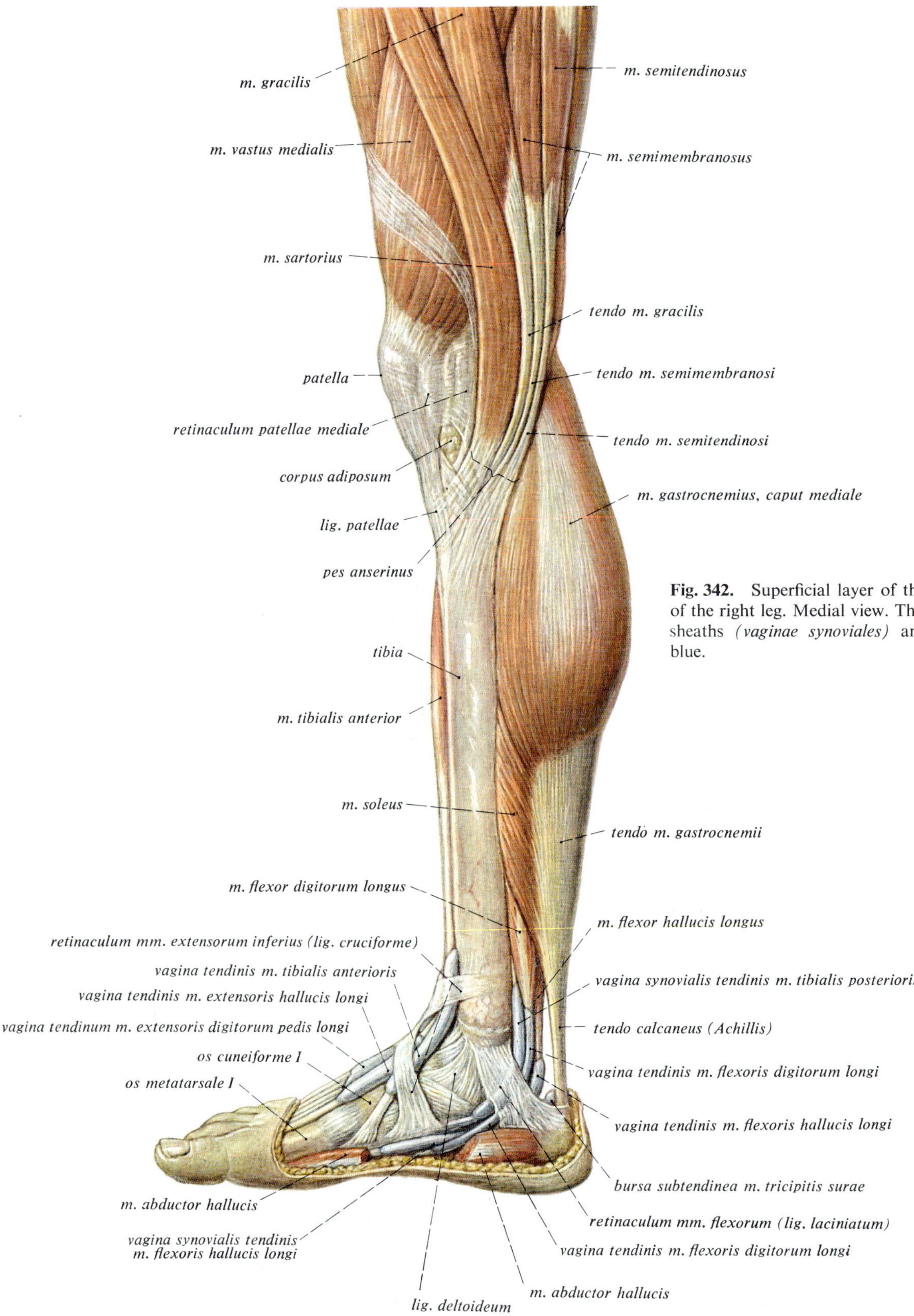

Fig. 342. Superficial layer of the muscles of the right leg. Medial view. The synovial sheaths *(vaginae synoviales)* are colored blue.

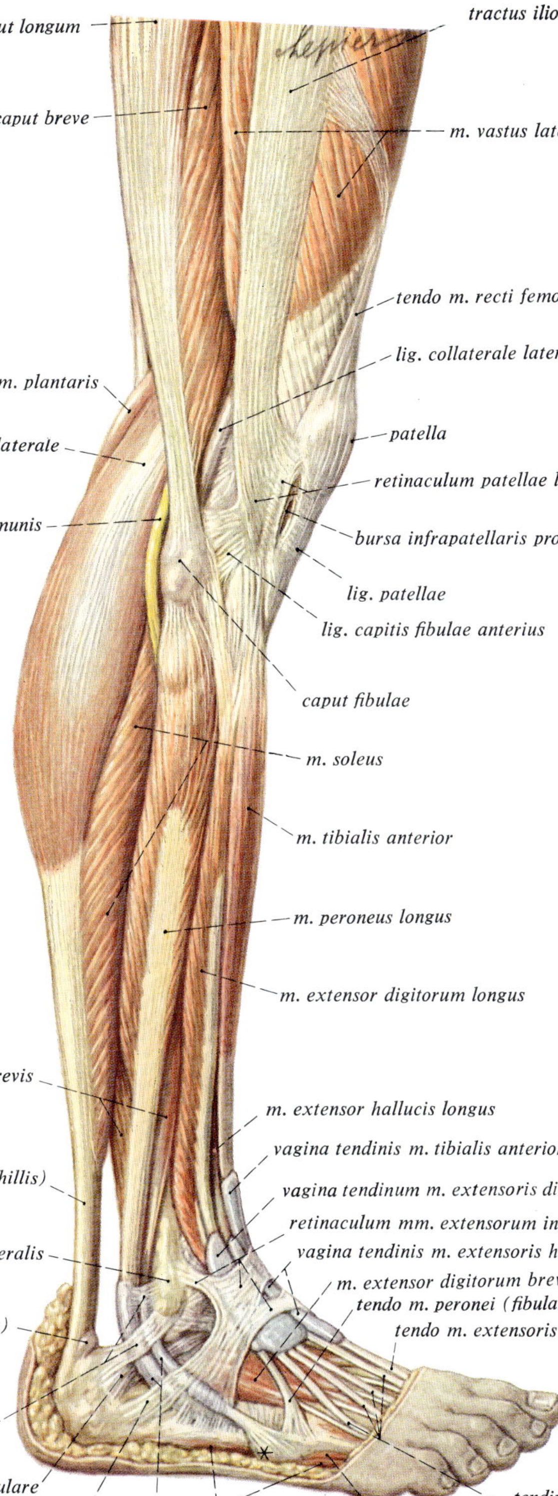

Fig. 343. The superficial layer of muscles of the right leg. Lateral view. The synovial sheaths *(vaginae synoviales)* are colored blue.

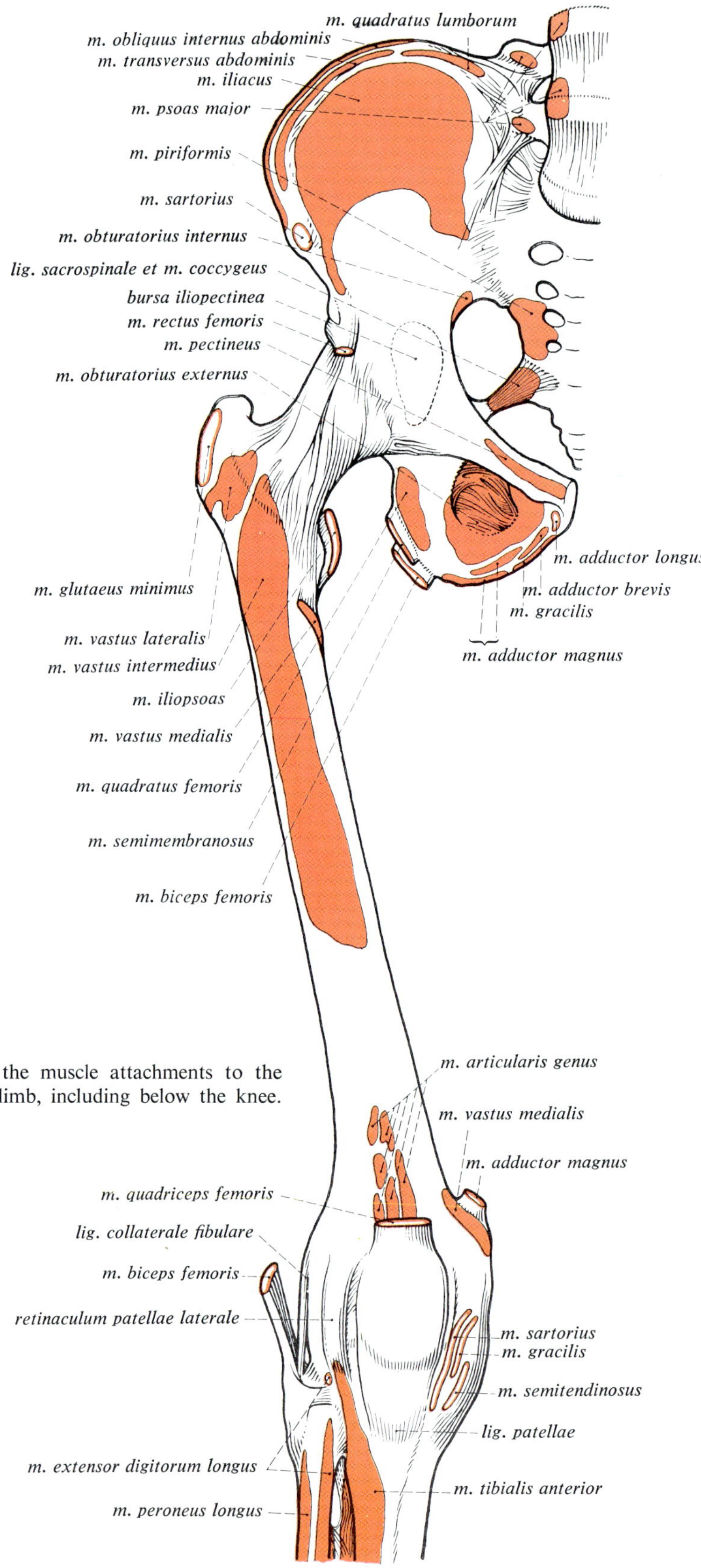

Fig. 344. Diagram of the muscle attachments to the pelvis and right lower limb, including below the knee. Ventral view.

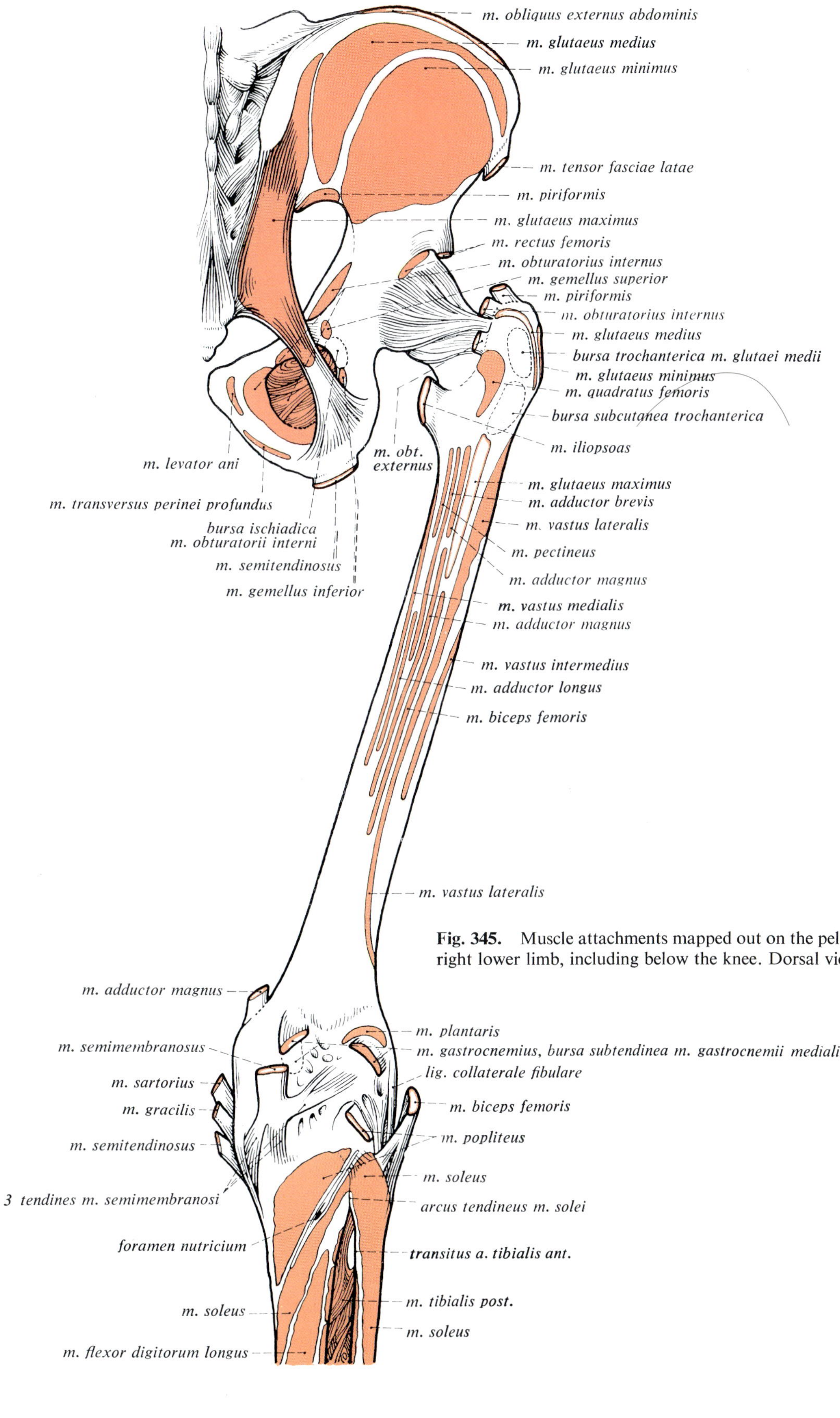

Fig. 345. Muscle attachments mapped out on the pelvis and right lower limb, including below the knee. Dorsal view.

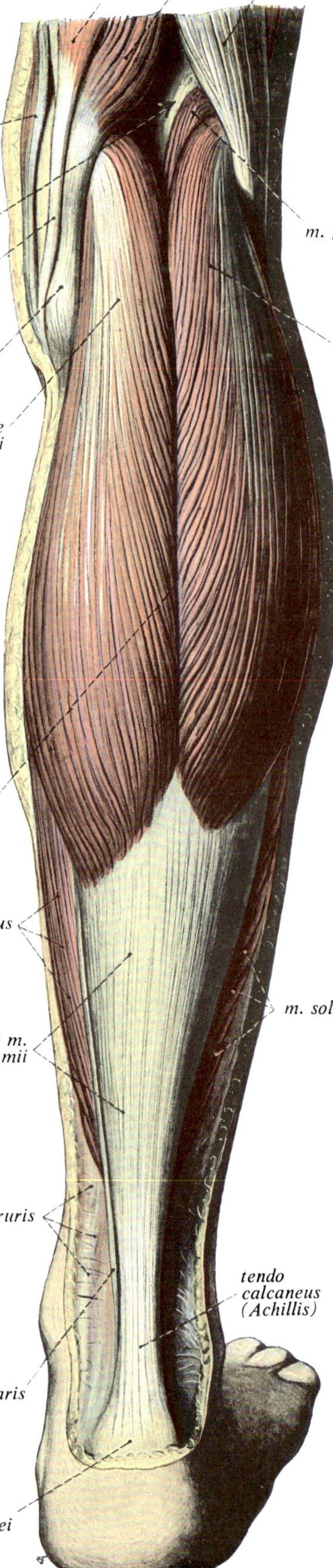
m. semitendinosus
m. semimembranosus
m. biceps femoris
m. gracilis
fossa poplitea
tendo m. semitendinosi
tendo m. semimembranosi
caput mediale m. gastrocnemii
m. plantaris
caput laterale m. gastrocnemii
sulcus inter capita m. gastrocnemii
m. soleus
tendo m. gastrocnemii
m. soleus
fascia cruris
tendo calcaneus (Achillis)
tendo m. plantaris
tuber calcanei

Fig. 346

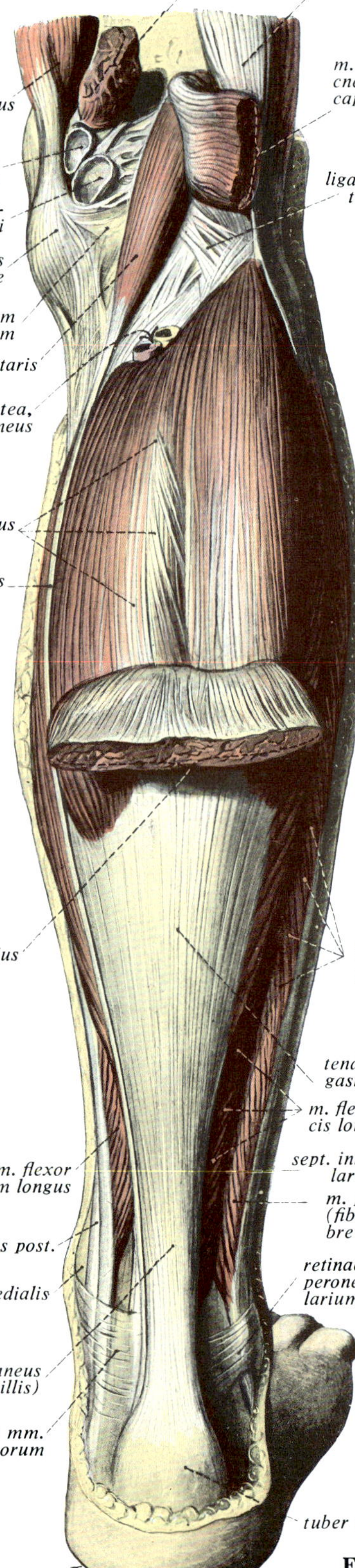
m. gastrocnemius, caput mediale
m. biceps femoris
m. gastrocnemius, caput laterale
m. semimembranosus
bursa subtendinea m. gastrocnemii medialis
ligamentum popliteum arcuatum
bursa m. semimembranosi
condylus medialis tibiae
lig. popliteum obliquum
m. plantaris
a. v. poplitea, arcus tendineus
m. soleus
tendo m. plantaris
m. gastrocnemius
m. peroneus (fibularis) longus
tendo m. gastrocnemii
m. flexor hallucis longus
sept. intermusculare posterius
m. flexor digitorum longus
m. peroneus (fibularis) brevis
tendo m. tibialis post.
retinaculum mm. peroneorum (fibularium) superius
malleolus medialis
tendo calcaneus (Achillis)
retinaculum mm. flexorum
tuber calcanei

Fig. 347

Muscles of the Posterior Compartment of the Leg (Figs. 341–343, 345–347)

Name	*Origin*	*Insertion*
1. m. gastrocnemius		
caput mediale (Fig. 345)	condylus medialis femoris; capsule of knee	Aponeurosis unites with the tendon of the m. soleus to form the tendo calcaneus (ACHIILLIS)
caput laterale	condylus lateralis femoris; capsule of knee	
2. m. soleus (with m. gastrocnemius, occasionally described as m. triceps surae)	Posterior surface of head and upper third of fibula; soleal line and middle third of medial border of tibia; arcus tendineus (transverse intermuscular septum) between the tibia and fibula	
3. m. plantaris	condylus lateralis femoris	Posterior part of calcaneus in front or side of the tendo calcaneus (with long thin tendon)
Nerve: n. tibialis		
Action: Plantar flexion of foot and tends to supinate it; The m. gastrocnemius points the toe (with Plantaris); flexes knee; braces knee and ankle joints when standing		
4. m. popliteus	Tendon from condylus lateralis femoris; somewhat from the ligamentum popliteum arcuatum	Posterior surface of tibia, proximal to soleal line (Fig. 353)
Nerve: n. tibialis		
Action: Flexes leg; rotates femur medially to help unlock dead center		

Note: The oblique origin of the *m. soleus* arises through an *arcus tendineus m. solei,* a fissure through this the vasa poplitea and *n. tibialis* leave the popliteal space distally and arrives in the deep region of the calf.

Fig. 346. Superficial view of the muscular components of the calf.

Fig. 347. Second layer of the calf muscles. The *m. gastrocnemius* is cut and reflected; the deeper layer of the *fascia cruralis* was removed up to the *retinacula.*

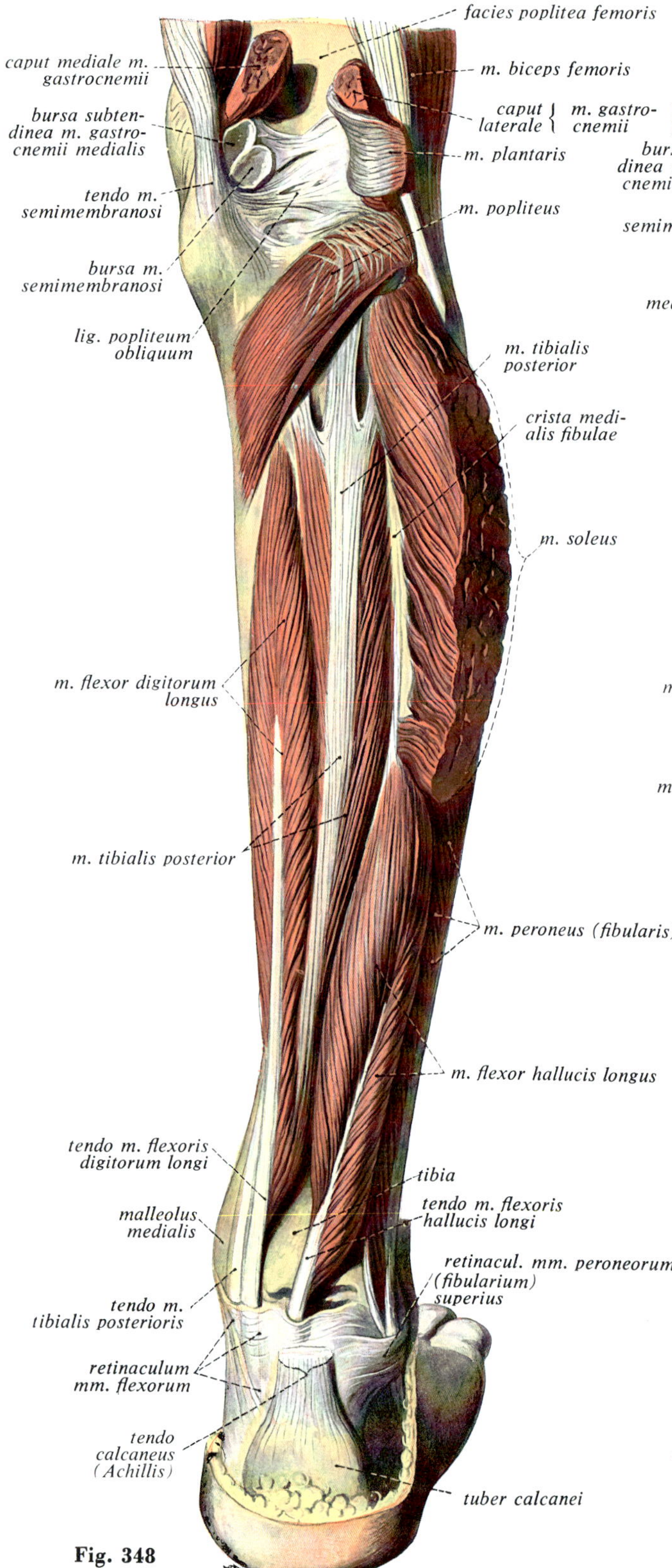
facies poplitea femoris
caput mediale m. gastrocnemii
m. biceps femoris
bursa subtendinea m. gastrocnemii medialis
caput laterale
m. gastrocnemii
m. plantaris
tendo m. semimembranosi
m. popliteus
bursa m. semimembranosi
lig. popliteum obliquum
m. tibialis posterior
crista medialis fibulae
m. soleus
m. flexor digitorum longus
m. tibialis posterior
m. peroneus (fibularis) longus
m. flexor hallucis longus
tendo m. flexoris digitorum longi
tibia
malleolus medialis
tendo m. flexoris hallucis longi
retinacul. mm. peroneorum (fibularium) superius
tendo m. tibialis posterioris
retinaculum mm. flexorum
tendo calcaneus (Achillis)
tuber calcanei

Fig. 348

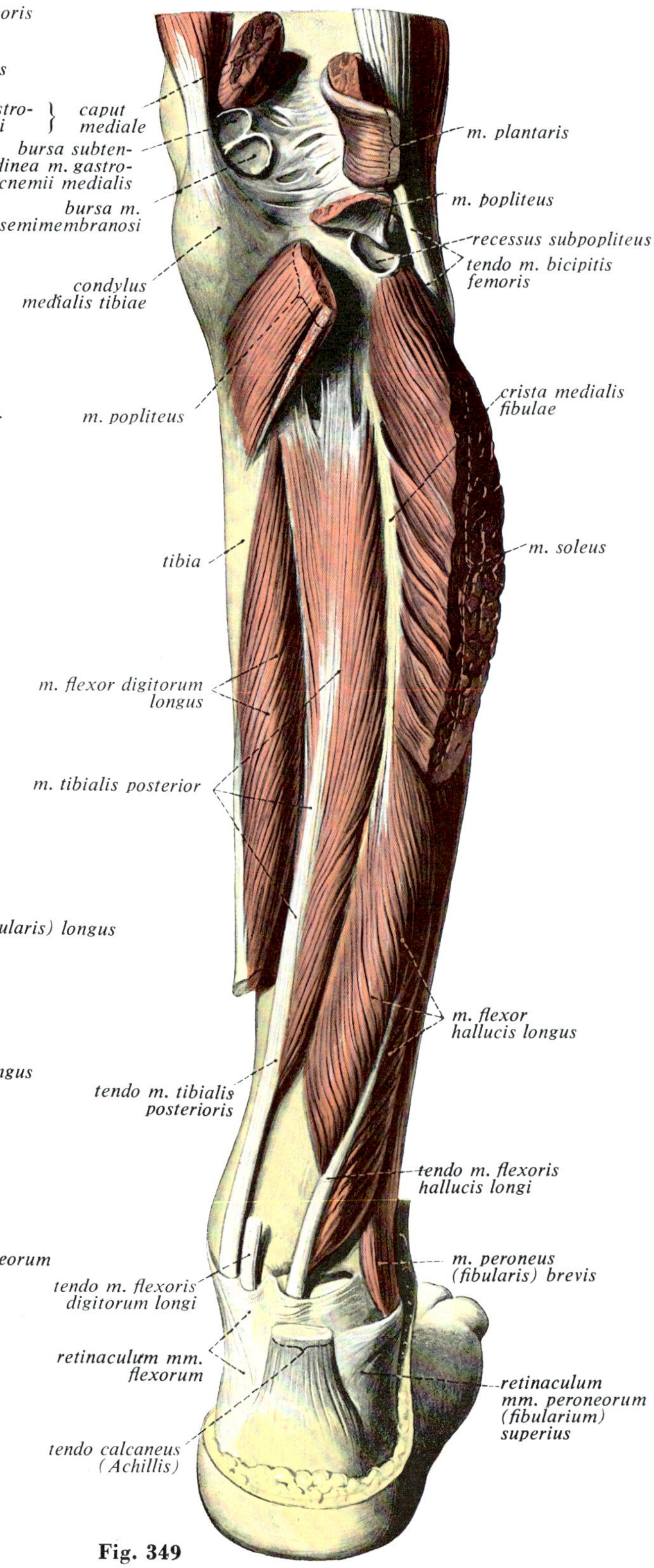
caput mediale
m. plantaris
bursa subtendinea m. gastrocnemii medialis
bursa m. semimembranosi
m. popliteus
recessus subpopliteus
tendo m. bicipitis femoris
condylus medialis tibiae
crista medialis fibulae
m. popliteus
tibia
m. soleus
m. flexor digitorum longus
m. tibialis posterior
m. flexor hallucis longus
tendo m. tibialis posterioris
tendo m. flexoris hallucis longi
m. peroneus (fibularis) brevis
tendo m. flexoris digitorum longi
retinaculum mm. flexorum
retinaculum mm. peroneorum (fibularium) superius
tendo calcaneus (Achillis)

Fig. 349

Muscles of the Posterior Compartment of the Leg (Deep Layers) (Figs. 348, 349, 353)

Name	*Origin*	*Insertion*
1. m. tibialis posterior	Posterior surface of the tibia (proximal part) membrana interossea cruris, medial surface of the fibula	tuberositas ossis navicularis; plantar surface of the 3 ossa cuneiformia, sustentaculum tali of the calcaneus, bases of ossa metatarsalia 2 to 4. (Fig. 354)
Action: Plantar flexes the foot, supinates (adducts and inverts)		
2. m. flexor digitorum longus	Posterior surface and interosseus margin of the tibia distal to soleal line with an arcus tendineus from distal third of the fibula	By 4 tendons into bases of distal phalanges of toes 2 to 5
Action: Flexes terminal phalanges of toes 2–5, assists in plantar flexion, supination and adduction of the foot		
3. m. flexor hallucis longus	Distal $^2/_3$ of posterior surface and margin of fibula, membrana interossea cruris, septum intermusculare posterius	Base of terminal phalanx of big toe
Nerve: n. tibialis for all three muscles		
Action: Flexes big toe, plantar flexion, supination, and adduction of foot		

Note: The *regio malleolaris medialis* contains from front to back: The tendons for the *mm. tibialis posterior* and *flexor digitorum longus*; the *vasa tibialia posterior*, the *n. tibialis* and, deep dorsally, the tendon of the *m. flexor hallucis longus*. A short tunnel is fashioned through the *retinaculum*, through which the structure of the deep calf region goes to the sole of the foot (Fig. 365).
The *regio malleolaris lateralis* contains the tendons of the *mm. peroneus longus* and *peroneus brevis*, which are fixed by a *retinaculum superius* and *inferius*.

◀ **Fig. 348.** Deeper muscles of the posterior compartment of the leg. The *mm. gastrocnemius*, the *soleus* and the *plantaris* were removed or reflected.

Fig. 349. Deepest layer of the muscular compartment of the calf. The *mm. popliteus* and *flexor digitorum longus* were transected.

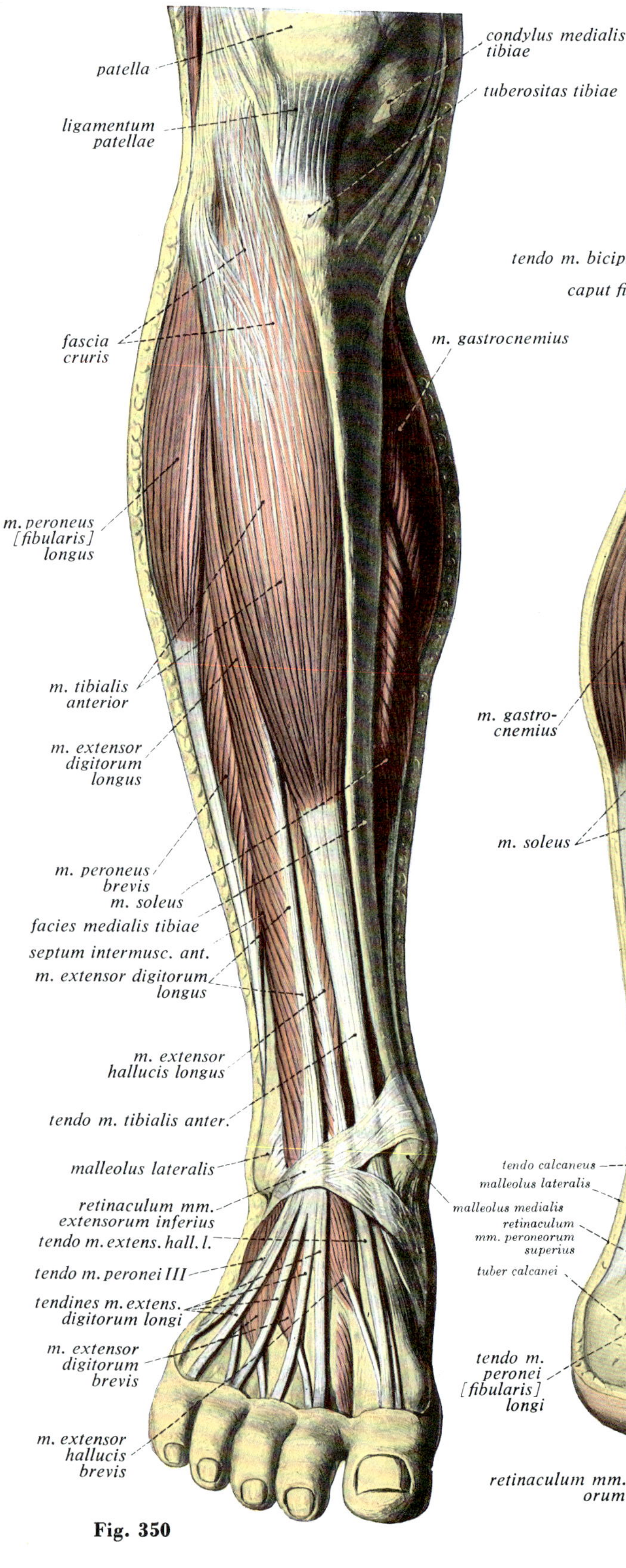

patella
condylus medialis tibiae
tuberositas tibiae
ligamentum patellae
fascia cruris
m. gastrocnemius
m. peroneus [fibularis] longus
m. tibialis anterior
m. extensor digitorum longus
m. peroneus brevis
m. soleus
facies medialis tibiae
septum intermusc. ant.
m. extensor digitorum longus
m. extensor hallucis longus
tendo m. tibialis anter.
malleolus lateralis
retinaculum mm. extensorum inferius
tendo m. extens. hall. l.
tendo m. peronei III
tendines m. extens. digitorum longi
m. extensor digitorum brevis
m. extensor hallucis brevis

Fig. 350

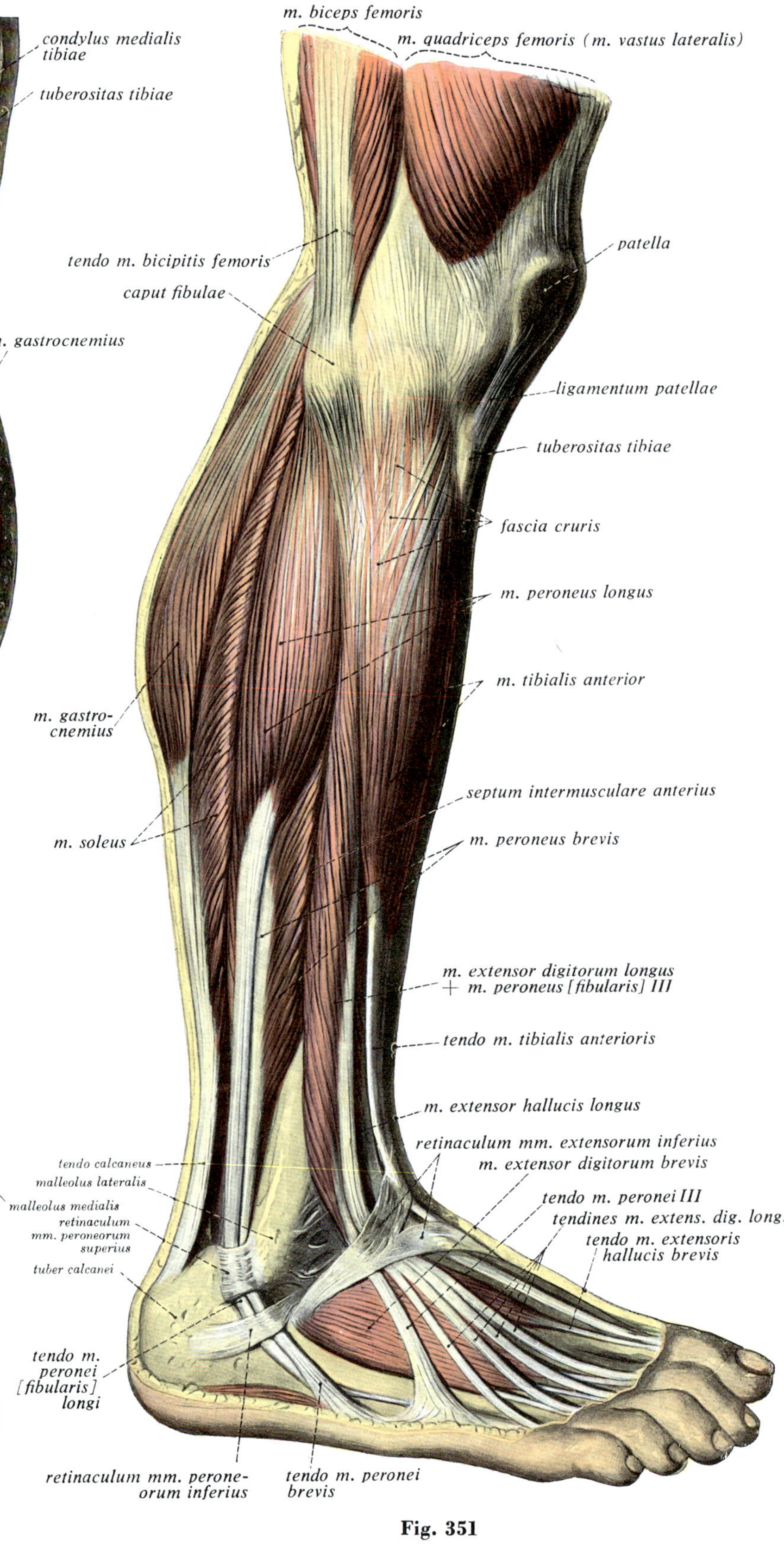

m. biceps femoris
m. quadriceps femoris (m. vastus lateralis)
tendo m. bicipitis femoris
patella
caput fibulae
ligamentum patellae
tuberositas tibiae
fascia cruris
m. peroneus longus
m. tibialis anterior
m. gastrocnemius
septum intermusculare anterius
m. soleus
m. peroneus brevis
m. extensor digitorum longus + m. peroneus [fibularis] III
tendo m. tibialis anterioris
m. extensor hallucis longus
retinaculum mm. extensorum inferius
m. extensor digitorum brevis
tendo calcaneus
malleolus lateralis
malleolus medialis
retinaculum mm. peroneorum superius
tendo m. peronei III
tendines m. extens. dig. long.
tendo m. extensoris hallucis brevis
tuber calcanei
tendo m. peronei [fibularis] longi
retinaculum mm. peroneorum inferius
tendo m. peronei brevis

Fig. 351

Muscles of the Anterior Compartment of the Leg (Figs. 350–352, 364)

Name	*Origin*	*Insertion*
1. m. tibialis anterior With long tendon running under the retinaculum of the mm. extensorum superius et inferius	epicondylus lateralis tibiae; upper half of lateral surface of tibia; membrana interossea; fascia cruris	Base of 1st metatarsal (medial edge); medial cuneiform (I) (plantar surface)

Nerve: ramus profundus n. peronei (fibularis) (L 4, 5; S 1)

Action: Dorsally flexes and supinates (adducts and inverts) the foot

2. m. extensor hallucis longus	Middle half of fibular and membrana interossea; fascia cruris	Base of distal phalanx of great toe
3. m. extensor digitorum longus Tendon fixed by the retinacula of the mm. extensorum superius et inferius	epicondylus lateralis tibiae; proximal ¾ of fibula; membrana interossea; fascia cruris; septum intermusculare anterius cruris	Tendons to 2nd and terminal phalanges of 4 lateral toes
4. m. peroneus (fibularis) tertius	Distal third of shaft of fibula; membrana interossea	Dorsal surface, fifth metatarsal bone (flat tendon)

Nerve: n. peroneus (fibular) (L 4, 5; S 1)

Action: Extends toes; dorsiflexes ankle joint at the same time the m. extensor digitorum longus pronates and abducts the foot; also the m. extensor hallucis longus supinates the foot

Muscles of the Lateral Compartment of the Leg (Figs. 350, 351, 353, 365)

1. m. peroneus (fibularis) longus The tendon is a cartilaginous thickening at the tuberositas ossis cuboidei	Head and upper $^2/_3$ of lateral surface and posterior margin of fibula; septum intermusculare	Long tendon ends on lateral side of the base of the 1st metatarsal bone and the lateral side of the medial cuneiform (Fig. 354)
2. m. peroneus brevis	Distal $^2/_3$ of the lateral surface and anterior margin of the fibula, septum intermusculare	Tuberosity at the base of the 5th metatarsal, tendon strip to little toe (Fig. 357)

Nerve: n. peroneus (fibularis) superficialis (L 4, 5; S 1)

Action: Both muscles pronates (everts and abducts) and plantar flexes the foot

Fig. 350. Muscles of the anterior compartments of the leg and the dorsum of the foot. The *retinaculum m. extensorum superius* was removed; the *retinaculum m. extensorum inferius* was retained.

Fig. 351. Muscles of the lower leg and dorsum of the foot, seen from the lateral side. The fascia was removed as far as the retinacula.

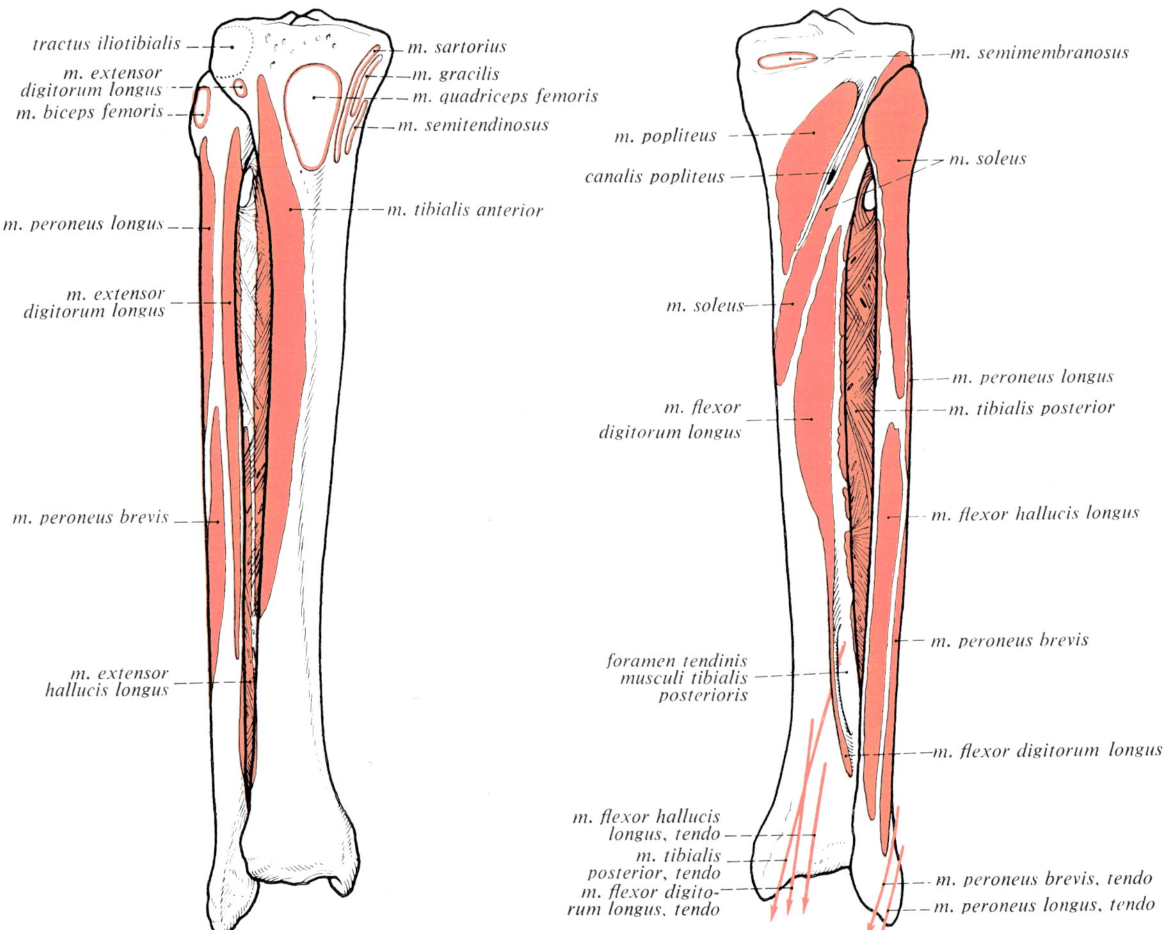

Figs. 352 and 353. Diagram of the muscle origins and insertions on the right *tibia* and *fibula*. Fig. 352. Ventral aspect. Fig. 353. Dorsal aspect.

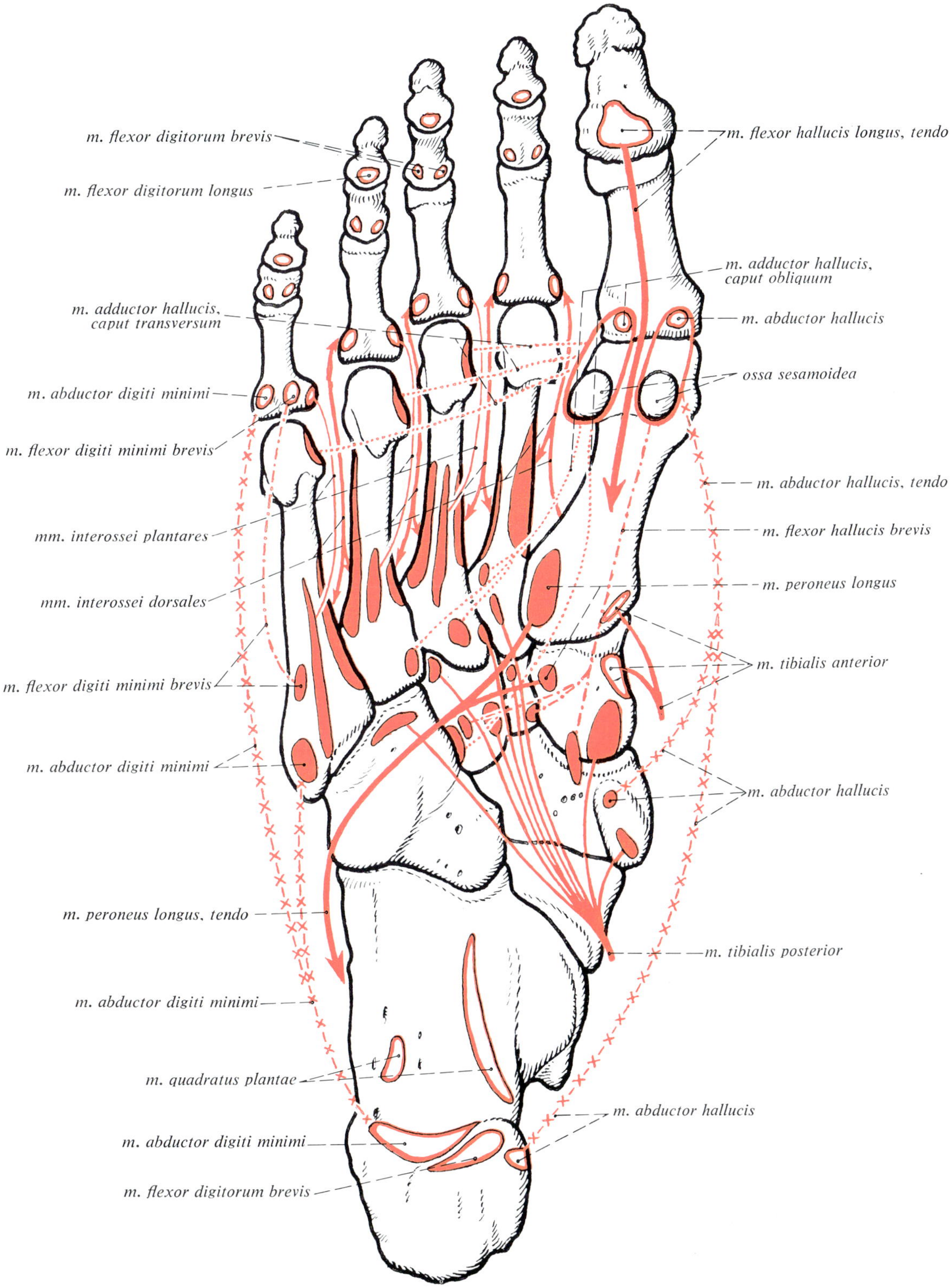

Fig. 354. Muscle origins and insertions mapped out on the sole of the right foot.

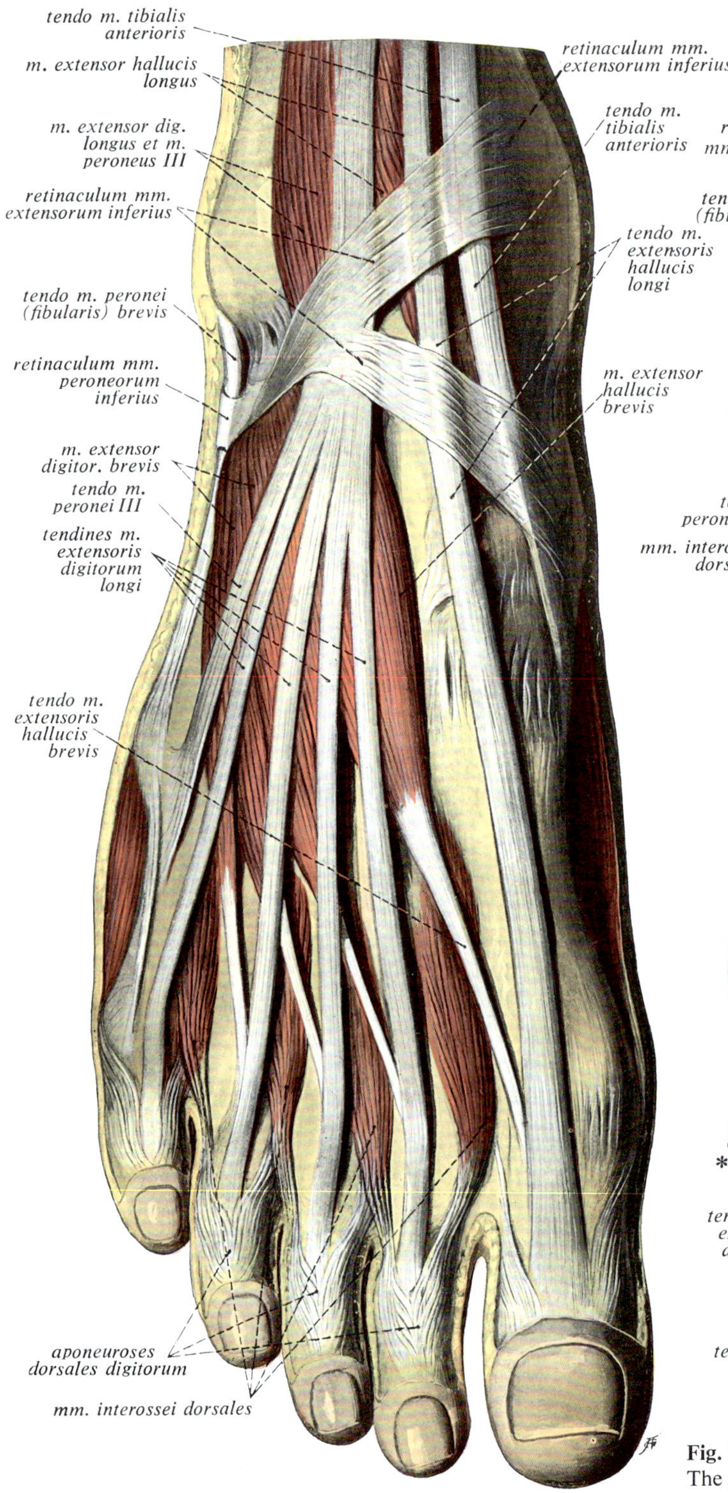

Fig. 355. Superficial muscles and the tendons of the dorsum of the foot.

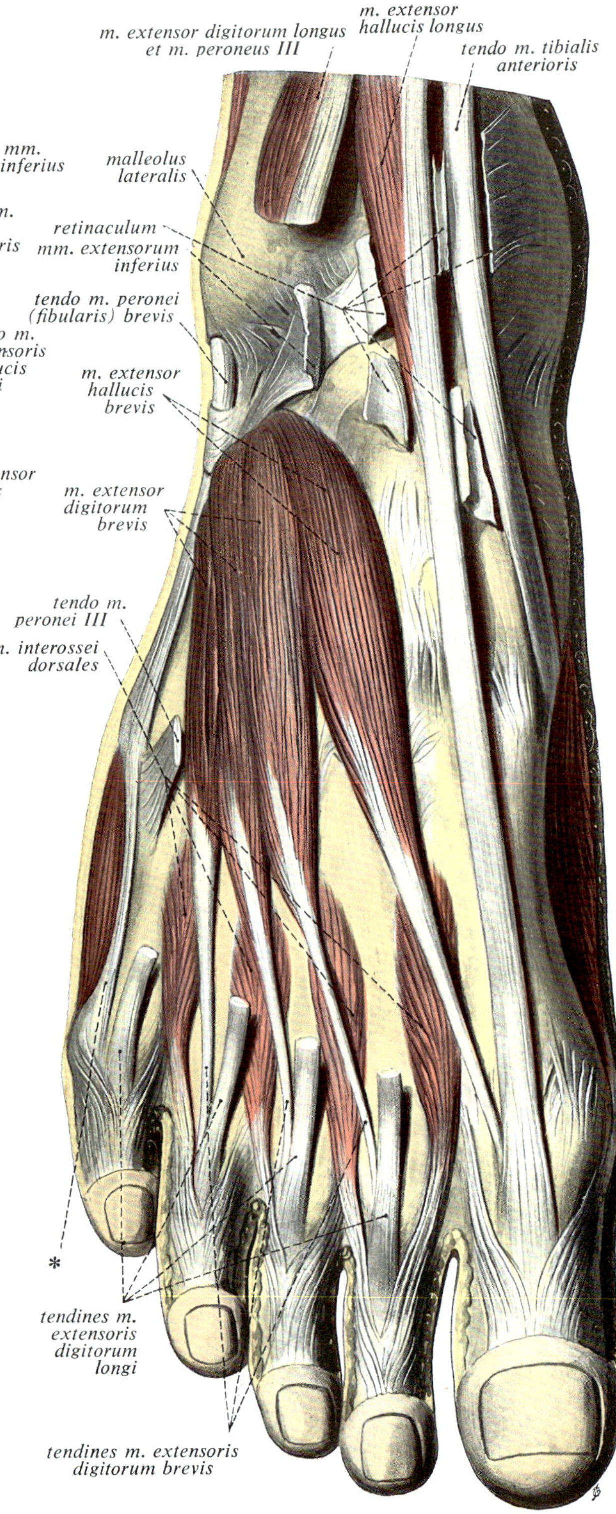

Fig. 356. Muscles and tendons of the dorsum of the foot. The *retinaculum* of the *mm. extensorum inferius* has been split. * The continuation of the tendon of the *m. peroneus (fibularis) brevis* on the small toe (var.).

Muscles of the Dorsum of the Foot (Figs. 355–357)

Name	*Origin*	*Insertion*
m. extensor digitorum brevis	facies lateralis et dorsalis calcanei	Dorsal aponeurosis of 3 middle toes (3 thin tendons)
m. extensor hallucis brevis	facies dorsalis calcanei	Base of 1st phalanx of big toe

Nerve: n. peroneus profundus (fibularis) (L 5; S 1)

Action: Extension of the toes (dorsiflexion)

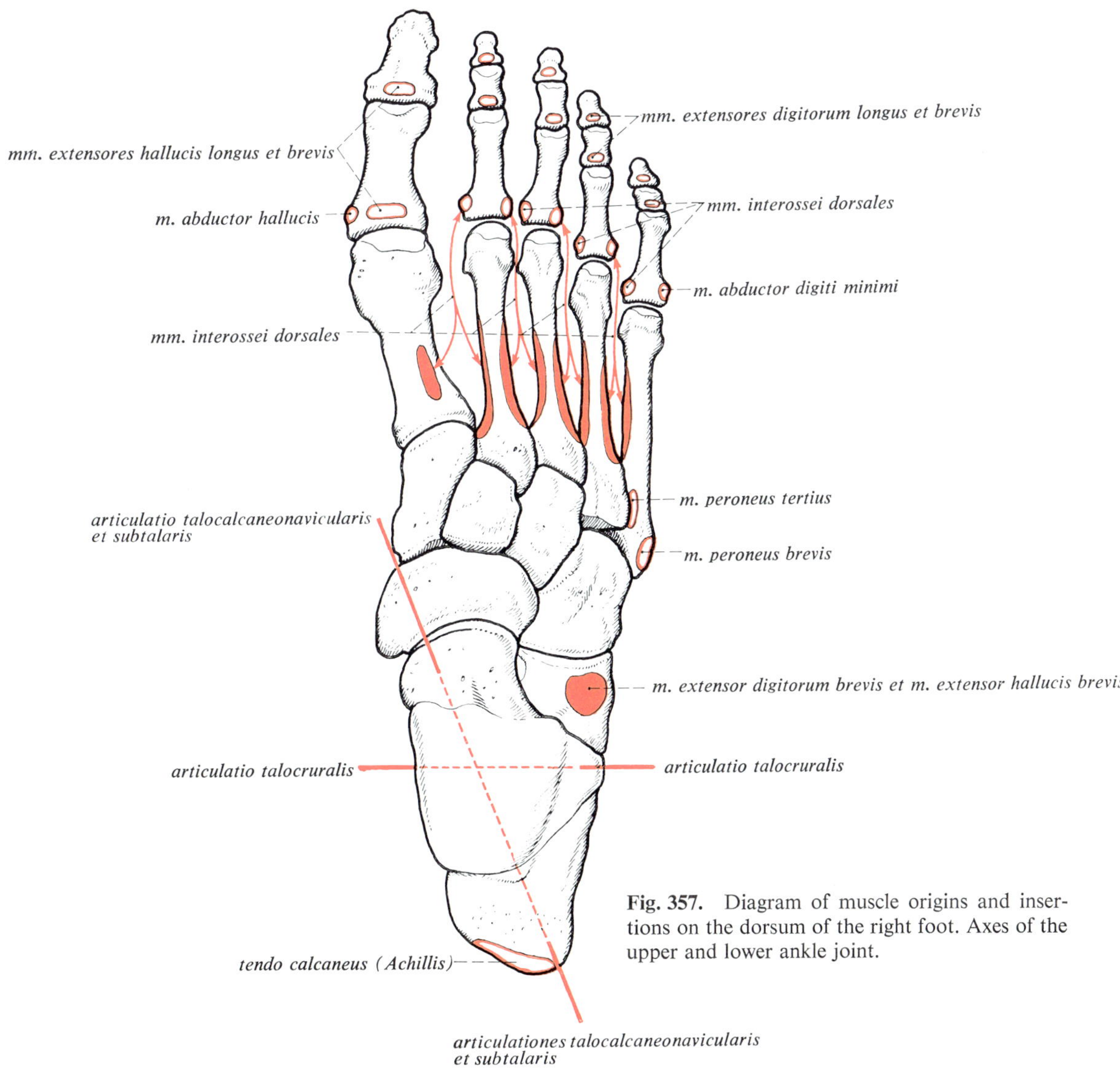

Fig. 357. Diagram of muscle origins and insertions on the dorsum of the right foot. Axes of the upper and lower ankle joint.

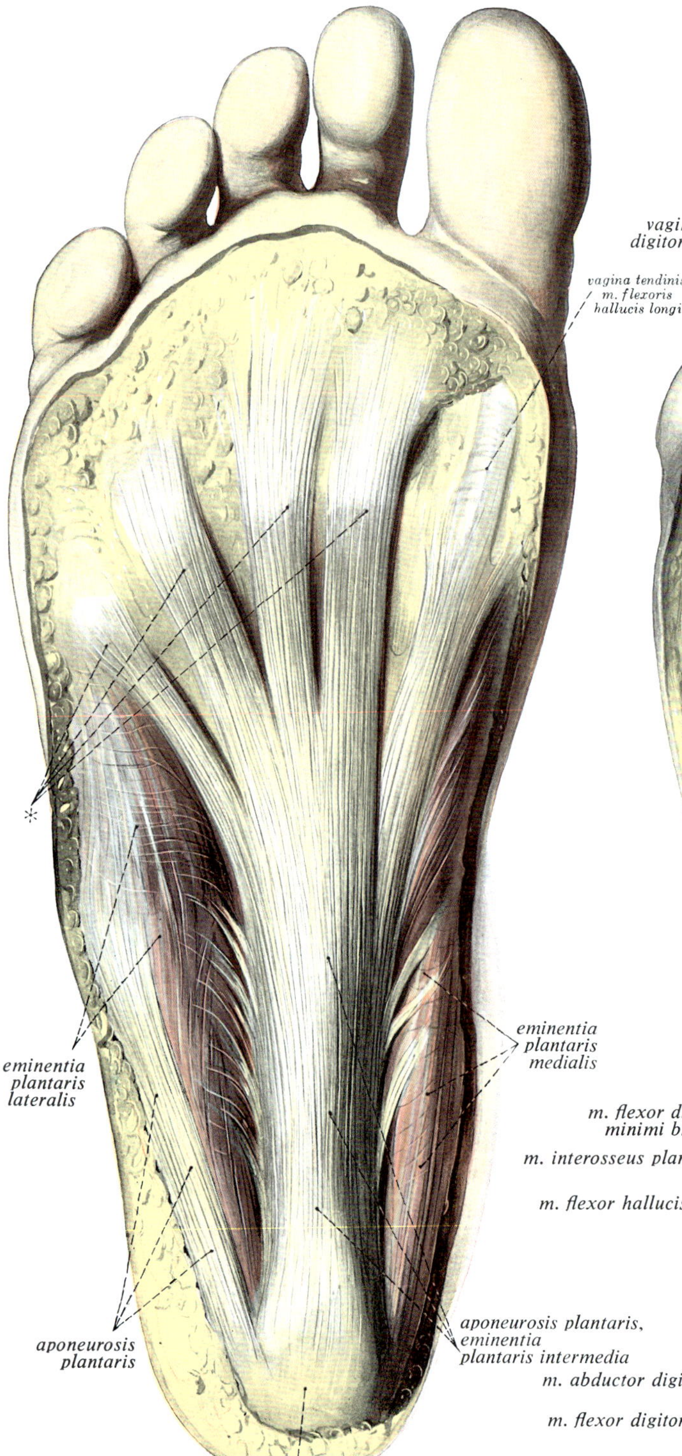
vagina tendinis m. flexoris hallucis longi
*
eminentia plantaris lateralis
eminentia plantaris medialis
aponeurosis plantaris
aponeurosis plantaris, eminentia plantaris intermedia
tuber calcanei

Fig. 358

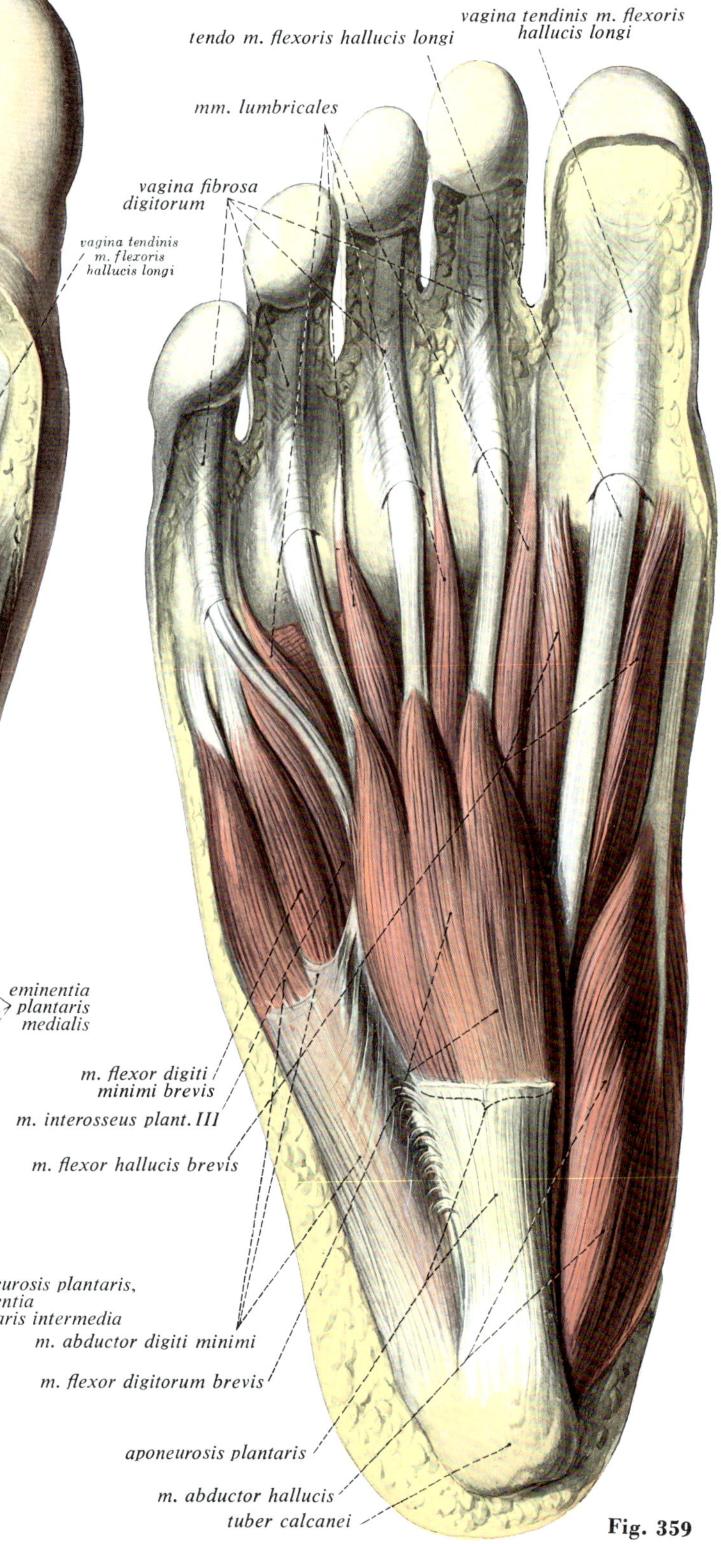
vagina tendinis m. flexoris hallucis longi
tendo m. flexoris hallucis longi
mm. lumbricales
vagina fibrosa digitorum
m. flexor digiti minimi brevis
m. interosseus plant. III
m. flexor hallucis brevis
m. abductor digiti minimi
m. flexor digitorum brevis
aponeurosis plantaris
m. abductor hallucis
tuber calcanei

Fig. 359

Muscles of the Sole of the Foot *(planta pedis)* (Figs. 354, 359–361)

Name	*Origin*	*Insertion*
m. flexor digitorum brevis Plantar muscle forms the eminentia plantaris intermedia	processus medialis tuberis calcanei and aponeurosis plantaris (medial part)	By 4 thin tendons (perforated by tendons of the m. flexor digitorum longus) on the middle phalanges of the 4 lateral toes
Nerve: n. plantaris medialis (L 4, 5)		
Action: Flexes middle phalanges of the toes		
m. quadratus plantae *(m. flexor accessorius)*	Two heads from plantar surface of calcaneus; ligamentum plantare longum	Lateral margin of tendon of m. flexor digitorum longus
Nerve: n. plantaris lateralis (S 1, 2)		
Action: Supports action of the m. flexor digitorum longus and corrects oblique direction of pull of its tendons		

Note: The muscle pattern on the sole of the foot is formed by 3 muscular eminences: *eminentiae plantares medialis, intermedia* and *lateralis.* In between are 2 longitudinal grooves: *sulci plantares medialis* and *lateralis.* The *sulci plantares medialis* and *lateralis* contain the *vasa plantaria lateralia* and *medialia* respectively and nerves having the same name (Fig. 358).
The *eminentia plantaris medialis* (compartment for the big toe) contains the belly of the the *m. abductor hallucis,* the tendon of the *m. flexor hallucis longus* and the *m. flexor hallucis brevis.* The *eminentia plantaris intermedia* (central compartment for the sole of the foot and is the thickest) contains the belly of the *m. flexor digitorum brevis,* which is covered by the *aponeurosis plantaris.* The *eminentia plantaris lateralis* (compartment for the small toe) contains the *mm. abductor digiti minimi* and *flexor digiti minimi brevis.*

Fig. 358. The plantar aponeurosis of the right foot. * Radiation of the digital slips of the plantar aponeurosis to the toes.

Fig. 359. The superficial musculature of the sole of the right foot. Part of the plantar aponeurosis is removed with the exception of the posterior part.

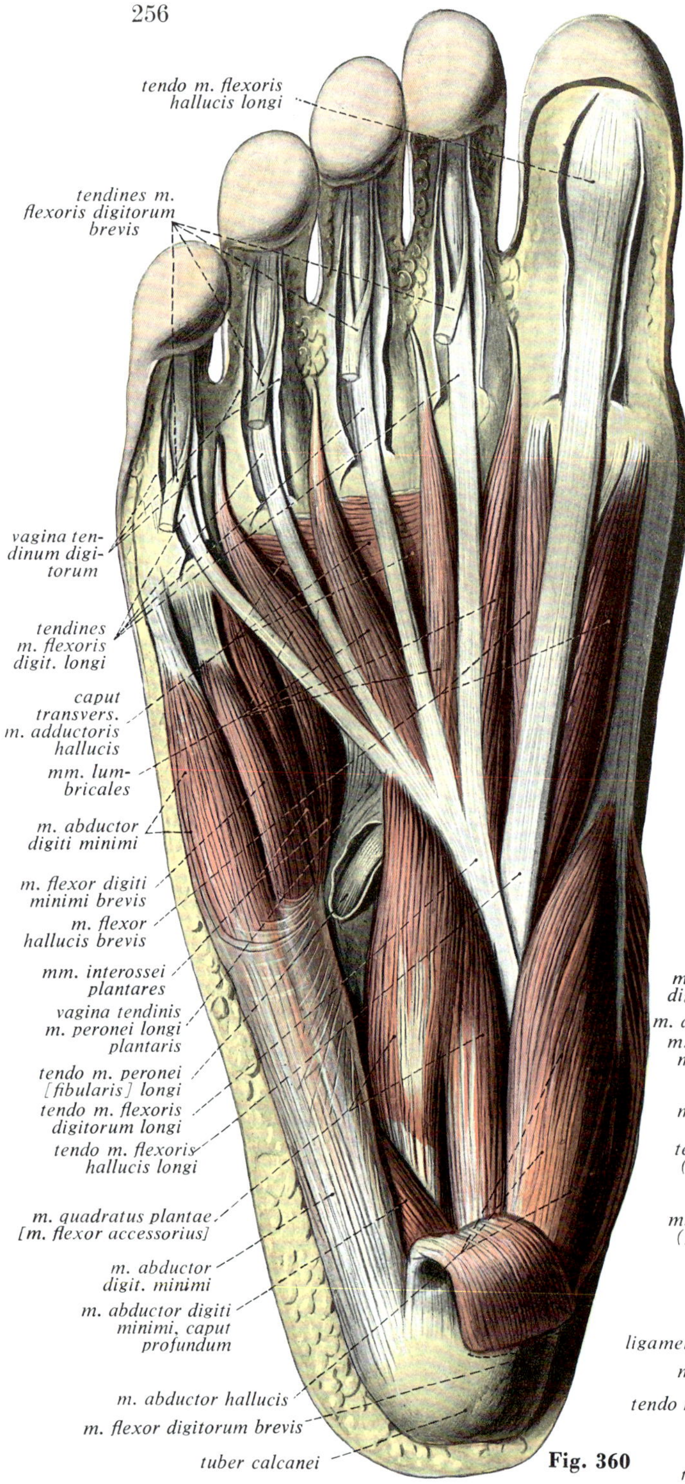

Fig. 360

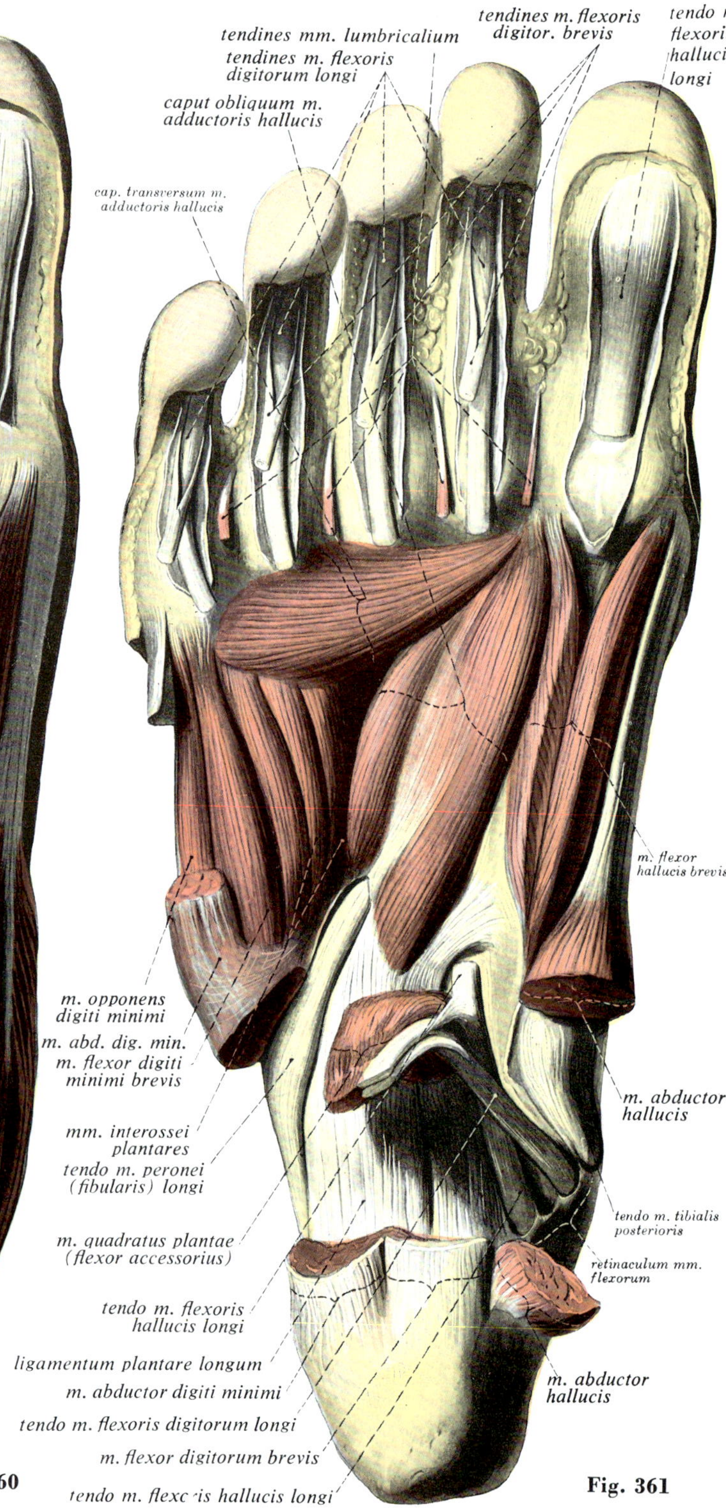

Fig. 361

Fig. 360. The middle layer of the musculature of the sole of the foot. Most of the *m. flexor digitorum brevis* was removed.

Fig. 361. Deep layer of the musculature of the sole of the foot. The following were transected: the tendons of the *mm. flexor digitorum brevis* and *longus, quadratus plantae (flexor accessorius), abductor digiti minimi, abductor hallucis* and *flexor hallucis longus*. The tendon sheath of the *m. peroneus (fibularis) longus* has been split for its entire length.

Muscles of the Great Toe (Figs. 359–361)

Name	*Origin*	*Insertion*
1. m. abductor hallucis Plantar muscle united to the eminentia plantaris medialis	processus medialis tuberis calcanei and aponeurosis plantaris	Base of proximal phalanx of great toe (Fig. 354)
2. m. flexor hallucis brevis	Plantar surface of cuboid and lateral cuneiform bones; tendon of m. tibialis posterior	Two heads on medial and lateral sides of proximal phalanx of big toe; sesamoid bones (Fig. 354)
3. m. adductor hallucis *caput obliquum*	Bases of metatarsal bones 2 to 4; sheath of tendon of m. peroneus longus	Lateral side of base of proximal phalanx of great toe; sesamoid bones (Fig. 354)
caput transversum	Metatarsophalangeal ligaments of the 3 lateral toes; deep transverse metatarsal ligament	

Nerve: For No. 1 and No. 2, the n. plantaris medialis; No. 3 (and sometimes No. 2) n. plantaris lateralis (S 1, 2)

Action: As the name implies: abducts, flexes, adducts big toe: above all, however, gives effective transverse and longitudinal tension to the arcus plantaris

Muscles of the Small Toe (Figs. 354, 359–361)

1. m. abductor digit minimi	processus medialis and lateralis tuberis calcanei; aponeurosis plantaris	Lateral side of proximal phalanx of small toe (and often into tuberositas of the 5th metatarsal bone)
2. m. flexor digiti minimi brevis	Base of 5th metatarsal bone; sheath of Peroneus longus tendon	Proximal phalanx of small toe
3. m. opponens digiti minimi (inconstant) (omitted by NA)		Lateral margin of 5th metatarsal

Nerve: n. plantaris lateralis

Action: As the name implies: abducts, flexes and opponed the small toe; above all, however, gives effectiv tension to the arcus plantaris

The *mm. lumbricales pedis* arise from the tendons of the *m. flexor digitorum longus*. The first one by a single head from the medial ridge of the first tendon (2nd toe) and the other three by two heads. They join the dorsal aponeurosis of the toes in the region of the metatarsophalangeal joints from the medial side. Most small bursae of the lumbricals are found at their insertion. The *n. plantaris medialis* (L 4, 5) supplies the first *m. lumbricalis* and the other three *mm. lumbricales* are supplied by the *n. plantaris lateralis* (S 1, 2).

Action: Flexes proximal phalanges, as in the hand.

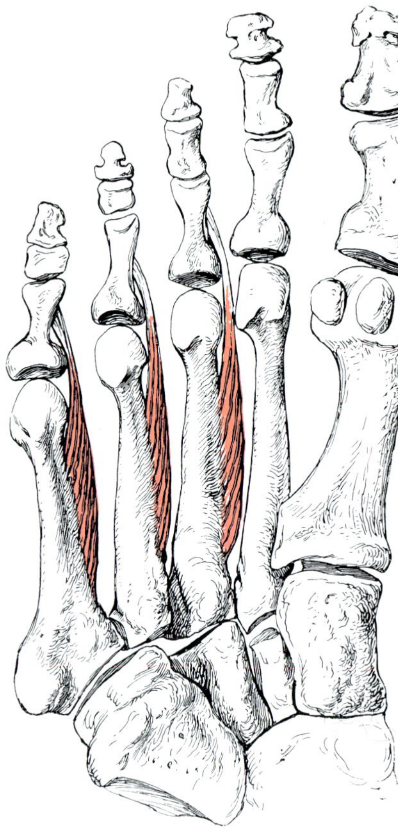

Fig. 362. *mm. interossei plantares.*

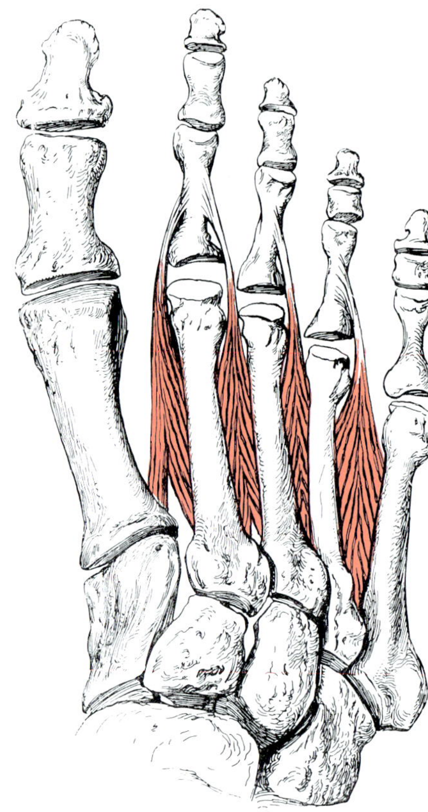

Fig. 363. *mm. interossei dorsales.*

The *mm. interossei* of the foot are arranged somewhat like those of the hand: There are four dorsal and three plantar muscles. The latter are relatively strong (stronger than the dorsal muscles of the foot) in contrast to those of the hand. All three Plantar muscles act in the same direction and arise from the medial border of the ossa metatarsalia III, IV, V, and all three are inserted in the dorsal aponeuroses of the toes of the same side. The relatively weak dorsal interosseus muscles arise by two heads as in the hand. The tendons (as in the hand) do not go in the same direction: I and II go to the second toe.

Nerve: *n. plantaris lateralis.*

Action: Similar to the muscles of the hand: Abduction, or else adduction and flexion.

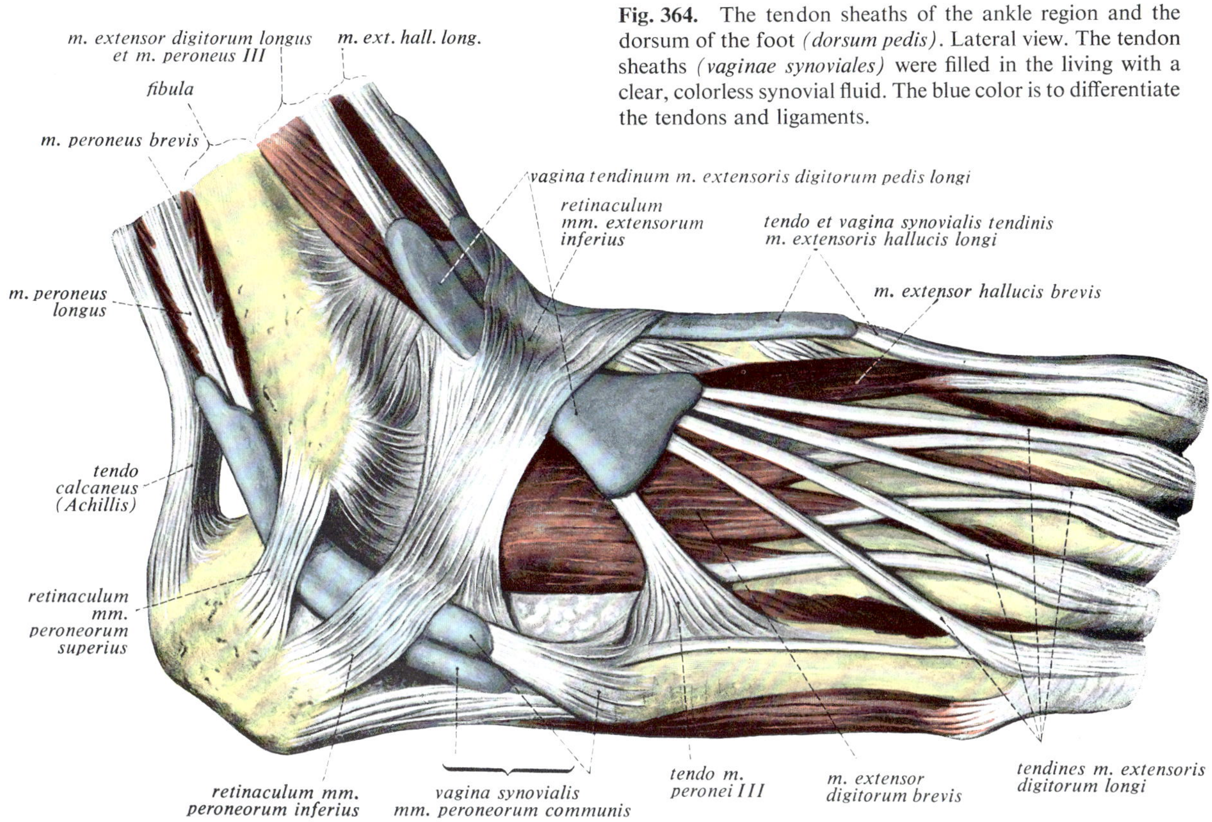

Fig. 364. The tendon sheaths of the ankle region and the dorsum of the foot *(dorsum pedis)*. Lateral view. The tendon sheaths *(vaginae synoviales)* were filled in the living with a clear, colorless synovial fluid. The blue color is to differentiate the tendons and ligaments.

Fig. 365. Tendon sheaths of the medial side of the ankle region and the sole and dorsum of the foot. Partially schematic. The *mm. abductor halluci* and the *flexor digitorum brevis* were partly removed.

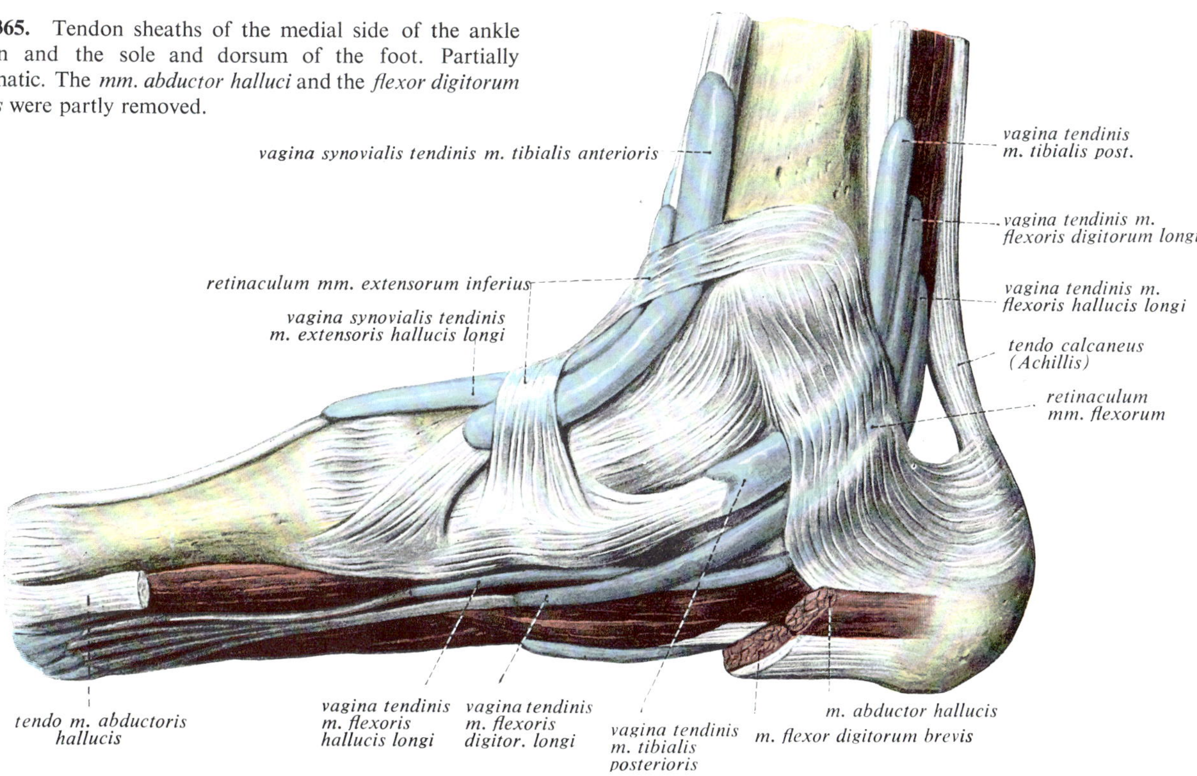

Subject Index (I. Latin/English, II. English/Latin)

(All numbers refer to the numbers of pages)
Names without an explanation in english or latin have no customary names in the corresponding language

I. Latin/English

A

Acetabulum 80–82
Acromion scapulae = Acromion 26, 27, 66, 109–111, 169, 197
Adminiculum lineae albae 160
Ala = Wing
– cristae galli = Wing of cristae galli 39, 54
– major ossis sphenoidalis = Great wing of sphenoid bone 31, 40, 45, 46, 61
– minor ossis sphenoidalis = Lesser wing of sphenoid bone 31, 39, 45, 46, 62
– ossis ilii = Wing of ilium 80–83
– vomeris = Wing of vomer 55, 56, 62
Angulus costae = Costal angle 22
– frontalis ossis parietalis = Frontal angle of parietal bone 53
– inferior scapulae = Inferior angle of scapula 66
– lateralis scapulae = Lateral angle of scapula 66
– mandibulae = Mandibular angle 59, 60, 104, 105
– mastoideus ossis parietalis = Mastoid angle (parietal bone) 53
– occipitalis ossis parietalis = Occipital angle of parietal bone 53
– sphenoidalis ossis parietalis = Sphenoidal angle of parietal bone 53
– sterni = Sternal angle 24
– subpubicus = Subpubic angle 119
– superior scapulae = Superior angle of scapula 66
Ansa tendinis m. digastrici = Ansa tendinis of digastric muscle 172
Antrum mastoideum = Mastoid antrum 49, 50
Anulus = Anulus (also ring)
– fibrosus (disci intervertebralis) = Anulus fibrosus (intervertebral disk) 98
– inguinalis profundus = Deep (or internal) abdominal ring 160
– – superficialis = Superficial (or external) abdominal ring 154, 159
– tympanicus = Tympanic ring 40, 49
Anus 165
Aorta 166, 176
Apertura externa aquaeductus vestibuli = External aperture of aqueduct of vestibule 47
– – canaliculi cochleae = External aperture of canaliculus of cochlea 48
Apertura interna canalis carotici = Internalaperture of carotid canal 50
– nasalis canalis incisivi = Nasal aperture of incisive canal 35
– piriformis = Piriform aperture 40
– sinus frontalis = Aperture of frontal sinus 52, 63
– – sphenoidalis = Aperture of sphenoidal sinus 46, 54, 63
Apex capitis fibulae = Apex of head of fibula 87
– ossis sacri = Apex of sacrum 20, 21
– partis petrosae ossis temporalis = Apex of petrous portion of temporal bone 47, 48
Aponeuroses tendinum digit. dorsales manus (aponeuroses m. extens. digit. manus) 212, 220, 223
Aponeurosis m. bicipitis brachii = Dicipital aponeurosis 190, 196, 198, 199, 202
– m. obliqui abdominis ext. = Aponeurosis of external oblique muscle of abdomen 141, 154, 159, 161, 162
– – – – int. = Aponeurosis of internal oblique muscle of abdomen 158, 161
– – transversi abdominis = Aponeurosis of transversal muscle of abdomen 161
– palatina m. tensoris veli palatini = Palatine aponeurosis of tensor muscle of veli palatini 188
– palmaris = Palmar aponeurosis 199, 213, 223
– plantaris = Plantar aponeurosis 254
Arcus = Arch
– alveolaris mandibulae = Alveolar arch of mandible 59
– anterior atlantis = Anterior arch of atlas 16, 96
– axis = Arch of axis 16
– costalis = Costal arch 25, 27, 162
– iliopectineus = Iliopectineal arch 166
– posterior atlantis = Posterior arch of atlas 16, 96
– pubis = Pubic arch 118, 124
– superciliaris ossis frontalis = Superciliary arch of frontal bone 51, 52
– tendineus m. psoatis = Tendinous arch of psoas muscle 166
– – (fasciae obturatoriae) m. levatoris ani = Tendinous arch of levator ani muscle 164
– – m. solei = Tendinous arch of soleus muscle 243
Arcus vertebrae = Vertebral arch 17–19, 99
– zygomaticus = Zygomatic arch 33, 37, 63, 104, 183
Area intercondylaris anterior tibiae = Anterior intercondylar area 87
– – posterior tibiae, Posterior intercondylar area 87
Arteria(e) = Artery(ies)
– axillaris = Axillary artery 174
– brachialis = Brachial artery 199
– carotis communis = Common carotid artery 169, 174–176, 185
– – externa = External carotid artery 175, 185
– – interna = Internal carotid artery 175
– collateralis ulnaris sup. = Superior ulnar collateral artery 199
– facialis = Facial artery 174
– femoralis = Femoral artery 228
– glutaea inferior = Inferior glutaeal artery 230
– – superior = Superior glutaeal artery 230
– iliaca externa = External iliac artery 228
– nutricia humeri = Nutritient artery of humerus 8
– (ae) perforantes = Perforating arteries 230
– poplitea = Popliteal artery 229
– pudenda interna = Internal pudendal artery 230
– radialis = Radial artery 199, 216
– subclavia = Subclavian artery 175, 176
– temporalis superficialis = Superficial temporal artery 181
– thoracica interna = Internal thoracic artery 176
– tibialis posterior = Posterior tibial artery 243
– ulnaris = Ulnar artery 199, 216
– vertebralis = Vertebral artery 150
Articulatio (nes) = Articulation (s) or Joint (s)
Articulations (Syndesmology) 93–137
Articulatio acromioclavicularis = Acromioclavicular articulation 109, 111
– atlantoaxialis lateralis = Lateral atlantoaxial articulation 94–96, 176
– – mediana = Medial atlantoaxial articulation 96, 187
– atlantooccipitalis = Atlantooccipital articulation 94, 95

Articulatio calcaneocuboidea = Calcaneocuboid articulation 135
– capitis costae = Articulation of head of rib 102
– (nes) carpometacarpeae = Carpometacarpal articulations 113–115
– – pollicis = Carpometacarpal articulation of thumb 113, 115
– (nes) costae = Costal articulations 102
– costotransversaria = Costotransverse articulation 102
– coxae = Articulation of hip 118–125
– cubiti = Cubital articulation (Elbow joint) 112, 113
– cuneonavicularis = Cuneonavicular articulation 135
– genus = Articulation of knee (Knee joint) 92, 126–129
– humeri = Articulation of shoulder (Shoulder joint) 109–111, 197
– humeroulnaris = Humeroulnar articulation 113
– incudomallearis = Incudomallear articulation 49
– (nes) intercarpeae = Intercarpal articulations 113
– (nes) manus = Articulations of the hand 113–115
– mediocarpea = Mediocarpal articulation 113
– (nes) metacarpophalangeae = Metacarpophalangeal articulations 72–75, 113–115
– radiocarpea = Radiocarpal articulation 113
– radioulnaris distalis = Distal radioulnar articulation 112, 113, 115
– sacroiliaca = Sacroiliac articulation 124
– sternoclavicularis = Sternoclavicular articulation 108, 174
– (nes) sternocostales = Sternocostal articulations 103
– subtalaris = Subtalar articulation 92, 133–135, 253
– talocalcaneonavicularis = Talocalcaneonavicular articulation 92, 133–135, 253
– talocruralis = Talocrural articulation (Ankle joint) 92, 130, 134, 253
– talonavicularis = Talonavicular articulation 135
– (nes) tarsometatarseae = Tarsometatarsal articulations 135
– tarsi transversus = *Chopart's* joint 92, 133, 134
– temporomandibularis = Temporomandibular articulation 104, 105, 183, 185, 186, 188
– (syndesmosis) tibiofibularis dist. = Distal tibiofibular articulation (syndesmosis) 128, 130
– tibiofibularis prox. = Proximal tibiofibular articulation 128, 130
Atlas 16, 17, 94–96
Auditory ossicles 49
Auris media = Middle ear 49, 50
Axis (Epistropheus) 16, 17, 96
– pelvis = Pelvic axis 124

B

Basis cranii externa = External base of cranium (skull) 36, 37, 188
– – interna = Internal base of cranium (skull) 38, 39
– mandibulae = Base of mandible 33, 188
– ossis sacri = Base of sacral bone 20, 21
– (es) ossium metacarpalium = Base of metacarpal bones 72, 73
– – metatarsalium = Base of metatarsal bones 88
– patellae = Base of patella 85
– phalangis (digit. manus) = Base of phalanx of fingers 72–75
– – (digit. pedis) = Base of phalanx of toes 88
Bones, characteristics of 8–11
Bones, classification of 8–11
Bulbus v. jugularis inferior = Inferior bulb of jugular vein 169
Bursa anserina = Anserine bursa 234
– bicipitoradialis = Bicipitoradial bursa 202
– coccygea subcutanea 229
– iliopectinea = Iliopectinal bursa 234
infrapatellaris profunda = Deep infrapatellar bursa 126, 128, 129, 241
– (ae) intermetacarpeae 212
– (ae) intermusculares mm. glutaeorum = Intermuscular gluteal bursae 230
– ischiadica m. obturatorii interni = Ischial bursa of internal obturator muscle 243
– m. latissimi dorsi subtendinea = Subtendinous bursa of latissimus dorsi muscle 196
– – pectoralis majoris 198
– – semimembranosi = Bursa of semimembranosus muscle 244
– – subscapularis subtendinea = Subtendinous bursa of subscapularis muscle 197
– subacromialis = Subacromial bursa 111, 197
– subcoracoidea 191, 198
– (ae) subcutaneae digitorum dorsales (manus) 212
– subcutanea infrapatellaris = Subcutaneous infrapatellar bursa 226, 227
– (ae) subcutaneae metacarpophalangeae dorsales 212
– subcutanea olecrani = Subcutaneous bursa of olecrani 113, 190
– – praepatellaris = Subcutaneous prepatellar bursa 128, 129, 226, 227
– – sacralis 229, 230
Bursa subcutanea spinae iliacae post. sup. 229, 230
– – trochanterica = Subcutaneous trochanteric bursa 243
– subdeltoidea = Subdeltoid bursa 191, 194, 197, 198
– subtendinea m. gastrocnemii medialis = Subtendinous bursa of medial head of gastrocnemius muscle 243, 244
– (ae) subtendineae m. sartorii = Subtendinous bursae of sartorius muscle 234
– – – tricipitis surae 240
– suprapatellaris = Suprapatellar bursa 126–129
– tendinis calcanei *(Achillis)* = Bursa of ialcaneol *(Achillis)* tendon 241
– trochanterica m. glutaei maximi = Trochanteric bursa of gluteus maximus muscle 142, 230, 236
– (ae) – (ae) – – medii = Trochanteric bursae of gluteus medius muscle 243

C

Calcaneus = Heel bone (also os calcis) 9, 10, 88–91, 130–133
Calvaria = Skullcap 41, 43
Canaliculi caroticotympanici = Caroticotympanic canaliculi 48
Canaliculus mastoideus = Mastoid canaliculus 37
Canalis adductorius = Abductor canal *(Hunteri)* 232
– caroticus = Carotid canal 37, 48–50, 176, 188
– carpi = Carpal canal 216, 218, 220
– condylaris = Condylar canal 37, 39, 44, 188
– facialis = Facial canal 49, 50
– hypoglossi = Hypoglossal canal 35, 37, 39, 44, 45, 95, 105, 176
– incisivus = Incisive canal 35, 55, 63
– infraorbitalis = Infraorbital canal 61, 62
– inguinalis = Inguinal canal 156
– musculotubarius = Musculotubal canal 48–50, 176
– nasolacrimalis = Nasolacrimal canal 58, 63
– nutricius = Nutritient canal of bone *(Haversian)* 8
– obturatorius = Obturator canal 164, 228, 234
– opticus = Optic canal 39, 45, 61, 62
– palatinus major = Greater palatine canal (palatomaxillary canal) 62
– pterygoideus = Pterygoid canal 46, 62
– pudendalis *(Alcock)* = Pudendal canal *(Alcock)* 165
– sacralis = Sacral canal 20, 21, 124, 164

Canalis semicircularis lateralis = Lateral semicircular canal 50
– tendinis m. flexoris carpi radialis 220
– vertebralis = Vertebral canal 25, 27
Capitulum humeri 68, 71
Caput = Head
– costae = Head of rib (capitulum costae) 22
– femoris = Head of femur 84, 85
– fibulae = Head of fibula 87
– humeri = Head of humerus 67, 68
– longum m. bicipitis brachii = Long head of biceps brachii muscle 109, 111, 197
– – – tricipitis brachii = Long head of triceps brachii muscle 110, 111, 197
– mandibulae = Head of mandible 59, 60
– radii = Head of radius (capitulum radii) 70, 71
– tali = Head of talus 88, 89
– ulnae = Head of ulna 69, 73
Carpus 72–75
Cartilago costalis = Costal cartilage 23, 103
– cricoidea = Cricoid cartilage 174
– thyroidea = Thyroid cartilage 174
Cavitis glenoidalis scapulae = Glenoid cavity of scapula 26, 61, 66, 111, 197
Cavum nasi = Nasal cavity 61–63
– thoracis = Thoracic cavity 166
– tympani = Tympanic cavity 49, 50
Cellulae ethmoidales = Bony ethmoid cells 51, 54, 61
– mastoideae = Mastoid cells 9, 49, 50
Centrum tendineum (diaphragmatis), Central tendon of diaphragm 160, 163, 166
– – perinei = Central tendon of perineum 165
Chewing muscles 183–188
Chiasma opticum = Optic chiasm 51
– tendinum = Tendon chiasma 216
Choanae 36, 37, 40
Chorda obliqua = Oblique cord of elbow joint 112, 201, 210
Circumferentia articularis radii = Articular circumference of head of radius 70, 112
– – ulnae = Articular circumference of head of ulna 69
Clavicula = Clavicle (collar bone) 25–27, 67, 169
Clivus 39, 105
Collum = Neck
– anatonicum humeri = Anatomical neck of humerus 67, 68
– chirurgicum humeri = Surgical neck of humeri 68, 191, 194
– costae = Neck of rib 22, 102
– femoris = Neck of femur 84, 85, 125
– mandibulae = Neck of mandible 60, 186
– radii = Neck of radius 70
Collum scapulae = Neck of scapula 66
– tali = Neck of talus 89
Columna vertebralis = Vertebral column (backbone) 15, 25–27, 97–100
Concha nasalis inferior = Inferior nasal concha 31, 61, 63
– – media = Middle nasal concha 31, 56, 61, 63
– – superior = Superior nasal concha 63
– sphenoidalis = Sphenoidal concha 54
Condylus lateralis femoris = Lateral condyle of femur 84, 85
– – tibiae = Lateral condyle of tibia 86, 87
– medialis femoris = Medial condyle of femur 84, 85
– medialis tibiae = Medial condyle of tibia 86
– occipitalis = Occipital condyle 33, 37, 44, 188
Conjugata (vera) = True conjugate diameter 79, 124
Connexus intertendineus (m. extensoris digit. manus) = 212, 214
Cornu = Horn
– coccygeum = Coccygeal cornu (horn of coccyx) 21
– majus ossis hyoidei = Greater horn of hyoid bone 60, 172, 187
– minus ossis hyoidei = Lesser horn of hyoid bone 60, 172, 187
Corpus = Corpus (see also body or shaft)
– adiposum buccae = Adipose body of check 169, 178, 183
– – infrapatellare = Infrapatellar fatty body 128
– costae = Shaft of rib 22
– femoris = Shaft of femur 84
– fibulae = Shaft of fibula 87
– humeri = Shaft of humerus 68
– mandibulae = Body of mandible 59
– ossis hyoidei = Body of hyoid bone 60
Costa (e) = Rib (s) 22, 23, 27
Coxa = Hip (or hip joint) 25, 80–83
Cranium 30–43
– (neonatus) = Skull (newborn) 40
– (neurocranium) = Skull (neurocranium) 32–35
– (splanchnocranium) = Skull (splanchnocranium) 32–35
Crista = Crest (also border, margin or ridge)
Crista capitis costae = Crest of head of rib 22
– colli costae = Crest of neck of rib 22
– conchalis maxillae = Conchal crest of maxilla 57
– – ossis palatini = Conchal crest of palatine bone 56, 57
– ethmoidalis maxillae = Ethmoidal crest of maxilla 57, 63
Crista ethmoidalis ossis palatini = Ethmoidal crest ofpalatine bone 56, 57, 63
– frontalis ossis frontalis = Frontal crest of frontal bone 39, 43, 52
– galli = 35, 39, 53, 61
– iliaca = Iliac crest 80–83, 142, 229, 230
– infratemporalis ossis sphenoidalis = Infratemporal crest of sphenoidal bone 37, 46, 186
– intertrochanterica femoris = Intertrochanteric crest of femur 84, 85
– lacrimalis anterior = Anterior lacrimal crest 57, 61, 62
– – posterior = Posterior lacrimal crest 61, 62
– medialis fibulae = Medial crest of fibula 87
– m. supinatoris ulnae = Crest of supinator muscle (ulna) 69
– nasalis maxillae = Nasal crest of maxilla 35
– obturatoria = Obturator crest 81, 82
– occipitalis externa = External occipital crest 42, 44
– – interna = Internal occipital crest 39, 44, 45
– orbitalis ossis sphenoidalis = Orbital crest of sphenoidal bone 46
– sacralis intermedia = Intermediate sacral crest 20, 21
– – lateralis = Lateral sacral crest 20
– – mediana = Medial sacral crest 20, 21, 122, 164
– sphenoidalis = Sphenoidal crest 46, 55
– tuberculi majoris humeri = Crest of larger tubercle of humerus 68
– – minoris humeri = Crest of lesser tubercle of humerus 68
Crus dextrum part. lumbal. diaphragmatis = Right diaphragmatic crus (lumbar portion) 166
– intermedium part. lumbal. diaphragmatis = Intermedial diaphragmatic crus (lumbar portion) 163, 166
– laterale diaphragmatis = Lateral diaphragmatic crus 163
– – anuli inguinalis superficialis, Lateral crus of superficial inguinal ring 159
– mediale part. lumbal. diaphragmatis, = Medial diaphragmatic crus (lumbar portion) 163, 166
– – anuli inguinalis superficialis = Medial crus of superficial inguinal ring 154, 159
– sinistrum part. lumbal. disphragmatis = Left diaphragmatic crus (lumbar portion) 166
Cupula pleurae = 166

D

Dens axis = (odontoid process of axis) 16, 17, 95, 96
Diameter aperturae pelvis inferioris 124
– diagonalis (conjugata diagonalis) 124
– mediana 79
– obliqua = Oblique diameter of pelvic inlet 79
Diameter pelvis = Pelvic diameter 79, 124
– transversa = Transverse diameter of pelvic inlet 79
Diaphragma = Diaphragm 160, 163
– oris = Oral diaphragm 172
– pelvis = Pelvic diaphragm 164, 165
– urogenitale = Urogenital diaphragm 164, 165
Diploe 10, 43
Discus articularis articulationis radioulnaris distalis = Articular disk of distal radioulnar articulation (joint) 112, 113, 115
– – – sternoclavicularis = Articular disk of sternoclavicular articulation (joint) 108, 174
– – – temporomandibularis = Articular disk of temporomandibular articulation (joint) 186
– interpubicus = Interpubic disk 118, 124
– intervertebralis = Intervertebral disk 96–98, 101
Dorsum sellae (turcicae) 35, 39, 46, 105
Ductus parotideus = Parotid, duct (*Stenon's* duct) 169, 178, 183, 185

E

Eminentia arcuata ossis temporalis = Arcuate eminence of temporal bone 35, 47–50
– iliopubica = Iliopectineal eminence 80, 82
– intercondylaris = Intercondylar eminence 86
– plantaris intermedia 254, 255
– – lateralis medialis 254, 255
– pyramidalis = Pyramidal eminence 49
Emissarium parietale = Parietal emissary 35
Epicondylus lateralis femoris = Lateral epicondyle of femur 84, 85
– – humeri = Lateral epicondyle of humerus 68, 112
– medialis femoris = Medial epicondyle of femur 68, 84, 85
– – humeri = Medial epicondyle of humerus 8, 112
Extremitas acromialis claviculae = Acromial extremity of clavicle 67
– sternalis claviculae = Sternal extremity of clavicle 67
– – costae = Sternal extremity of rib 22

F

Facies = Facies (also facet or surface)
– anterior lateralis humeri = Anterolateral surface of humerus 68
– – medialis humeri = Anteromedial surface of humerus 68
– – partis petrosae = Anterior surface of petrous part of temporal bone 48
– – radii = Anterior surface of radius 71
– – ulnae = Anterior surface of ulna 71
– articularis acromialis claviculae = Acromial articular facet of clavicle 67
– – acromii scapulae = Acromial articular facet of scapula 66, 111
– – anterior axis = Anterior articular facet of axis 16
– – calcanea anterior tali = Anterior calcaneal articular facet of talus 89
– – – media tali = Medial calcaneal articular facet of talus 89
– – posterior tali = Posterior calcaneal articular facet of talus 89
– – capitis costae = Superior costal facets 22
– – – fibulae = Articular facet of head of fibula 87
– – carpea radii = Carpal articular facet of radius 70, 112
– – cuboidea (calcanei) = Cuboid articular facet of calcaneus 90
– – fibularis tibiae = Fibular articular facet of tibia 86
– – inferior tibiae = Inferior articular facet of tibia 86, 87
– – – vertebrae = Inferior articular facets of vertebrae 19
– – malleolaris fibulae = Malleolar articular facet of fibula 87
– – – tibiae = Malleolar articular facet of tibia 86
– – navicularis tali = Navicular articular facet of talus 89
– – patellae = Articular facet of patella 85, 127, 128
– – posterior axis = Posterior articular facet of odontoid process of axis 16
– – sternalis claviculae = Sternal articular facet of clavicle 67
– – superior axis = Superior articular faiet of axis 16
– – – tibiae = Superior articular facet of tibia 86
– – – vertebrae = Superior articular facets of vertebrae 97
– – – talaris anterior calcanei = Anterior articular facet for talus of calcaneus 90
– – – media calcanei = Middle articular facet for talus of calcaneus 90
– – – posterior calcanei = Posterior articular facet for talus of calcaneus 90
Facies articularis tuberculic ostae = Articular facet of tubercle of rib 22
– auricularis ossis ilii = Auricular surface of ilium 82, 83
– – – sacri = Auricular surface of sacrum 20, 21
– cerebralis alae majoris ossis sphenoidalis = Cerebral surface of greater wings of sphenoid bone 46
– – partis squamosae ossis temporalis = Cerebral surface of squamous part of temporal bone 47
– costalis scapulae = Costal surface of scapula 66
– dorsalis ossis sacri = Dorsal surface of sacrum 20
– – scapulae = Dorsal surface of scapula 66
– inferior partis petrosae = Inferior surface of petrous part of temporal bone 48
– infratemporalis maxillae = Infratemporal surface of maxilla 57
– lateralis fibulae = Lateral surface of fibula 87
– – radii = Lateral surface of radius 71
– – tibiae = Lateral surface of tibia 86
– lunata (acetabuli) = Articular surface of hip bone 81, 82, 125
– malleolaris lateralis trochleae tali = Malleolar facet of lateral surface of talus 89
– maxillaris laminae perpendicularis ossis palatini = Maxillar surface of perpendicular plate of palatine bone 56
– – – – – sphenoidalis = Maxillar surface of perpendicular plate of sphenoid bone 46
medialis fibulae = Medial surface of fibula 87
– – tibiae = Medial surface of tibia 86
– – ulnae = Medial surface of ulna 71
– nasalis maxillae = Nasal surface of maxilla 57
– orbitalis alae majoris ossis sphenoidalis = Orbital surface of greater wing of sphenoid bone 31, 46, 61
– – maxillae = Orbital surface of maxilla 57
– orbitalis partis orbitalis ossis frontalis = Orbital surface of orbital part of frontal bone 51, 52
– – ossis sphenoidalis = Orbital surface of sphenoid bone 54
– – – zygomatici = Orbital surface of zygomatic bone 61
– patellaris femoris = Patellar surface of femur 84, 85, 127
– pelvina ossis sacri = Pelvis surface of sacrum 21
– poplitea femoris = Popliteal surface of femur 84
– posterior fibulae = Posterior surface of fibula 87

Facies posterior humeri = Posterior surface of humerus 68
– – partis petrosae = Posterior surface of petrous parts of temporal bone 39
– – tibiae = Posterior surface of tibia 86
– – ulnae = Posterior surface of ulna 71
– symphysialis ossis pubis = Symphyseal surface of pubic bone 82, 83
– temporalis alae majoris = Temporal surface of greater wing of sphenoid bone 46
Falx inguinalis = Inguinal falx 160
Fascia antebrachii = Antebrachial fascia 190, 196, 199, 202, 213
– axillaris = Axillary fascia 190
– brachii = Brachial fascia 154, 190, 199
– cervicalis = Cervical fascia 173
– –, lamina superficialis = Superficial lamina of cervical fascia 168, 173
– –, – praetrachealis = Pretracheal lamina of cervical fascia 173, 174
– clavipectoralis = Clavipectoral fascia 154, 174
– cruris = Crural fascia 227, 244, 248
– diaphragmatis pelvis inferior = Inferior fascia of pelvic diaphragm 165
– – urogenitalis inferior = Inferior fascia of urogenital diaphragm 165
– infraspinata = Infraspinous fasciia 192
– lata 226
– obturatoria = Obturator fascia 164, 165
– pectinea = Pectineal fascia 226
– temporalis = Temporal fascia 183
– thoracolumbalis = Thoracolumbar fascia 141, 142, 144, 148, 152, 153
– transversalis = Transverse fascia 153, 161
Fasciculi mamillotendinei (musculorum dorsi) 146
– transversi aponeurosis palmaris = Superficial transverse ligaments of palm 213
Femur = Thigh bone 10, 84, 85, 125
Fenestra cochleae = Round window 49
– vestibuli = Oval window 48–50
Fibrae intercrurales = Intercrural fibers of inguinal canal 154, 159, 162
Fibrocartilago basalis = Basilar fibrocartilage 188
Fibula 87, 128, 241
Fissura orbitalis inferior = Inferior orbital fissure 31, 37, 61
– – superior = Superior orbital fissure (anterior lacerate foramen) 31, 39, 45, 46, 51, 61
– petrooccipitalis = Petrooccipital fissure 39
– petrosquamosa = Petrosquamous fissure 39, 48
Fissura petrotympanica ossis temporalis = Petrotympanic fissure of temporalbone 47, 48, 50
– sphenopetrosa = Sphenopetrosal fissure 39
– tympanomastoidea = Tympanomastoid fissure 47, 50
Fonticulus = Fontanelle
– anterior = Anterior fontanelle 40
– anterolateralis = Anterolateral fontanelle 40
– posterior = Posterior fontanelle 40
– posterolateralis = Posterolateral fontanelle 40
Foramen (-ina)
– (-ina) alveolaria maxillae = Dental foramina of maxilla 57, 63
– caecum ossis frontalis = Foramen cecum of frontal bone 35, 39, 52
– costotransversarium = Costotransverse foramen 16, 17
– ethmoidale anterius ossis frontalis = Anterior ethmoidal foramen of frontal bone 51, 61
– – posterius ossis frontalis = Posterior ethmoidal foramen of frontal bone 51, 61, 62
– incisivum = Incisive foramen 35, 37, 58
– infraorbitale = Infraorbital foramen 31, 57
– infrapiriforme 230, 236, 237
– intervertebrale = Intervertebral foramen 15, 98
– ischiadicum majus = Greater sciatic foramen 120, 122, 237
– – minus = Lesser sciatic foramen 120, 122, 237
– jugulare = Jugular foramen (or: posterior lacerate f.) 37, 39, 188
– lacerum = Middle lacerate foramen 37, 39
– magnum 37, 39, 44, 45
– mandibulae = Mandibular foramen 60, 172
– mastoideum = Mastoid foramen 35, 37, 39, 47, 48
– mentale = Mental foramen 31, 39, 59, 172, 178
– obturatum = Obturator foramen 81–83
– ovale ossis sphenoidalis = Oval foramen of sphenoid bone 37, 39, 45, 63
– palatinum majus = Greater palatine foramen 37, 56, 58
– (-ina) palatina minora = Lesser palatine foramina 58
– parietale = Parietal foramen 41, 42, 53
– rotundum 39, 45, 46, 62
– (-ina) sacralia dorsalia = Posterior sacral foramina 20
– (-ina) – pelvina = Anterior sacral foramina 20
Foramen sphenopalatinum = Sphenopalatine foramen 62, 63
– spinosum ossis sphenoidalis = Spinous foramen of sphenoid bone 37, 39, 45
– stylomastoideum = Stylomastoid foramen 37, 48, 49
– supraorbitale = Supraorbital foramen 31, 52
– suprapiriforme = Suprapiriform foramen 230, 236, 237
– transversarium = Transverse foramen 14, 16, 17
– v. cavae = Vena caval foramen 160, 163, 166
– vertebrale = Vertebral foramen 16, 17, 19, 102
– zygomaticofaciale = Zygomaticofacial foramen 54, 61, 63
– zygomaticoorbitale = Zygomaticoorbital foramen 54, 62
– zygomaticotemporale = Zygomaticotemporal foramen 54
Fossa acetabuli = Acetabular fossa 80–82, 125, 165
– axillaris = Axillary fossa 2
– canina = Canine fossa 57
– condylaris ossis occipitalis = Condylar fossa of occipital bone 44
– coronoidea humeri = Coronoid fossa of humerus 68, 113
– cranii anterior = Anterior cranial fossa 39
– – media = Middle cranial fossa 39
– – posterior = Posterior cranial fossa 39
– digastrica mandibulae = Digastric fossa of mandible 60, 172
– glandulae lacrimalis = Fossa for lacrimal gland 55
– hypophysialis = Hypophyseal fossa 39, 45, 51, 187
– iliaca = Iliac fossa 82, 83
– infraclavicularis = Infraclavicular fossa 168
– infraspinata = Infraspinous fossa 66
– infratemporalis = Infratemporal fossa 63
– intercondylaris = Intercondylar fossa of femur 84, 85
– jugularis = Jugular fossa 4, 37, 48, 168
– malleoli lateralis = Fossa of lateral malleolus 87
– mandibularis ossis temporalis = Mandibular fossa of temporal bone 37, 47, 48
– occipitalis cerebellaris = Cerebellar fossa of occipital bone 45
– – inferior = Inferior occipital fossa 44
– – superior = Superior occipital fossa 44
– olecrani = Olecranon fossa 8, 68, 113
– poplitea = Popliteal fossa 3, 226, 227, 236, 244

Fossa pterygoidea = Pterygoid fossa of sphenoid bone 35, 46
– pterygopalatina = Pterygopalatine fossa 62, 63
– radialis humeri = Radial fossa of humerus 68
– scaphoidea ossis sphenoidalis = Scaphoid fossa of sphenoid bone 46
– subarcuata ossis temporalis = Subarcuate fossa of temporal bone 39, 47, 48
– supraclavicularis major = Greater supraclavicular fossa 168, 173
– – minor = Lesser supraclavicular fossa 4, 168, 173
– supraspinata = Supraspinous fossa 66
– temporalis = Temporal fossa 32, 33
– trochanterica = Trochanteric fossa 84, 85
Fossula petrosa = Petrosal fossula 37, 48
Fovea = Fovea (also facet)
– articularis inferior atlantis = Inferior articular facet of atlas 16
– – superior atlantis = Superior articular facet of atlas 16
– capitis femoris = Fovea of head of femur 84, 85
– – radii = Fovea of head of radius 70
– costalis inferior vertebrae = Inferior costal facet of vertebrae 18
– – superior vertebrae = Superior costal facet of vertebrae 18, 19
– – transversalis = Transverse costal facet 18, 19
– dentis atlantis = Dental facet of atlas 16
– pterygoidea proc. condylaris, mandibulae = Pterygoid facet of condylar process of mandible (scaphoid fossa) 59
– sublingualis = Sublingual fossa 60
– submandibularis = Submandibular fossa 60
– trochlearis ossis frontalis = Trochlear fossa of frontal bone 51
Foveola radialis 216
Foveolae ethmoidales ossis frontalis 51
– granulares = Granular pits 43, 52
Funiculus spermaticus = Spermatic cord 154, 158, 226

G

Galea aponeurotica = Tendinous galea 178, 181, 183, 185
Glabella 51, 52
Glandula(e) palatina(e) = Palatine gland(s) 187
– parotis = Parotid gland 169, 174, 175, 178, 183
– – accessoria = Accessory parotid gland 169, 183
– sublingualis = Sublingual gland 187
Glandula(e) submandibularis = Submandibular gland 169, 174, 175, 183
– thyroidea = Thyroid gland 169, 174

H

Hamulus = Hamulus (also hook)
Hamulus ossis hamati = Hook of hamate bone 73, 74, 115
– pterygoideus = Pterygoid hamulus 35, 37, 46, 62, 63, 105, 187, 188
Head (Muscles) 168–188
Helix 173
Hernia femoralis = Femoral hernia 233
Hiatus aorticus diaphragmatis = Aortic hiatus of diaphragm 163, 166
– canalis n. petrosi majoris = Hiatus of facial canal for greater petrosal nerve 48
– maxillaris = Maxillary hiatus 63
– (o)esophageus = Esophageal hiatus 166
– sacralis = Sacral hiatus 20, 21
– saphenus = Saphenous hiatus 226
– scalenus = Scalene hiatus 174–176
– tendineus adductorius = Tendinous hiatus (adductorius) 232, 234, 239
– urogenitalis et ani 164
Humerus 8, 11, 67, 68, 71, 198
Hypothenar = Hypothenar eminence 219

I

Impressio lig. costoclavicularis = Impression of costoclavicular ligament 67
– (nes) digitatae = Digitate impressions 35, 39, 49
Incisura = Incisure (also notch)
– acetabuli = Acetabular notch 81
– clavicularis sterni = Clavicular notch of sternum 24
– costalis = Costal notch 24
– ethmoidalis ossis frontalis = Ethmoid notch of frontal bone 51
– fibularis tibiae = Fibular notch of tibia 86
– frontalis ossis frontalis = Frontal notch of frontal bone 52
– ischiadica major = Greater sciatic notch 81, 83
– – minor = Lesser sciatic notch 81, 83
– jugularis ossis occipitalis = Jugular notch of occipital bone 45
– – sterni = Jugular notch of sternum 24
– lacrimalis maxillae = Lacrimal notch of maxilla 57
– mandibulae = Mandibular notch 59, 60
– mastoidea ossis temporalis = Mastoid notch of temporal bone 37, 42, 47, 48
– nasalis maxillae = Nasal notch of maxilla 57
Incisura parietalis ossis temporalis = Parietal notch of temporal bone 47, 48
– poplitea extensoria femoris 85
– – flexoria femoris 85
– pterygoidea = Pterygoid notch 46
– radialis ulnae = Radial notch of ulna 69
– scapulae = Scapular notch 66
– sphenopalatina ossis palatini = Sphenopalatine notch of palatine bone 56, 57
– supraorbitalis ossis frontalis = Supraorbital notch of frontal bone 51, 55
– trochlearis ulnae = Trochlear notch of ulna 69, 70
– ulnaris radii = Ulnar notch of radius 70
– vertebralis inferior = Inferior vertebral notch 18
Inclinatio pelvis = Pelvic incline 78, 79, 124
Incus = Anvil 49
Intersectiones (inscriptiones) tendineae m. recti abdom. = Tendinous intersections of rectus abdominis muscle 156, 158, 160

J

Joint (s) (Syndesmology) or articulation (s) 93–137
Juga = Ridges
– alveolaria mandibulae = Alveolar ridges of mandible 59
– – maxillae = Alveolar ridges of maxilla 57
– cerebralia = Cerebral ridges of cranium 39, 49

L

Labium = Lip
– externum cristae iliacae = External lip of iliac crest 82
– internum cristae iliacae = Internal lip of iliac crest 81–83
– laterale lineae asperae femoris = Lateral lip of linea aspera of femur 84, 85
– mediale lineae asperae femoris = Medial lip of linea aspera of femur 84, 85
Labrum = Lip
– acetabulare = Acetabular lip 125
– glenoidale = Glenoid lip 111, 197
Labyrinthus ethmoidalis = Ethmoidal labyrinth 54, 55, 61, 63
Lacertus fibrosus 198, 199
Lacuna musculorum 233
– vasorum 233
Lamina = Lamina (also layer or plate)
– cribrosa ossis ethmoidalis = Cribriform plate of ethmoid bone 35, 39, 54, 55, 63

Lamina externa = Outer table of bones of skull 10, 43
– horizontalis ossis palatini = Horizontal plate of palatine bone 37, 40, 55, 56, 58
– interna = Inner table of bones of skull 10, 43
– lateralis processus pterygoidei = Lateral plate of pterygoid process 35, 37, 46, 58, 62, 104, 105
– medialis processus pterygoidei = Medial plate of pterygoid process 35, 37, 46, 58, 63
– orbitalis ossis ethmoidalis = Orbital plate of ethmoid bone 54, 61, 62
– perpendicularis ossis ethmoidalis = Perpendicular plate of ethmoid bone 34, 54, 55, 61
– – – palatini = Perpendicular plate of palatine bone 56, 57, 63
– praetrachealis fasciae cervicalis = Pretracheal layer of cervical fascia 173
– superficialis fasciae cervicalis = Superficial layer of cervical fascia 173
– tragi (auris externae) 173
Ligamentum (a) = Ligament (s) 93–137
– (a) alaria (axis) = Alar ligaments of axis 95
– acromioclaviculare = Acromioclavicular ligament 109, 110, 111, 197
– anulare radii = anular ligament of radius 112
– anococcygeum = Anococcygeal ligament 165
– apicis dentis (axis) = Apical dental ligament of axis 95, 187
– arcuatum laterale (diaphragmatis) = Lateral arcuate ligament of diaphragm 163, 166
– – mediale (diaphragmatis) = Medial arcuate ligament of diaphragm 163
– – pubis = Arcuate ligament of pubis 118, 119, 122–124, 165
– auriculare anterius = Anterior auricular ligament 173
– – superius = Superior auricular ligament 173
– bifurcatum = Bifurcate ligament 132
– calcaneocuboideum dorsale = Dorsal calconeocuboid ligament 132, 133
– – (ligamenti bifurcati) = Calcaneocuboid ligament (part of bifurcate l.) 132
– – plantare = Plantar calcaneocuboid ligament 136, 137
– calcaneofibulare = Calcaneofibular ligament 130, 132, 134, 136
– calcaneonaviculare (lig. bifurcati) = Calcaneonavicular ligament (part of bifurcate l.) 132
Ligamentum calcaneonaviculare plantare = Plantar calcaneonavicular ligament 131, 133, 136, 137
– capitis costae intraarticulare = Intraarticular ligament of head of rib 98
– – – radiatum 97, 102
– – femoris = Ligament of head of femur 124, 125
– – fibulae anterius = Anterior ligament of head of fibula 127, 128, 241
– – – posterius = Posterior ligament of head of fibula 126
– carpi palmare (volare) 216, 218
– – radiale 220
– – radiatum = Radiate carpal ligament 115, 220
– – ulnare 220
– collaterale = Collateral ligament (finger) 114
– – fibulare = Collateral fibular ligament 126, 127, 129, 242, 243
– – carpi radiale = Radial carpal collateral ligament 113
– – radiale = Radial collateral ligament 112
– (a) collateralia (artic. interphal. manus) = Collateral ligaments of interphalangeal articulations 114
– – (– metacarpophalangeae) = Collateral ligaments of metacarpophalangeal articulations 114, 115
– conoideum (lig. coracoclavicularis) = Conoid ligament (part of coracoclavicular l.) 108, 109, 111, 197, 198
– coracoacromiale = Coracoacronial ligament 109, 110, 111, 197
– coracoclaviculare = Coracoclavicular ligament 109, 110, 197
– coracohumerale = Coracohumeral ligament 109, 110, 197
– costotransversarium = Costotransverse ligament 97–100, 102, 148, 152
– – laterale = Lateral costotransverse ligament 97–99, 102, 152
– – superius = Superior costotransverse ligament 97–99, 102, 148
– (a) costoxiphoidea = Costoxiphoid ligaments 154
– cricothyroideum = Cricothyroid ligament 174
– cruciatum anterius (art. genus) = Anterior cruciate ligament of knee 127
– – posterius (art. genus) – Posterior cruciate ligament of knee 127
– cruciforme atlantis = Cruciform ligament of atlas 95
– – (cruris) = Cruciform ligament (cruris) 240, 241
– (a) cuneonaviculare (ia) dorsale (ia) = Dorsal cuneonavicular ligaments 132, 133
– (a) cuneonaviculare (ia) plantare (ia) = Plantar cuneonavicular ligaments 136
Ligamentum deltoideum = Deltoid ligament 130, 131, 134
– flavum = Flaval ligament (yellow l.) 98–100, 102
– fundiforme penis = Fundiform ligament of penis 154, 162
– (a) glenohumerale (ia) = Glenohumeral ligaments 109
– iliofemorale = Iliofemoral ligament 118–121, 125, 166
– iliolumbale = Iliolumbal ligament 118–121, 123, 166
– inguinale = Inguinal ligament 118–122, 156, 159, 160, 166, 226, 228, 232
– (a) intercarpeum (a) dorsale (ia) = Dorsal intercarpal ligaments 114
– interclaviculare = Interclavicular ligament 108, 169
– (a) intercuneiforme (ia) dorsale (ia) = Dorsal intercuneiform ligaments 133
– interfoveolare = Interfoveolar ligament 160
– interspinale = Interspinal ligament 98, 148
– intertransversarium = Intertransverse ligament 97, 99, 148
– ischiofemorale = Ischiofemoral ligament 80–83, 125, 230
– lacunare = Lacunar ligament 121, 228
– laterale (art. temporomandibularis) = Lateral ligament of temporomandibular articulation 104, 183, 185
– longitudinale anterius (columnae vertebral.) = Anterior longitudinal ligament (vertebral column) 94, 97, 118–121, 166
– – posterius (columnae vertebral.) = Posterior longitudinal ligament (vertebral column) 101
– (a) metacarpeum (a) dorsale (ia) = Dorsal metacarpal ligaments 114
– – interosseum (a) = Interosseous metacarpal ligaments 113
– – palmarium (a) = Palmar metacarpal ligaments 115
– – transversum profundum = Deep transverse metacarpal ligament 115, 216, 220
– – – superficiale = Superficial transverse metacarpal ligament 213
– (a) metatarseum (a) dorsale (ia) = Dorsal metatarsal ligaments 132, 135–137
– – interosseum (a) = Interosseous metatarsal ligaments 135
– – plantare (ia) = Plantar metatarsal ligaments 137
– – transversum profundum = Deep transverse metatarsal ligament 132, 136, 137
– – – superficiale = Superficial transverse metatarsal ligament 136
– nuchae 142, 144, 146, 175

Ligamentum (a) palmarium (interphalang.) = Palmar ligaments 115
– (a) palmaria = Palmar ligaments 115
– palpebrale mediale = Medial palpebral ligament 169, 178, 183
– patellae = Patellar ligament 126–129, 232, 234, 238, 248
– (a) pelvis = Pelvic ligaments 118–124
– pisohamatum = Pisohamate ligament 115, 220
– pisometacarpeum = Pisometacarpal ligament 115
– plantare longum = Long plantar ligament 131, 132, 134, 136, 256
– (a) plantaria = Plantar ligaments 131, 132, 134, 136, 137
– popliteum arcuatum = Arcuate popliteal ligament 126, 244
– – obliquum = Oblique popliteal ligament 126, 244, 246
– pterygospinale = Pterygospinal ligament 105, 188
– pubicum superius = Superior pubic ligament 118–120
– pubofemorale = Pubofemoral ligament 125
– radiocarpeum dorsale = Dorsal radiocarpal ligament 114
– – palmare = Palmar radiocarpal ligament 115, 218, 220
– reflexum 154, 159, 162
– sacrococcygeum dorsale profundum = Deep dorsal sacrococcygeal ligament 122
– – – superficiale = Superficial dorsal sacrococcygeal ligament 122, 123
– – laterale = Lateral sacrococcygeal ligament 120, 124
– – ventrale = Ventral sacrococcygeal ligament 118, 120, 124, 164
– (a) sacroiliacum (a) dorsale (ia) = Dorsal sacroiliac ligaments 123, 124
– – interosseum (a) = Interosseous sacroiliac ligaments 124, 164
– – ventrale (ia) = Ventral sacroiliac ligaments 118–120, 124, 164
– sacrospinale = Sacrospinal ligament 122–124, 164, 166, 230, 232, 242
– sacrotuberale = Sacrotuberal ligament 122–124, 142, 164, 165, 166, 228, 230, 236
– sphenomandibulare = Sphenomandibular ligament 105, 187
– sternoclaviculare anterius = Anterior sternoclavicular ligament 108
– sternocostale intraarticulare = Intraarticular sternocostal ligament 103
– (a) – (ia) radiatum (a) = Radiate sternocostal ligaments 108
– stylohyoideum = Stylohyoid ligament 172, 173, 187, 188
– stylomandibulare = Stylomandibular ligament 104, 105, 187, 188
– supraspinale = Supraspinous ligament 99, 123
Ligamentum suspensorium penis = Suspensory ligament of penis 154
– talocalcaneum interosseum = Interosseous talocalcaneal ligament 133, 135
– – laterale = Lateral talocalcaneal ligament 132
– – mediale = Medial talocalcaneal ligament 130
– – posterius = Posterior talocalcaneal ligament 130
– talofibulare anterius = Anterior talofibular ligament 128, 132
– – posterius = Posterior talofibular ligament 130
– (a) tarsi interosseum (a) = Interosseous ligaments of tarsus 135
– (a) tarsi plantare (ia) = Plantar ligaments of tarsus 137
– (a) tarsometatarseum (a) dorsale (ia) = Dorsal tarsometatarsal ligaments 131–133
– tarsometatarseum interosseum = Interosseous tarsometatarsal ligaments 135
– – plantare = Plantar tarsometatarsal ligament 136, 137
– thyrohyoideum medianum = Median thyrohyoid ligament 174
– tibiofibulare anterius = Anterior tibiofibular ligament 128, 132
– – posterius = Posterior tibiofibular ligament 130
– transversum acetabuli = Transverse ligament of acetabulum 125, 165
– – atlantis = Transverse ligament of atlas 96
– – genus = Transverse ligament of knee 127
– – perinei = Transverse perineal ligament 165
– – scapulae = Transverse ligament of scapula 109, 110, 198
– trapezoideum (lig. coracoclavicularis) = Trapezoid ligament (part of coracoclavicular l.) 109, 111, 197, 198
– ulnocarpeum palmare = Palmar ulnocarpal ligament 115, 220
Linea alba 154, 159–162
– arcuata = Arcuate line 83, 158, 160
– – ossis ischii = Arcuate line of sciatic bone 83
– aspera femoris 84, 85, 239
– epiphyseos = Epiphyseal line 8, 71, 75, 76, 91
– glutaea anterior = Anterior gluteal line 81
– – inferior = Inferior gluteal line 81
– – posterior = Posterior gluteal line 81
– intercondylaris femoris = Intercondylar line of femur 84
– intermedia cristae iliacae = Intermediate line of iliac crest 81–83
– intertrochanterica = Intertrochanteric line 84, 85
– muscularis = Muscular line (of scapula) 66
Linea musculi solei 86
– mylohyoidea = Mylohyoid line 60, 172
– nuchae inferior = Inferior nuchal line 37, 42, 44
– – superior = Superior nuchal line 37, 42, 44
– – suprema = Supreme nuchal line 44
– obliqua mandibulae = Oblique line of mandible 59
– pectinea femoris = Pectineal line of femur 84, 85
– semilunaris = Semilunar line 158
– *spighelli* = Linea semilunaris 158
– temporalis inferior ossis parietalis = Inferior temporal line of parietal bone 41, 53
– – – – temporalis = Inferior temporal line of temporal bone 47
– – ossis frontalis = Temporal line of frontal bone 52
– – superior ossis parietalis = Superior temporal line of temporal bone 41, 53
– terminalis (pelvis) 20, 120, 164, 166
– (ae) transversae ossis sacri = Transverse lines of sacrum 20
– trapezoidea = Trapezoid line 67
Lingula mandibulae = Lingula of mandible 60, 105
– sphenoidalis = Lingula of sphenoid bone 45, 46
Lower limb (Joints and ligaments) 92, 118–137
– – (Muscles) 225–259
– – (Osteology) 84 92

M

Malleolus lateralis = Lateral malleolus 87, 128, 130, 134
– medialis = Medial malleolus 86, 87, 248
Malleus = (Hammer) 49
Mandibula = Mandible 31, 33, 40, 59, 60, 172
Manubrium sterni = Manubrium of sternum 24, 25, 103, 108, 160
Margo = Margin (also border or crest)
– anterior fibulae = Anterior crest of fibula 87
– – radii = Anterior border of radius 71
– – tibiae = Anterior border of tibia 86
– – ulnae = Anterior margin of ulna 71
– frontalis alae majoris ossis sphenoidalis = Frontal margin of greater wing of sphenoid bone 46
– – ossis parietalis = Frontal margin of parietal bone 53
– infraorbitalis = Infraorbital margin (of maxilla) 31, 54, 57
– interosseus fibulae = Interosseous border of fibula 87
– – radii = Interosseous border of radius 70, 71

Margo interosseus tibiae = Interosseous border of tibia 86
– – ulnae = Interosseous border of ulna 69, 71
– lacrimalis maxillae = Lacrimal border of maxilla 57
– lambdoideus ossis occipitalis = Lambdoid margin of occipital bone 44, 45
– lateralis humeri = Lateral border of humerus 68
– – scapulae = Lateral border of scapula 66
– mastoideus ossis occipitalis = Mastoid margin of occipital bone 44, 45
– medialis humeri = Medial border of humerus 68
– – scapulae = Medial (vertebral) border of scapula 66
– – tibiae = Medial border of tibia 86
– occipitalis ossis parietalis = Occipital margin of parietal bone 53
– – – temporalis = Occipital margin of temporal bone 47, 48
– parietalis alae majoris ossis sphenoidalis = Parietal margin of great wing of sphenoid bone 45, 46
– – ossis frontalis = Parietal margin of frontal bone 52
– – – temporalis = Parietal margin of temporal bone 47
– posterior fibulae = Posterior border of fibula 87
– – partis petrosae ossis temporalis = Posterior margin of petrosal part of temporal bone 47, 48
– – radii = Posterior border of radius 71
– – ulnae = Posterior margin of ulna 71
– sagittalis ossis parietalis = Sagittal margin of parietal bone 53
– sphenoidalis ossis frontalis = Sphenoidal margin of frontal bone 52
– – – temporalis = Sphenoidal margin of temporal bone 47, 48
– squamosus ossis parietalis = Squamous margin of parietal bone 53
– – alae majoris ossis sphenoidalis = Squamous margin of great wing of sphenoid bone 45, 46
– superior partis petrosae ossis temporalis = Superior margin of petrosal part of temporal bone 39, 47
– – scapulae = Superior border of scapula 66
– supraorbitalis = Supraorbital margin of frontal bone 31, 51, 52
– zygomaticus alae majoris ossis sphenoidalis = Zygomatic margin of great wing of sphenoid bone 46
Massa lateralis atlantis = Lateral mass of atlas 16
Maxilla 30–37, 57, 58, 61–63
Meatus acusticus externus = External acoustic meatus 33, 37, 47, 48, 50, 104
– – internus = Internal acoustic meatus 35, 39, 47
– nasi inferior = Inferior nasal meatus 61, 63
– – medius = Middle nasal meatus 63
– – superior = Superior nasal meatus 63
Medulla ossium = Bone marrow 8
Membrana atlantooccipitalis anterior = Anterior atlantooccipital membrane 94, 176, 187
– – posterior = Posterior atlanto-occipital membrane 94, 150, 187
– interossea antebrachii = Interosseous membrane of forearm 71, 112, 210, 211
– – cruris = Interosseous membrane of leg 128
– obturatoria = Obturator membrane 118, 119, 124, 125, 166
– tectoria = Tectorial membrane 94, 96
– tympani = Tympanic membrane 49
Meniscus lateralis art. genu 92, 127–129
– medialis art. genu 92, 127, 129
Mesotendineum 216
Metacarpus 72–76, 113–115
Metatarsus 88, 89, 91, 132–137
Mimetic musculature 178–185
Musculus (li) = Muscle (s) (see also sheath or tendon of m.)
– (i) abdominis = Abdominal musculature 154–160
– abductor digiti minimi (manus) = Abductor muscle of little finger 212, 215, 216, 219, 220, 223, 224
– – – – (pedis) = Abductor muscle of little toe 241, 251, 253, 254, 256, 257
– abductor hallucis = Abductor muscle of great toe 240, 251, 253, 254, 256, 257
– – pollicis brevis = Short abductor múscle of thumb 213, 215, 216, 218, 220, 221, 223, 224
– – – longus = Long abductor muscle of thumb 192, 199, 202, 204, 206, 208, 209, 211, 212, 214, 224
– adductor brevis = Short adductor muscle 230, 234, 235, 236, 242, 243
– – hallucis = Adductor muscle of great toe 251, 253, 254, 256, 257
– – longus = Long adductor muscle 228, 232, 234, 235, 242, 243
– – magnus = Great adductor muscle 228–230, 234, 236, 239, 242, 243
– – minimus = Smallest adductor muscle 230, 234, 236
– – pollicis = Adductor muscle of thumb 192, 215, 216, 218, 220, 221, 223, 224
– anconeus = Anconeus muscle 192, 194, 195, 200, 206, 208, 211
Musculus articularis cubiti = Articular muscle of elbow 201, 210, 211
– – genus = Articular muscle of knee 126, 242
– auricularis anterior = Anterior auricular muscle 169, 171, 181
– – posterior = Posterior auricular muscle 171
– – superior = Superior auricular muscle 173
– biceps brachii = Biceps muscle of arm 112, 141, 142, 196–198, 199, 201, 206, 210
– – femoris = Biceps muscle of thigh 229, 230, 236–239, 241–243, 248, 250
– brachialis = Brachial muscle 112, 141, 192, 194, 196–202, 210, 211
– brachioradialis = Brachioradial muscle 192, 194, 199–202, 204, 206, 207, 208, 210, 211, 224
– buccinator = Buccinator muscle 169, 178, 182, 183, 185, 187
– coccygeus = Coccygeal muscle 164, 165, 228, 242
– coracobrachialis = Coracobrachial muscle 162, 191, 196–198, 201
– corrugator supercilii = Superciliary corrugator muscle 178, 179, 183
– cremaster = Cremaster muscle 154, 156, 162
– cricothyroideus = Cricothyroid muscle 174
– deltoideus = Deltoid muscle 191–194, 196–198, 200, 201
– depressor anguli oris = Depressor muscle of angle of mouth 168, 169, 178, 181–183, 185
– – labii inferioris = Depressor muscle of lower lip 169, 178, 181–183, 185
– – septi = Depressor muscle of nasal septum 178, 180
– – supercilii = Superciliary depressor muscle 178, 179, 181–183
– digastricus = Digastric muscle 162, 169, 170, 172–176, 185, 187, 188
– (i) dorsi = Dorsal muscles 142–153
– epicranius = Epicranial muscle 169, 178, 181, 183, 185
– erector spinae = Erector muscle of spine 144, 146, 147, 152, 153
– extensor carpi radialis brevis = Short radial extensor muscle of wrist 192, 194, 200, 201, 206–208, 210–212
– – – – longus = Long radial extensor muscle of wrist 192, 194, 196, 200, 201, 206–208, 210 bis 212
– – – ulnaris = Ulnar extensor muscle of wrist 200, 206–208, 211, 212
– – digiti minimi = Extensor muscle of little finger 206–208, 211, 212, 214
– – digitorum (manus) = Extensor muscle of fingers 192, 200, 206, 207, 211, 212, 214

Musculus extensor digitorum brevis (pedis) = Short extensor muscle of toes 241, 248, 252, 253, 259
– – – longus (pedis) = Long extensor muscle of toes 92, 241, 242, 248–250, 252, 253, 259
– – hallucis brevis = Short extensor muscle of great toe 248, 252, 253, 259
– – – longus = Long extensor muscle of great toe 92, 240, 241, 248 bis 250, 253, 259
– – indicis = Extensor muscle of index finger 208, 209, 211, 212, 214, 223
– – pollicis brevis = Short extensor muscle of thumb 192, 199, 206, 208, 209, 211, 212, 214
– extensor pollicis longus = Long extensor muscle of thumb 192, 206, 208, 209, 211, 212, 214, 223
– flexor carpi radialis = Radial flexor muscle of wrist 192, 198, 199, 201 bis 204, 210, 224
– – – ulnaris = Ulnar flexor muscle of wrist 199, 201–204, 206, 208, 210, 211, 216, 224
– – digiti minimi brevis (manus) = Short flexor muscle of little finger 216, 218–220, 223, 224
– – – – (pedis) = Short flexor muscle of little toe 251, 254, 256, 257
– – digitorum brevis (pedis) = Short flexor muscle of toes 251, 254–256
– – – longus (pedis) = Long flexor muscle of toes 92, 240, 243, 244, 246, 247, 250, 251, 256
– – – profundus = Deep flexor muscle of fingers 201, 204, 205, 210, 211, 220, 224
– – – superficialis = Superficial flexor muscle of fingers 199, 201–204, 210, 216, 224
– – hallucis brevis = Short flexor muscle of great toe 251, 254, 256, 257
– – – longus = Long flexor muscle of great toe 92, 240, 246, 247, 250, 251, 254, 256, 259
– – pollicis brevis = Short flexor muscle of thumb 216, 218, 220, 221, 223, 224
– – – longus = Long flexor muscle of thumb 192, 199, 202, 204, 205, 210
– gastrocnemius = Gastrocnemius muscle 229, 236, 239–241, 243–245, 248
– gemellus inferior = Inferior gemellus muscle 142, 230, 231, 236, 243
– – superior = Superior gemellus muscle 142, 230, 231, 236, 243
– genioglossus = Genioglossus muscle 172, 187, 188
– geniohyoideus = Geniohyoid muscle 170, 172, 187, 188
Musculus glutaeus maximus = Greatest gluteal muscle 141, 142, 228–231, 236, 238, 242, 243
– – medius = Middle gluteal muscle 142, 230, 231, 236, 243
– – minimus = Least gluteal muscle 230, 231, 236, 242, 243
– gracilis = Gracilis muscle 228–230, 232, 234–236, 242, 243, 250
– helicis major = Larger muscle of helix 173
– – minor = Smoller muscle of helix 173
– hyoglossus = Hyoglossus muscle 162, 187
– iliacus = Iliac muscle 166, 228, 232, 242
– iliocostalis cervicis = Iliocastal muscle of neck 146, 147, 175
– lumborum = Iliocostal muscle of loin 146
– – thoracis = Iliocostal muscle of thorax 144, 146, 147, 152
– iliopsoas = Iliopsoas muscle 166, 228, 232, 234, 242, 243
– (i) infrahyoidei = Infrahyoid musculature 169, 171, 174, 175
– infraspinatus = Infraspinous muscle 110, 141, 142, 144, 191, 193, 194, 197, 200
– intercostalis cervicis = Cervical intercostal muscle 176
– (i) intercostales externi = External intercostal muscles 146, 148, 152, 156, 158, 162, 166, 174
– – interni = Internal intercostal muscles 148, 150, 152, 156, 158, 160, 166
– – intimi = Innermost intercostal muscles 148, 152
– interossei dorsales (manus) = Dorsal interosseous muscles of hand 192, 208, 212–214, 216, 218, 222–224
– – – (pedis) = Dorsal interosseous muscles of foot 251–253, 258
– – palmares = Palmar interosseous muscles 216, 218, 220, 222–224
– – plantares = Plantar interosseous muscles 251, 253, 256, 258
– interspinales cervicis = Interspinal muscles of neck 148, 150
– – lumborum = Interspinal muscles of loin 148
– intertransversarii anteriores cervicis= Anterior intertransverse muscles of neck 176
– – laterales lumborum = Lateral intertransverse muscles of loin 148, 152
– – mediales lumborum = Medial intertransverse muscles of loin 148, 152
– – posteriores cervicis = Posterior intertransverse muscles of neck 148, 150
– – thoracis = Intertransverse muscles of thorax 148, 152
Musculus latissimus dorsi = Latissimus-muscle of back 141–144, 153, 162, 191, 198, 200, 201
– levator anguli oris = Levator muscle of angle of mouth 169, 178, 182, 183
– – ani = Levator ani muscle 164, 165, 243
– (i) levatores costarum = Levator muscles of ribs 146, 148, 150, 152
– – – breves = Short levator muscles of ribs 148, 152
– – – longi = Long levator muscles of ribs 148, 152
– levator labii superioris = Levator muscle of upper lip 169, 178, 181–183
– – – – alaeque nasi = Levator muscle of upper lip and ala of nose 178, 181–183
– – scapulae = Levator muscle of scapula 141–144, 146, 162, 169, 176, 192, 198, 200
– – veli palatini = Levator muscle of velum palatini 187, 188
– longissimus capitis = Longissimus muscle of head 146–148, 175, 176, 188
– – cervicis = Longissimus muscle of neck 146–148, 175
– – thoracis = Longissimus muscle of thorax 144, 146, 147, 152
– longus capitis = Long muscle of head 176, 177, 188
– – colli = Long muscle of neck 166, 176, 177
– (i) lumbricales (manus) = Lumbrical muscles of hand 215–218, 223
– – (pedis) = Lumbrical muscles of foot 254, 256
– masseter = Masseter muscle 183–185, 188
– mentalis = Chin muscle 169, 178, 181–183, 185
– (i) multifidi = Multifidus muscles 148–150, 152
– mylohyoideus = Mylohyoid muscle 162, 169, 170, 172–174, 187, 188
– nasalis = Nasal muscle 169, 178, 180, 181, 183, 185
– obliquus capitis inferior = Inferior oblique muscle of head 148, 150, 151
– – – superior = Superior oblique muscle of head 148, 150, 151, 188
– – externus abdominis = External oblique muscle of abdomen 141, 142, 144, 153–162, 243
– – internus abdominis = Internal oblique muscle of abdomen 146, 148, 156–158, 160–162, 242
– obturatorius externus = External obturator muscle 230, 235, 236, 242, 243
– – internus = Internal obturator muscle 165, 228, 230, 231, 236, 242, 243
– occipitofrontalis = Occipitofrontal muscle 169, 178, 180, 181, 183, 185

Musculus omohyoideus = Omohyoid muscle 141, 162, 169, 171, 173–175, 200, 201
– opponens digiti minimi (manus) = Opposing muscle of little finger 215, 218–220, 223, 224
– – – – (pedis) = Opposing muscle of little toe 241, 256, 257
– – pollicis = Opposing muscle of thumb 215, 216, 218, 220, 221, 223, 224
– orbicularis oculi = Orbicular muscle of eye 169, 178, 179, 181, 183, 185
– – oris = Orbicular muscle of mouth 169, 178, 181–183, 187
– palmaris brevis = Short palmar muscle 199, 213, 223
– – longus = Long palmar muscle 199, 203, 213, 216
– pectineus = Pectineal muscle 232, 234, 235, 242, 243
– pectoralis major = Greater pectoral muscle 141, 154, 162, 169, 174, 191, 192, 197, 198, 200, 201
– – minor = Smaller pectoral muscle 162, 191, 192, 197, 198, 201
– peroneus (fibularis) brevis = Short peroneal (fibular) muscle 92, 132, 241, 246, 248–250, 253
– – – longus = Long peroneal (fibular) muscle 92, 241, 242, 244, 246, 248–251, 256
– – – tertius = Third peroneal muscle 241, 248, 249, 252, 253, 259
– piriformis = Piriform muscle 142, 228, 230–232, 236, 242, 243
– plantaris = Plantar muscle 229, 238, 239, 241, 243–245
– popliteus = Popliteal muscle 126, 129, 243, 245, 246, 250
– procerus = Procerus muscle 178, 179, 183
– pronator quadratus = Quadrate pronator muscle 199, 202, 204, 210, 218, 220
– – teres = Round pronator muscle 192, 198, 199, 201–204, 210, 211
– psoas major = Greater psoas muscle 153, 166, 228, 232, 242
– psoas minor = Smaller psoas muscle 166, 228
– pterygoideus lateralis = Lateral pterygoid muscle 184, 186–188
– – medialis = Medial pterygoid muscle 184, 186–188
– pyramidalis = Pyramidal muscle 156, 158, 159
– quadratus femoris = Quadrate muscle of thigh 142, 230, 231, 236, 242, 243
– – lumborum = Quadrate muscle of loin 153, 163, 164, 166, 242
– – plantae (flexor accessorius) = Quadrate muscle of sole 251, 255, 256
– quadriceps femoris = Quadriceps muscle of thigh 232–234, 242, 250
Musculus rectococcygeus = Rectococcygeal muscle 164
– rectus abdominis = Straight muscle of abdomen 156, 158–161
– – capitis anterior = Anterior straight muscle of head 176, 177, 188
– – – lateralis = Lateral straight muscle of head 150, 151, 176, 188
– – – posterior major = Greater posterior straight muscle of head 148, 150, 151, 188
– – – – minor = Smaller posterior straight muscle of head 148, 150, 151, 188
– – femoris = Straight muscle of thigh 125, 232–234, 242, 243
– rhomboideus major = Greater rhomboid muscle 142–144, 198, 200
– – minor = Lesser rhomboid muscle 142–144, 198, 200
– risorius = Risorius muscle 168, 178, 181–183
– (i) rotatores = Rotator muscles 148, 149, 152
– – breves = Short rotator muscles 148, 149, 152
– – longi = Long rotator muscles 148, 149, 152
– – thoracis = Rotator muscles of thorax 148, 149, 152
– sacrococcygeus ventralis = Ventral sacrococcygeal muscle 164, 228
– sartorius = Sartorius muscle 141, 228, 229, 232, 233, 240, 242, 243, 250
– scalenus anterior = Anterior scalene muscle 162, 165, 169, 175–177
– – medius = Middle scalene muscle 141, 144, 150, 166, 168, 169, 175–177, 192
– – posterior = Posterior scalene muscle 141, 144, 146, 148, 150, 162, 166, 176, 177, 192
– semimembranosus = Semimembranous muscle 229, 230, 236, 237, 239, 240, 242–244, 250
– semispinalis capitis = Semispinal muscle of head 142, 144, 146, 148, 150, 169, 175, 185, 188
– – cervicis = Semispinal muscle of neck 146, 148, 150, 175
– – thoracis = Semispinal muscle of thorax 148, 152
– semitendinosus = Semitendinous muscle 228–230, 236, 237, 240, 242–244, 250
– serratus anterior = Anterior serratus muscle 141, 154–156, 162, 191, 192, 198, 201
– – posterior inferior = Inferior posterior serratus muscle 144–146
– – – superior = Superior posterior serratus muscle 142, 144, 145
– soleus = Soleus muscle 240, 241, 243–246, 248
Musculus sphincter ani externus = External sphincter muscle of anus 65
– spinalis thoracis = Spinal muscle of thorax 144, 146, 147, 152
– splenius capitis = Splenius muscle of head 142, 144–146, 148, 150, 162, 175, 181, 185, 188
– – cervicis = Splenius muscle of neck 142, 144–146, 169, 175, 176, 192
– sternocleidomastoideus = Sternocleidomastoid muscle 141, 142, 154, 169, 171, 173, 174, 181, 183, 188, 192
– sternohyoideus = Sternohyoid muscle 162, 169, 171, 173–175, 185, 192, 200
– sternothyroideus = Sternothyroid muscle 160, 162, 169, 171, 174, 175, 185
– styloglossus = Styloglossus muscle 185, 187, 188
– stylohyoideus = Stylohyoid muscle 162, 169, 170, 172–175, 185, 187, 188, 200
– stylopharyngeus = Stylopharyngeal muscle 187, 188
– subclavius = Subclavius muscle 162, 174, 197, 198, 200, 201
– (i) subcostales = Subcostal muscles 166
– subscapularis = Subscapular muscle 162, 191, 193, 198, 201
– supinator = Supinator muscle 199, 201, 204, 208–211
– (i) suprahyoidei = Suprahyoid musculature 170, 172, 174, 188
– supraspinatus 110, 142, 144, 191, 193, 197, 198, 200, 201
– temporalis = Temporal muscle 184, 185, 188
– temporoparietalis = Temporoparietal muscle 169, 178, 180, 181, 183
– tensor fasciae latae = Tensor muscle of fascia lata 141, 226, 231, 232, 236, 238, 243
– – veli palatini = Tensor muscle of velum palatini 187, 188
– teres major = Teres major muscle 141, 142, 144, 191–194, 196, 198, 200, 201
– – minor = Teres minor muscle 141, 142, 144, 191–194, 197, 200
– thyrohyoideus = Thyrohyoid muscle 162, 169, 171, 174, 185
– tibialis anterior = Anterior tibial muscle 92, 131, 240–242, 248–251
– – posterior = Posterior tibial muscle 92, 131, 137, 243, 246, 247, 250, 251
– tragicus 173
– transversus abdominis = Transverse muscle of abdomen 148, 153, 157, 158, 160, 161, 166, 242
– – perinei profundus = Deep transverse muscle of perineum 165, 243
– – – superficialis = Superficial transverse muscle of perineum 165

Musculus transversus thoracis = Transverse muscle of thorax 160
– trapezius = Trapezius muscle 141 bis 144, 169, 188, 192, 200, 201
– triceps brachii = Triceps muscle of arm 110, 111, 141, 142, 191, 192, 194–198, 200, 201, 211
– vastus intermedius = Intermediate great muscle 233, 234, 242, 243
– – lateralis = Lateral great muscle 232–234, 238, 242, 243
– – medialis = Medial great muscle 232–234, 240, 242, 243
– zygomaticus major = Greater zygomatic muscle 169, 178, 181–183, 188
– – minor = Smaller zygomatic muscle 169, 178, 181–183, 188
Myology 139–259

N

Nares = Nostrils 4
Neck (Muscles) 141–151, 162, 168–177
Nervus auricularis magnus = Great auricular nerve 168
– facialis = Facial nerve 179
– glutaeus inferior = Inferior gluteal nerve 230
– ischiadicus = Sciatic nerve 142, 230
– medianus = Median nerve 199, 216, 223
– musculocutaneus = Musculocutaneous nerve 196, 197
– peroneus communis = Common peroneal nerve 229, 241
– tibialis = Tibial nerve 229
– ulnaris = Ulnar nerve 199, 216
– vagus = Vagus nerve 185
Nuchal musculature 150, 151
Nucleus pulposus = Pulpy nucleus 98

O

Olecranon ulnae 69–71, 192, 194
Orbita 61, 62
Os (sa) = Bone (s)
– capitatum = Capitate bone 72–76, 113–115
– (sa) carpi = Carpal bones 72–76, 113–115
– coccygis = Coccygeal bone 15, 21, 25, 165
– coxae = Hip bone 25, 80–83
– cuboideum = Cuboid bone 88–91, 135
– cuneiforme intermedium = Intermediate cuneiform bone 88–91
– – laterale = Lateral cuneiform bone 88–91
– – mediale = Medial cuneiform bone 88–91
– ethmoidale = Ethmoid bone 35, 54, 55, 61–63
– frontale = Frontal bone 30–35, 39, 51, 52, 55, 61, 62
Os hamatum = Hamate bone 72–76, 113, 114
– hyoideum = Hyoid bone 60, 162, 169, 172, 174, 185, 187
– ilium = Ilium 25, 80–83, 164
– incisivum = Incisive bone 40
– interparietale = Interparietal bone 42
– ischii = Ischium 25, 80–83
– lacrimale = Lacrimal bone 30–33, 61, 62
– lunatum = Lunate bone 72–76, 113, 115
– (sa) manus = Bones of hand 72–76
– (sa) metacarpalia = Metacarpal bones 72–76, 113–115
– (sa) metatarsalia = Metatarsal bones 88–91
– nasale = Nasal bone 30–35, 61, 62
– naviculare = Navicular bone 88–91, 135
– occipitale = Occipital bone 33–42, 44, 45
– palatinum = Palatine bone 35, 56–58
– parietale = Parietal bone 31–43, 53
– (sa) pedis = Bones of foot 88–91
– pisiforme = Pisiform bone 72–75, 115
– pubis = Pubic bone (pubis) 80–83, 160, 164, 165
– sacrum = Sacrum 15, 20, 21, 164, 165
– scaphoideum (naviculare) = Scaphoid bone 72–75, 113, 114
– (sa) sesamoidea (manus) = Sesamoid bones (hand) 73–75, 88, 115, 220
– (sa) – (pedis) = Sesamoid bones (foot) 88, 251
– sphenoidale = Sphenoid bone 31, 34–39, 45, 46, 55–58, 63, 105
– (sa) suturarum = Sutural bones 42
– (sa) tarsi = Tarsal bones 88–91, 135
– temporale = Temporal bone 9, 32–35, 47–50
– trapezium (multangulum majus) = Trapezium bone 72–75, 113
– trapezoideum (multangulum) minus = Trapezoid bone 72–75, 113, 114
– triquetrum = Triquetral (or triangular) bone 72–76, 113, 114
– zygomaticum = Zygomatic bone 31, 33, 40, 54, 61, 104
Ostium canalis nasofrontalis 63
Osteology 7–92

P

Palatum durum = Hard palate 58, 187
Palma manus = Palm of hand 2, 3, 213, 215
Pars alveolaris mandibulae = Alveolar part of mandible 59
– anularis vaginae fibrosae digiti manus 216, 220
– basilaris ossis occipitalis = Basilar part of occipital bone 44
Pars costalis diaphragmatis = Costal part of diaphragm 163
– cruciforme vaginae fibrosae digiti manus 216, 220
– lateralis ossis occipitalis = Lateral part of occipital bone 44, 45
– – – sacri = Lateral part of sacrum 20, 21
– lumbalis diaphragmatis = Lumbar part of diaphragm 163
– mastoidea ossis temporalis = Mastoid part of temporal bone 47
– nasalis ossis frontalis = Nasal part of frontal bone 52
– orbitalis ossis frontalis = Orbital part of frontal bone 52
– petrosa ossis temporalis = Petrosal part of temporal bone 35, 39, 40, 47, 48, 50
– sacralis lineae terminalis = Sacral part of terminal line 20
– squamosa ossis temporalis = Squamous part of temporal bone 33, 35, 39, 40, 47–49, 61
– sternalis diaphragmatis = Sternal part of diaphragm 163
– tibiocalcanearis ligamenti deltoidei = Tibiocalcaneal part of deltoid ligament 130, 131
– tibionavicularis ligamenti deltoidei = Tibionavicular part of deltoid ligament 131
– tibiotalaris anterior ligamenti deltoidei = Anterior tibiotalar part of deltoid ligament 131
– – posterior ligamenti deltoidei = Posterior tibiotalar part of deltoid ligament 130, 131
– tympanica ossis temporalis = Tympanic part of temporal bone 47–50
Patella = Knee cap (also: knee pan) 85, 126, 128, 232, 240, 241
Pecten ossis pubis 81, 82
Pediculus arcus vertebrae = Pedicle of vertebral arch 18, 19, 101
Pelvic girdle (Joints and ligaments) 118–125
– – (Muscles) 164–166
– – (Osteology) 25, 78–83
Pelvis 78, 79, 118–124
Perineum 5
Periosteum 8
Pes anserinus 234, 240
Phalanges digitorum manus 72–76
– – pedis 88, 89, 91
Planta pedis = Sole of foot 3, 254, 256
Planum nuchale = Nuchal plane 42, 44
– occipitale = Occipital plane 44
Platysma 154, 168, 169, 178, 181
Plexus brachialis = Brachial plexus 169, 174, 175, 185
– parotideus = Parotid plexus 179
Plica (e) = Fold (s)
– alaris = Alar folds 127
– synovialis infrapatellaris = Infrapatellar synovial fold 127

Porus acusticus externus = External acoustic pore 33
– – internus = Internal acoustic pore 39, 47
Processus accessorius vertebrae = Accessory process of vertebrae 18, 19
– alveolaris maxillae = Alveolar process of maxilla 31, 57, 61, 62
– articularis inferior vertebrae = Inferior articular process of vertebrae 16, 18, 19
– – superior vertebrae = Superior articular process of vertebrae 16–20
– clinoideus anterior = Anterior clinoid process 39, 45, 46
– – medius = Middle clinoid process 45
– – posterior = Posterior clinoid process 39, 45, 46
– condylaris mandibulae = Condylar process of mandible 33, 59, 60, 104, 172
– coracoideus scapulae = Coracoid process of scapula 26, 66, 109–111, 197
– coronoideus mandibulae = Coronoid process of mandible 33, 59, 60, 104, 172
– – ulnae = Coronoid process of ulna 69, 71
– costarius = Costal process 19
– ethmoidalis conchae nasalis inferioris = Ethmoidal process of inferior nasal concha 63
– falciformis lig. sacrotuberalis = Falciform process of sacrotuberal ligament 123
– frontalis maxillae = Frontal process of maxilla 57
– – ossis zygomatici = Frontal process of zygomatic bone 33, 54
– – ossis occipitalis = Intrajugular process of occipital bone 39, 45
– – – temporalis = Intrajugular process of temporal bone 35, 47, 48
– jugularis ossis occipitalis = Jugular process of occipital bone 39, 44, 45
– lateralis tali = Lateral process of talus 89
– – tuberis calcanei = Lateral process of toberosity of calcaneus 88, 90
– mamillaris vertebrarum = Mamillary process of vertebrae 18, 19
– mastoideus = Mastoid process 33, 37, 42, 47–50
– medialis tuberis calcanei = Medial process of tuberosity of calcaneus 88, 90
– orbitalis ossis palatini = Orbital process of palatine bone 56, 61, 62
– palatinus maxillae = Palatine process of maxilla 37, 40, 55, 57, 58, 61
– posterior tali = Posterior process of talus 89
– pterygoideus ossis sphenoidalis = Pterygoid process of sphenoid bone 37, 40, 46, 58, 62, 63, 104, 105
Processus pyramidalis ossis palatini = Pyramidal process of palatine bone 37, 56, 58, 63
– sphenoidalis ossis palatini = Sphenoid process of palatine bone 56
– spinosus = Spinous process 16–19, 153
– styloideus ossis temporalis = Styloid process of temporal bone 9, 32–37, 47–50, 104, 105, 185, 187
– – radii = Styloid process of radius 70, 72–75
– – ulnae = Styloid process of ulna 69, 70, 72–75, 114
– temporalis ossis zygomatici = Temporal process of zygomatic bone 54
– transversus vertebrae = Transverse process of vertebrae 16–18, 21, 102
– uncinatus ossis ethmoidalis = Uncinate process of ethmoid bone 54, 63
– vaginalis ossis sphenoidalis = Vaginal process of sphenoid bone 46
– xyphoideus = Xyphoid process 24, 160
– zygomaticus maxillae = Zygomatic process of maxilla 37, 57, 62
– – ossis frontalis = Zygomatic process of frontal bone 31, 52
– – ossis temporalis = Zygomatic process of temporal bone 37, 47, 48, 104
Prominentia canalis semicircularis lateralis = Prominence of lateral semicircular canal 50
Promontorium ossis sacri = Promontory of sacrum 15, 27, 79, 124, 232
– – temporalis = Promontory of temporal bone 49, 50, 71
Protuberantia mentalis = Mental protuberance 33, 59, 172
– occipitalis externa = External occipital protuberance 35, 37, 42, 44, 142, 188
– – interna = Internal occipital protuberance 39, 44, 45

R

Radius 70, 71, 112
Ramus = Branch
– inferior ossis pubis = Inferior branch of pubis 80–83, 160
– mandibulae = Branch of mandible 60
– ossis ischii = Branch of ischium 80–83
– superior ossis pubis = Superior branch of pubis 80, 82, 83, 160
Raphe mylohyoidea = Mylohyoid raphe 172
– pterygomandibularis = Pterygomandibular raphe 187
Recessus epitympanicus = Epitympanic recess 49
Regio (nes) = Region (s)
– (nes) corporis = Regions of the body 2–5
– cubiti = Cubital region 2, 3, 71, 72
– malleolaris medialis = Medial malleolar region 2, 247
– – lateralis = Lateral malleolar region 2, 247
Retinaculum extensorum = Retinaculum of extensors 192, 206, 208, 212, 214
– flexorum = Retinaculum of flexors 213, 215, 216, 218, 220
– mm. extensorum inferius = Inferior retinaculum of extensor muscles 227, 240, 241, 248, 252, 259
– – – superius = Superior retinaculum of extensor muscles 227
– – flexorum (ligamentum laciniatum) = Retinaculum of flexor muscles (latiniate ligament) 240, 244, 259
– – peroneorum (fibularium) inferius = Inferior retinaculum of peroneus muscles 241, 248, 252, 259
– – (–) superius = Superior retinaculum of peroneus muscles 241, 246, 248, 259
– patellae laterale = Lateral retinaculum of patella 126, 241, 242
– – mediale = Medial retinaculum of patella 126, 240
Ring (also anulus)
Rostrum sphenoidale = Sphenoidal rostrum 46
Rudimenta costae = Costal rudiments 14, 18, 19

S

Scapula 25–27, 66, 111
Sella turcica (Fossa hypophysialis) = Hypophyseal fossa 35, 39, 45, 105
Semicanalis m. tensoris tympani = Semicanal of tensor tympani muscle 49
– tubae auditivae = Semicanal of auditory tube 49
Septum intermusculare anterius cruris = Anterior intermuscular septum of leg 248
– – brachii laterale = External intermuscular septum of arm 190, 192, 194, 206, 208 211
– – – mediale = Internal intermuscular septum of arm 190, 196, 198, 199, 202, 204, 211
– – posterius cruris = Posterior intermuscular septum of leg 242
– nasi = Nasal septum 55, 187
– – osseum = Bony septum of nose 31, 35, 55, 56
Shoulder Girdle (Joints and Ligaments) 108–111
– – (Osteology) 25–27, 66, 67

Sinus frontalis = Frontal sinus 35, 51, 61, 63, 187
– maxillaris = Maxillary sinus 58, 61, 62
– paranasales = Paranasal air sinus 51, 61–63
– sigmoideus = Sigmoid sinus 50
– sphenoidalis = Sphenoidal sinus 35, 46, 51, 55, 62, 63, 105, 187
– tarsi = Tarsal sinus 89
Skull (Joints and ligaments) 94–96, 104, 105
– (Osteology) 30–63
Spatium axillare laterale (quadrangulare) = Quadrangular space 142, 191, 195
– axillare mediale (triangulare) = Triangular space 142, 191, 195
– praetracheale = Pretracheal space 174
Spina ethmoidalis ossis sphenoidalis = Ethmoidal spine of sphenoid bone 45
– iliaca anterior inferior = Inferior anterior iliac spine 81–83, 165
– – – superior = Superior anterior iliac spine 25, 81–83, 118, 121, 141, 154, 156, 159, 165, 228, 232
– – posterior inferior = Inferior posterior iliac spine 81, 83
– – – superior = Superior posterior iliac spine 81, 83, 122, 141, 165, 230
– ischiadica = Ischial spine 25, 81–83, 165
– mentalis = Mental spine 60, 172
– m. genioglossi = Spine for genioglossus muscle 60, 172
– – recti lateralis = Spine for lateral straight muscle of eyeball 62
– nasalis anterior maxillae = Anterior nasal spine of maxilla 31, 33, 57, 63
– ossis frontalis = Nasal spine of frontal bone 51, 52
– – posterior ossis palatini = Posterior nasal spine of palatine bone 37, 56–58
– ossis sphenoidalis = Spine of sphenoid bone 37, 46, 63, 105
– (ae) palatinae = Palatine spines 58
– scapulae = Spine of scapula 66, 110, 141, 192
– suprameatum = Suprameatal spine 47
– trochlearis (Var.) ossis frontalis = Trochlear spine of frontal bone (variation) 51
Squama frontalis = Squamous part of frontal bone 31, 33, 52
– occipitalis = Squamous part of occipital bone 33, 40, 44
– temporalis = Squamous part of temporal bone 32–35, 39, 40, 47, 49, 61–63
Stapes = Stirrup 49
Sternum 9, 10, 24, 103
Substantia spongiosa = Spongy bone 8, 10, 11
Sulcus (i) = Sulcus (i) (see also groove)
– (i) arteriosi = Arterial sulci (intracranial) 35, 39, 43, 48, 53
Sulcus arteriae subclaviae costae I = Sulcus for subclavian artery (and vein) 22
– – temporalis mediae = Sulcus for middle temporal artery 47
– – vertebralis atlantis = Sulcus for vertebral artery of atlas 16, 94
– bicipitalis medialis = Medial bicipital groove 190
– calcanei = Calcaneal sulcus 90
– caroticus ossis sphenoidalis = Carotid sulcus of sphenoid bone 39, 45, 46
– costae = Costal sulcus 22
– infraorbitalis = Infraorbital sulcus of maxilla 57, 61, 62
– intertubercularis humeri = Intertubercular sulcus of humerus 67, 68
– lacrimalis maxillae = Lacrimal sulcus of maxilla 57
– malleolaris lateralis = Lateral malleolar sulcus 87
– – medialis = Medial malleolar sulcus 86
– mylohyoideus = Mylohyoid sulcus 60, 105
– n. petrosi majoris = Sulcus for greater petrosal nerve 39, 47, 48
– – – minoris = Sulcus for lesser petrosal nerve 39, 47, 48
– – radialis = Sulcus for radial n. 68
– – spinalis = Sulcus for spinal nerve 17
– – ulnaris = Groove for ulnar nerve 67, 68
– obturatorius = Obturator sulcus of pubis 83
– opticus ossis sphenoidalis = Optic sulcus of sphenoid bone 45
– palatinus major ossis palatini = Great palatine sulcus of palatine bone 56
– popliteus = Popliteal sulcus 85
– pterygopalatinus ossis sphenoidalis = Pterygopalatine sulcus of sphenoid bone 46
– sagittalis ossis parietalis = Sagittal sulcus of parietal bone 53
– sinus petrosi inferioris ossis occipitalis = Sulcus of inferior petrosal sinus of occipital bone 39, 47, 48
– – – – – temporalis = Sulcus of inferior petrosal sinus of temporal bone 39, 47, 48
– – – superioris = Sulcus of superior petrosal sinus 39
– – sagittalis superioris ossis frontalis = Sulcus of superior sagittal sinus of frontal bone 39, 43, 52
– – – – – occipitalis = Sulcus of superior sagittal sinus of occipital bone 44
Sulcus sinus sigmoidei ossis occipitalis = Sulcus of sigmoid sinus of occipital bone 39, 44, 45
– – – partis petrosae ossis temporalis = Sulcus of sigmoid sinus of petrosal parts of temporal bone 48
– – transversi ossis occipitalis = Sulcus of transverse sinus of occipital bone 39, 44, 45
– tali = Sulcus of talus 89
– tendinis m. flexoris hallucis longi calcanei 90, 136
– – – – – – tali 89
– tendinum mm. peroneorum (fibularium) calcanei = Sulcus of tendous of peroneus muscles 90
– tendinis m. peronei (fibularis) longi ossis cuboidei = Sulcus of tendon of peroneus longus muscle 88
– tubae auditivae 46
– venae subclaviae costae I = Sulcus for subclavian vein (and artery) 22
Sustentaculum tali = Sustentaculum of talus 88–90, 131
Sutura coronalis = Coronal suture 31, 33, 35, 40, 41, 43
– frontalis = Frontal suture 40
– frontoethmoidalis = Frontoethmoidal suture 39
– frontolacrimalis = Frontolacrimal suture 31
– frontomaxillaris = Frontomaxillary suture 31, 61
– frontonasalis = Frontonasal suture 31
– frontozygomatica = Frontozygomatic suture 33
– incisiva = Incisive suture 37, 58
– infraorbitalis = Infraorbital suture 61, 62
– internasalis = Internasal suture 31
– lacrimoethmoidalis = Lacrimoethmoidal suture 62
– lacrimomaxillaris = Lacrimomaxillary suture 33
– lambdoidea = Lambdoid suture 33, 35, 37, 40–43
– nasomaxillaris = Nasomaxillary suture 31, 33
– occipitalis transversa (Var.) = Transverse occipital suture (variation) 40, 42
– occipitomastoidea = Occipitomastoid suture 33, 37, 39, 42
– palatina mediana = Median palatine suture 37, 58
– – transversa = Transverse palatine suture 37, 57, 58
– parietomastoidea = Parietomastoid suture 33, 42
– sagittalis = Sagittal suture 40–43
– sphenofrontalis = Sphenofrontal suture 31, 33, 39, 62
– sphenosquamosa = Sphenosquamous suture 33, 39

Sutura sphenozygomatica
= Sphenozygomatic suture 31, 33
– squamosa = Squamous sutura 33, 35
– temporozygomatica
= Temporozygomatic sutura 33
– zygomaticomaxillaris
= Zygomaticomaxillary suture 31, 61
Symphysis pubica = Pubic symphysis 123, 124, 159, 160, 165, 166, 228
Synchondrosis (es) sacrales = Sacral synchondrosis 21
– sphenooccipitalis = Sphenooccipital synchondrosis 39, 45
– sternalis = Sternal synchondrosis 24, 103, 108
– sternocostalis costae I
= Sternocostal synchondrosis 103
Syndesmology 93–137
Syndesmosis (articulatio) tibiofibularis
= Tibiofibular syndesmosis (articulation) 128, 130, 134
Synostosis epiphysialis = Epiphyseal synostosis 8
– vertebrae = Vertebral synostosis 14

T

Talus = Ankle bone 88–91, 134, 135
Tarsus 88–91, 135
Tegmen tympani = Roof of tympanon 48
Tendo = Tendon (see also muscle or sheath)
Tendo calcaneus *(Achillis)* = Calcancal tendon *(Achillis)* 240, 241, 244, 259
Thenar = Thenar eminence 221
Thorax = Chest 25–27
Thorax (Joints and ligaments) 94–103
Tibia 11, 86, 87, 128, 240
Tonsilla pharyngea = Pharyngeal tonsil 187
Torus tubarius 187
Tractus angularis fasciae cervicalis 173
– iliotibialis = Iliotibial tract 141, 226, 229, 238, 241, 250
Trigonum = Trigone (also triangle)
– caroticum = Carotide trigone 4
– deltoideopectorale *(Mohrenheim)*
= Deltoideopectoral trigone *(Mohrenheim)* 2, 4, 154, 168, 169, 174
– femorale = Femoral trigone 2
– lumbale = Lumbar trigone 141, 142, 144, 153
– lumbocostale = Lumbocostal trigone 163
– omoclaviculare = Omoclavicular trigone (also: subclavian triangle) 4, 173
– retromolare = Retromolar trigone 60
– sternocostale = Sternocostal trigone 163
– submandibulare = Submandibular trigone 4
Trochanter major = Greater trochanter 84, 85, 118, 122, 123, 125, 166, 230, 236
– minor = Lesser trochanter 84, 85, 166, 230, 234
Trochlea humeri = Trochlea of humerus 67, 68, 113
– peronealis (fibularis) = Peroneal trochlea of calcaneus 89, 90
– tali = Trochlea of talus 88, 89
Truncus brachiocephalicus
= Brachiocephalic trunk 176
Trunk (Muscles) 141–166
– (Osteology) 14–27
Tuber = Tuber (also tubercle or tuberosity)
– calcanei = Tuberosity of calcaneus 88–90, 130–132, 254
– frontale = Frontal eminence 40, 52
– ischiadicum = Ischial tuberosity 25, 80–83, 122, 165, 236
– parietale = Parietal eminence 40, 41, 53
Tuberculum anterius atlantis
= Anterior tubercle of atlas 16, 17
– – axis = Anterior tubercle of axis 16
– – proc. transversum = Anterior tubercle of transverse process 17
– – vertebrarum cervicalium
= Anterior tubercle of cervical vertebrae 17
– articulare ossis temporalis
= Articular tubercle of temporal bone 37, 47, 48, 186
– caroticum vertebrae cervicalis VI
= Carotid tubercle of sixth cervical vertebra 166, 176
– conoideum = Conoid tubercle 67
– costae = Tubercle of rib 22, 102
– infraglenoidale = Infraglenoid tubercle 66
– intercondylare laterale tibiae
= Lateral intercondylar tubercle of tibia 87
– – mediale tibiae = Medial intercondylar tubercle of tibia 87
– jugulare ossis occipitalis = Jugular tubercle of occipital bone 39, 44, 45
– laterale processus posterioris tali
= Lateral eminence of posterior process of talus 89
– majus humeri = Greater tubercle of humerus 67, 68, 110
– mediale processus posterioris tali
= Medial eminence of posterior process of talus 89
– mentale = Mental tubercle 59, 172
– minus humeri = Lesser tubercle of humerus 67, 68
– m. scaleni anterioris = Tubercle of anterior scalene muscle 22
– obturatorium anterius = Anterior obturator tubercle 81
– – posterius = Posterior obturator tubercle 81–83
– pharyngeum = Pharyngeal tubercle 37
Tuberculum posterius atlantis =
Posterior tubercle of atlas 16, 17, 148
– – processus transversum = Posterior tubercle of transverse process 17
– – vertebrarum cervicalium
= Posterior tubercle of cervical vertebrae 17
– pubicum = Pubic tubercle of pubic bone 81–83, 121, 164–166, 232
– sellae = Tubercle of sella turcica 39, 45
Tuberositas deltoidea = Deltoid tuberosity of humerus 68
– glutaea = Gluteal tuberosity of femur 85, 125
– iliaca = Iliac tuberosity 82, 83
– masseterica = Masseteric tuberosity 59, 104
– m. glutaei maximi = Tuberosity for greatest gluteal muscle 81
– m. scaleni medii = Tuberosity for middle scalene muscle 22
– ossis cuboidei = Tuberosity of cuboid bone 88
– – metatarsalis V = Tuberosity of fifth metatarsal bone 88, 89
– – – hallucis = Tuberosity of metatarsal bone of great toe 88
– – navicularis = Tuberosity of navicular bone 88, 90
– – scaphoidei = Tuberosity of scaphoid bone 74
– phalangis distalis (digit. manus)
= Distal tuberosity of fingers 72–74
– pterygoidea = Pterygoid tuberosity of mandible 60
– radii = Tuberosity of radius 70
– sacralis = Tuberosity of sacrum 20, 21
– tibiae = Tuberosity of tibia 86, 87, 126–128, 248
– ulnae = Tuberosity of ulna 69

U

Ulna 69–71, 112, 113
Umbilicus 141, 154, 160
Upper limb (Joints and ligaments) 109–115
– – (Muscles) 190–224
– – (Osteology) 68–76

V

Vagina = Sheath (see also muscle or tendon s.)
– fibrosa digit. (manus)
= Fibrous sheaths of fingers 220
– – – (pedis) = Fibrous sheaths of toes 254
– (ae) fibrosae tendin. mm. flex. digit. manus 216
– m. recti abdominis = Sheath of straight abdominal muscle 154, 156 158, 160, 161, 192
– processus styloidei = Vaginal process of styloid 37, 42, 47, 48, 50

Vagina synovialis communis mm. flexorum 215, 216
- (ae) synoviales digit. manus = Synovial sheaths of tendons of fingers 212, 214–216, 220, 223
- synovialis intertubercularis = Synovial sheath of intertubercular groove 109, 111, 196, 198
- - mm. peroneorum communis 241, 259
- - tendinis m. abductoris pollicis longi 215, 216
- - - - flexoris carpi radialis 215, 216
- - - - - hallucis longi 216, 240, 254, 259
- tendinis m. extensoris carpi ulnaris 212, 214
- - - - digiti minimi (manus) 212, 214
- - - - hallucis longi 240, 241, 259
- - - - pollicis longi 212, 214
- - - flexoris pollicis longi 215, 216
- - - peronei longi plantaris 256
- - - tibialis anterioris 240, 241, 259
- - - - posterioris 240, 259
Vagina tendinum mm. abductoris pollicis longi et extensoris pollicis brevis 212, 214
- (ae) tendinum m. extensoris digit. (pedis) longi 240, 241, 259
- - - flexoris digit. (pedis) longi 240, 259
Vena (e) = Vein (s)
- axillaris = Axillary vein 174
- basilica = Basilic vein 190
- brachiocephalica = Brachiocephalic veins 176
- cava inferior = Inferior cava vein 176
- cephalica = Cephalic vein 154, 169, 174, 190, 197
- facialis = Facial vein 174
- femoralis = Femoral vein 228
- iliaca externa = External iliac vein 228
- jugularis anterior = Anterior jugular vein 168
- - externa = External jugular vein 168, 173
- - interna = Internal jugular vein 169, 174, 175, 185
Vena poplitea = Popliteal vein 229
- saphena magna = Great saphenous vein 226, 228
- - parva = Small saphenous vein 229
- subclavia = Subclavian vein 175, 176
- temporalis superficialis = Superficial temporal veins 181
- thoracica interna = Internal thoracic vein 176
- ulnaris = Ulnar vein 216
Vertebra prominens = Seventh cervical vertebra 17, 25, 142
Vertebrae cervicales = Cervical vertebrae 14–17, 25–27
- coccygeae = Coccygeal vertebrae 14, 15, 21, 165
- lumbales = Lumbal vertebrae 11, 14, 15, 19
- sacrales = Sacral vertebrae 14, 15, 20, 21
- thoracicae = Thoracic vertebrae 14, 15, 18, 19, 25–27
Vertebral column (Joints and ligaments) 97–103
Vinculum tendinum = Vincula of tendons of fingers 220, 223
Vomer 31, 35, 37, 40, 55, 56, 61, 105

II. English/Latin

A

Abdominal musculature = Musculi abdominis 154–160
Acetabulum 80–82
Acromion (scapulae) = Acromion 26, 27, 66, 109–111, 169, 197
Adminiculum lineae albae 160
Ala = Wing
Angle = Angulus
-, costal = Angulus costae 22
-, mandibular = Angulus mandibulae 59, 60, 104, 105
- of parietal bone, frontal = Angulus frontalis ossis parietalis 53
- - - -, occipital = Angulus occipitalis ossis parietalis 53
- - - -, mastoid = Angulus mastoideus ossis parietalis 53
- - - -, sphenoidal = Angulus sphenoidalis ossis parietalis 53
- of scapula, inferior = Angulus inferior scapulae 66
- - -, lateral = Angulus lateralis scapulae 66
- - -, superior = Angulus superior scapulae 66
-, sternal = Angulus sterni 24
-, subpubic = Angulus subpubicus 119
Ankle bone = Talus 88–91, 134, 135
Ansa tendinis of digastric muscle = Ansa tendinis m. digastrici 172
Antrum, mastoid = Antrum mastoideum 49, 50
Anulus (also ring) = Anulus
- fibrosus (intervertebral disk) = Anulus fibrosus (disci intervertebralis) 98
Anus 165
Anvil = Incus 49
Aorta 166, 176
Aperture of aqueduct of vestibule, external = Apertura externa aquaeductus vestibuli 47
- of canaliculus of cochlea, external = Apertura externa canaliculi cochleae 48
- of carotid canal, internal = Apertura interna canalis carotici 50
- of incisive canal, nasal = Apertura nasalis canalis incisivi 35
- of frontal sinus = Apertura sinus frontalis 52, 63
-, piriform = Apertura piriformis 40
- of sphenoidal sinus = Apertura sinus sphenoidalis 46, 54, 63
Apex of head of fibula = Apex capitis fibulae 87
- of petrous portion of temporal bone = Apex partis petrosae ossis temporalis 47, 48
- of sacrum = Apex ossis sacri 20, 21
Aponeuroses tendinum digitales dorsales manus (aponeuroses m. extens. digit. manus) 212, 220, 223
Aponeurosis, bicipital = Aponeurosis m. bicipitis brachii 190, 196, 198, 199, 202
- of external oblique muscle of abdomen = Aponeurosis m. obliqui abdominis externus 141, 154, 159, 161, 162
- of internal oblique muscle of abdomen = Aponeurosis m. obliqui abdominis internus 158, 161
-, palmar = Aponeurosis palmaris 199, 213, 223
-, plantar = Aponeurosis plantaris 254
- of tensor muscle of veli palatini, palatine = Aponeurosis palatina m. tensoris veli palatini 188
- of transversal muscle of abdomen = Aponeurosis m. transversi abdominis 161
Arch = Arcus
- of atlas, anterior = Arcus anterior atlantis 16, 96
- - -, posterior = Arcus posterior atlantis 16, 96
- of axis = Arcus axis 16
-, costal = Arcus costalis 25, 27, 162
- of frontal bone, superciliary = Arcus superciliaris ossis frontalis 51, 52
-, iliopectineal = Arcus iliopectineus 166
- of mandible, alveolar = Arcus alveolaris mandibulae 59

Arch, pubic = Arcus pubis 118, 124
–, tendinous of levator ani muscle = Arcus tendineus (fasciae obturatoriae) m. levatoris ani 164
–, – of psoas muscle = Arcus tendineus m. psoatis 166
–, – of soleus muscle = Arcus tendineus m. solei 243
–, vertebral = Arcus vertebrae 17–19, 99
–, zygomatic = Arcus zygomaticus 33, 37, 63, 104, 183
Area, intercondylar, anterior = Area intercondylaris anterior tibiae 87
–, –, posterior = Area intercondylaris posterior tibiae 87
Artery (ies) = Arteria (ae)
–, axillary = Arteria axillaris 174
–, brachial = Arteria brachialis 199
–, carotid, common = Arteria carotis communis 169, 174–176, 185
–, –, external = Arteria carotis externa 175, 185
–, –, internal = Arteria carotis interna 175
–, facial = Arteria facialis 174
–, femoral = Arteria femoralis 228
–, glutaeal, inferior = Arteria glutaea inferior 230
–, –, superior = Arteria glutaea superior 230
–, iliac, external = Arteria iliaca externa 228
–, nutritient of humerus = Arteria nutricia humeri 8
– (ies), perforating = Arteriae perforantes 230
–, popliteal = Arteria poplitea 229
–, pudendal, internal = Arteria pudenda interna 230
–, radial = Arteria radialis 199, 216
–, subclavian = Arteria subclavia 175, 176
–, temporal, superficial = Arteria temporalis superficialis 181
–, thoracic, internal = Arteria thoracica interna 176
–, tibial, posterior = Arteria tibialis posterior 243
–, ulnar = Arteria ulnaris 199, 216
–, – collateral, superior = Arteria collateralis ulnaris sup. 199
–, vertebral = Arteria vertebralis 150
Articulation (s) (Syndesmology) 93–137
Articulation (s) (see also joint or synchondrosis) = Articulatio (nes)
–, acromioclavicular = Articulatio acromioclavicularis 109, 111
–, atlantoaxial, lateral = Articulatio atlantoaxialis lateralis 94–96, 176
–, –, medial = Articulatio atlanto-axialis 96, 187
–, atlantooccipital = Articulatio atlantooccipitalis 94, 95
–, calcaneocuboid = Articulatio calcaneocuboidea 135
Articulation (s), carpometacarpal = Articulationes carpometacarpeae 113–115
–, – of thumb = Articulatio carpo-metacarpea pollicis 113, 115
–, costal = Articulationes costae 102
–, costotransverse = Articulatio costotransversaria 102
–, cubital (elbow joint) = Articulatio cubiti 112, 113
–, cuneonavicular = Articulatio cuneonavicularis 135
– (s) of the hand = Articulationes manus 113–115
– of head of rib = Articulatio capitis costae 102
– of hip (hip joint) = Articulatio coxae 118–125
–, humeroulnar = Articulatio humeroulnaris 113
–, incudomallear = Articulatio incudomallearis 49
– (s), intercarpal = Articulationes intercarpeae 113
– of knee (knee joint) = Articulatio genus 92, 126–129
–, mediocarpal = Articulatio mediocarpea 113
– (s), metacarpophalangeal = Articulationes metacarpophalangeae 72–75, 113–115
–, radiocarpal = Articulatio radiocarpea 113
–, radioulnar, distal = Articulatio radioulnaris distalis 112, 113, 115
–, sacroiliac = Articulatio sacroiliaca 124
– of shoulder (shoulder joint) = Articulatio humeri 109–111, 197
–, sternoclavicular = Articulatio sternoclavicularis 108, 174
–, sternocostal = Articulationes sternocostales 103
–, subtalar = Articulatio subtalaris 92, 133–135, 253
–, talocalcaneonavicular = Articulatio talocalcaneonavicularis 92, 133–135, 253
–, talocrural (ankle joint) = Articulatio talocruralis 92, 130, 134, 253
–, talonavicular = Articulatio talonavicularis 135
– (s), tarsometatarsal = Articulationes tarsometatarseae 135
–, temporomandibular = Articulatio temporomandibularis 104, 105, 183, 185, 186, 188
–, tibiofibular (syndesmosis), distal = Articulatio (syndesmosis) tibiofibularis distales 128, 130
–, –, proximal = – tibiofibularis proximalis 128, 130
Atlas 16, 17, 94–96
Auditory ossicles 49
Axis (Epistropheus) 16, 17, 96
Axis, pelvic = Axis pelvis 124

B

Backbone (vertebral column) = Columna vertebralis 15, 25–27, 97–100
Base of cranium (skull), external = Basis cranii externa 36, 37, 188
– – – –, internal = Basis cranii interna 38, 39
– of mandible = Basis mandibulae 33, 188
– of metacarpal bones = Bases ossium metacarpalium 72, 73
– of metatarsal bones = Bases ossium metatarsalium 88
– of patella = Basis patellae 85
– of phalanx of fingers = Basis phalangis (digit. manus) 72–75
– – – of toes = Basis phalangis (digit. pedis) 88
– of sacral bone = Basis ossis sacri 20, 21
Body (see also corpus or shaft) = Corpus
–, adipose b. of cheek = Corpus adiposum buccae 169, 178, 183
– of hyoid bone = Corpus ossis hyoidei 60
–, infrapatellar fatty b. = Corpus adiposum infrapatellare 128
– of mandible = Corpus mandibulae 59
Bone (s) called also os (sa)
Bones, characteristics of 8–11
–, classification of 8–11
–, individual (see under individual names)
Bone marrow = Medulla ossium 8
Bone, spongy 8, 10, 11
Border (also crest, margin or ridge) = Crista
Border (also crest or margin) = Margo
–, anterior b. of radius = Margo anterior radii 71
–, anterior b. of tibia = Margo anterior tibiae 86
–, interosseous b. of fibula = Margo interosseus fibulae 87
–, – – of radius = Margo inter-osseus radii 70, 71
–, – – of tibia = Margo interosseus tibiae 86
–, – – of ulna = Margo interosseus ulnae 69, 71
–, lacrimal b. of maxilla = Margo lacrimalis maxillae 57
–, lateral b. of humerus = Margo lateralis humeri 68
–, – – of scapula = Margo lateralis scapulae 66
–, medial b. of humerus = Margo medialis humeri 68
–, – (vertebral) b. of scapula = Margo medialis scapulae 66
–, – b. of tibia = Margo medialis tibiae 86

Border, posterior b. of fibula = Margo posterior fibulae 87
–, – – of radius = Margo posterior radii 71
–, superior b. of scapula = Margo superior scapulae 66
Branch = Ramus
– of ischium = Ramus ossis ischii 80–83
– of mandible = Ramus mandibulae 60
– of pubis, inferior = Ramus inferior ossis pubis 80–83, 160
– – –, superior = Ramus superior ossis pubis 80, 82, 83, 160
Bulb of jugular vein, inferior = Bulbus v. jugularis inferior 169
Bursa, anserine = Bursa anserina 234
–, bicipitoradial = Bursa bicipitoradialis 202
– of calcaneal *(Achillis)* tendon = Bursa tendinis calcanei *(Achillis)* 241
– coccygea subcutanea 229
– (ae), gluteal, intermuscular = Bursae intermusculares mm. glutaeorum 230
–, iliopectinal = Bursa iliopectinea 234
–, infrapatellar, deep = Bursa infrapatellaris profunda 126, 128, 129, 241
–, –, subcutaneous = Bursa subcutanea infrapatellaris 226, 227
– (ae) intermetacarpeae 212
–, ischial b. of (internal) obturator muscle = Bursa ischiadica m. obturatorii interni 243
– m. pectoralis majoris 198
– of olecrani, subcutaneous = Bursa subcutanea olecrani 113, 190
–, prepatellar, subcutaneous = Bursa subcutanea praepatellaris 128, 129, 226, 227
– of semimembranosus muscle = Bursa m. semimembranosi 244
–, subacromial = Bursa subacromialis 111, 197
–, subcoracoid = Bursa subcoracoides 191, 198
– (ae) subcutaneae digitorum dorsales (manus) 212
– – metacarpophalangeae dorsales 212
– subcutanea sacralis 229, 230
– – spinae iliacae post. sup. 229, 230
–, subdeltoid = Bursa subdeltoidea 191, 194, 197, 198
–, subtendinous b. (of medial head) of gastrocnemius muscle = Bursa subtendinea m. gastrocnemii medialis 243, 244
–, – – of latissimus dorsi muscle = Bursa m. latissimi dorsi subtendinea 196
–, – – of sartorius muscle = Bursae subtendineae m. sartorii 234
Bursa, subtendinous b. of subscapularis muscle = Bursa m. subscapularis subtendinea 197
–, – – of triceps surae muscle = Bursa subtendinea m. tricipitis surae 240
–, suprapatellar = Bursa suprapatellaris 126–129
– trochanteric b. of gluteus maximus trochanterica m. glutaei maximi 142, 230, 236
–, – – – – medius muscle = Bursae trochantericae m. glutei medii 243
–, –, subcutaneous = Bursa subcutanea trochanterica 243

C

Calcaneus (Heel bone) = Calcaneus 9, 10, 88–91, 130–133
Canaliculi, caroticotympanic = Canaliculi caroticotympanici 48
Canaliculus, mastoid = Canaliculus mastoideus 37
Canal, adductor *(Hunteri)* = Canalis adductorius 232
–, carotid = Canalis caroticus 37, 48–50, 176, 188
–, carpal = Canalis carpi 216, 218, 220
–, condylar = Canalis condylaris 37, 39, 44, 188
–, facial = Canalis facialis 49, 50
–, hypoglossal = Canalis hypoglossi 35, 37, 39, 44, 45, 95, 105, 176
–, incisive = Canalis incisivus 35, 55, 63
–, infraorbital = Canalis infraorbitalis 61, 62
–, inguinal = Canalis inguinalis 156
–, musculotubal = Canalis musculotubarius 48–50, 176
–, nasolacrimal = Canalis nasolacrimalis 58, 63
–, nutritient c. of bone *(Haversian)* = Canalis nutricius 8
–, obturator = Canalis obturatorius 164, 228, 234
–, optic = Canalis opticus 39, 45, 61, 62
–, palatine, greater (palatomaxillary canal) = Canalis palatinus major 62
–, pterygoid = Canalis pterygoideus 46, 62
–, pudendal *(Alcock)* = Canalis pudendalis *(Alcock)* 165
–, sacral = Canalis sacralis 20, 21, 124, 164
–, semicircular, lateral = Canalis semicircularis lateralis 50
–, vertebral = Canalis vertebralis 25, 27
Canalis tendinis m. flexoris carpi radialis 220
Capitulum humeri 68, 71
Caput (see head)
Carpus 72–75
Cartilage, costal = Cartilago costalis 23, 103
–, cricoid = Cartilago cricoidea 174
–, thyroid = Cartilago thyroidea 174
Cavity, glenoid c. of scapula = Cavitas glenoidalis scapulae 26, 61, 66, 111, 197
–, thoracic = Cavum thoracis 166
–, tympanic = Cavum tympani 49, 50
Cells, ethmoid, bony = Cellulae ethmoidales 51, 54, 61
–, mastoid = Cellulae mastoideae 9, 49, 50
Central tendon of diaphragm = Centrum tendineum (diaphragmatis) 160, 163, 166
– – of perineum = Centrum tendineum perinei 165
Chest = Thorax 25–27
Chewing muscles 183–188
Chiasm optic = Chiasma opticum 51
Chiasma tendon = Chiasma tendinum 216
Chin muscle = Musculus mentalis 169, 178, 181-183, 185
Choanae 36, 37, 40
Chopart's joint = Articulatio tarsi transversus 92, 133, 134
Circumference, articular c. of head of radius = Circumferentia articularis radii 70, 112
–, – – of head of ulna = Circumferentia articularis ulnae 69
Clavicle (collar bone) = Clavicula 25–27, 67, 169
Clivus 39, 105
Collar bone (clavicle) = Clavicula 25–27, 67, 169
Column, vertebral (backbone) = Columna vertebralis 15, 25–27, 97–100
Concha, nasal, inferior = Concha nasalis inferior 31, 61, 63
–, –, middle = Concha nasalis 31, 54, 61, 63
–, –, superior = Concha nasalis superior 63
–, sphenoidal = Concha sphenoidalis 54
Condyle of femur, lateral = Condylus lateralis femoris 84, 85
– – –, medial = Condylus medialis femoris 84, 85
–, occipital = Condylus occipitalis 33, 37, 44, 188
– of tibia, lateral = Condylus lateralis tibiae 86, 87
– – –, medial = Condylus medialis tibiae 86
Connexus intertendineus (m. extensoris digit. manus) 212, 214
Cord, oblique c. of elbow joint = Chorda obliqua 112, 201, **210**
Corpus (see also body or shaft) = Corpus

Costal rudiments = Rudimenta costae 14, 18, 19
Cranium 30–43
Crest (also border, margin or ridge) = Crista (or margo)
–, conchal c. of maxilla = Crista conchalis maxillae 57
–, – – of palatine bone = Crista conchalis ossis palatini 56, 57
–, ethmoidal c. of maxilla = Crista ethmoidalis maxillae 57, 63
–, – – of palatine bone = Crista ethmoidalis ossis palatini 56, 57, 63
– of fibula, anterior = Margo anterior fibulae 87
– – –, medial = Crista medialis fibulae 87
–, frontal c. of frontal bone = Crista frontalis ossis frontalis 39, 43, 52
– of head of rib = Crista capitis costae 22
–, iliac = Crista iliaca 80–83, 142, 229, 230
–, infratemporal c. of sphenoidal bone = Crista infratemporalis ossis sphenoidalis 37, 46, 186
–, intertrochanteric c. of femur = Crista intertrochanterica femoris 84, 85
–, lacrimal, anterior = Crista lacrimalis anterior 57, 61, 62
–, –, posterior = Crista lacrimalis posterior 61, 62
–, nasal c. of maxilla = Crista nasalis maxillae 35
– of neck of rib = Crista colli costae 22
–, obturator = Crista obturatoria 81, 82
–, occipital, external = Crista occipitalis externa 42, 44
–, –, internal = Crista occipitalis interna 39, 44, 45
–, orbital c. of sphenoidal bone = Crista orbitalis ossis sphenoidalis 46
–, sacral, intermediate = Crista sacralis intermedia 20, 21
–, –, lateral = Crista sacralis 20
–, –, medial = Crista sacralis mediana 20, 21, 122, 164
–, sphenoidal = Crista sphenoidalis 46, 55
– of supinator muscle (ulna) = Crista m. supinatoris ulnae 69
– of (larger) tubercle of humerus = Crista tuberculi majoris humeri 68
– of (lesser) tubercle of humerus = Crista tuberculi minoris humeri 68
Crista galli 35, 39, 53, 61
Crus, diaphragmatic (lumbar portion), intermedial = Crus intermedium part. lumbal. diaphragmatis 163, 166
–, diaphragmatic, lateral = Crus laterale diaphragmatis 163
–, – (lumbar portion), left = Crus sinistrum part. lumbal. diaphragmatis 166
Crista, diaphragmatic (lumbar portion), medial = Crus mediale part. lumbal. diaphragmatis 163, 166
–, – – –, right = Crus dextrum part. lumbal diaphragmatis 166
– of superficial inguinal ring, lateral = Crus laterale anuli inguinalis superficialis 159
– – – – –, medial = Crus mediale anuli inguinalis superficialis 154, 159
Cupula pleurae 166

D

Dens axis (odontoid process of axis) 16, 17, 95, 96
Diameter aperturae pelvis inferioris 124
– diagonalis (conjugata diagonalis) 124
– mediana 79
–, oblique d. of pelvic inlet = Diameter obliqua 79
–, pelvic = Diameter pelvis 79, 124
–, transverse d. of pelvic inlet = Diameter transversa 79
–, true conjugate = Conjugata (vera) 79, 124
Diaphragm = Diaphragma 160, 163
–, oral = Diaphragma oris 172
–, pelvic = Diaphragma pelvis 164, 165
–, urogenital = Diaphragma urogenitale 164, 165
Diploe 10, 43
Disk, articular d. of (distal) radioulnar articulation (joint) = Discus articularis articulationis radioulnaris distalis 112, 113, 115
–, – – of sternoclavicular articulation (joint) = Discus articularis articulationis sternoclavicularis 108, 174
–, – – of temporomandibular articulation (joint) = Discus articularis articulationis temporomandibularis 186
–, interpubic = Discus interpubicus 118, 124
–, intervertebral = Discus intervertebralis 96–98, 101
Dorsal muscles = Musculi dorsi 142–153
Dorsum sellae (turcicae) 35, 39, 46, 105
Duct, parotid (*Stenon's* duct) = Ductus parotideus 169, 178, 183, 185

E

Ear, middle = Auris media 49, 50
Elbow Joint = Articulatio cubiti 112, 113
Eminence (see also tuber or tuberculum)
Eminence = Eminentia
–, arcuate e. of temporal bone = Eminentia arcuata ossis temporalis 35, 47–50
Eminence, frontal = Tuber frontale 40, 52
–, hypothenar = Hypothenar
–, iliopectineal = Eminentia iliopubica 80, 82
–, intercondylar = Eminentia intercondylaris 86
–, parietal = Tuber parietale 40, 41, 53
– of posterior process of talus, lateral = Tuberculum laterale processus posterioris tali 89
– – – – – –, medial = Tuberculum mediale processus posterioris tali 89
–, pyramidal = Eminentia pyramidalis 49
–, thenar = Thenar 221
Eminentia plantaris intermedia 254, 255
– – lateralis medialis 254, 255
Emissary, parietal = Emissarium parietale 35
Epicondyle of femur, lateral = Epicondylus lateralis femoris 68, 84, 85, 112
– – –, medial = Epicondylus medialis femoris 68, 84, 85
– – humerus, medial = Epixondylus medialis humeri 8, 112
Extremity of clavicle, acromial (external) = Extremitas acromialis claviculae 67
– – –, sternal = Extremitas sternalis claviculae 67
– of rib, sternal = Extremitas sternalis costae 22

F

Facet (also facies, fovea or surface) = Facies
–, articular f. of atlas, inferior = Fovea articularis inferior atlantis 16
–, – – – –, superior = Fovea articularis superior atlantis 16
–, – – of axis, anterior = Facies articularis anterior axis 16
–, – – – –, superior = Facies articularis superior axis 16
–, – – (anterior, middle, posterior) of calcaneus (for talus) = Facies articularis talaris (anterior, medius, posterior) calcanei 90
–, – – of calcaneus, cuboid = Facies articularis cuboidea (calcanei) 90
–, – – of clavicle, acromial = Facies articularis acromialis claviculae 67
–, – – of clavicle, sternal = Facies articularis sternalis claviculae 67
–, – – (of head) of fibula = Facies articularis capitis fibulae 87
–, – – of fibula, malleolar = Facies articularis malleolaris fibulae 87

Facet, articular f, of odontoid process of axis, posterior = Facies articularis posterior axis 16
–, – – of patella = Facies articularis patellae 85, 127, 128
–, – – of radius, carpal = Facies articularis carpea radii 70, 112
–, – – (of tubercle) of rib = Facies articularis tuberculi costae 22
–, – – of scapula, acromial = Facies articularis acromii scapulae 66, 111
–, – – of talus, anterior calcaneal = Facies anticularis calcanea anterior tali 89
–, – – – –, medial calcaneal = Facies articularis calcanea media tali 89
–, – – – –, posterior calcaneal = Facies articularis calcanea posterior tali 89
–, – – – –, navicular = Facies articularis navicularis tali 89
–, – – of tibia, fibular = Facies articularis fibularis tibiae 86
–, – – – –, inferior = Facies articularis inferior tibiae 86, 87
–, – – – –, malleolar = Facies articularis malleolaris tibiae 86
–, – – – –, superior = Facies articularis superior tibiae 86
–, – – of vertebrae, inferior = Facies articularis inferior vertebrae 19
–, – – – –, superior = Facies articularis superior vertebrae 97
– (s),–, costal, superior = Facies articulares capitis costae 22
–, costal f. of vertebrae, inferior = Fovea costalis inferior vertebrae 18
–, – – – –, superior = Fovea costalis superior vertebrae 18, 19
–, – transverse = Fovea costalis transversalis 18, 19
–, dental f. of atlas = Fovea dentis atlantis 16
–, malleolar f. of lateral surface of talus = Facies malleolaris lateralis trochleae tali 89
–, pterygoid f. of condylar process of mandible (scaphoid fossa) = Fovea pterygoidea proc. condylaris mandibulae 59
Facies (also facet or surface) = Facies
Falx, inguinal = Falx inguinalis 160
Fascia, antebrachial = Fascia antebrachii 190, 196, 199, 202, 213
–, axillary = Fascia axillaris 190
–, brachial = Fascia brachii 154, 190, 199
–, cervical = Fascia cervicalis 173
–, –, pretracheal lamina = Fascie cervicalis, lamina praetrachealis 173, 174
Fascia, cervical superficial lamina = Fascia cervicalis, lamina superficialis 168, 173
–, clavipectoral = Fascia clavipectoralis 154, 174
–, crural = Fascia cruris 227, 244, 248
– of (pelvic) diaphragm, inferior f. = Fascia diaphragmatis pelvis inferior 165
– of (urogenital) diaphragm, inferior f. = Fascia diaphragmatis urogenitalis inferior 165
–, infraspinous = Fascia infraspinata 192
–, lata 226
–, obturator = Fascia obturatoria 164, 165
–, pectineal = Fascia pectinea 226
–, temporal = Fascia temporalis 183
–, thoracolumbar = Fascia thoracolumbalis 141, 142, 144, 148, 152, 153
–, transverse = Fascia transversalis 153, 161
Fasciculi mamillotendinei (musculorum dorsi) 146
Femur (thigh bone) 10, 84, 85, 125
Fibres, intercrural f. of inguinal canal = Fibrae intercrurales 154, 159, 162
Fibrocartilage, basilar = Fibrocartilago basalis 188
Fibula 87, 128, 241
Fissure (s) (see also grooves or sulci) = Fissura
–, orbital, inferior = Fissura orbitalis inferior 31, 37, 61
–, –, superior (anterior lacerate foramen) = Fissura orbitalis superior 31, 39, 45, 46, 51, 61
–, petrooccipital = Fissura petrooccipitalis 39
–, petrosquamous = Fissura petrosquamosa 39, 48
–, petrotympanic f. of temporal bone = Fissura petrotympanica ossis temporalis 47, 48, 50
–, sphenopetrosal = Fissura sphenopetrosa 39
–, tympanomastoid = Fissura tympanomastoidea 47, 50
Fold (s) = Plica (e)
– (s), alar = Plica alaris 127
– (s), synovial fold, infrapatellar = Plicae synovialis infrapatellaris 127
Fontanelle = Fonticulus
–, anterior = Fonticulus anterior 40
–, anterolateral = Fonticulus anterolateralis 40
–, posterior = Fonticulus posterior 40
–, posterolateral = Fonticulus posterolateralis 40
Foramen cecum of frontal bone = Foramen caecum ossis frontalis 35, 39, 52
–, costotransverse = Foramen costotransversarium 16, 17
Foramen (ina), dental f. of maxilla = Foramina alveolaria maxillae 57, 63
–, ethmoidal f. of frontal bone, anterior = Foramen ethmoidale anterius ossis frontalis 51, 61
–, – – – – –, posterior = Foramen ethmoidale posterius ossis frontalis 51, 61, 62
–, incisive = Foramen incisivum 35, 37, 58
–, infraorbital = Foramen infraorbitale 31, 57
– infrapiriforme 230, 236, 237
–, intervertebral = Foramen intervertebrale 15, 98
–, jugular (or: posterior lacerate f.) = Foramen jugulare 37, 39, 188
, lacerate, middle = Foramen lacerum 37, 39
–, magnum 37, 39, 44, 45
–, mandibular = Foramen mandibulae 60, 172
–, mastoid = Foramen mastoideum 35, 37, 39, 47, 48
–, mental = Foramen mentale 31, 39, 59, 172, 178
–, obturator = Foramen obturatum 81–83
–, oval f. of sphenoid bone = Foramen ovale ossis sphenoidalis 37, 39, 45, 63
–, palatine, greater = Foramen palatinum majus 37, 56, 58
– (ina), –, lesser = Foramina palatina minora 58
–, parietal = Foramen parietale 41, 42, 53
– rotundum 39, 45, 46, 62
– (ina), sacral, anterior = Foramina pelvina 20
– (ina), –, posterior = Foramina sacralia dorsalia 20
–, sciatic, greater = Foramen ischiadicum majus 120, 122, 237
–, –, lesser = Foramen ischiadicum minus 120, 122, 237
–, sphenopalatine = Foramen sphenopalatinum 62, 63
–, spinous f. of sphenoid bone = Foramen spinosum ossis sphenoidalis 37, 39, 45
–, stylomastoid = Foramen stylomastoideum 37, 48, 49
–, supraorbital = Foramen supraorbitale 31, 52
–, suprapiriform = Foramen suprapiriforme 230, 236, 237
–, transverse = Foramen transversarium 14, 16, 17
–, vena caval = Foramen v. cavae 160, 163, 166
–, vertebral = Foramen vertebrale 16, 17, 19, 102
–, zygomaticofacial = Foramen zygomaticofaciale 54, 61, 63
–, zygomaticoorbital = Foramen zygomaticoorbitale 54, 62

Foramen, zygomaticotemporal = Foramen zygomaticotemporale 54
Fossa, acetabular = Fossa acetabuli 80–82, 125, 165
–, axillary = Fossa axillaris 2
–, canine = Fossa canina 57
–, cerebellar f. of occipital bone = Fossa occipitalis cerebellaris 45
–, condylar f. of occipital bone = Fossa condylaris ossis occipialis 44
–, coronoid f. of humerus = Fossa coronoidea humeri 68, 113
–, cranial, anterior = Fossa cranii anterior 39
–, –, middle = Fossa cranii media 39
–, –, posterior = Fossa cranii posterior 39
–, digastric f. of mandible = Fossa digastrica mandibulae 60, 172
–, hypophyseal = Sella turcica (Fossa hypophysialis) 35, 39, 45, 51, 105, 187
–, iliac = Fossa iliaca 82, 83
–, infraclavicular = Fossa infraclavicularis 168
–, infraspinous = Fossa infraspinata 66
–, infratemporal = Fossa infratemporalis 63
–, intercondylar f. of femur = Fossa intercondylaris 84, 85
–, jugular = Fossa jugularis 4, 37, 48, 168
– for lacrimal gland = Fossa glandulae lacrimalis 55
– of (lateral) malleolus = Fossa malleoli lateralis 87
–, mandibular f. of temporal bone = Fossa mandibularis ossis temporalis 37, 47, 48
–, occipital, inferior = Fossa occipitalis inferior 44
–, –, superior = Fossa occipitalis superior 44
–, olecranon = Fossa olecrani 8, 68, 113
–, popliteal = Fossa poplitea 3, 226, 227, 236, 244
–, pterygoid f. of sphenoid bone = Fossa pterygoidea 35, 46
–, pterygopalatine = Fossa pterygopalatina 62, 63
–, radial f. of humerus = Fossa radialis humeri 68
–, scaphoid f. of sphenoid bone = Fossa scaphoidea ossis sphenoidalis 46
–, subarcuate f. of temporal bone = Fossa subarcuata ossis temporalis 39, 47, 48
–, supraclavicular, greater = Fossa supraclavicularis major 168, 173
–, –, lesser = Fossa supraclavicularis 4, 168, 173
–, supraspinous = Fossa supraspinata 66
–, temporal = Fossa temporalis 32, 33
–, trochanteric = Fossa trochanterica 84, 85
Fossula, petrosal = Fossula petrosa 37, 48
Fovea (also facet) = Fovea (or fossa)
– (of head) of femur = Fovea capitis femoris 84, 85
– (of head) of radius = Fovea capitis radii 70
–, sublingual = Fossa sublingualis 60
–, submandibular = Fossa submandibularis 60
– trochlear f. of frontal bone = Fossa trochlearis ossis frontalis 51
Foveola radialis 216
Foveolae ethmoidales ossis frontalis 51

G

Galea, tendinous = Galea aponeurotica 178, 181, 183, 185
Glabella 51, 52
Gland (s), palatine = Glandula (e) palatina (e) 187
–, parotid = Glandula parotis 169, 174, 175, 178, 183
–, –, accessory = Glandula parotis accessoria 169, 183
–, sublingual = Glandula sublingualis 187
–, submandibular = Glandula submandibularis 169, 174, 175, 183
–, thyroid = Glandula thyroidea 169, 174
Granular pits = Foveolae granulares
Groove (s) (see also fissures or sulcus)
–, bicipital, medial = Sulcus bicipitalis medialis 190
– for ulnar nerve = Sulcus n. ulnaris 67, 68

H

Hammer = Malleus
Hamulus (also hook) = Hamulus
–, pterygoid = Hamulus pterygoideus 35, 37, 46, 62, 63, 105, 187, 188
Head (Muscles) 168–188
Head = Caput
– of rib (capitulum costae) = Caput costae 22
– of femur = Caput femoris 84, 85
– of fibula = Caput fibulae 87
– of humerus = Caput humeri 67, 68
– of biceps brachii muscle, long = Caput longum m. bicipitis brachii 109, 111, 197
– of triceps brachii muscle, long = Caput longum m. tricipitis brachii 110, 111, 197
– of mandible = Caput mandibulae 59, 60
– of radius (capitulum radii) = Caput radii 70, 71
– of talus = Caput tali 88, 89
– of ulna = Caput ulnae 69, 73
Heel bone (also os calcis) = Calcaneus 9, 10, 88–91, 130–133
Helix 173
Hernia, femoral = Hernia femoralis 233
Hiatus (also aperture) = Hiatus
–, aortic h. of diaphragm = Hiatus aorticus diaphragmatis 163, 166
–, esophageal = Hiatus (o) esophageus 166
– of facial canal for greater petrosal nerve = Hiatus canalis n. petrosi majoris 48
–, maxillary = Hiatus maxillaris 63
–, sacral = Hiatus sacralis 20, 21
–, saphenous = Hiatus saphenus 226
–, scalene = Hiatus scalenus 174–176
–, tendinous (adductorius) = Hiatus tendineus adductorius 232, 234, 239
–, urogenital and anal = Hiatus urogenitalis et ani 164
Hip (or hip joint) = Coxa 25, 80–83, 118–125
Hook (also hamulus) = Hamulus
– of hamate bone = Hamulus ossis hamati 73, 74, 115
Horn = Cornu
– of coccyx (coccygeal cornu) = cornu coccygeum 21
– of hyoid bone, greater = Cornu majus ossis hyoidei 60, 172, 187
– – – –, lesser = Cornu minus ossis hyoidei 60, 172, 187
Humerus 8, 11, 67, 68, 71, 198
Hypothenar eminence = Hypothenar 219

I

Impression (s) = Impressio (nes)
– of costoclavicular ligament = Impressio lig. costoclavicularis 67
– (s), digitate = Impressiones digitatae 35, 39, 49
Incisure (see also notch) = Incisura
Incisura poplitea extensoria femoris 85
– poplitea flexoria femoris 85
Incline, pelvic = Inclinatio pelvis 78, 79, 124
Infrahyoid musculature = Musculi infrahyoidei 169, 171, 174, 175
Intersections, tendinous i. of rectus abdominis muscle = Intersectiones (inscriptiones) tendineae m. recti abdom. 156, 158, 160

J

Joint (s) (see articulation or synchondrosis)
Joint (s) (Syndesmology) 93–137

K

Knee cap (also knee pan) = Patella 85, 126, 128, 232, 240, 241
– joint = Articulatio genus 92, 126–129
– pan (also knee cap) = Patella 86, 126, 128, 232, 240, 241

L

Labyrinth, ethmoidal = Labyrinthus ethmoidalis 54, 55, 61, 63
Lacertus fibrosus 198, 199
Lacuna musculorum 233
– vasorum 233
Lamina (also layer or plate) = Lamina
– tragi (auris externae) 173
Layer (also lamina or plate) = Lamina
–, pretracheal l. of cervical fascia = Lamina praetrachealis faciae cervicalis 173
–, superficial l. of cervical fascia = Lamina superficialis fasciae cervicalis 173
Ligament (s) = Ligamentum (a) 93–137
–, acromioclavicular = Ligamentum acromioclaviculare 109, 110, 111, 197
– (s), alar l. of axis = Ligamenta alaria (axis) 95
–, anococcygeal = Ligamentum anococcygeum 165
–, anular l. of radius = Ligamentum anulare radii 112
–, apical dental l. of axis = Ligamentum apicis dentis (axis) 95, 187
–, arcuate (lateral) l. of diaphragm = Ligamentum arcuatum laterale (diaphragmatis) 163, 166
–, – (medial) l. of diaphragm = Ligamentum arcuatum mediale (diaphragmatis) 163
–, – l. of pubis = Ligamentum arcuatum pubis 118, 119, 122–124, 165
–, auricular, anterior = Ligamentum auriculare anterius 173
–, –, superior = Ligamentum auriculare superius 173
–, bifurcate = Ligamentum bifurcatum 132
–, calcaneocuboid (part of bifurcate l.) = Ligamentum calcaneocuboideum (ligamenti bifurcati) 132
–, –, dorsal = Ligamentum calcaneocuboideum dorsale 132, 133
–, –, plantar = Ligamentum calcaneocuboideum plantare 136, 137
–, calcaneofibular = Ligamentum calcaneofibulare 130, 132, 134, 136
–, calcaneonavicular (part of bifurcate l.) = Ligamentum calcaneonaviculare (lig. bifurcati) 132
–, –, plantar = Ligamentum calcaneonaviculare plantare 131, 133, 136, 137
–, carpal, radiate = Ligamentum carpi radiatum 115, 220
–, collateral, fibular = Ligamentum collaterale fibulare 126, 127, 129, 242, 243
– (s), – (fingers) = Ligamenta collateralia 114
Ligament (s), collaterale l. of interphalangeal articulations = Ligamenta collateralia (artic. interphal. manus) 114
– (s), – – of metacarpophalangeal articulations = Ligamenta collateralis artic. metacarpophalangeae 114, 115
–, –, radial = Ligamentum collaterale radiale 112
–, –, – carpal = Ligamentum collaterale carpi radiale 113
–, conoid (part of coracoclavicular l.) = Ligamentum conoideum (lig. coracoclavicularis) 108, 109, 111, 197, 198
–, coracoacromial = Ligamentum coracoacromiale 109, 110, 111, 197
–, coracoclavicular = Ligamentum coracoclaviculare 109, 110, 197
–, coracohumeral = Ligamentum coracohumerale 109, 110, 197
– costotransverse = Ligamentum costotransversarium 97–100, 102, 148, 152
–, –, lateral = Ligamentum costotransversarium laterale 97–99, 102, 152
–, –, superior = Ligamentum costotransversarium superius 97–99, 102, 148
– (s), costoxiphoid = Ligamenta costoxiphoidea 154
–, cricothyroid = Ligamentum cricothyroideum 174
–, cruciate l. of knee, anterior = Ligamentum cruciatum anterius (art. genus) 127
–, – – – –, posterior = Ligamentum cruciatum posterius (art. genus) 127
–, cruciform l. of atlas = Ligamentum cruciforme atlantis 95
–, – (cruris) = Ligamentum cruciforme (cruris) 240, 241
– (s), cuneonavicular, dorsal = Ligamentum (a) cuneonaviculare (ia) dorsale (ia) 132, 133
–, –, plantar = Ligamentum (a) cuneonaviculare (ia) plantare (ia) 136
–, deltoid = Ligamentum deltoideum 130, 131, 134
–, flaval (yellow l.) = Ligamentum flavum 98–100, 102
–, fundiform l. of penis = Ligamentum fundiforme penis 154, 162
– (s), glenohumeral = Ligamentum (a) glenohumerale (ia) 109
– of head of femur = Ligamentum capitis femoris 124, 125
– – – of fibula, anterior = Ligamentum capitis fibulae anterius 127, 128, 241
– – – – –, posterior = Ligamentum capitis fibulae posterius 126
Ligament, (intraarticular) l. of head of rib = Ligamentum capitis costae intraarticulare 98
–, (radiate) l. of head of rib = Ligamentum capitis costae radiatum 97, 102
–, iliofemoral = Ligamentum iliofemorale 118–121, 125, 166
–, iliolumbal = Ligamentum iliolumbale 118–121, 123, 166
–, inguinal = Ligamentum inguinale 118–122, 156, 159, 160, 166, 226, 228, 232
– (s), intercarpal, dorsal = Ligamentum (a) intercarpeum (a) dorsale (ia) 114
–, interclavicular = Ligamentum interclaviculare 108, 169
– (s), intercuneiform, dorsal = Ligamentum (a) intercuneiforme (ia) dorsale (ia) 133
–, interfoveolar = Ligamentum interfoveolare 160
–, interspinal = Ligamentum interspinale 98, 148
–, intertransverse = Ligamentum intertransversarium 97, 99, 148
–, ischiofemoral = Ligamentum ischiofemorale 80–83, 125, 230
–, lacunar = Ligamentum lacunare 121, 228
–, lateral l. of temporomandibular articulation = Ligamentum laterale (art. temporomandibularis) 104, 183, 185
–, longitudinal (vertebral column), anterior = Ligamentum longitudinale anterius (columnae vertebral.) 94, 97, 118–121, 166
–, – – –, posterior = Ligamentum longitudinale posterius (columnae vertebral.) 101
– (s), metacarpal, dorsal = Ligamentum (a) metacarpeum (a) dorsale (ia) 114
– (s), –, interosseous = Ligamenta metacarpea interossea 113
– (s), –, palmar = Ligamenta metacarpea palmaria 115
–, – (deep) transverse = Ligamentum metacarpeum transversum profundum 115, 216, 220
–, –, (superficial) transverse = Ligamentum metacarpeum transversum superficiale 213
– (s), metatarsal, dorsal = Ligamentum (a) metatarseum (a) dorsale (ia) 132, 135–137
– (s), –, interosseous = Ligamentum (a) metatarseum (a) interosseum (a) 135
– (s), –, plantar = Ligamentum (a) metatarseum (a) plantare (ia) 137
–, –, (deep) transverse = Ligamentum metatarseum transversum profundum 132, 136, 137

Ligament, metatarsal, (superficial) transverse = Ligamentum metatarseum transversum superficiale 136
– (s), palmar = Ligamenta palmaria 115
–, palpebral, medial = Ligamentum palpebrale mediale 169, 178, 183
–, patellar = Ligamentum patellae 126–129, 232, 234, 238, 248
– (s), pelvic = Ligamenta pelvis 118–124
–, pisohamate = Ligamentum pisohamatum 115, 220
–, pisometacarpal = Ligamentum pisometacarpeum 115
– (s), plantar = Ligamenta plantaria 131, 132, 134, 136, 137
–, –, long = Ligamentum plantare longum 131, 132, 134, 136, 256
–, popliteal, arcuate = Ligamentum popliteum arcuatum 126, 244
–, –, oblique = Ligamentum popliteum obliquum 126, 244, 246
–, pterygospinal = Ligamentum pterygospinale 105, 188
–, pubic, superior = Ligamentum pubicum superius 118–120
–, pubofemoral = Ligamentum pubofemorale 125
–, radiocarpal, dorsal = Ligamentum radiocarpeum dorsale 114
–, –, palmar = Ligamentum radiocarpeum palmare 115, 218, 220
–, reflex *(Gimbernati)* = Ligamentum reflexum 154, 159, 162
–, sacrococcygeal, deep dorsal = Ligamentum sacrococcygeum dorsale profundum 122
–, –, lateral = Ligamentum sacrococcygeum laterale 120, 124
–, –, superficial dorsal = Ligamentum sacrococcygeum dorsale superficiale 122, 123
–, –, ventral = Lig. sacrococcygeum ventrale 118, 120, 124, 164
– (s), sacroiliac, dorsal = Ligamentum (a) sacroiliacum (a) dorsale (ia) 123, 124
– (s), –, interosseous = Ligamentum (a) sacroiliacum (a) interosseum (a) 124, 164
– (s), –, ventral = Ligamentum (a) sacroiliacum (a) ventrale (ia) 118–120, 124, 164
–, sacrospinal = Ligamentum sacrospinale 122–124, 164, 166, 230, 232, 242
–, sacrotuberal = Ligamentum sacrotuberale 122–124, 142, 164, 165, 166, 228, 230, 236
–, sphenomandibular = Ligamentum sphenomandibulare 105, 187
–, sternoclavicular, anterior = Ligamentum sternoclaviculare anterius 108
Ligament, sternocostal, intraarticular = Ligamentum sternocostale intraarticulare 103
– (s), –, radiate = Ligamentum (a) sternocostale (ia) radiatum (a) 108
–, stylohyoid = Ligamentum stylohyoideum 172, 173, 187, 188
–, stylomandibular = Ligamentum stylomandibulare 104, 105, 187, 188
–, supraspinous = Ligamentum supraspinale 99, 123
–, suspensory l. of penis = Ligamentum suspensorium penis 154
–, talocalcaneal, interosseous = Ligamentum talocalcaneum interosseum 133, 135
–, –, lateral = Ligamentum talocalcaneale laterale 132
–, –, medial = Ligamentum talocalcaneale mediale 130
–, –, posterior = Ligamentum talocalcaneale posterius 130
–, talofibular, anterior = Ligamentum talofibulare anterius 128, 132
–, –, posterior = Ligamentum talofibulare posterius 130
– (s) tarsometatarsal, dorsal = Ligamentum (a) tarsometatarseum (a) dorsale (ia) 131–133
– (s), –, interosseous = Ligamentum (a) tarsometatarseum (a) interosseum (a) 135
–, –, plantar = Ligamentum tarsometatarseum plantare 136, 137
– (s) of tarsus, interosseous = Ligamentum (a) tarsi interosseum (a) 135
– (s) – –, plantar = Ligamentum (a) tarsi plantare (ia) 137
–, thyrohyoid, median = Ligamentum thyrohyoideum medianum 174
–, tibiofibular, anterior = Ligamentum tibiofibulare anterius 128, 132
–, –, posterior = Ligamentum tibiofibulare posterius 130
–, transverse l. of acetabulum = Ligamentum transversum acetabuli 125, 165
–, – – of atlas = Ligamentum transversum atlantis 96
–, – – of knee = Ligamentum transversum genus 127
– (s), – – of palm, superficial = Fasciculi transversi aponeurosis palmaris 213
–, –, perineal (pelvic) = Ligamentum transversum perinei 165
–, – l. of scapula = Ligamentum transversum scapulae 109, 110, 198
–, trapezoid (part of coracoclavicular l.) = Ligamentum trapezoideum (lig. coracoclavicularis) 109, 111, 197, 198
–, ulnocarpal, palmar = Ligamentum ulnocarpeum palmare 115, 220
Ligamentum carpi palmare (volare) 216, 218
– – radiale 220
– – ulnare 220
– nuchae 142, 144, 146, 175
Line (or linea) = Linea
–, arcuate l. of pelvis = Linea arcuata pelvis 83
–, – – of rectus sheath = Linea arcuata vaginae m. recti abdominis 158, 160
–, – – of sciatic bone = Linea arcuata ossis ischii 83
–, epiphyseal = Linea epiphyseos 8, 71, 75, 76, 91
–, gluteal, anterior = Linea glutaea anterior 81
–, –, inferior = Linea glutaea inferior 81
–, –, posterior = Linea glutaea posterior
–, intercondylar l. of femur = Linea intercondylaris femoris 84
–, intermediate l. of iliac crest = Linea intermedia cristae iliacae 81–83
–, intertrochanteric = Linea intertrochanterica 84, 85
–, muscular (of scapula) = Linea muscularis 66
–, mylohyoid = Linea mylohyoidea 60, 172
–, nuchal, inferior = Linea nuchae inferior 37, 42, 44
–, –, superior = Linea nuchae superior 37, 42, 44
–, –, supreme = Linea nuchae suprema 44
–, oblique l. of mandible = Linea obliqua mandibulae 59
–, pectineal l. of femur = Linea pectinea femoris 84, 85
–, semilunar = Linea semilunaris 158
– of *spighelli* = semilunar line 158
–, temporal l. of frontal bone =Linea temporalis ossis frontalis 52
–, (inferior) temporal l. of parietal bone = Linea temporalis inferior ossis parietalis 41, 53
–, – – – of temporal bone = Linea temporalis inferior ossis temporalis 47
–, (superior) temporal l. of temporal bone = Linea temporalis superior ossis parietalis 41, 53
– (s), transverse l. of sacrum = Linea (ae) transverse ossis sacri 20
–, trapezoid = Linea trapezoidea 67
Linea alba 154, 159–162
– aspera femoris 84, 85, 239
– musculi solei 86
– terminalis (pelvis) 20, 120, 164, 166
Lingula of mandible = Lingula mandibulae 60, 105
– of sphenoid bone = Lingula sphenoidalis 45, 46
Lip = Labium or labrum
–, acetabular = Labrum acetabulare 125

Lip, glenoid = Labrum glenoidale 111, 197
- of iliac crest, external = Labium externum cristae iliacae 82
- - - -, internal = Labium internum cristae iliacae 81–83
- of linea aspera of femur, lateral = Labium laterale lineae asperae femoris 84, 85
- - - - - -, medial = Labium mediale lineae asperae femoris 84, 85
Lower limb (Joints and ligaments) 92, 118–137
- - (Muscles) 226–259
- - (Osteology) 84–92

M

Malleolus, lateral = Malleolus lateralis 87, 128, 130, 134
–, medial = Malleolus medialis 86, 87, 248
Malleus (Hammer) = Malleus 49
Mandible = Mandibula 31, 33, 40, 59, 60, 172
Manubrium of sternum = Manubrium sterni 24, 25, 103, 108, 160
Margin (also border, crest or ridge) = Crista
Margin (also border or crest) = Margo
–, anterior m. of ulna = Margo anterior ulnae 71
–, frontal m. of parietal bone = Margo frontalis ossis parietalis 53
–, - - of (greater) wing of sphenoid bone = Margo frontalis alae majoris ossis sphenoidalis 46
–, infraorbital m. (of maxilla) = Margo infraorbitalis 31, 54, 57
–, lambdoid m. of occipital bone = Margo lambdoideus ossis occipitalis 44, 45
–, mastoid m. of occipital bone = Margo mastoideus ossis occipitalis 44, 45
–, occipital m. of parietal bone = Margo occipitalis ossis parietalis 53
–, - - of temporal bone = Margo occipitalis ossis temporalis 47, 48
–, parietal m. of frontal bone = Margo parietalis ossis frontalis 52
–, - - of temporal bone = Margo parietalis ossis temporalis 47
–, - - of (great) wing of sphenoid bone = Margo parietalis alae majoris ossis sphenoidalis 45, 46
–, posterior m. of petrosal part of temporal bone = Margo posterior partis petrosae ossis temporalis 47, 48
–, - - of ulna = Margo posterior ulnae 71
–, sagittal m. of parietal bone = Margo sagittalis ossis parietalis 53
Margin, sphenoidal m. of frontal bone = Margo sphenoidalis ossis frontalis 52
–, - - of temporal bone = Margo sphenoidalis ossis temporalis 47, 48
–, squamous m. of parietal bone = Margo squamosus ossis parietalis 53
–, - - of (great) wing of sphenoid bone = Margo squamosus alae majoris ossis sphenoidalis 45, 46
–, superior m. of petrosal part of temporal bone = Margo superior partis petrosae ossis temporalis 39, 47
–, supraorbital m. of frontal bone = Margo supraorbitalis 31, 51, 52
–, zygomatic m. of (great) wing of sphenoid bone = Margo zygomaticus alae majoris ossis sphenoidalis 46
Mass = Massa
–, lateral m. of atlas = Massa lateralis atlantis 16
Maxilla 30–37, 57, 58, 61–63
Meatus, acoustic, external = Meatus acusticus externus 33, 37, 47, 48, 50, 104
–, –, internal = Meatus acusticus internus 35, 39, 47
–, nasal, inferior = Meatus nasi inferior 61, 63
–, –, middle = Meatus nasi medius 63
–, –, superior = Meatus nasi superior 63
Membrane, atlantooccipital, anterior = Membrana atlantooccipitalis anterior 94, 176, 187
–, –, posterior = Membrana atlantooccipitalis posterior 94, 150, 187
–, interosseous m. of forearm = Membrana interossea antebrachii 71, 112, 210, 211
–, - - of leg = Membrana interossea cruris 128
–, obturator = Membrana obturatoria 118, 119, 124, 125, 166
–, tectorial = Membrana tectoria 94, 96
–, tympanic = Membrana tympani 49
Meniscus lateralis art. genu 92, 127–129
- medialis art. genu 92, 127, 129
Mesotendineum 216
Metacarpus 72–76, 113–115
Metatarsus 88, 89, 91, 132–137
Mimetic musculature 178–185
Middle ear = Auris media 49, 50
Muscle (s) (see also sheath or tendon of m.) = Musculus (li)
–, abductor m. of great toe = Musculus abductor hallucis 240, 251, 253, 254, 256, 257
–, - - of little finger = Musculus abductor digiti minimi (manus) 212, 215, 216, 219, 220, 223, 224
–, - - of little toe = Musculus abductor digiti minimi (pedis) 241, 251, 253, 254, 256, 257
Muscle, (long) abductor m. of thumb = Musculus abductor pollicis longus 192, 199, 202, 204, 206, 208, 209, 211, 212, 214, 224
–, (short) abductor m. of thumb = Musculus abductor pollicis brevis 213, 215, 216, 218, 220, 221, 223, 224
–, adductor, great = Musculus adductor magnus 228–230, 234, 236, 239, 242, 243
–, – m. of great toe = Musculus adductor hallucis 251, 253, 254, 256, 257
–, –, long = Musculus adductor longus 228, 232, 234, 235, 242, 243
–, –, short = Musculus adductor brevis 230, 234, 235, 236, 242, 243
–, –, smallest = Musculus adductor minimus 230, 234, 236
–, – m. of thumb = Musculus adductor pollicis 192, 215, 216, 218, 220, 221, 223, 224
–, anconeus = Musculus anconeus 192, 194, 195, 200, 206, 208, 211
–, articular m. of elbow = Musculus articularis cubiti 201, 210, 211
–, - - of knee = Musculus articularis genus 126, 242
–, auricular, anterior = Musculus auricularis anterior 169, 171, 181
–, –, posterior = Musculus auricularis posterior 171
–, –, superior = Musculus auricularis superior 173
–, biceps m. of arm = Musculus biceps brachii 112, 141, 192, 196–198, 199, 201, 206, 210
–, - - of thigh = Musculus biceps femoris 229, 230, 236–239, 241–243, 248, 250
–, brachial = Musculus brachialis 112, 141, 192, 194, 196–202, 210, 211
–, brachioradial = Musculus brachioradialis 192, 194, 199–202, 204, 206, 207, 208, 210, 211, 224
–, buccinator = Musculus buccinatorius 169, 178, 182, 183, 185, 187
–, coccygeal = Musculus coccygeus 164, 165, 228, 242
–, coracobrachial = Musculus coracobrachialis 162, 191, 196–198, 201
–, corrugator superciliary = Musculus corrugator supercillii 178, 179, 183
–, cremaster = Musculus cremaster 154, 156, 162
–, cricothyroid = Musculus cricothyroideus 174
–, deltoid = Musculus deltoideus 191–194, 196–198, 200, 201
–, depressor m. of angle of mouth = Musculus depressor anguli oris 168, 169, 178, 181–183, 185
–, - - of lower lip = Musculus depressor labii inferioris 169, 178, 181–183, 185

Muscle, depressor m. of nasal septum = Musculus depressor septi 178, 180
–, – superciliary = Musculus depressor supercilii 178, 179, 181–183
–, digastric = Musculus digastricus 162, 169, 170, 172–176, 185, 187, 188
–, epicranial = Musculus epicranius 169, 178, 181, 183, 185
–, erector m. of spine = Musculus erector spinae 144, 146, 147, 152, 153
–, extensor m. of fingers = Musculus extensor digitorum (manus) 192, 200, 206, 207, 211, 212, 214
–, – – of great toe, long = Musculus extensor hallucis longus 92, 240, 241, 248–250, 253, 259
–, – – – – – –, short = Musculus extensor hallucis brevis 248, 252, 253, 259
–, – – of index finger = Musculus extensor indicis 208, 209, 211, 212, 214, 223
–, – – of little finger = Musculus extensor digiti minimi 206–208, 211, 212, 214
–, – – of thumb, long = Musculus extensor pollicis longus 192, 206, 208, 209, 211, 212, 214, 223
–, – – – – –, short = Musculus extensor pollicis brevis 192, 199, 206, 208, 209, 211, 212, 214
–, – – of toes, long = Musculus extensor digitorum longus (pedis) 92, 241, 242, 248–250, 252, 253, 259
–, – – – – –, short = Musculus extensor digitorum brevis (pedis) 241, 248, 252, 253, 259
–, – – of wrist, (long) radial = Musculus extensor carpi radialis longus 192, 194, 196, 200, 201, 206–208, 210–212
–, – – – – –, (short) radial = Musculus extensor carpi radialis brevis 192, 200, 201, 206–208, 210–212
–, – – – – –, ulnar = Musculus extensor carpi ulnaris 200, 206–208, 211, 212
–, flexor m. of fingers, deep = Musculus flexor digitorum profundus 201, 204, 205, 210, 211, 220, 224
–, – – – – –, superficial = Musculus flexor digitorum superficialis 199, 201–204, 210, 216, 224
–, – – of great toe, long = Musculus flexor hallucis longus 92, 240, 246, 247, 250, 251, 254, 256, 259
–, – – – – – –, short = Musculus flexor hallucis brevis 251, 254, 256, 257
–, – – of little finger, short = Musculus flexor digiti minimi brevis (manus) 216, 218–220, 223, 224
Muscle, flexor m. of little toe, short = Musculus flexor digiti minimi (pedis) 251, 254, 256, 257
–, – – of thumb, long = Musculus flexor pollicis longus 192, 299, 202, 204, 205, 210
–, – – – – –, short = Musculus flexor pollicis brevis 216, 218, 220, 221, 223, 224
–, – – of toes, long = Musculus flexor digitorum longus (pedis) 92, 240, 243, 244, 246, 247, 250, 251, 256
–, – – – – –, short = Musculus flexor digitorum brevis (pedis) 251, 254–256
–, flexor m. of wrist, radial = Musculus flexor carpi radialis 192, 198, 199, 201–204, 210, 224
–, – – – – –, ulnar = Musculus flexor carpi ulnaris 199, 201–204, 206, 208, 210, 211, 216, 224
–, gastrocnemius = Musculus gastrocnemius 229, 236, 239–241, 243–245, 248
–, gemellus, inferior = Musculus gemellus inferior 142, 230, 231, 236, 243
–, –, superior = Musculus gemellus superior 142, 230, 231, 236, 243
–, genioglossus = Musculus genioglossus 172, 187, 188
–, geniohyoid = Musculus geniohyoideus 170, 172, 187, 188
–, gluteal, greatest = Musculus glutaeus maximus 141, 142, 228–231, 236, 238, 242, 243
–, –, least = Musculus glutaeus minimus 230, 231, 236, 242, 243
–, –, middle = Musculus glutaeus medius 142, 230, 231, 236, 243
–, gracilis = Musculus gracilis 228–230, 232, 234–236, 242, 243, 250
–, great, intermediate = Musculus vastus intermedius 233, 234, 242, 243
–, –, lateral = Musculus vastus lateralis 232–234, 238, 242, 243
–, –, medial = Musculus vastus medialis 232–234, 240, 242, 243
– of helix, larger = Musculus helicis major 173
– – –, smaller = Musculus helicis minor 173
–, hyoglossus = Musculus hyoglossus 162, 187
–, iliac = Musculus iliacus 166, 228, 232, 242
–, iliocostal m. of loin = Musculus iliocostalis lumborum 146
–, – – of neck = Musculus iliocostalis cervicis 146, 147, 175
–, – – of thorax = Musculus iliocostalis thoracis 144, 146, 147, 152
–, iliopsoas = Musculus iliopsoas 166, 228, 232, 234, 242, 243
Muscle infraspinous = Musculus infraspinatus 110, 141, 142, 144, 191, 193, 194, 197, 200
–, intercostal, cervical = Musculus intercostalis cervicis 176
– (s), –, external = Musculi intercostales externi 146, 148, 152, 156, 158, 162, 166, 174
–, –, innermost = Musculi intercostales intimi 148, 152
– (s), –, internal = Musculi intercostales interni 148, 150, 152, 156, 158, 160, 166
– (s), interosseous m. of hand dorsal = Musculi interossei dorsales (manus) 192, 208, 212–214, 216, 218, 222–224
– (s), – – of foot, dorsal = Musculi interossei dorsales (pedis) 251–253, 258
– (s), –, palmar = Musculi interossei palmares 216, 218, 220, 222–224
– (s), –, plantar = Musculi interossei plantares 251, 253, 256, 258
– (s), interspinal m. of loin = Musculi interspinales lumborum 148
– (s), – – of neck = Musculi interspinales cervicis 148, 150
– (s), intertransverse m. of loin, lateral = Musculi intertransversarii laterales lumborum 148, 152
– (s), – – – –, medial = Musculi intertransversarii mediales lumborum 148, 152
– (s), – – of neck, anterior = Musculi intertransversarii anteriores cervicis 176
– (s), – – of neck, posterior = Musculi intertransversarii posteriores cervicis 148, 150
– (s), – – of thorax = Musculi intertransversarii thoracis 148, 152
–, latissimus m. of back = Musculus latissimus dorsi 141–144, 153, 162, 191, 198, 200, 201
–, levator m. of angle of mouth = Musculus levator anguli oris 169, 178, 182, 183
–, – ani = Musculus levator ani 164, 165, 243
– (s), – m. of ribs = Musculi levatores costarum 146, 148, 150, 152
– (s), – – – –, long = Musculi levatores costarum longi 148, 152
– (s), – – – –, short = Musculi levatores costarum breves 148, 152
–, – – scapula = Musculus levator scapulae 141–144, 146, 162, 169, 176, 192, 198, 200
–, – – of upper lip = Musculus levator labii superioris 169, 178, 181–183

Muscle, levator m. of upper lip and ala of nose = Musculus levator labii superioris alaeque nasi 178, 181–183
–, – – of velum palatini = Musculus levator veli palatini 187, 188
–, long m. of head = Musculus longus capitis 176, 177, 188
–, long m. of neck = Musculus longus colli 166, 176, 177
–, longissimus m. of head = Musculus longissimus capitis 146–148, 175, 176, 188
–, – – of neck = Musculus longissimus cervicis 146–148, 175
–, – – of thorax = Musculus longissimus thoracis 144, 146, 147, 152
– (s), lumbrical m. of hand = Musculi lumbricales (manus) 215–218, 223
– (s), – – of foot = Musculi lumbricales (pedis) 254, 256
–, masseter = Musculus masseter 183–185, 188
–, mental (chin m.) = Musculus mentalis
– (s), multifidus = Musculi multifidi 148–150, 152
–, mylohyoid = Musculus mylohyoideus 162, 169, 170, 172–174, 187, 188
–, nasal = Musculus nasalis 169, 178, 180, 181, 183, 185
–, oblique muscle of abdomen, external = Musculus obliquus externus abdominis 141, 142, 144, 153–162, 243
–, – – – –, internal = Musculus obliquus internus abdominis 146, 148, 156–158, 160–162, 242
–, – – of head, inferior = Musculus obliquus capitis inferior 148, 150, 151
–, – – – –, superior = Musculus obliquus capitis superior 148, 150, 151, 188
–, obturator, external = Musculus obturatorius externus 230, 235, 236, 242, 243
–, –, internal = Musculus obturator internus 165, 228, 230, 231, 236, 242, 243
–, occipitofrontal = Musculus occipitofrontalis 169, 178, 180, 181, 183, 185
–, omohyoid = Musculus omohyoideus 141, 162, 169, 171, 173–175, 200, 201
–, opposing m. of little finger = Musculus oppenens digiti minimi (manus) 215, 218–220, 223, 224
–, – – of little toe = Musculus opponens digiti minimi 241, 256, 257
–, – – of thumb = Musculus oppenens pollicis 215, 216, 218, 220, 221, 223, 224
Muscle, orbicular m. of eye = Musculus orbicularis oculi 169, 178, 179, 181, 183, 185
–, – – of mouth = Musculus orbicularis oris 169, 178, 181–183, 187
–, palmar, long = Musculus palmaris longus 199, 203, 213, 216
–, –, short = Musculus palmaris brevis 199, 213, 223
–, pectineal = Musculus pectineus 232, 234, 235, 242, 243
–, pectoral, greater = Musculus pectoralis major 141, 154, 162, 169, 174, 191, 192, 197, 198, 200, 201
–, –, smaller = Musculus pectoralis minor 162, 191, 192, 197, 198, 201
–, peroneal (fibular), long = Musculus peroneus (fibularis) longus 92, 241, 242, 244, 246, 248–251, 256
–, – –, short = Musculus peroneus (fibularis) brevis 92, 132, 241, 246, 248–250, 253
–, – –, third = Musculus peroneus (fibularis) tertius 241, 248, 249, 252, 253, 259
–, piriform = Musculus piriformis 142, 228, 230–232, 236, 242, 243
–, plantar = Musculus plantaris 229, 238, 239, 241, 243–245
–, popliteal = Musculus popliteus 126, 129, 243, 245, 246, 250
–, procerus = Musculus procerus 178, 179, 183
–, pronator, quadrate = Musculus pronator quadratus 199, 202, 204, 210, 218, 220
–, –, round = Musculus pronator teres 192, 198, 199, 201–204, 210, 211
–, psoas, greater = Musculus psoas major 153, 166, 228, 232, 242
–, –, smaller = Musculus psoas minor 166, 228
–, pterygoid, lateral = Musculus pterygoideus lateralis 184, 186–188
–, –, medial = Musculus pterygoideus medialis 184, 186–188
–, pyramidal = Musculus pyramidalis 156, 158, 159
–, quadrate m. of loins = Musculus quadratus lumborum 153, 163, 164, 166, 242
–, – – of sole = Musculus quadratus plantae (flexor accessorius) 251, 255, 256
–, – – of thigh = Musculus quadratus femoris 142, 230, 231, 236, 242, 243
–, quadriceps m. of thigh = Musculus quadriceps femoris 232–234, 242, 250
–, rectococcygeal = Musculus rectococcygeus 164
–, rhomboid, greater = Musculus rhomboideus major 142–144, 198, 200
–, –, lesser = Musculus rhombrideus minor 142–144, 198, 200
Muscle, risorius = Musculus risorius 168, 178, 181–183
– (s) rotator = Musculi rotatores 148, 149, 152
– (s), –, long = Musculi rotatores longi 148, 149, 152
– (s), –, short = Musculi rotatores breves 148, 149, 152
– (s), – m. of thorax = Musculi rotatores thoracis 148, 149, 152
–, sacrococcygeal, ventral = Musculus sacrococcygeus ventralis 164, 228
–, sartorius = Musculus sartorius 141, 228, 229, 232, 233, 240, 242, 243, 250
–, scalene, anterior = Musculus scalenus anterior 162, 165, 169, 175–177
–, –, middle = Musculus scalenus medius 141, 144, 150, 166, 168, 169, 175–177, 192
–, –, posterior = Musculus scalenus posterior 141, 144, 146, 148, 150, 162, 166, 176, 177, 192
–, semimembranous = Musculus semimembranosus 229, 230, 236, 237, 239, 240, 242–244, 250
–, semispinal m. of head = Musculus semispinalis capitis 142, 144, 146, 148, 150, 169, 175, 185, 188
–, – – of neck = Musculus semispinalis 146, 148, 150, 175
–, – – of thorax = Musculus semispinalis thoracis 148, 152
–, semitendinous = Musculus semitendinosus 228–230, 236, 237, 240, 242–244, 250
–, serratus, anterior = Musculus serratus anterior 141, 154–156, 162, 191, 192, 198, 201
–, –, posterior inferior = Musculus serratus posterior inferior 144–146
–, –, – superior = Musculus serratus posterior superior 142, 144, 145
–, soleus = Musculus soleus 240, 241, 243–246, 248
–, sphincter m. of anus, external = Musculus sphincter ani externus 165
–, spinal m. of thorax = Musculus spinalis thoracis 144, 146, 147, 152
–, splenius m. of head = Musculus splenius capitis 142, 144–146, 148, 150, 162, 175, 181, 185, 188
–, – – of neck = Musculus splenius cervicis 142, 144–146, 169, 175, 176, 192
–, sternocleidomastoid = Musculus sternocleidomastoideus 141, 142, 154, 169, 171, 173, 174, 181, 183, 188, 192
–, sternohyoid = Musculus sternohyoideus 162, 169, 171, 173–175, 185, 192, 200
–, sternothyroid = Musculus sternothyroideus 160, 162, 169, 171, 174, 175, 185

Muscle, straight m. of abdomen = Musculus rectus abdominis 156, 158–161
–, – – of head, anterior = Musculus rectus capitis anterior 176, 177, 178
–, – – of head, lateral = Musculus rectus capitis lateralis 150, 151, 176, 188
–, – – – –, greater posterior = Musculus rectus capitis posterior major 148, 150, 151, 188
–, – – – –, smaller posterior = Musculus rectus capitis posterior minor 148, 150, 151, 188
–, – – of thigh = Musculus rectus femoris 125, 232–234, 242, 243
–, styloglossus = Musculus styloglossus 185, 187, 188
–, stylohyoid = Musculus stylohyoideus 162, 169, 170, 172–175, 185, 187, 188, 200
–, stylopharyngeal = Musculus stylopharyngeus 187, 188
–, subclavius = Musculus subclavius 162, 174, 197, 198, 200, 201
– (s), subcostal = Musculi subcostales 166
–, subscapular = Musculus subscapularis 162, 191, 193, 198, 201
–, supinator = Musculus supinator 199, 201, 204, 208–211
–, supraspinous = Musculus supraspinatus 110, 142, 144, 191, 193, 197, 198, 200, 201
–, temporal = Musculus temporalis 184, 185, 188
–, temporoparietal = Musculus temporoparietalis 169, 178, 180, 181, 183
–, tensor m. of fascia lata = Musculus tensor fasciae latae 141, 226, 231, 232, 236, 238, 243
–, – – of velum palatini = Musculus tensor veli palatini 187, 188
–, teres major = Musculus teres major 141, 142, 144, 191–194, 196, 198, 200, 201
–, – minor = Musculus teres minor 141, 142, 144, 191–194, 197, 200
–, thyrohyoid = Musculus thyrohyoideus 162, 169, 171, 174, 185
–, tibial, anterior = Musculus tibialis anterior 92, 131, 240–242, 248–251
–, –, posterior = Musculus tibialis posterior 92, 131, 137, 243, 246, 247, 250, 251
–, tragicus 173
–, transverse m. of abdomen = Musculus transversus abdominis 148, 153, 157, 158, 160, 161, 166, 242
–, (deep) transverse m. of perineum = Musculus transversus perinei profundus 165, 243
Muscle, (superficial) transverse m. of perineum = Musculus transversus perinei superficialis 165
–, transverse m. of thorax = Musculus transversus thoracis 160
–, trapezius = Musculus trapezius 141–144, 169, 188, 192, 200, 201
–, triceps m. of arm = Musculus triceps brachii 110, 111, 141, 142, 191, 192, 194–198, 200, 201, 211
–, zygomatic, greater = Musculus zygomaticus major 169, 178, 181–183, 188
–, –, smaller = Musculus zygomaticus minor 169, 178, 181–183, 188
Myology 139–259

N

Nasal cavity = Cavum nasi 61–63
Neck (Muscles) 141–151, 162, 168–177
Neck = Collum
–, anatomical n. of humerus = Collum anatonicum humeri 67, 68
– of femur = Collum femoris 84, 85, 125
– of mandible = Collum mandibulae 60, 186
– of radius = Collum radii 70
– of rib = Collum costae 22, 102
– of scapula = Collum scapulae 66
–, surgical n. of humeri = Collum chirurgicum humeri 68, 191, 194
– of talus = Collum tali 89
Nerve (s) = Nervus (i)
–, auricular, great = Nervus auricularis magnus 168
–, facial = Nervus facialis 179
–, gluteal, inferior = Nervus glutaeus inferior 230
–, median = Nervus medianus 199, 216, 223
–, musculocutaneous = Nervus musculocutaneus 196, 197
–, peroneal, common = Nervus peroneus communis 229, 241
–, sciatic = Nervus ischiadicus 142, 230
–, tibial = Nervus tibialis 229
–, ulnar = Nervus ulnaris 199, 216
–, vagus = Nervus vagus 185
Nostrils = Nares 4
Notch (also incisure) = Incisura
–, acetabular = Incisura acetabuli 81
–, clavicular n. of sternum = Incisura clavicularis sterni 24
–, costal = Incisura costalis 24
–, ethmoid n. of frontal bone = Incisura ethmoidalis ossis frontalis 51
–, fibular n. of tibia = Incisura fibularis tibiae 86
–, frontal n. of frontal bone = Incisura frontalis ossis frontalis 52
–, jugular n. of occipital bone = Incisura jugularis ossis occipitalis 45
–, – – of sternum = Incisura jugularis sterni 24
Notch, lacrimal n. of maxilla = Incisura lacrimalis maxillae 57
–, mandibular n. = Incisura mandibulae 59, 60
–, mastoid n. of temporal bone = Incisura mastoidea ossis temporalis 37, 42, 47, 48
–, nasal n. of maxilla = Incisura nasalis maxillae 57
–, parietal n. of temporal bone = Incisura parietalis ossis temporalis 47, 48
–, pterygoid = Incisura pterygoidea 46
–, radial n. of ulna = Incisura radialis ulnae 69
–, scapular = Incisura scapulae 66
–, sciatic, greater = Incisura ischiadica major 81, 83
–, –, lesser = Incisura ischiadica minor 81, 83
–, sphenopalatine n. of palatine bone = Incisura sphenopalatina ossis palatini 56, 57
–, supraorbital n. of frontal bone = Incisura supraorbitalis ossis frontalis 51, 55
–, trochlear n. of ulna = Incisura trochlearis ulnae 69, 70
–, ulnar n. of radius = Incisura ulnaris radii 70
–, vertebral, inferior = Incisura vertebralis inferior 18
Nuchal musculature 150, 151
Nucleus, palpous = Nucleus pulposus 98

O

Olecranon ulnae 69–71, 192, 194
Orbita 61, 62
Os (sa) see also bone (s)
–, calcis (also heel bone) = Calcaneus
–, capitate = Os capitatum 72–76, 113–115
– (sa), carpal = Ossa carpi 72–76, 113–115
–, coccygeal = Os coccygis 15, 21, 25, 165
–, coxae 25, 80–83
–, cuboid = Os cuboideum 88–91, 135
–, cuneiform, intermediate = Os cuneiforme intermedium 88–91
–, –, lateral = Os cuneiforme laterale 88–91
–, –, medial = Os cuneiforme mediale 88–91
–, ethmoid = Os ethmoidale 35, 54, 55, 61–63
– (sa) of foot = Ossa pedis 88–91
–, frontal = Os frontale 30–35, 39, 51, 52, 55, 61, 62
–, hamate = Os hamatum 72–76, 113, 114
– (sa) of hand = Ossa manus 72–76
–, hyoid = Os hyoideum 60, 162, 169, 172, 174, 185, 187
–, ilium = Os ilium 25, 80–83, 164
–, incisive = Os incisivum 40
–, interparietal = Os interparietale 42

Os, ischium = Os ischii 25, 80–83
–, lacrimal = Os lacrimale 30–33, 61, 62
–, lunate = Os lunatum 72–76, 113, 115
– (sa), metacarpal = Ossa metacarpalia 72–76, 113–115
– (sa), metatarsal = Ossa metatarsalia 88–91
–, nasal = Os nasale 30–35, 61, 62
–, navicular = Os naviculare 88–91, 135
–, occipital = Os occipitale 33–42, 44, 45
–, palatine = Os palatinum 35, 56–58
–, parietal = Os parietale 31–43, 53
–, pisiform = Os pisiforme 72–75, 115
–, pubic (pubis) = Os pubis 80–83, 160, 164, 165
–, sacrum 15, 20, 21, 164, 165
–, scaphoid = Os scaphoideum (naviculare) 72–75, 113, 114
– (sa), sesamoid (hand) = Ossa sesamoidea (manus) 73–75, 88, 115, 220
– (sa), sesamoid (foot) = Ossa sesamoidea (pedis) 88, 251
–, sphenoid = Os sphenoidale 31, 34–39, 45, 46, 55–58, 63, 105
– (sa), sutural = Ossa suturarum 42
– (sa), tarsal = Ossa tarsi 88–91, 135
–, temporal = Os temporale 9, 32–35, 47–50
–, trapezium = Os trapezium (multangulum majus) 72–75, 113
–, trapezoid = Os trapezoideum (multangulum minus) 72–75, 113, 114
–, triquetral (or triangular) = Os triquetrum 72–76, 113, 114
–, zygomatic = Os zygomaticum 31, 33, 40, 54, 61, 104
Osteology 7–92
Ostium canalis nasofrontalis 63

P

Palate, hard = Palatum durum 58, 187
Palm of hand = Palma manus 2, 3, 213, 215
Pars (also part or portion) = Pars
–, alveolar p. of mandible = Pars alveolaris mandibulae 59
– anularis vaginae fibrosae digiti manus 216, 220
–, basilar p. of occipital bone = Pars basilaris ossis occipitalis 44
–, costal p. of diaphragm = Pars costalis diaphragmatis 163
– cruciforme vaginae fibrosae digiti manus 216, 220
–, lateral p. of occipital bone = Pars lateralis ossis occipitalis 44, 45
–, – – of sacrum = Pars lateralis ossis sacri 20, 21
–, lumbar p. of diaphragm = Pars lumbalis diaphragmatis 163
Pars, mastoid p. of temporal bone = Pars mastoidea ossis temporalis 47
–, nasal p. of frontal bone = Pars nasalis ossis frontalis 52
–, orbital p. of frontal bone = Pars orbitalis ossis frontalis 52
–, petrosal p. of temporal bone = Pars petrosa ossis temporalis 35, 39, 40, 47, 48, 50
–, sacral p. of terminal line = Pars sacralis lineae terminalis 20
–, squamous p. of temporal bone = Pars squamosa ossis temporalis 33, 35, 39, 40, 47–49
–, sternal p. of diaphragm = Pars sternalis diaphragmatis 163
–, tibiocalcaneal p. of deltoid ligament = Pars tibiocalcanearis ligamenti deltoidei 130, 131
–, tibionavicular p. of deltoid ligament = Pars tibionavicularis ligamenti deltoidei 131
–, (anterior) tibiotalar p. of deltoid ligament = Pars tibiotalaris anterior ligamenti deltoidei 131
–, (posterior) tibiotalar p. of deltoid ligament = Pars tibiotalaris posterior ligamenti deltoidei 130, 131
–, tympanic p. of temporal bone = Pars tympanica ossis temporalis 47–50
Part (also pars or portion) = Pars
Patella (also knee cap or knee pan) = Patella 85, 126, 128, 232, 240, 241
Pecten ossis pubis 81, 82
Pedicle of vertebral arch = Pediculus arcus vertebrae 18, 19, 101
Pelvic girdle (Joints and ligaments) 118–125
– – (Muscles) 164–166
– – (Osteology) 25, 78–83
Pelvis 78, 79, 118–124
Perineum 5
Periosteum 8
Pes anserinus 234, 240
Phalanges digitorum manus 72–76
– – pedis 88, 89, 91
Pits, granular = Foveolae granulares 43, 52
Plane, nuchal = Planum nuchale 42, 44
–, occipital = Planum occipitale 44
Plate (also lamina or layer) = Lamina
–, cribriform p. of ethmoid bone = Lamina cribrosa ossis ethmoidalis 35, 39, 54, 55, 63
–, horizontal p. of palatine bone = Lamina horizontalis ossis palatini 37, 40, 55, 56, 58
–, lateral p. of pterygoid process = Lamina lateralis processus pterygoidei 35, 37, 46, 58, 62, 104, 105
–, medial p. of pterygoid process = Lamina medialis processus pterygoidei 35, 37, 46, 58, 63
Plate, orbital p. of ethmoid bone = Lamina orbitalis ossis ethmoidalis 54, 61, 62
–, perpendicular p. of ethmoid bone = Lamina perpendicularis ossis ethmoidalis 34, 54, 55, 61
–, – – of palatine bone = Lamina perpendicularis ossis palatini 56, 57, 63
Platysma 154, 168, 169, 178, 181
Plexus, brachial = Plexus brachialis 169, 174, 175, 185
–, parotid = Plexus parotideus 179
Pore, acoustic, external = Porus acusticus externus 33
–, –, internal = Porus acusticus internus 39, 47
Process, accessory p. of vertebrae = Processus accessorius vertebrae 18, 19
–, alveolar p. of maxilla = Processus alveolaris maxillae 31, 57, 61, 62
–, articular p. of vertebrae, inferior = Processus articularis inferior vertebrae 16, 18, 19
–, – – – –, superior = Processus articulares superior vertebrae 16–20
–, clinoid, anterior = Processus clinoideus anterior 39, 45, 46
–, –, middle = Processus clinoideus medius 45
–, –, posterior = Processus clinoideus posterior 39, 45, 46
–, condylar p. of mandible = = Processus condylaris mandibulae 33, 59, 60, 104, 172
–, coracoid p. of scapula = Processus coracoideus scapulae 26, 66, 109–111, 197
–, coronoid process of mandible = Processus coronoideus mandibulae 33, 59, 60, 104, 172
–, – – of ulna = Processus coronoideus ulnae 69, 71
–, costal = Processus costarius 19
–, ethmoidal p. of inferior nasal concha = Processus ethmoidalis conchae nasalis inferioris 63
–, falciform p. of sacrotuberal ligament = Processus falciformis lig. sacrotuberalis 123
–, frontal p. of maxilla = Processus frontalis maxillae 57
–, – – of zygomatic bone = Processus frontalis ossis zygomatici 33, 54
–, intrajugular process of occipital bone = Processus frontalis ossis occipitalis 39, 45
–, – – of temporal bone = Processus frontalis ossis temporalis 35, 47, 48
–, jugular p. of occipital bone = = Processus jugularis ossis occipitalis 39, 44, 45

Process, lateral p. of talus = Processus lateralis tali 89
–, – – of tuberosity of calcaneus = Processus lateralis tuberis calcanei 88, 90
–, mamillary p. of vertebrae = Processus mamillaris vertebrarum 18, 19
–, mastoid p. = Processus mastoideus 33, 37, 42, 47–50
–, medial p. of tuberosity of calcaneus = Processus medialis tuberis calcanei 88, 90
–, orbital p. of palatine bone = Processus orbitalis ossis palatini 56, 61, 62
–, palatine p. of maxilla = Processus palatinus maxillae 37, 40, 55, 57, 58, 61
–, posterior p. of talus = Processus posterior tali 89
–, pterygoid p. of sphenoid bone = Processus pterygoideus ossis sphenoidalis 37, 40, 46, 58, 62, 63, 104, 105
–, pyramidal p. of palatine bone = Processus pyramidalis ossis palatini 37, 56, 58, 63
–, sphenoid p. of palatine bone = Processus sphenoidalis ossis palatini 56
–, spinous = Processus spinosus 16–19, 153
–, styloid p. of radius = Processus styloides radii 70, 72–75
–, – – of temporal bone = Processus styloideus ossis temporalis 9, 32–37, 47–50, 104, 105, 185, 187
–, – – of ulna = Processus styloides ulnae 69, 70, 72–75, 114
–, temporal p. of zygomatic bone = Processus temporalis ossis zygomatici 54
–, transverse p. of vertebrae = Processus transversus vertebrae 16–18, 21, 102
–, uncinate p. of ethmoid bone = Processus uncinatus ossis ethmoidalis 54, 63
–, vaginal p. of sphenoid bone = Processus vaginalis ossis sphenoidalis 46
– xyphoid = Processus xyphoideus 24, 160
–, zygomatic p. of frontal bone = Processus zygomaticus ossis frontalis 31, 52
–, – – of maxilla = Processus zygomaticus maxillae 37, 57, 62
–, – – of temporal bone = Processus zygomaticus ossis temporalis 37, 47, 48, 104
Prominence of (lateral) semicircular canal = Prominentia canalis semicircularis lateralis 50
Promontory of sacrum = Promontorium ossis sacri 15, 27, 79, 124, 232
– of temporal bone = Promontorium ossis temporalis 49, 50, 71
Protuberance, mental = Protuberantia mentalis 33, 59, 172
–, occipital, external = Protuberantia occipitalis externa 35, 37, 42, 44, 142, 188
–, –, internal = Protuberantia occipitalis interna 39, 44, 45
Pubis = Os pubis 80–83, 160, 164, 165

R

Radius 70, 71, 112
Raphe, mylohyoid = Raphe mylohyoidea 172
–, pterygomandibular = Raphe pterygomandibularis 187
Recess (es) = Recessus
–, epitympanic = Recessus epithympanicus 49
Region (s) = Regio (nes)
– of the body = Regiones corporis 2–5
–, cubital = Regio cubiti 2, 3, 71, 72
–, malleolar, medial = Regio malleolaris medialis 2, 247
–, –, lateral = Regio malleolaris lateralis 2, 247
Retinaculum of extensor muscles = Retinaculum extensorum 192, 206, 208, 212, 214
– – – –, inferior = Retinaculum mm. extensorum inferius 227, 240, 241, 248, 252, 259
– – – –, superior = Retinaculum mm. extensorum superius 227
– of flexors = Retinaculum flexorum 213, 215, 216, 218, 220
– of flexor muscles (laciniate ligament) = Retinaculum mm. flexorum (ligamentum laciniatum) 240, 244, 259
– of patella, lateral = Retinaculum patellae laterale 126, 241, 242
– – –, medial = Retinaculum patellae mediale 126, 240
– of peroneus muscles, inferior = Retinaculum mm. peroneorum (fibularium) inferius 241, 248, 252, 259
– – – –, superior = Retinaculum mm. peroneorum (fibularium) superior 241, 246, 248, 259
Rib (s) = Costa (e) 22, 23, 27
Ridge (also border, crest or margin) = Crista
Ridge (s) = Jugum (a)
– (s), alveolar r. of mandible = Juga alveolaria mandibulae 59
– (s), – – of maxilla = Juga alveolaria maxillae 57
– (s), cerebral r. of cranium = Juga cerebralia 39, 49
Ring (also anulus) = Anulus
–, abdominal r., deep (or internal) = Anulus inguinalis profundus 160
–, – –, superficial (or external) = Anulus inguinalis superficialis 154, 159
–, tympanic = Anulus tympanicus 40, 49
Roof of tympanon = Tegmen tympani 48
Rostrum, sphenoidal = Rostrum sphenoidale 46

S

Sacrum = Os sacrum 15, 20, 21, 164, 165
Scapula 25–27, 66, 111
Semicanal of auditory tube = Semicanalis tubae auditivae 49
– – tensor tympani muscle = Semicanalis m. tensoris tympani 49
Septum, intermuscular (external) of arm = Septum intermusculare brachii laterale 190, 192, 194, 206, 208, 211
–, – (internal) of arm = Septum intermusculare brachii mediale 190, 196, 198, 199, 202, 204, 211
–, – (anterior) of leg = Septum intermusculare anterius cruris 248
–, – (posterior) of leg = Septum intermusculare posterius cruris 242
–, nasal = Septum nasi 55, 187
– of nose, bony = Septum nasi osseum 31, 35, 55, 56
Shaft (see also body or corpus) = Corpus
– of femur = Corpus femoris 84
– of fibula = Corpus fibulae 87
– of humerus = Corpus humeri 68
– of rib = Corpus costae 22
Sheath (see also muscle or tendon s.) = Vagina
– (s), fibrous s. of fingers = Vagina fibrosa digit. (manus) 220
–, – – of toes = Vagina fibrosa digit. (pedis) 254
– of straight abdominal muscle = Vagina m. recti abdominis 154, 156, 158, 160, 161, 192
– of styloid = Vagina processus styloidei 37, 42, 47, 48, 50
–, (common) synovial s. of flexor muscle = Vagina synovialis communis mm. flexorum 215, 216
– (s), – – of tendons of fingers = Vaginae synoviales digit. manus 212, 214–216, 220, 223
–, – – of intertubercular groove = Vagina synovialis intertubercularis 109, 111, 196, 198
–, – – of peroneal muscles = Vagina synovialis mm. peroneorum communis 241, 259

Sheath, tendon s. of (long) abductor muscle of the thumb = Vagina synovialis tendinis m. abductoris pollicis longi 215, 216
–, – – of flexor carpi radial muscle = Vagina synovialis tendinis m. flexoris carpi radialis 215, 216
–, – – of (long) flexor muscle of the great toe = Vagina synovialis tendinis m. flexoris hallucis longi 216, 240, 254, 259
–, – – of extensor carpi ulnar muscle = Vagina tendinis m. extensoris carpi ulnaris 212, 214
–, – – – – minimi muscle (hand) = Vagina tendinis m. extensoris digiti minimi (manus) 212, 214
–, – – of (long) extensor muscle of the great toe = Vagina tendinis m. extensoris hallucis longi 240, 241, 259
–, – – – – – – of the thumb = Vagina tendinis m. extensoris pollicis longi 212, 214
–, – – of (long) flexor muscle of the great toe = Vagina tendinis m. flexoris pollicis longi 215, 216
–, – – of peroneus longus muscle = Vagina tendinis m. peronei longi plantaris 256
–, – – of tibialis muscle, anterior = Vagina tendinis m. tibialis anterioris 240, 241, 259
–, – – – – –, posterior = Vagina tendinis m. tibialis posterior 240, 259
– (s), – – of (long) abductor and (short) extensor muscles of the thumb = Vagina tendinum mm. abductoris pollicis longi et extensoris pollicis brevis 212, 214
– (s), – – of (long) extensor digitorum muscle (foot) = Vaginae tendinum m. extensoris digit. (pedis) longi 240, 241, 259
– (s), – – of (long) flexor digitorum muscle (foot) = Vaginae tendinum m. flexoris digit. (pedis) 240, 259
Shoulder Girdle (Joints and Ligaments) 108–111
– – (Osteology) 25–27, 66, 67
Sinus, frontal = Sinus frontalis 35, 51, 61, 63, 187
–, maxillary = Sinus maxillaris 58, 61, 62
–, paranasal air s. = Sinus paranasales 51, 61–63
–, sigmoid = Sinus sigmoideus 50
–, sphenoidal = Sinus sphenoidalis 35, 46, 51, 55, 62, 63, 105, 187
Sinus, tarsal = Sinus tarsi 89
Skull (Joints and ligaments) 94–96, 104, 105
– (neurocranium) = Cranium (neurocranium) 32–35
– (newborn) = Cranium (neonatus) 40
– (Osteology) 30–63
– (splanchnocranium) = Cranium (splanchnocranium) 32–35
Skullcap = Calvaria 41, 43
Sole of foot = Planta pedis 3, 254, 256
Space = Spatium
–, pretracheal = Spatium praetracheale 174
–, quadrangular = Spatium axillare laterale (quadrangulare) 142, 191, 195
–, triangular = Spatium axillare mediale (triangulare) 142, 191, 195
Spermatic cord = Funiculus spermaticus 154, 158, 226
Spina (s) = Spina (ae)
–, ethmoidal s. of sphenoid bone = Spina ethmoidalis ossis sphenoidalis 45
–, iliac, anterior inferior = Spina iliaca anterior inferior 81–83, 165
–, –, anterior superior = Spina iliaca anterior superior 25, 81–83, 118, 121, 141, 154, 156, 159, 165, 228, 232
–, –, posterior inferior = Spina iliaca posterior inferior 81, 83
–, –, posterior superior = Spina iliaca posterior superior 81, 83, 122, 141, 165, 230
–, ischial = Spina ischiadica 25, 81–83, 165
–, mental = Spina mentalis 60, 172
– for (lateral straight) muscle of eyeball = Spina m. recti lateralis 62
– for (genioglossus) muscle = Spina m. genioglossi 60, 172
–, nasal s. of frontal bone = Spina nasalis ossis frontalis 51, 52
–, (anterior) nasal s. of maxilla = Spina nasalis anterior maxillae 31, 33, 57, 63
–, (posterior) nasal s. of palatine bone = Spina nasalis posterior ossis palatini 37, 56–58
– (s), palatine = Spina palatinae 58
– of scapula = Spina scapulae 66, 110, 141, 192
– of sphenoid bone = Spina ossis sphenoidalis 37, 46, 63, 105
–, suprameatal = Spina suprameatum 47
–, trochlear s. of frontal bone (variation) = Spina trochlearis (Var.) ossis frontalis 51
Spongy bone = Substantia spongiosa 8, 10, 11
Squamous part of frontal bone = Squama frontalis 31, 33, 52
Squamous part of occipital bone = Squama occipitalis 33, 40, 44
– – of temporal bone = Squama temporalis 32–35, 39, 40, 47, 49, 61–63
Sternum 9, 10, 24, 103
Stirrup = Stapes 49
Sulcus (i) (see also fissures or grooves) = Sulcus (i)
–, arterial (intracranial) = Sulci arteriosi 35, 39, 43, 48, 53
–, calcaneal = Sulcus calcanei 90
–, carotid s. of sphenoid bone = Sulcus caroticus ossis sphenoidalis 39, 45, 46
–, costal = Sulcus costae 22
–, infraorbital s. of maxilla = Sulcus infraorbitalis 57, 61, 62
–, intertubercular s. of humerus = Sulcus intertubercularis humeri 67, 68
–, lacrimal s. of maxilla = Sulcus lacrimalis maxillae 57
–, malleolar, lateral = Sulcus malleolaris lateralis 87
–, –, medial = Sulcus malleolaris medialis 86
–, mylohyoid = Sulcus mylohyoideus 60, 105
–, obturator s. of pubis = Sulcus obturatorius 83
–, optic s. of sphenoid bone = Sulcus opticus ossis sphenoidalis 45
–, (great) palatine s. of palatine bone = Sulcus palatinus major ossis palatini 56
– for (greater) petrosal nerve = Sulcus n. petrosi majoris 39, 47, 48
– for (lesser) petrosal nerve = Sulcus n. petrosi minoris 39, 47, 48
– of (inferior) petrosal sinus of occipital bone = Sulcus sinus petrosi inferioris ossis occipitalis 39, 47, 48
– – – – – of temporal bone = Sulcus sinus petrosi inferioris ossis temporalis 39, 47, 48
– of (superior) petrosal sinus = Sulcus sinus petrosi superioris 39
–, popliteal = Sulcus popliteus 85
–, pterygopalatine s. of sphenoid bone = Sulcus pterygopalatinus ossis sphenoidalis 46
– for radial n. = Sulcus n. radialis 68
–, sagittal s. of parietal bone = Sulcus sagittalis ossis parietalis 53
– of (superior) sagittal sinus of frontal bone = Sulcus sinus sagittalis superioris ossis frontalis 39, 43, 52
– – – – – of occipital bone = Sulcus sinus sagittalis superioris ossis occipitalis 44
– of sigmoid sinus of occipital bone = Sulcus sinus sigmoidei ossis occipitalis 39, 44, 45

Sulcus of sigmoid sinus of petrosal parts of temporal bone = Sulcus sinus sigmoidei partis petrosae ossis temporalis 48
– for spinal nerve = Sulcus n. spinalis 17
– for subclavian artery (and vein) = Sulcus arteriae subclaviae costae I 22
– – – vein (and artery) = Sulcus venae subclaviae costae I 22
– of talus = Sulcus tali 89
– for (middle) temporal artery = Sulcus arteriae temporalis mediae 47
– tendinis m. flexoris hallucis longi calcanei 90, 136
– – – – – – tali 89
– (i) of tendons of peroneus muscles = Sulci tendinum mm. peroneorum (fibularium) calcanei 90
– of tendon of peroneus longus muscle = Sulcus tendinis m. peronei (fibularis) longi ossis cuboidei 88
– of transverse sinus of occipital bone = Sulcus sinus transversi ossis occipitalis 39, 44, 45
– tubae auditivae 46
– for vertebral artery of atlas = Sulcus arteriae vertebralis atlantis 16, 94
Suprahyoid musculature = Musculi suprahyoidei 170, 172, 174, 188
Surface (also facet or facies) = Facies
–, anterior s. of radius = Facies anterior radii 71
–, – – of petrous part of temporal bone = Facies anterior partis petrosae 48
–, – – of ulna = Facies anterior ulnae 71
–, anterolateral s. of humerus = Facies anterior lateralis humeri 68
–, anteromedial s. of humerus = Facies anterior medialis humeri 68
–, articular s. (lunate) of hip bone = Facies lunata (acetabuli) 81, 82, 125
–, auricular s. of ilium = Facies auricularis ossis ilii 82, 83
–, – – of sacrum = Facies auricularis ossis sacri 20, 21
–, cerebral s. of greater wings of sphenoid bone = Facies cerebralis alae majoris ossis sphenoidalis 46
–, – – of squamous part of temporal bone = Facies cerebralis partis squamosae ossis temporalis 47
–, costal s. of scapula = Facies costalis scapulae 66
–, dorsal s. of sacrum = Facies dorsalis ossis sacri 20
–, – – of scapula = Facies dorsalis scapulae 66
Surface, inferior s. of petrous part of temporal bone = Facies inferior partis petrosae 48
–, infratemporal s. of maxilla = Facies infratemporalis maxillae 57
–, lateral s. of fibula = Facies lateralis fibulae 87
–, – – of radius = Facies lateralis radii 71
–, – – of tibia = Facies lateralis tibiae 86
–, maxillar s. of perpendicular plate of palatine bone = Facies maxillaris laminae perpendicularis ossis palatini 56
–, – – – – – of sphenoid bone = Facies maxillaris laminae perpendicularis 46
–, medial s. of fibula = Facies medialis fibulae 87
–, – – of tibia = Facies medialis tibia 86
–, – – of ulna = Facies medialis ulnae 71
–, nasal s. of maxilla = Facies nasalis maxillae 57
–, orbital s. of greater wing of sphenoid bone = Facies orbitalis alae majoris ossis sphenoidalis 31, 46, 61
–, – – of maxilla = Facies orbitalis maxillae 57
–, – – of orbital part of frontal bone = Facies orbitalis partis orbitalis ossis frontalis 51, 52
–, – – of sphenoid bone = Facies orbitalis ossis sphenoidalis 54
–, – – of zygomatic bone = Facies orbitalis ossis zygomatici 61
–, patellar s. of femur = Facies patellaris femoris 84, 85, 127
–, pelvic s. of sacrum = Facies pelvina ossis sacri 21
–, popliteal s. of femur = Facies poplitea femoris 84
–, posterior s. of fibula = Facies posterior fibulae 87
–, – – of humerus = Facies posterior humeri 68
–, – – of petrous parts of temporal bone = Facies posterior partis petrosae 39
–, – – of tibia = Facies posterior tibiae 86
–, – – of ulna = Facies posterior ulnae 71
–, symphyseal s. of pubic bone = Facies symphysialis ossis pubis 82, 83
–, temporal s. of greater wing of sphenoid bone = Facies temporalis alae majoris 46
Sustentaculum of talus = Sustentaculum tali 88–90, 131
Suture, coronal = Sutura coronalis 31, 33, 35, 40, 41, 43
–, frontal = Sutura frontalis 40
–, frontoethmoidal = Sutura frontoethmoidalis 39
–, frontolacrimal = Sutura frontolacrimalis 31
–, frontomaxillary = Sutura frontomaxillaris 31, 61
–, frontonasal = Sutura frontonasalis 31
–, frontozygomatic = Sutura frontozygomatica 33
–, incisive = Sutura incisiva 37, 58
–, infraorbital = Sutura infraorbitalis 61, 62
–, internasal = Sutura internasalis 31
–, lacrimoethmoidal = Sutura lacrimoethmoidalis 62
–, lacrimomaxillary = Sutura lacrimomaxillaris 33
–, lambdoid = Sutura lambdoidea 33, 35, 37, 40–43
–, nasomaxillary = Sutura nasomaxillaris 31, 33
–, occipital, transverse (variation) = Sutura occipitalis transversa (Var.) 40, 42
–, occipitomastoid = Sutura occipitomastoidea 33, 37, 39, 42
–, palatine, median = Sutura palatina mediana 37, 58
–, –, transverse = Sutura palatina transversa 37, 57, 58
–, parietomastoid = Sutura parietomastoidea 33, 42
–, sagittal = Sutura sagittalis 40–43
–, sphenofrontal = Sutura sphenofrontalis 31, 33, 39, 62
–, sphenosquamous = Sutura sphenosquamosa 33, 39
–, sphenozygomatic = Sutura sphenozygomatica 31, 33
–, squamous = Sutura squamosa 33, 35
–, temporozygomatic = Sutura temporozygomatica 33
–, zygomaticomaxillary = Sutura zygomaticomaxillaris 31, 61
Symphysis, pubic = Symphysis pubica 123, 124, 159, 160, 165, 166, 228
Synchondrosis (see also articulation or joint)
–, sacral = Synchondrosis (es) sacrales 21
–, sphenooccipital = Synchondrosis sphenooccipitalis 39, 45
–, sternal = Synchondrosis sternalis 24, 103, 108
–, sternocostal = Synchondrosis sternocostalis costae I 103
Syndesmology 93–137
Syndesmosis (articulation), tibiofibular = Syndesmosis (articulatio) tibiofibularis 128, 130, 134

Synostosis, epiphyseal = Synostosis epiphysialis 8
–, vertebral = Synostosis vertebrae 14

T

Table of skull bone (inner, outer) = Lamina interna et externa ossium cranii 10, 43
Talus (ankle bone) = Talus 88–91, 134, 135
Tarsus 88–91, 135
Tendon (see also muscle or sheath = Tendo
–, calcaneal *(Achilles)* = Tendon calcaneus *(Achilles)* 240, 241, 244, 259
Thenar eminence = Thenar 221
Thigh bone = Femur 10, 84, 85, 125
Thorax (Joints and ligaments) 94–103
Tibia 11, 86, 87, 128, 240
Tonsil, pharyngeal = Tonsilla pharyngea 187
Torus tubarius 187
Tract = Tractus
–, iliotibial = Tractus iliotibialis 141, 226, 229, 238, 241, 250
– angularis fasciae cervicalis 173
Triangle (also trigone) = Trigonum
Trigone (also triangle) = Trigonum
–, carotide = Trigonum caroticum 4
–, deltoideopectoral *(Mohrenheim)* = Trigonum deltoideopectorale *(Mohrenheim)* 2, 4, 154, 168, 169, 174
–, femoral = Trigonum femorale 2
–, lumbar = Trigonum lumbale 141, 142, 144, 153
–, lumbocostal = Trigonum lumbocostale 163
–, omoclavicular (also subclavian triangle) = Trigonum omoclaviculare 4, 173
–, retromolar = Trigonum retromolare 60
–, sternocostal = Trigonum sternocostale 163
–, submandibular = Trigonum submandibulare 4
Trochanter, greater = Trochanter major 84, 85, 118, 122, 123, 125, 166, 230, 236
–, lesser = Trochanter minor 84, 85, 166, 230, 234
Trochlea of calcaneus, peroneal = Trochlea peronealis (fibularis) 89, 90
– of humerus = Trochlea humeri 67, 68, 113
– of talus = Trochlea tali 88, 89
Trunk, brachiocephalic = Truncus brachiocephalicus 176
Trunk (Muscles) 141–166
– (Osteology) 14–27
Tuber (also tubercle or tuberosity) = Tuber
Tubercle (also tuber or tuberosity) = Tuberculum
–, articular t. of temporal bone = Tuberculum articulare ossis temporalis 37, 47, 48, 186
– of atlas, anterior = Tuberculum anterius atlantis 16, 17
– – –, posterior = Tuberculum posterius atlantis 16, 17, 148
– of axis, anterior = Tuberculum anterius axis 16
– of cervical vertebrae, anterior = Tuberculum anterius vertebrarum cervicalium 17
– – – –, posterior = Tuberculum posterius vertebrarum cervicalium 17
–, carotid t. of sixth cervical vertebra = Tuberculum caroticum vertebrae cervicalis VI 166, 176
–, conoid = Tuberculum conoideum 67
– of humerus, greater = Tuberculum majus humeri 67, 68, 110
– – –, lesser = Tuberculum minus humeri 67, 68
–, infraglenoid = Tuberculum infraglenoidale 66
–, intercondylar t. of tibia, medial = Tuberculum intercondylare mediale tibiae 87
–, – – – –, lateral = Tuberculum intercondylare laterale tibiae 87
–, jugular t. of occipital bone = = Tuberculum jugulare ossis occipitalis 39, 44, 45
–, mental = Tuberculum mentale 59, 172
–, obturator, anterior = Tuberculum obturatorium anterius 81
–, –, posterior = Tuberculum obturatorium posterius 81–83
–, pharyngeal = Tuberculum pharyngeum 37
–, pubic t. of pubic bone = Tuberculum pubicum 81–83, 121, 164–166, 232
– of rib = Tuberculum costae 22, 102
– of (anterior) scalene muscle = Tuberculum m. scaleni anterioris 22
– of sella turcica = Tuberculum sellae 39, 45
– of transverse process, anterior = Tuberculum anterius proc. transversum 17
– – – –, posterior = Tuberculum posterius processus transversum 17
Tuberosity (also tubercle or tuber) = Tuberositas
– of calcaneus = Tuber calcanei 88–90, 130–132, 254
– of cuboid bone = Tuberositas ossis cuboidei 88
–, deltoid t. of humerus = Tuberositas deltoidea 68
Tuberosity, (distal) t. of fingers = Tuberositas phalangis distalis (digit. manus) 72–74
–, gluteal t. of femur = Tuberositas glutaea 85, 125
– for (greatest) gluteal muscle = Tuberositas m. glutaei maximi 81
–, iliac = Tuberositas iliaca 82, 83
–, ischial = Tuber ischiadicum 25, 80–83, 122, 165, 236
–, masseteric = Tuberositas masseterica 59, 104
– of (fifth) metatarsal bone = Tubersitas ossis metatarsalis V 88, 89
– of metatarsal bone of great toe = Tuberositas ossis metatarsalis hallucis 88
– for (middle) scalene muscle = Tuberositas m. scaleni medii 22
– of navicular bone = Tuberositas ossis navicularis 88, 90
–, pterygoid t. of mandible = Tuberositas pterygoidea 60
– of radius = Tuberositas radii 70
– of sacrum = Tuberositas sacralis 20, 21
– of scaphoid bone = Tuberositas ossis scaphoidei 74
– of tibia = Tuberositas tibiae 86, 87, 126–128, 248
– of ulna = Tuberositas ulnae 69
Tympanic membrane = Membrana tympani 49

U

Ulna 69–71, 112, 113
Umbilicus 141, 154, 160
Upper limb (Joints and ligaments) 109–115
– – (Muscles) 190–224
– – (Osteology) 68–76

V

Vagina (see also muscle, sheath or tendon) = Vagina
– (ae) fibrosae tendin. mm. flex. digit. manus 216
Vein (s) = Vena (e)
–, axillary = Vena axillaris 174
–, basilic = Vena basilica 190
–, brachiocephalic = Vena brachiocephalica 176
–, cava, inferior = Vena cava inferior 176
–, cephalic = Vena cephalica 154, 169, 174, 190, 197
–, facial = Vena facialis 174
–, femoral = Vena femoralis 228
–, iliac, external = Vena iliaca externa 228
–, jugular, anterior = Vena jugularis anterior 168
–, –, external = Vena jugularis externa 168, 173

Vein, jugular, internal = Vena jugularis interna 169, 174, 175, 185
–, popliteal = Vena poplitea 229
–, saphenous, great = Vena saphena magna 226, 228
–, –, small = Vena saphena parva 229
–, subclavian = Vena subclavia 175, 176
–, temporal, superficial = Vena temporalis superficialis 181
–, thoracic, internal = Vena thoracica interna 176
–, ulnar = Vena ulnaris 216
Vertebra, (seventh) cervical = Vertebra prominens 17, 25, 142
Vertebrae, cervical = Vertebrae cervicales 14–17, 25–27
–, coccygeal = Vertebrae coccygeae 14, 15, 21, 165
Vertebrae, lumbal = Vertebrae lumbales 11, 14, 15, 19
–, sacral = Vertebrae sacrales 14, 15, 20, 21
–, thoracic = Vertebrae thoracicae 14, 15, 18, 19, 25–27
Vertebral column (backbone) = Columna vertebralis 15, 25–27, 97–100
– – (Joints and ligaments) 97–103
Vincula of tendons of fingers = Vinculum tendinum 220, 223
Vomer 31, 35, 37, 40, 55, 56, 61, 105

W

Window = Fenestra
–, oval = Fenestra vestibuli 48–50
Window, round = Fenestra cochleae 49
Wing = Ala
– of cristae galli = Ala cristae galli 39, 54
– of ilium = Ala ossis ilii 80–83
– of sphenoid bone, great = Ala major ossis sphenoidalis 31, 40, 45, 46, 61
– – – –, lesser = Ala minor ossis sphenoidalis 31, 39, 45, 46, 62
– of vomer = Ala vomeris 55, 56, 62

X

Yellow ligament = Ligamentum flavum 98–100, 102

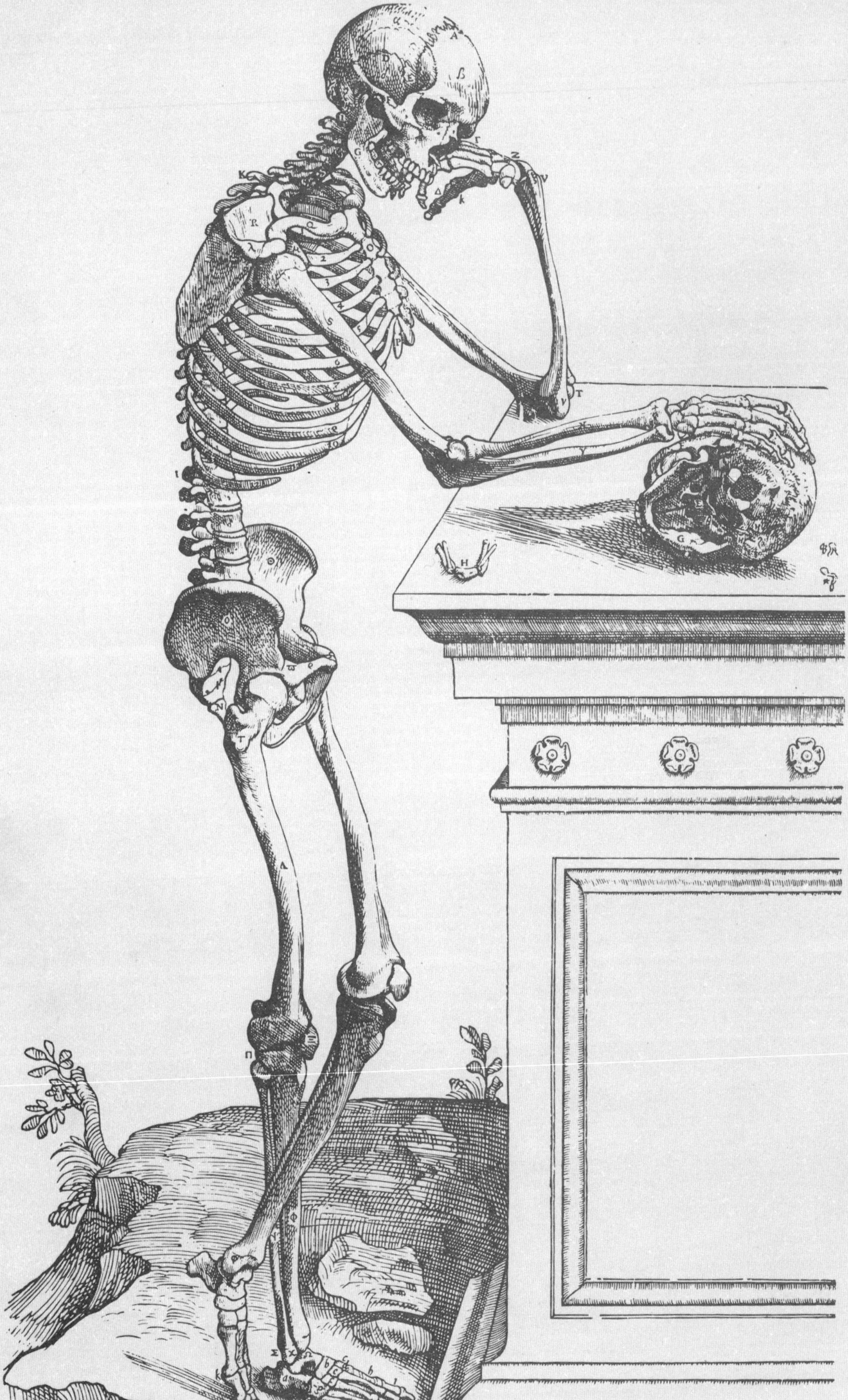